TEXTBOOK OF RHEUMATOLOGY

VOLUME 2

FOUNDATIONS, INFECTIONS, AND OBSTRUCTIVE LUNG DISEASES

Dr. Anand Anerao

ALLIED HEALTH PRESS

Textbook of Rheumatology Volume 2

Foundations, Infections, and Obstructive Lung Diseases

Author: **Dr. Anand Anerao**

Allied Health Press
4164 Lakeshore Road
Burlington ON L7L 1A4
Canada
www.alliedhealthpress.com
Email: orders@arclereducation.com

ISBN: 978-1-77956-859-5

ABOUT THE AUTHOR

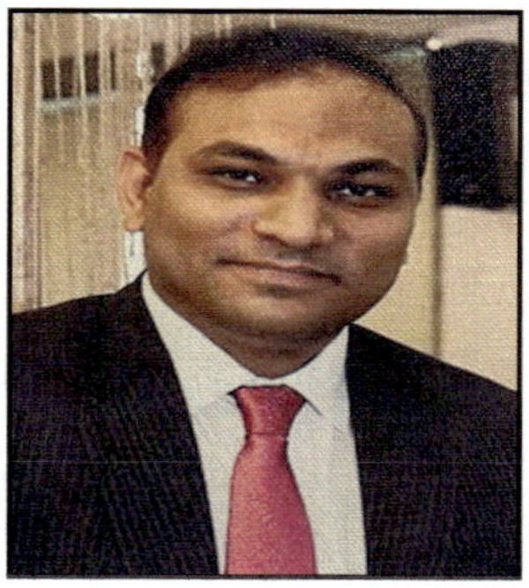

Dr. Anand Anerao is currently an Associate Professor at Parbhani Medical College. After completing his MBBS in 2001 from Indira Gandhi Medical College, Nagpur, he pursued his master's degree in Orthopedic Surgery from Shivaji University in 2007. Following his MS, he completed a fellowship in Arthroscopy from Kamineni Hospital, Hyderabad in 2009. He served as a Medical Officer at Sub-District Hospital, Gangakhed, for three years (2009-2012). Additionally, he has been in private practice for the past 18 years.

Brief Table of Contents

1. Rheumatoid Arthritis (RA)	1
2. Systemic Lupus Erythematosus (SLE)	29
3. Spondyloarthritides	59
4. Sjogren's Syndrome	85
5. Systemic Sclerosis (Scleroderma)	113
6. Idiopathic Inflammatory Myopathies	141
7. Vasculitides	171
8. Gout and Pseudogout	199
9. Osteoarthritis	225
10. Calcium and Bone Metabolism Disorders	255
11. Juvenile Idiopathic Arthritis (JIA)	285
12. Therapeutics in Rheumatology	313
Index	335

Getting Started with This Book

Chapter Openers

A list of Chapter Outline is presented providing a brief Introduction to what will be covered in the chapter.

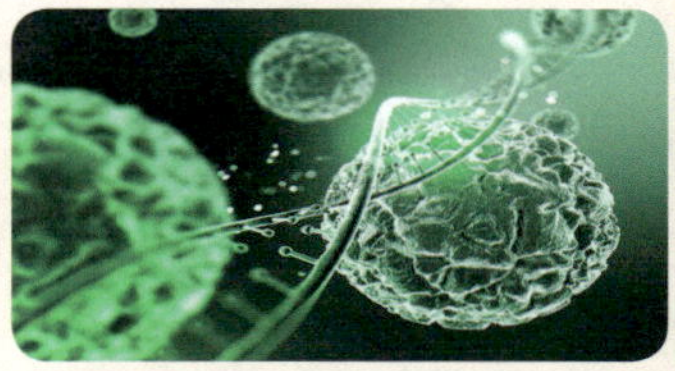

LEARNING OBJECTIVES

After studying this chapter, you will be able to:

1. Discuss the scientific method in biology;
2. Explain the cell theory;
3. Discuss the genetics and heredity;
4. Evolution and natural selection;
5. Focus on ecology and ecosystems;
6. Learn about human biology;
7. Evaluate the plant biology;
8. Explain the microbiology;
9. Focus on current trends in biology.

Introduction

Often referred to as the science of life, biology is a broad field of study aimed at comprehending the several kinds of life on Earth, from tiny creatures to sophisticated multicellular entities. Comprising several subfields, including molecular biology, ecology, and evolutionary biology, each of which advances our knowledge of living systems, this field clarifies the mechanisms controlling life events, including development, reproduction, and interaction with the surroundings, which is the central goal of biology. Moreover, biology fills in the void between the natural sciences and medicine by offering a necessary understanding of health, illness, and the interactions between organisms and their environments. Dealing with urgent global issues such as climate change, biodiversity loss, and new diseases depends on an awareness of these complex biological interactions, therefore highlighting the critical part biology plays in modern civilization. Fundamentally, biology explores and tests ideas about the living world using the scientific method. Through methodical observation and experimentation,

1.1. The Scientific Method in Biology

Learning Outcome

1. Describe the steps of the scientific method;
2. Focus on hypothesis formation;
3. Learn about experimental design.

Learning Outcomes

The beginning of each section of every chapter contains a set of Learning Outcomes that inform students of concepts they should understand. These outcomes help students understand what they should be able to do if they have mastered the material in that section.

Test Your Knowledge

Throughout each chapter, Test Your Knowledge cues you to note which topics have been covered and to self-test your understanding of the material presented.

Test Your Knowledge

1. Explain why correlation does not imply causation in scientific experiments.
2. How does the scientific method help reduce the influence of personal opinions in research?

Chapter Summary

The Summary Section appear at the end of each chapter and summarize main concepts covered throughout the chapter. These points provide key concepts in an engaging and meaningful way.

Summary

The investigation of biological principles highlights the importance of a comprehensive view of life by reflecting the intricate interactions that occur within living systems. The complexity of biology goes beyond individual species or systems, as this essay highlights; it also includes the interactions that mold ecosystems and affect biodiversity. Researchers can conduct in-depth analyses of metabolomic data using sophisticated technologies like MetaboAnalyst, which offer insights into the molecular mechanisms underlying these interactions. As demonstrated by the developments in MetaboAnalyst, for example, the integration of diverse omics data promotes a thorough understanding of metabolic pathways and helps identify important biological markers necessary for research on development and disease (Chong et al., 2018). Additionally, the phenomenon of ecological invasions is a key component of biological research and a vital field of study. The introduction of non-native species into unfamiliar habitats has significant ramifications and calls for multidisciplinary management strategies. Examining the origins and effects of these biological incursions, invasion science has become a crucial field that highlights the need to comprehend ecological dynamics and community interactions. As interest in biological invasions increases, new findings are emerging that put conventional ecological theories and practices to the test. The importance of incorporating various scientific viewpoints is shown by this developing discipline, which also highlights how invasive species shape ecosystems and advances our knowledge of ecological resilience (David et al., 2013). When taken as a whole, these discoveries from invasion science and metabolomics highlight the value of multidisciplinary biology research. Fostering cross-disciplinary collaboration and utilizing technological breakthroughs to improve our comprehension of intricate biological interactions are crucial as we look to the future of biological research. In addition to deepening our understanding of the complexities of life, this method lays the groundwork for tackling urgent environmental issues. Future studies can ensure the continued relevance of biology in a world that is constantly changing by acknowledging the interconnection of biological systems and opening the door to creative solutions that support sustainability and biodiversity conservation. We might imagine a thorough comprehension of life that serves both academia and society at large through ongoing investigation and integration of scientific knowledge.

Knowledge Assessment

The chapter includes material designed to review and reinforce each content. It includes Critical Thinking Questions to help test of your understanding of information presented in the chapter and Short answer Questions to review your understanding of the key concepts presented in the chapter.

Critical Thinking Questions

1. **Who is known as the "Father of Modern Biology"?**
   a. Aristotle
   b. Charles Darwin
   c. Gregor Mendel
   d. Louis Pasteur
2. **What is the basic unit of life?**
   a. Atom
   b. Molecule
   c. Cell
   d. Organism
3. **Which branch of biology studies the interaction of organisms with their environment?**
   a. Genetics
   b. Ecology
   c. Physiology
   d. Botany
4. **Which macromolecule is the main source of energy for living organisms?**
   a. Proteins
   b. Lipids
   c. Carbohydrates
   d. Nucleic acids
5. **DNA is primarily responsible for which function in living organisms?**
   a. Energy production
   b. Protein synthesis
   c. Storing genetic information
   d. Regulating body temperature

Short Answer Questions

1. What is biology, and why is it important to study biology?
2. What are the three main domains of life, and how are they different from one another?
3. Define homeostasis and give an example of how it works in living organisms.
4. What is the cell theory, and why is it fundamental to biology?
5. How do autotrophs and heterotrophs differ in the way they obtain energy?
6. What is the scientific method, and how is it applied in biological research?
7. Discuss how biology helps address global challenges such as climate change, disease, and food security.
8. Explain the levels of biological organization from the smallest unit to the largest. Provide examples at each level.
9. Describe the relationship between structure and function in biology, giving specific examples from cells or organs.
10. How has the discovery of genetics shaped our understanding of inheritance and variation among organisms?

Supplementary Materials

Key Terms: A list of key terms is given for quick reference

KEY TERMS FROM THIS CHAPTER

Annotation enrichment analysis	Biological structure	Cell
Cell theory	Cellular structure	Ecology
Ecosystems	Genetics	Human biology
Microbiology	Natural selection	Organism
Plant biology		

Further Resources: Recommendations for additional readings, websites, and multimedia resources.

References

1. Argelaguet, R., Velten, B., Arnol, D., Dietrich, S., Zenz, T., Marioni, J. C., Buettner, F., et al. (2018). Multi-omics factor analysis—A framework for unsupervised integration of multi-omics data sets. *Molecular Systems Biology, 14*. https://doi.org/10.15252/msb.20178124.
2. Bacher, S., Blackburn, T. M., Essl, F., & Genovesi, P. (2017). *Socio-Economic Impact Classification of Alien Taxa (SEICAT)*. https://core.ac.uk/download/286567949.pdf (accessed on 8th March 2025).
3. Barnett, R., Brace, S., Cucchi, T., & Dobney, K. (2013). *Divergent Evolutionary Processes Associated with Colonization of Offshore Islands.* https://core.ac.uk/download/20664364.pdf (accessed on 8th March 2025).

Detailed Table of Contents

List of Figures *xvii*
Preface *xxxi*

CHAPTER 1

Rheumatoid Arthritis (RA) 1

Introduction 1
1.1. Causes and Risk Factors of Rheumatoid Arthritis 2
1.1.1. Genetic Predisposition 2
1.1.2. Environmental Triggers 3
1.1.3. Hormonal Influences 3
1.1.4. Age-Related Factors 4
1.1.5. Gender Differences 4
1.1.6. Lifestyle Factors (e.g., Smoking, Diet) 5
1.1.7. Infections and Autoimmune Responses 5
1.1.8. Family History of Autoimmune Diseases 5
1.1.9. Socioeconomic Factors 6
1.2. Symptoms and Diagnosis of Rheumatoid Arthritis 7
1.2.1. Common Physical Symptoms 7
1.2.2. Joint-Specific Symptoms 8
1.2.3. Systemic Symptoms 8
1.2.4. Early Signs of RA 8
1.2.5. Diagnostic Criteria (e.g., ACR/EULAR) 9
1.2.6. Laboratory Tests (e.g., RF, anti-CCP) 9
1.2.7. Imaging Techniques (e.g., X-Rays, MRI) 10
1.2.8. Differential Diagnosis 10
1.2.9. Importance of Early Diagnosis 11
1.3. Treatment Options for Rheumatoid Arthritis 12
1.3.1. Pharmacological Treatments 12
1.3.2. Non-Steroidal Anti-Inflammatory Drugs (NSAIDs) 13
1.3.3. Disease-Modifying Antirheumatic Drugs (DMARDs) 13
1.3.4. Biologic Therapies 14
1.3.5. Corticosteroids 14
1.3.6. Physical Therapy and Rehabilitation 14
1.3.7. Lifestyle Modifications 15
1.3.8. Complementary and Alternative Therapies 15
1.3.9. Importance of a Multidisciplinary Approach 16
1.4. Living with Rheumatoid Arthritis 17
1.4.1. Coping Strategies 17
1.4.2. Impact on Daily Activities 17
1.4.3. Psychological Effects 18
1.4.4. Support Systems and Resources 18
1.4.5. Role of Patient Education 19
1.4.6. Managing Flares and Remission 19
1.4.7. Nutrition and Dietary Considerations 20
1.4.8. Exercise and Physical Activity 20
1.4.9. Long-Term Outlook and Prognosis 21
Summary 22
References 24

CHAPTER 2

Systemic Lupus Erythematosus (SLE) 29

Introduction 29

2.1. Pathophysiology of SLE **30**
2.1.1. Immune System Dysfunction 30
2.1.2. Genetic Factors Contributing to SLE 31
2.1.3. Environmental Triggers 31
2.1.4. Role of Hormones in SLE 32
2.1.5. Mechanisms of Autoimmunity 33
2.1.6. Inflammatory Processes Involved 33
2.1.7. Organ Systems Affected by SLE 33
2.1.8. Differences Between SLE and Other Autoimmune Diseases 34
2.1.9. Current Research on Pathophysiology 35
2.2. Clinical Manifestations of SLE **36**
2.2.1. Common Symptoms of SLE 36
2.2.2. Cutaneous Manifestations 36
2.2.3. Musculoskeletal Symptoms 37
2.2.4. Renal Involvement in SLE 37
2.2.5. Neurological Symptoms 38
2.2.6. Hematological Abnormalities 38
2.2.7. Cardiovascular Complications 39
2.2.8. Gastrointestinal Manifestations 40
2.2.9. Variability of Symptoms Among Patients 40
2.3. Diagnosis of SLE **41**
2.3.1. Criteria for SLE Diagnosis 41
2.3.2. Role of Laboratory Tests 41
2.3.3. Importance of Clinical History 42
2.3.4. Differential Diagnosis Considerations 42
2.3.5. Use of Imaging Studies 43
2.3.6. Challenges in Diagnosing SLE 43
2.3.7. Role of Biomarkers in Diagnosis 43
2.3.8. Importance of Multidisciplinary Approach 44
2.3.9. Advances in Diagnostic Techniques 45
2.4. Treatment and Management of SLE **46**
2.4.1. Overview of Treatment Goals 46
2.4.2. Pharmacological Treatments 47
2.4.3. Non-Pharmacological Interventions 47
2.4.4. Role of Lifestyle Modifications 48
2.4.5. Management of Flares 48
2.4.6. Importance of Patient Education 49
2.4.7. Monitoring Disease Progression 49
2.4.8. Psychological Support for Patients 50
2.4.9. Future Directions in SLE Treatment 50
Summary **51**
References **53**

CHAPTER 4

Spondyloarthritides 59

Introduction **59**
3.1. Types of Spondyloarthritides **60**
3.1.1. Ankylosing Spondylitis 60
3.1.2. Psoriatic Arthritis 61
3.1.3. Reactive Arthritis 61
3.1.4. Enteropathic Arthritis 62
3.1.5. Undifferentiated Spondyloarthritis 62
3.1.6. Juvenile Spondyloarthritis 63
3.1.7. Non-Radiographic Axial Spondyloarthritis 63
3.2. Pathophysiology **64**
3.2.1. Genetic Factors and HLA-B27 65
3.2.2. Immune System Involvement 65
3.2.3. Inflammatory Processes 65
3.2.4. Role of Cytokines 66
3.2.5. Bone Remodeling and Erosion 66
3.2.6. Extra-Articular Manifestations 67
3.2.7. Environmental Triggers 67
3.2.8. Interaction Between Genetics and Environment 68
3.2.9. Current Research on Pathophysiology 69
3.3. Diagnosis **70**
3.3.1. Clinical Evaluation and History 70
3.3.2. Physical Examination Techniques 70
3.3.3. Imaging Studies (X-Rays, MRI) 71
3.3.4. Laboratory Tests (Blood Tests, Markers) 71
3.3.5. Differential Diagnosis 72
3.3.6. Role of Rheumatologists 72
3.3.7. Diagnostic Criteria 72
3.3.8. Challenges in Diagnosis 73
3.3.9. Importance of Early Diagnosis 73
3.4. Treatment and Management **75**
3.4.1. Pharmacological Treatments (NSAIDs, DMARDs) 75
3.4.2. Biologic Therapies 76
3.4.3. Physical Therapy and Exercise 76

3.4.4. Lifestyle Modifications 76
3.4.5. Surgical Options 77
3.4.6. Pain Management Strategies 78
3.4.7. Role of Patient Education 78
3.4.8. Multidisciplinary Approach 79
3.4.9. Future Directions in Treatment 79
Summary **80**
References **82**

CHAPTER 5

Sjogren's Syndrome 85

Introduction **85**
4.1. Pathophysiology of Sjogren's Syndrome **86**
4.1.1. Immune System Involvement 86
4.1.2. Role of Exocrine Glands 87
4.1.3. Mechanisms of Glandular Dysfunction 87
4.1.4. Genetic Factors Contributing to the Disease 88
4.1.5. Environmental Triggers 88
4.1.6. Inflammatory Processes 89
4.1.7. Differences Between Primary and Secondary Sjogren's 89
4.1.8. Impact on Salivary and Lacrimal Glands 90
4.2. Symptoms and Diagnosis **91**
4.2.1. Common Symptoms of Sjogren's Syndrome 91
4.2.2. Ocular Manifestations 92
4.2.3. Oral Manifestations 92
4.2.4. Fatigue and Systemic Symptoms 92
4.2.5. Diagnostic Criteria 93
4.2.6. Laboratory Tests for Diagnosis 93
4.2.7. Imaging Studies and Their Relevance 94
4.2.8. Differential Diagnosis 94
4.2.9. Challenges in Diagnosing Sjogren's Syndrome 95
4.3. Treatment and Management **96**
4.3.1. Overview of Treatment Options 96
4.3.2. Symptomatic Relief for Dry Eyes 97
4.3.3. Management of Dry Mouth 97
4.3.4. Pharmacological Treatments 98
4.3.5. Role of Lifestyle Modifications 98
4.3.6. Importance of Regular Monitoring 99
4.3.7. Multidisciplinary Approach to Care 100
4.3.8. Patient Education and Support 100
4.3.9. Emerging Therapies and Research 101
4.4. Complications and |Comorbidities **101**
4.4.1. Potential Complications of Sjogren's Syndrome 101
4.4.2. Increased Risk of Lymphoma 102
4.4.3. Association with Other Autoimmune Diseases 102
4.4.4. Impact on Quality of Life 103
4.4.5. Psychological Effects of the Disease 103
4.4.6. Oral Health Complications 104
4.4.7. Musculoskeletal Manifestations 105
4.4.8. Neurological Complications 105
4.4.9. Long-Term Prognosis 105
Summary **107**
References **109**

CHAPTER 6

Systemic Sclerosis (Scleroderma) 113

Introduction **113**
5.1. Pathophysiology of Systemic Sclerosis **114**
5.1.1. Immune System Dysfunction 114
5.1.2. Role of Fibrosis in Scleroderma 115
5.1.3. Vascular Changes and Endothelial Damage 115
5.1.4. Genetic Factors and Susceptibility 116
5.1.5. Environmental Triggers 117
5.1.6. Pathways of Collagen Production 117
5.1.7. Impact of Inflammation 118
5.1.8. Organ Involvement Mechanisms 118
5.1.9. Current Research on Pathophysiology 118
5.2. Clinical Manifestations **119**
5.2.1. Skin Changes and Symptoms 119
5.2.2. Gastrointestinal Complications 120
5.2.3. Pulmonary Involvement 120
5.2.4. Cardiac Manifestations 121
5.2.5. Renal Implications 121
5.2.6. Musculoskeletal Symptoms 121
5.2.7. Neurological Effects 122
5.2.8. Raynaud's Phenomenon 122
5.2.9. Quality of Life Considerations 123
5.3. Diagnosis and Assessment **124**

5.3.1. Clinical Evaluation Techniques 124
5.3.2. Laboratory Tests and Biomarkers 125
5.3.3. Imaging Studies Utilized 125
5.3.4. Differential Diagnosis Considerations 126
5.3.5. Role of Skin Biopsy 126
5.3.6. Assessment of Organ Function 126
5.3.7. Use of Scoring Systems 127
5.3.8. Importance of Multidisciplinary Approach 127
5.3.9. Challenges in Early Diagnosis 128
5.4. Treatment and Management 129
5.4.1. Pharmacological Interventions 129
5.4.2. Non-Pharmacological Therapies 130
5.4.3. Role of Physical Therapy 130
5.4.4. Management of Specific Symptoms 130
5.4.5. Importance of Patient Education 131
5.4.6. Psychological Support and Counseling 131
5.4.7. Emerging Therapies and Clinical Trials 132
5.4.8. Lifestyle Modifications 133
5.4.9. Long-term Management Strategies 133
Summary 134
References 136

CHAPTER 6

Idiopathic Inflammatory Myopathies 141

Introduction 141
6.1. Types of Idiopathic Inflammatory Myopathies 142
6.1.1. Polymyositis 142
6.1.2. Dermatomyositis 143
6.1.3. Inclusion Body Myositis 143
6.1.4. Necrotizing Autoimmune Myopathy 144
6.1.5. Overlap Myositis 144
6.1.6. Juvenile Idiopathic Inflammatory Myopathy 145
6.1.7. Classification Criteria 145
6.1.8. Differences in Clinical Features 146
6.1.9. Prognosis for Each Type 146
6.2. Pathophysiology and Mechanisms 147
6.2.1. Immune System Involvement 148
6.2.2. Role of Autoantibodies 148
6.2.3. Muscle Fiber Damage 149
6.2.4. Inflammatory Processes 149
6.2.5. Genetic Predispositions 150
6.2.6. Environmental Triggers 150
6.2.7. Role of Cytokines and Chemokines 151
6.2.8. Muscle Regeneration and Repair Mechanisms 151
6.2.9. Current Research on Pathophysiological Mechanisms 152
6.3. Diagnosis and Assessment 153
6.3.1. Clinical Evaluation and History 153
6.3.2. Laboratory Tests and Biomarkers 154
6.3.3. Electromyography (EMG) 154
6.3.4. Muscle Biopsy Techniques 155
6.3.5. Imaging Studies (MRI, CT) 155
6.3.6. Differential Diagnosis Considerations 156
6.3.7. Role of Multidisciplinary Teams 156
6.3.8. Challenges in Early Diagnosis 157
6.3.9. Advances in Diagnostic Technologies 157
6.4. Treatment and Management Strategies 158
6.4.1. Corticosteroids and Immunosuppressants 158
6.4.2. Physical Therapy and Rehabilitation 159
6.4.3. Role of Biologic Therapies 160
6.4.4. Nutritional Considerations 160
6.4.5. Management of Comorbidities 161
6.4.6. Patient Education and Support 161
6.4.7. Long-term Monitoring and Follow-up 162
6.4.8. Emerging Therapies and Clinical Trials 162
6.4.9. Impact of Treatment on Quality of Life 163
Summary 164
References 166

CHAPTER 7

Vasculitides 171

Introduction 171
7.1. Classification of Vasculitides 172
7.1.1. Large Vessel Vasculitides 172
7.1.2. Medium Vessel Vasculitides 173
7.1.3. Small Vessel Vasculitides 173
7.1.4. Primary vs. Secondary Vasculitides 174

7.1.5. Systemic vs. Localized Vasculitides 174
7.1.6. Granulomatous vs. Non-granulomatous Vasculitides 174
7.1.7. Classification Criteria and Guidelines 175
7.1.8. Role of the American College of Rheumatology 176
7.1.9. Importance of Accurate Classification 176
7.2. Pathophysiology of Vasculitides 177
7.2.1. Immune System Involvement 177
7.2.2. Genetic Predispositions 178
7.2.3. Environmental Triggers 178
7.2.4. Inflammatory Processes 179
7.2.5. Vascular Damage Mechanisms 179
7.2.6. Role of Cytokines and Chemokines 180
7.2.7. Endothelial Dysfunction 180
7.2.8. Organ Involvement and Complications 181
7.3. Clinical Manifestations and Diagnosis 182
7.3.1. Common Symptoms Across Types 182
7.3.2. Organ-specific Manifestations 183
7.3.3. Laboratory Tests and Biomarkers 183
7.3.4. Imaging Techniques for Diagnosis 183
7.3.5. Biopsy and Histopathological Findings 184
7.3.6. Differential Diagnosis Considerations 185
7.3.7. Role of Rheumatologists in Diagnosis 185
7.3.8. Challenges in Early Diagnosis 186
7.3.9. Importance of Patient History and Examination 186
7.4. Treatment and Management Strategies 187
7.4.1. Corticosteroids in Treatment 187
7.4.2. Immunosuppressive Therapies 188
7.4.3. Biologic Agents and Targeted Therapies 188
7.4.4. Supportive Care and Symptom Management 189
7.4.5. Role of Multidisciplinary Teams 189
7.4.6. Monitoring for Treatment Efficacy 190
7.4.7. Long-term Management Strategies 190
7.4.8. Patient Education and Self-management 191
7.4.9. Future Directions in Treatment Research 191
Summary 192
References 194

CHAPTER 8

Gout and Pseudogout 199

Introduction 199
8.1. Pathophysiology of Gout 200
8.1.1. Mechanism of Uric Acid Production 200
8.1.2. Role of Purines in Gout 201
8.1.3. Crystal Formation in Joints 201
8.1.4. Inflammatory Response to Crystals 202
8.1.5. Genetic Factors Influencing Gout 202
8.1.6. Risk Factors associated with Gout 202
8.1.7. Stages of Gout Development 203
8.1.8. Common Sites of Gout Attacks 203
8.1.9. Long-term Effects of Untreated Gout 204
8.2. Pathophysiology of Pseudogout 205
8.2.1. Mechanism of Calcium Pyrophosphate Dihydrate (CPPD) Crystal Formation 205
8.2.2. Role of Calcium Metabolism in Pseudogout 206
8.2.3. Inflammatory Response to CPPD Crystals 206
8.2.4. Genetic Predisposition to Pseudogout 206
8.2.5. Risk Factors Associated with Pseudogout 207
8.2.6. Common Sites of Pseudogout Attacks 207
8.2.7. Stages of Pseudogout Development 208
8.2.8. Differences in Symptoms compared to Gout 208
8.2.9. Long-term Effects of Untreated Pseudogout 209
8.3. Diagnosis and Treatment of Gout 210
8.3.1. Clinical Symptoms and Physical Examination 210
8.3.2. Laboratory Tests for Uric Acid Levels 211
8.3.3. Imaging Techniques for Diagnosis 211
8.3.4. Acute Treatment Options for Gout Attacks 211
8.3.5. Long-term Management Strategies 212
8.3.6. Dietary Modifications and Lifestyle Changes 212
8.3.7. Medications used in Gout Treatment 213
8.3.8. Role of Patient Education in Management 214
8.3.9. Importance of Regular Follow-up 214
8.4. Diagnosis and Treatment of Pseudogout 215
8.4.1. Clinical Symptoms and Physical Examination 215
8.4.2. Laboratory Tests for CPPD Crystals 216
8.4.3. Imaging Techniques for Diagnosis 216

8.4.4. Acute Treatment Options for Pseudogout Attacks 217
8.4.5. Long-term Management Strategies 217
8.4.6. Dietary Modifications and Lifestyle Changes 218
8.4.7. Medications used in Pseudogout Treatment 218
8.4.8. Role of Patient Education in Management 218
8.4.9. Importance of Regular Follow-up 219
Summary **220**
References **222**

CHAPTER 9

Osteoarthritis 225

Introduction **225**
9.1. Causes and Risk Factors **226**
9.1.1. Age as a Primary Risk Factor 226
9.1.2. Genetic Predisposition 227
9.1.3. Obesity and its Effects 227
9.1.4. Joint Injuries and Trauma 227
9.1.5. Gender Differences in Prevalence 228
9.1.6. Occupational Hazards 228
9.1.7. Lifestyle Factors (e.g., Diet, Exercise) 229
9.1.8. Comorbid Conditions (e.g., Diabetes) 229
9.1.9. Environmental Factors 230
9.2. Symptoms and Diagnosis **231**
9.2.1. Common Symptoms of Osteoarthritis 231
9.2.2. Pain Characteristics 232
9.2.3. Stiffness and Its Implications 232
9.2.4. Swelling and Inflammation 232
9.2.5. Physical Examination Techniques 233
9.2.6. Imaging Methods (e.g., X-rays, MRIs) 233
9.2.7. Laboratory Tests and Biomarkers 234
9.2.8. Differential Diagnosis 234
9.2.9. Importance of Early Diagnosis 235
9.3. Treatment Options **235**
9.3.1. Non-pharmacological Interventions 236
9.3.2. Pharmacological Treatments 236
9.3.3. Physical Therapy and Rehabilitation 236
9.3.4. Surgical Options (e.g., Joint Replacement) 237
9.3.5. Alternative therapies (e.g., Acupuncture) 237
9.3.6. Lifestyle Modifications 238
9.3.7. Role of Nutrition in Management 238
9.3.8. Patient Education and Self-management 239
9.3.9. Emerging Treatments and Research 239
9.4. Impact on Daily Life **241**
9.4.1. Effects on Mobility and Physical Activity 241
9.4.2. Psychological Impact (e.g., Depression, Anxiety) 242
9.4.3. Social Implications and Relationships 242
9.4.4. Economic Burden on Individuals and Healthcare 243
9.4.5. Work-Related Challenges 243
9.4.6. Coping Strategies for Patients 244
9.4.7. Support Systems and Resources 244
9.4.8. Community and Family Involvement 245
9.4.9. Long-term Outlook for Patients 245
Summary **246**
References **248**

CHAPTER 10

Calcium and Bone Metabolism Disorders 255

Introduction **255**
10.1. Calcium Homeostasis **256**
10.1.1. Mechanisms of Calcium Absorption in the Intestines 256
10.1.2. Role of Vitamin D in Calcium Metabolism 257
10.1.3. Hormonal Regulation of Calcium Levels 257
10.1.4. Calcium Storage in Bones 258
10.1.5. Calcium Release from Bones 258
10.1.6. Factors Affecting Calcium Homeostasis 259
10.1.7. Consequences of Disrupted Calcium Homeostasis 259
10.1.8. Diagnostic Methods for Assessing Calcium Levels 260
10.1.9. Importance of Maintaining Calcium Balance 260
10.2. Osteoporosis **261**
10.2.1. Definition and Types of Osteoporosis 261
10.2.2. Risk Factors for Developing Osteoporosis 262
10.2.3. Symptoms and Clinical Manifestations 262
10.2.4. Pathophysiology of Bone Loss 262

10.2.5. Diagnostic Criteria and Imaging Techniques 263
10.2.6. Treatment Options and Management Strategies 263
10.2.7. Role of Calcium and Vitamin D in Prevention 264
10.2.8. Lifestyle Modifications to Reduce Risk 265
10.2.9. Impact of Osteoporosis on Quality of Life 265
10.3. Osteomalacia and Rickets 266
10.3.1. Definition and Differences between Osteomalacia and Rickets 266
10.3.2. Causes and Risk Factors for Osteomalacia 267
10.3.3. Causes and Risk Factors for Rickets 267
10.3.4. Symptoms and Clinical Features of Both Conditions 267
10.3.5. Pathophysiological Mechanisms Involved 268
10.3.6. Diagnostic Approaches and Laboratory Tests 269
10.3.7. Treatment Options and Nutritional Interventions 269
10.3.8. Long-term Consequences of Untreated Conditions 270
10.3.9. Public Health Implications and Prevention Strategies 270
10.4. Hypercalcemia and Hypocalcemia 272
10.4.1. Definition and Causes of Hypercalcemia 272
10.4.2. Definition and Causes of Hypocalcemia 273
10.4.3. Symptoms Associated with Hypercalcemia 273
10.4.4. Symptoms associated with Hypocalcemia 274
10.4.5. Diagnostic Methods for Hypercalcemia and Hypocalcemia 274
10.4.6. Treatment Options for Hypercalcemia 275
10.4.7. Treatment Options for Hypocalcemia 275
10.4.8. Role of Calcium Supplements in Management 276
10.4.9. Importance of Monitoring Calcium Levels in at-risk Populations 276
Summary 279
References 282

CHAPTER 11

Juvenile Idiopathic Arthritis (JIA) 285

Introduction 285
11.1. Causes and Risk Factors 286
11.1.1. Genetic Predisposition 287
11.1.2. Environmental Triggers 287
11.1.3. Immune System Dysfunction 287
11.1.4. Role of Infections 288
11.1.5. Family History of Autoimmune Diseases 288
11.1.6. Gender Differences in Incidence 289
11.1.7. Socioeconomic Factors 289
11.1.8. Ethnic Variations in Prevalence 290
11.2. Symptoms and Diagnosis 291
11.2.1. Common Symptoms of Juvenile Idiopathic Arthritis 291
11.2.2. Types of Juvenile Idiopathic Arthritis and their Specific Symptoms 291
11.2.3. Diagnostic Criteria for Juvenile Idiopathic Arthritis 292
11.2.4. Role of Physical Examinations 292
11.2.5. Importance of Medical History 293
11.2.6. Laboratory Tests and Imaging Studies 294
11.2.7. Differential Diagnosis Considerations 294
11.2.8. Challenges in Diagnosing Juvenile Idiopathic Arthritis 295
11.2.9. Early Signs to Watch For 295
11.3. Treatment Options 296
11.3.1. Overview of Treatment Goals 296
11.3.2. Nonsteroidal Anti-inflammatory Drugs (NSAIDs) 297
11.3.3. Disease-modifying Antirheumatic Drugs (DMARDs) 297
11.3.4. Biologic Therapies 297
11.3.5. Corticosteroids 298
11.3.6. Physical Therapy and Rehabilitation 298
11.3.7. Role of Nutrition and Lifestyle Changes 299
11.3.8. Pain Management Strategies 299
11.3.9. Importance of Multidisciplinary Care 300
11.4. Living with JIA 301

11.4.1. Psychological Impact on Children and Families 301
11.4.2. Coping Strategies for Patients 302
11.4.3. Support Systems and Resources 302
11.4.4. Educational Accommodations for Affected Children 302
11.4.5. Social Implications and Peer Relationships 303
11.4.6. Transitioning to Adult Care 303
11.4.7. Long-term Health Considerations 304
11.4.8. Advocacy and Awareness Efforts 304
11.4.9. Personal Stories and Testimonials 305
Summary **306**
References **308**

CHAPTER 12

Therapeutics in Rheumatology **313**

Introduction **313**
12.1. Pharmacological Treatments **314**
12.1.1. Nonsteroidal Anti-Inflammatory Drugs (NSAIDs) 314
12.1.2. Disease-Modifying Antirheumatic Drugs (DMARDs) 315
12.1.3. Biologic Response Modifiers 315
12.1.4. Corticosteroids 315
12.1.5. Analgesics and Pain Management 316
12.1.6. Targeted Synthetic DMARDs 316
12.1.7. Combination Therapy Approaches 317
12.1.8. Side Effects and Risks of Pharmacological Treatments 317
12.2. Non-Pharmacological Interventions **318**
12.2.1. Physical Therapy and Rehabilitation 318
12.2.2. Occupational Therapy 319
12.2.3. Dietary Modifications and Nutrition 319
12.2.4. Exercise and Lifestyle Changes 320
12.2.5. Complementary and Alternative Medicine 320
12.2.6. Patient Education and Self-Management 321
12.2.7. Psychological Support and Counseling 321
12.2.8. Role of Support Groups 322
12.2.9. Integrative Approaches in Rheumatology 322
12.3. Advances in Research and Technology **323**
12.3.1. Genetic Research in Rheumatology 323
12.3.2. Biomarkers for Disease Monitoring 324
12.3.3. Advances in Imaging Techniques 324
12.3.4. Telemedicine in Rheumatology 325
12.3.5. Artificial Intelligence and Machine Learning 325
12.3.6. Clinical Trials and Their Importance 326
12.3.7. Personalized Medicine Approaches 326
12.3.8. Innovations in Drug Development 327
12.3.9. Future Research Directions 327
Summary **328**
References **330**

Index **335**

LIST OF FIGURES

Figure 1.1. Rheumatoid arthritis (RA)

Figure 1.2. Understanding genetic predisposition plays a crucial role in unraveling the complex etiology of rheumatoid arthritis (RA)

Figure 1.3. The influence of hormones on the development and progression of rheumatoid arthritis (RA) is a significant area of investigation, particularly as it pertains to the disparities observed between genders

Figure 1.4. The progression and symptomatology of RA often manifest differently across genders; women frequently report greater pain and fatigue, while men may experience a more aggressive disease course

Figure 1.5. Chronic inflammation in RA can be influenced by the host's microbiota, which, through a process of co-evolution, forms a symbiotic relationship with the immune system

Figure 1.6. Socioeconomic status, which encompasses income, education, and occupation, can affect access to healthcare resources, thereby altering treatment outcomes and quality of life for RA patients

Figure 1.7. The hallmark symptoms are joint pain, often accompanied by swelling and stiffness, particularly in the mornings or after periods of inactivity

Figure 1.8. Systemic symptoms can manifest as fatigue, fever, and malaise, often resulting from the underlying autoimmune process that characterizes the disease

Figure 1.9. The integration of composite indices to measure disease activity is critical in steering treatment strategies toward target outcomes, such as remission or low disease activity

Figure 1.10. X-rays have long been utilized to visualize joint damage and erosions characteristic of RA

Figure 1.11. Early diagnosis allows for the prompt initiation of disease-modifying treatments, which can significantly improve clinical outcomes and enhance the quality of life for patients

Figure 1.12. The pharmacological treatment of rheumatoid arthritis (RA) is critical in managing symptoms and slowing disease progression

Figure 1.13. The management of rheumatoid arthritis (RA) primarily involves the use of disease-modifying antirheumatic drugs (DMARDs), which are essential for slowing disease progression and alleviating joint damage

Figure 1.14. In the management of rheumatoid arthritis (RA), corticosteroids play a pivotal role due to their potent anti-inflammatory properties

Figure 1.15. Lifestyle modifications play a crucial role in the management of rheumatoid arthritis (RA), influencing both symptom relief and overall quality of life

Figure 1.16. The complexity of RA necessitates not only pharmacological interventions but also support from specialists such as physical therapists, occupational therapists, and dietitians

Figure 1.17. Coping strategies play a crucial role in managing the emotional and physical challenges associated with rheumatoid arthritis (RA)

Figure 1.18. Managing chronic pain and disability often leads to debilitating psychological distress, including heightened levels of anxiety and depression, which can significantly impede patients' ability to respond to treatment effectively

Figure 1.19. Effective patient education plays a crucial role in the management of rheumatoid arthritis (RA), significantly influencing clinical outcomes and empowering patients to take an active role in their treatment

Figure 1.20. Understanding the role of nutrition in managing rheumatoid arthritis (RA) is increasingly recognized as vital for improving patient outcomes

Figure 1.21. The chronic nature of RA means that symptoms can persist over time, leading to potential disability and reduced quality of life

Figure 2.1. Systemic lupus erythematosus

Figure 2.2. The immune system dysfunction observed in systemic lupus erythematosus (SLE) underscores the complex interplay between metabolic disturbances and autoimmunity

Figure 2.3. Understanding the role of environmental triggers in the pathogenesis of Systemic Lupus Erythematosus (SLE) is critical for developing targeted therapeutic strategies

Figure 2.4. The discovery of Toll-like receptors (TLRs) significantly enhances our understanding of this phenomenon, as TLRs can initiate innate and adaptive immune responses upon encountering pathogen-associated molecules

Figure 2.5. Systemic lupus erythematosus (SLE) is a multifaceted autoimmune disorder that impacts various organ systems, significantly complicating its clinical presentation

Figure 2.6. SLE is characterized by diverse clinical manifestations, often resulting in multi-organ damage, which complicates management options for affected individuals

Figure 2.7. Systemic Lupus Erythematosus (SLE) patients experience fatigue, joint pain, and skin rashes, particularly the characteristic butterfly rash across the cheeks and nose

Figure 2.8. Patients report a range of musculoskeletal issues, including arthralgia, myalgia, and even inflammatory arthritis, which contribute to substantial morbidity

Figure 2.9. Neurological symptoms in patients with Systemic Lupus Erythematosus (SLE) can significantly impact their quality of life, presenting a complex challenge for diagnosis and management

Figure 2.10. Cardiovascular complications are a significant concern for patients with systemic lupus erythematosus (SLE), as they contribute markedly to morbidity and mortality within this population

Figure 2.11. Some patients may experience audiovestibular symptoms like sensorineural hearing loss, which can occur in a fluctuating or progressive manner

Figure 2.12. Accurate identification of these criteria is crucial, given that early diagnosis can significantly influence patient outcomes and treatment efficacy

Figure 2.13. Understanding a patient's complete medical background, including prior infections and hematological status, can guide clinicians in tailoring therapeutic interventions effectively

Figure 2.14. Imaging studies play a crucial role in the assessment and management of Systemic Lupus Erythematosus (SLE)

Figure 2.15. The identification and utilization of biomarkers play a crucial role in the diagnosis and management of Systemic Lupus Erythematosus (SLE), a complex autoimmune disorder

Figure 2.16. The utilization of advanced magnetic resonance imaging (MRI) technologies, which facilitate more precise evaluations of neuropsychiatric manifestations in SLE patients

Figure 2.17. The management of Systemic Lupus Erythematosus (SLE) necessitates a comprehensive overview of treatment goals aimed at optimizing patient outcomes and minimizing disease-related morbidity

Figure 2.18. Structured exercise has emerged as a particularly effective adjunctive therapy, showing significant benefits in reducing fatigue and improving functional capacity

Figure 2.19. Employing a treat-to-target (T2T) strategy, clinicians can adjust therapies to meet predefined objectives that aim for low disease activity or remission, thus reducing the frequency and severity of flares

Figure 2.20. Monitoring disease progression in systemic lupus erythematosus (SLE) is critical for effective management and treatment outcomes, as the condition can lead to severe organ damage and complications

Figure 3.1. Spondyloarthritides

Figure 3.2. Ankylosing spondylitis (AS)

Figure 3.3. Reactive arthritis, a form of *spondyloarthritis*, typically arises following an infection, often in the genitourinary or gastrointestinal tract

Figure 3.4. Undifferentiated *Spondyloarthritis* (uSpA)

Figure 3.5. Non-radiographic axial *spondyloarthritis*

Figure 3.6. An understanding of genetic factors, particularly the role of the HLA-B27 antigen, is crucial for elucidating the pathophysiology of spondyloarthritides (SpA)

Figure 3.7. Inflammatory processes play a crucial role in the pathophysiology of spondyloarthritides, characterized by significant joint inflammation that leads to both acute symptoms and chronic structural changes

Figure 3.8. Bone remodeling, a dynamic process crucial for maintaining skeletal integrity, is significantly altered in conditions like spondyloarthritides

Figure 3.9. Microbial infections are thought to provoke reactions in genetically predisposed individuals, highlighting the interaction between environmental agents and host genetics, particularly concerning the HLA-B27 allele

Figure 3.10. A summarized illustration of the mendelian randomization causal association assessment between Ankylosing Spondylitis (exposure) and the need for a second-line therapy in Crohn's disease (outcome)

Figure 3.11. Lower back pain is particularly prevalent among patients consulting general practitioners, often complicating the assessment due to its benign and mechanical nature in many cases

Figure 3.12. X-rays are traditionally utilized to assess structural changes in the spine and sacroiliac joints, offering a visual representation of characteristic alterations associated with spinal fusion and inflammation

Figure 3.13. Accurate identification of the subtype of *spondyloarthritis* is crucial for effective management and intervention

Figure 3.14. The diagnostic criteria for spondyloarthritides (SpA) have evolved significantly in recent years, reflecting advancements in both clinical practice and scientific understanding

Figure 3.15. The importance of early diagnosis in spondyloarthritides cannot be overstated, as timely identification of these conditions significantly influences the overall management and prognosis of affected patients

Figure 3.16. The management of spondyloarthritides, particularly ankylosing spondylitis (AS), often involves pharmacological treatments such as nonsteroidal anti-inflammatory drugs (NSAIDs) and disease-modifying antirheumatic drugs (DMARDs)

Figure 3.17. Physical therapy and exercise play crucial roles in the management of spondyloarthritides (SpA), providing patients with effective strategies for maintaining mobility and alleviating pain

Figure 3.18. Surgical interventions may involve procedures such as spinal fusion or decompression, aimed at addressing severe structural deformities or debilitating pain linked to inflammation and arthritis

Figure 3.19. Effective patient education plays a crucial role in the management of spondyloarthritides, as informed patients are better equipped to engage in their treatment processes and mitigate associated complications

Figure 3.20. The future directions in the treatment of spondyloarthritides promise to be transformative, emphasizing the integration of targeted therapies and personalized medicine

Figure 4.1. Sjogren's syndrome

Figure 4.2. The role of invariant natural killer T cells (iNKT), which modulate immune activity and contribute to inflammation within the affected tissues, suggesting their potential as biomarkers for disease progression

Figure 4.3. Infiltration of lymphocytes into exocrine glands, leading to significant architectural changes and impaired glandular function

Figure 4.4. Factors such as exposure to certain chemicals, infections, and even climate conditions can exacerbate the autoimmune responses seen in affected individuals

Figure 4.5. Secondary Sjögren's is associated with other autoimmune conditions, such as rheumatoid arthritis or lupus, complicating the clinical presentation and management due to the interplay of multiple autoimmune processes

Figure 4.6. Sjogren's Syndrome, an autoimmune disorder characterized by the dysfunction of exocrine glands, primarily manifests through a distinctive set of symptoms

Figure 4.7. Patients often experience xerostomia, or dry mouth, which arises from decreased saliva production, leading to difficulties in chewing, swallowing, and speaking

Figure 4.8. a Lacrimal Schirmer test, b Salivary Schirmer test 1. c Salivary Schirmer test 2

Figure 4.9. Emerging fields such as oculomics have begun to highlight the relevance of ocular imaging in identifying systemic disease markers associated with Sjögren's Syndrome

Figure 4.1.0. Immunoglobulin G4-related diseases have emerged as complex multi-organ conditions characterized by an autoimmune reaction that targets salivary glands, making identification crucial since these disorders were previously regarded as mere variants of Sjögrens syndrome

Figure 4.11. Symptomatic relief for xerostomia and dry eye involves the use of over-the-counter artificial saliva substitutes and prescription medications such as pilocarpine, which stimulate saliva production

Figure 4.12. Dry mouth remedies

Figure 4.13. Maintaining hydration and utilizing humidifiers can alleviate the discomfort associated with dry mucous membranes, while regular use of artificial tears can provide symptomatic relief

Figure 4.14. Regular monitoring is crucial for managing Sjogren's Syndrome, as it allows healthcare providers to track the progression of the disease and promptly address emerging complications

Figure 4.15. Effective patient education and support are crucial components in managing Sjögren's Syndrome, a complex autoimmune condition characterized by symptoms such as dryness, fatigue, and pain

Figure 4.16. The chronic inflammation associated with the syndrome may lead to increased risks of ocular surface diseases, including keratoconjunctivitis sicca, which can significantly impair vision and diminish quality of life

Figure 4.17. Patients with Sjögren's frequently exhibit comorbid conditions such as rheumatoid arthritis, systemic lupus erythematosus, and thyroid disorders, suggesting a shared underlying immunological mechanism

Figure 4.18. Patients often experience anxiety and depression, primarily due to the chronic discomfort caused by symptoms such as xerostomia and xerophthalmia, which can lead to social withdrawal and a sense of isolation

Figure 4.19. Joint pain, stiffness, and inflammation are commonly reported symptoms, affecting approximately 30–50% of individuals with this autoimmune condition

Figure 5.1. Systemic sclerosis, commonly known as scleroderma, represents a complex and severe autoimmune disorder characterized by aberrant connective tissue production and extensive fibrosis

Figure 5.2. The immune system dysfunction observed in systemic sclerosis (scleroderma) significantly contributes to the disease's pathological progression and severity

Figure 5.3. The vascular changes observed in systemic sclerosis (scleroderma) significantly contribute to the disease's complex pathophysiology, particularly through endothelial damage

Figure 5.4. The genetic landscape of systemic sclerosis (scleroderma) reveals significant insights into the hereditary factors contributing to disease susceptibility

Figure 5.5. Central to this fibrotic process are various growth factors, notably transforming growth factor beta (TGF-β), connective tissue growth factor (CTGF), and platelet-derived growth factor (PDGF), which promote the differentiation of fibroblasts into myofibroblasts

Figure 5.6. Understanding the mechanisms underlying organ involvement in systemic sclerosis (scleroderma) is crucial for improving patient outcomes, as this multifaceted disease often affects various internal organs, with the gastrointestinal tract being the most commonly involved

Figure 5.7. Patients may experience skin thickening and tightness, often referred to as sclerodactyly, which affects the fingers and can severely limit mobility

Figure 5.8. Pulmonary involvement is a critical concern in systemic sclerosis (SSc), significantly impacting patient morbidity and mortality

Figure 5.9. In systemic sclerosis (scleroderma), renal implications are particularly concerning, as renal crisis represents a potentially life-threatening manifestation of the disease

Figure 5.10. Cognitive dysfunction, neuropathy, and erectile dysfunction (ED) frequently emerge as complications, highlighting the multi-systemic impact of SSc on neurological health

Figure 5.11. The quality of life for individuals diagnosed with systemic sclerosis (scleroderma) is significantly compromised due to the multifaceted nature of the disease, which encompasses both physical and psychological dimensions

Figure 5.12. Nailfold video capillaroscopy (NVC)

Figure 5.13. Nailfold video capillaroscopy (NVC) stands as the gold standard for visualizing capillary alterations, enabling direct observation of microvascular remodeling specific to scleroderma patients

Figure 5.14. The role of skin biopsy in the diagnosis and management of systemic sclerosis (scleroderma) is paramount, offering critical insights into the pathophysiological changes associated with the disease

Figure 5.15. Most established method is the modified Rodnan Skin Score (MRSS), which quantitatively measures skin thickening and serves as a critical indicator of disease progression

Figure 5.16. Patients often exhibit nonspecific signs such as fatigue, joint pain, and skin changes, which can easily lead to misdiagnosis or delayed recognition of the underlying condition

Figure 5.17. Nifedipine is recommended as a first-line therapy for RP, while sildenafil and bosentan serve as effective second-line treatments for patients experiencing severe and refractory cases

Figure 5.18. Physical therapy interventions focus on improving mobility, reducing pain, and enhancing overall physical function, which can be significantly compromised due to the disease's symptoms

Figure 5.19. Effective patient education plays a pivotal role in managing systemic sclerosis (scleroderma), particularly given the complexity of this chronic condition

Figure 5.20. Clinical trials are integral to assessing the safety and efficacy of these innovative approaches, including immunosuppressive therapies and potential antifibrotic agents

Figure 5.21. Effective long-term management strategies for Systemic Sclerosis (Scleroderma) necessitate a multidisciplinary approach that encompasses pharmacological interventions, physical therapies, and psychological support

Figure 6.1. Idiopathic Inflammatory Myopathies (IIM) represent a diverse group of autoimmune diseases characterized by muscle inflammation, weakness, and varying degrees of muscle damage

Figure 6.2. Polymyositis (PM) is a prominent subtype of idiopathic inflammatory myopathies characterized by symmetrical proximal muscle weakness and inflammation

Figure 6.3. Inclusion body myositis (IBM) stands out as a distinct form of idiopathic inflammatory myopathy, predominantly affecting older adults, typically those over the age of 50

Figure 6.4. Overlap myositis

Figure 6.5. The classification of idiopathic inflammatory myopathies (IIM) has been significantly advanced through the implementation of the EULAR/ACR criteria, which were established by a consortium of experts aimed at improving diagnostic accuracy

Figure 6.6. Understanding the prognosis for each type of idiopathic inflammatory myopathy (IIM), primarily polymyositis and dermatomyositis, is critical for patient management and care optimization

Figure 6.7. The pathophysiology of idiopathic inflammatory myopathies (IIMs) is marked by a complex interplay of autoimmune mechanisms that lead to muscle inflammation and damage

Figure 6.8. Autoantibodies can serve as important biomarkers that not only assist in confirming the diagnosis of various subtypes, such as polymyositis and dermatomyositis, but also help in predicting disease progression and treatment response

Figure 6.9. The inflammatory processes underlying idiopathic inflammatory myopathies (IIMs) are complex and multifaceted, involving a myriad of cellular and molecular interactions

Figure 6.10. The role of environmental triggers in the onset and progression of idiopathic inflammatory myopathies (IIM) presents a complex interplay of factors that warrant careful examination

Figure 6.11. Macrophages, as central players in muscle inflammation, have dual roles; they can exacerbate damage through the release of proinflammatory cytokines and reactive oxygen species while also facilitating tissue repair and regeneration

Figure 6.12. Electromyography (EMG) and magnetic resonance imaging (MRI) also play crucial roles in identifying characteristic muscle inflammation

Figure 6.13. In the diagnosis and management of idiopathic inflammatory myopathies (IIMs), laboratory tests and biomarkers play a crucial role in enhancing understanding and tailoring treatment strategies

Figure 6.14. Muscle biopsy techniques play a crucial role in the diagnosis and management of idiopathic inflammatory myopathies (IIM)

Figure 6.15. Accurate differential diagnosis in idiopathic inflammatory myopathies (IIM) is critical due to the clinical and pathological similarities these conditions share with other neuromuscular disorders

Figure 6.16. Symptoms such as muscle weakness, fatigue, and dysphagia are often non-specific and can overlap with other conditions, delaying accurate identification

Figure 6.17. Corticosteroids and immunosuppressants play a pivotal role in mitigating the autoimmune response that characterizes these conditions

Figure 6.18. Mechanism of action of abatacept

Figure 6.19. Physical and mental health in this population are significantly impaired, particularly in individuals with additional comorbidities, which can exacerbate their overall health status

Figure 6.20. Effective long-term monitoring and follow-up of patients with idiopathic inflammatory myopathies (IIM) are crucial for optimizing treatment outcomes and enhancing quality of life

Figure 6.21. The interplay between chronic inflammatory processes and muscle integrity necessitates preventive strategies to maintain muscle health and ward off complications

Figure 7.1. Systemic vasculitides

Figure 7.2. Large vessel vasculitides represent a significant subset of vasculitis disorders that primarily affect the major arteries, notably the aorta and its major branches

Figure 7.3. Small vessel vasculitides represent a distinct group of disorders characterized by inflammation of the small blood vessels, leading to a diverse array of clinical manifestations

Figure 7.4. Systemic vasculitides, such as Granulomatosis with Polyangiitis (GPA) or Eosinophilic Granulomatosis with Polyangiitis (EGPA), involve widespread inflammatory responses that can affect multiple organ systems, leading to significant morbidity and mortality if left untreated

Figure 7.5. The classification of vasculitides is foundational for accurate diagnosis and treatment, given the heterogeneous nature of these conditions

Figure 7.6. Accurate classification of vasculitides is crucial for effective diagnosis and management, as it directly influences therapeutic strategies and patient outcomes

Figure 7.7. Granulomatosis with polyangiitis (GPA)

Figure 7.8. The interaction between neutrophils and environmental stressors has been shown to amplify vascular inflammation, contributing to vascular damage and disease progression

Figure 7.9. A key player in this process is the subset of CD4(+) T cells known as effector memory T (T-EM) cells

Figure 7.10. Endothelial dysfunction is a crucial factor in the pathogenesis of vasculitides, characterized by an imbalance between endothelial injury and repair

Figure 7.11. Dermatological symptoms, including rashes and purpura, are frequently observed across various forms of vasculitis, highlighting the condition's impact on skin integrity and vascular health

Figure 7.12. Laboratory diagnostics are essential for distinguishing between various types of vasculitides

Figure 7.13. In the context of vasculitides, biopsy and histopathological findings serve as crucial elements in accurately diagnosing conditions such as granulomatosis with polyangiitis (GPA) and cryoglobulinaemic vasculitis

Figure 7.14. Rheumatologists play a critical role in the diagnosis and management of vasculitides, particularly in distinguishing conditions such as granulomatosis with polyangiitis (GPA) from other autoimmune disorders

Figure 7.15. Understanding the patients' prior health conditions, including infections or autoimmune disorders, can offer insights into potential triggers for these complex diseases

Figure 7.16. Judicious use of corticosteroids, coupled with careful monitoring of blood pressure, may alleviate symptoms while addressing underlying inflammatory processes

Figure 7.17. Therapies aimed at interleukin-5 have shown promise in treating eosinophilic granulomatosis with polyangiitis and hyper eosinophilic syndrome

Figure 7.18. Cogans syndrome

Figure 7.19. Cryoglobulinaemia

Figure 8.1. Gout and pseudogout

Figure 8.2. Uric acid production is a crucial biochemical process that influences the pathophysiology of gout, a form of inflammatory arthritis marked by elevated levels of this metabolite in the bloodstream

Figure 8.3. The formation of crystals in joints is a central aspect of both gout and pseudogout, where the presence of monosodium urate (MSU) and calcium pyrophosphate dihydrate (CPPD) crystals, respectively, leads to significant inflammatory responses

Figure 8.4. Gout, a complex form of inflammatory arthritis, is significantly influenced by genetic factors that predispose individuals to hyperuricemia—the primary cause of gouty attacks

Figure 8.5. The progression of gout typically unfolds in a series of distinct stages, each characterized by specific physiological changes and clinical manifestations

Figure 8.6. Chronic, untreated gout often results in recurrent acute attacks, which, if persistent, may progress to chronic gouty arthritis characterized by joint deformities and severe disability

Figure 8.7. The formation of calcium pyrophosphate dihydrate (CPPD) crystals is a complex biochemical process that highlights the interplay between metabolic conditions and mineral deposition

Figure 8.8. The inflammatory response to calcium pyrophosphate dihydrate (CPPD) crystals is a critical aspect of pseudogout, mirroring the pathophysiological mechanisms observed in gout with monosodium urate crystals

Figure 8.9. The emergence of pseudogout, a form of inflammatory arthritis, is closely linked to various risk factors that can predispose individuals to the condition

Figure 8.10. The body may exhibit asymptomatic crystal deposition in joint cartilage, often unnoticed until precipitating factors, such as trauma or surgery, trigger an inflammatory response

Figure 8.11. Chronic joint inflammation may result in persistent pain, stiffness, and reduced mobility, leading to functional impairments and potentially causing an increased risk of falls and fractures in older adults

Figure 8.12. The clinical symptoms and physical examination of gout and pseudogout share notable similarities, yet they are distinct conditions requiring careful differentiation to ensure appropriate management

Figure 8.13. The analysis of bone markers (BMs) in synovial fluid and serum represents another dimension in imaging diagnostics, providing insights into the underlying pathophysiology of arthropathies such as gout and pseudogout

Figure 8.14. Effective long-term management strategies for gout and pseudogout are essential to alleviate the burden these conditions impose on patients' quality of life

Figure 8.15. For long-term management, urate-lowering therapy such as allopurinol or febuxostat is often prescribed to maintain serum urate levels within the target range, preventing future episodes and potential joint damage

Figure 8.16. Regular follow-up care is paramount in effectively managing gout and pseudogout, as it fosters a continuous dialogue between patients and healthcare providers, ensuring timely adjustments to treatment plans

Figure 8.17. The clinical symptoms associated with gout and pseudogout share notable similarities, particularly the sudden onset of joint pain, swelling, and redness, typically affecting the lower extremities

Figure 8.18. The diagnosis of gout and pseudogout has evolved significantly with advancements in imaging techniques, enhancing the accuracy of clinical assessments

Figure 8.19. Effective long-term management strategies for gout and pseudogout are crucial to mitigate the recurring pain and inflammation associated with these conditions

Figure 8.20. Medications used in pseudogout treatment

Figure 8.21. Regular follow-up appointments are paramount in the management of gout and pseudogout, as they facilitate ongoing assessment and adjustment of treatment plans

Figure 9.1. Osteoarthritis

Figure 9.2. As individuals age, the risk of developing osteoarthritis significantly increases, making age a primary risk factor for this degenerative joint disease

Figure 9.3. The prevalence of obesity has reached alarming levels globally, significantly impacting public health and contributing to various chronic conditions, including osteoarthritis

Figure 9.4. Gender differences significantly influence the prevalence of osteoarthritis, with emerging evidence highlighting a higher susceptibility in women compared to men

Figure 9.5. Engaging in regular physical activity enhances joint mobility and strengthens the muscles surrounding the affected joints, thereby reducing stress on the cartilage

Figure 9.6. Environmental factors play a pivotal role in the development and progression of osteoarthritis (OA), with dietary patterns emerging as a significant influence

Figure 9.7. Common manifestations include persistent joint pain, stiffness, and swelling, particularly after periods of inactivity or excessive use

Figure 9.8. Stiffness is a hallmark symptom of osteoarthritis (OA) that significantly affects patients' mobility and quality of life

Figure 9.9. An effective physical examination is paramount in the evaluation and management of osteoarthritis, as it provides critical insights into the condition's progression and the patient's functional limitations

Figure 9.10. Effective differential diagnosis is crucial in the accurate identification of osteoarthritis, as its symptoms frequently overlap with those of various other musculoskeletal disorders

Figure 9.11. Non-pharmacological interventions have gained recognition as vital components in the management of osteoarthritis (OA), addressing both the physical and psychological dimensions of the condition

Figure 9.12. Physical therapy and rehabilitation play a critical role in managing osteoarthritis (OA), significantly enhancing patients' quality of life

Figure 9.13. Alternative therapies, such as acupuncture, have emerged as potential adjuncts in the management of osteoarthritis (OA), particularly for alleviating pain

Figure 9.14. The management of osteoarthritis (OA) significantly benefits from targeted nutritional interventions, which play a crucial role in mitigating symptoms and improving patients' quality of life

Figure 9.15. Traditionally, therapies have centered around symptom management with non-steroidal anti-inflammatory drugs and physical interventions, which often fail to address the underlying disease progression

Figure 9.16. As joint degeneration progresses, individuals often experience increased pain and stiffness, which can severely limit their ability to engage in physical activities

Figure 9.17. The social implications of osteoarthritis extend far beyond the physical limitations commonly associated with the condition

Figure 9.18. Employees afflicted with osteoarthritis (OA) often encounter significant work-related challenges that can hinder their performance and overall job satisfaction

Figure 9.19. The management of osteoarthritis (OA) is significantly enhanced by robust support systems and resources that empower patients in their treatment decisions

Figure 10.1. Disorders in calcium homeostasis can lead to significant skeletal issues, resulting in conditions such as osteoporosis, osteomalacia, and various forms of metabolic bone disease

Figure 10.2. The mechanisms of calcium absorption in the intestines are complex and highly regulated, playing a critical role in maintaining bone health and overall mineral balance

Figure 10.3. The hormonal regulation of calcium levels is crucial for maintaining bone health and overall metabolic functions, particularly in conditions that alter calcium homeostasis

Figure 10.4. The release of calcium from bones is a crucial physiological process that underpins numerous metabolic functions within the body

Figure 10.5. Hypercalcemia

Figure 10.6. The maintenance of calcium balance is crucial for both skeletal and systemic health, as calcium plays a key role in bone formation and remodeling

Figure 10.7. Osteoporosis is a metabolic bone disorder characterized by decreased bone density and structural deterioration of bone tissue, leading to increased fracture risk

Figure 10.8. The symptoms and clinical manifestations of calcium and bone metabolism disorders are diverse and can significantly impact patient quality of life

Figure 10.9. The accurate diagnosis of calcium and bone metabolism disorders necessitates a comprehensive understanding of both diagnostic criteria and advanced imaging techniques

Figure 10.10. Calcium and vitamin D are pivotal in the prevention of bone metabolism disorders, particularly in enhancing bone density and overall skeletal health

Figure 10.11. Individuals with osteoporosis often experience fractures, which can lead to chronic pain, loss of mobility, and decreased independence

Figure 10.12. Osteomalacia

Figure 10.13. Rickets, a condition characterized by impaired bone mineralization, primarily stems from deficiencies in vitamins, calcium, and phosphate

Figure 10.14. Importance of magnesium in bone health

Figure 10.15. Effective management of calcium and bone metabolism disorders necessitates a multifaceted approach encompassing both treatment options and nutritional interventions

Figure 10.16. Calcium plays a pivotal role in maintaining bone density, and deficiencies can lead to osteoporosis, elevating the risk of fractures and associated health complications in the aging population

Figure 10.17. Hypercalcemia, characterized by elevated levels of calcium in the bloodstream, poses significant clinical implications and can result from various underlying conditions

Figure 10.18. Hypercalcemia, characterized by elevated calcium levels in the blood, presents a range of symptoms that can profoundly affect an individual's health and quality of life

Figure 10.19. Diagnostic methods for hypercalcemia and hypocalcemia

Figure 10.20. In cases where hypoparathyroidism is confirmed, synthetic parathyroid hormone (PTH) replacement therapy is becoming increasingly recognized as a viable option, particularly beneficial for patients with chronic hypoparathyroidism following neck surgery

Figure 10.21. Menopause and bone loss

Figure 11.1. Juvenile Idiopathic Arthritis (JIA)

Figure 11.2. Genetic predispositions play a significant role; children with a family history of autoimmune diseases exhibit a higher likelihood of developing JIA

Figure 11.3. Immune system dysfunction is a central aspect of Juvenile Idiopathic Arthritis (JIA), characterized by an inappropriate immune response that targets the body's own joint tissues

Figure 11.4. The significance of a family history of autoimmune diseases emerges as a critical factor in understanding the etiology of Juvenile Idiopathic Arthritis (JIA)

Figure 11.5. Understanding the socioeconomic factors influencing juvenile idiopathic arthritis (JIA) is crucial for developing effective treatment and intervention strategies

Figure 11.6. Commonly reported symptoms include persistent joint pain, swelling, and stiffness, particularly notable in the morning or after periods of inactivity

Figure 11.7. The classification of JIA relies heavily on a comprehensive assessment which distinguishes it from other rheumatic diseases, highlighting the importance of accurate diagnostic methods

Figure 11.8. The importance of medical history in the context of Juvenile Idiopathic Arthritis (JIA) cannot be overstated, as it serves as a foundational element for effective diagnosis and treatment planning

Figure 11.9. Juvenile dermatomyositis

Figure 11.10. Early detection can significantly affect long-term outcomes, as timely treatment may prevent irreversible joint damage

Figure 11.11. Biologic agents, along with non-corticosteroid systemic immunomodulatory therapies, have transformed the therapeutic landscape, enhancing patient outcomes and quality of life

Figure 11.12. In the management of Juvenile Idiopathic Arthritis (JIA), Nonsteroidal Anti-Inflammatory Drugs (NSAIDs) play a pivotal role in alleviating pain and inflammation

Figure 11.13. The advent of biologic therapies has revolutionized the treatment landscape for Juvenile Idiopathic Arthritis (JIA), offering targeted interventions that significantly improve patient outcomes

Figure 11.14. The role of physical therapy and rehabilitation is paramount in the management of Juvenile Idiopathic Arthritis (JIA), aiming to enhance mobility, function, and overall quality of life

Figure 11.15. Effective pain management strategies for Juvenile Idiopathic Arthritis (JIA) are essential in enhancing the quality of life for affected children and their families

Figure 11.16. Children diagnosed with JIA often experience feelings of isolation and anxiety, as their condition may set them apart from peers, leading to a perception of their family as different from others

Figure 11.17. Effective management of Juvenile Idiopathic Arthritis (JIA) hinges significantly on robust support systems and resources

Figure 11.18. Healthy siblings in families with a JIA diagnosis often perceive their familial dynamic as distinct from peers, leading to feelings of isolation and a forfeiture of typical childhood experiences, such as spending quality time with friends or engaging in shared activities

Figure 11.19. Chronic inflammation associated with JIA can lead to joint damage and functional impairments, which may affect mobility and overall quality of life as patients transition into adulthood

Figure 11.20. Personal stories and testimonials play a crucial role in understanding the lived experiences of those affected by Juvenile Idiopathic Arthritis (JIA), shedding light on the challenges and triumphs faced by children and their families

Figure 12.1. Nonsteroidal Anti-Inflammatory Drugs (NSAIDs) stand out as cornerstone treatments due to their efficacy in managing symptoms associated with inflammatory conditions such as osteoarthritis (OA)

Figure 12.2. Biologic response modifiers represent a significant advancement in the treatment landscape of rheumatology

Figure 12.3. Effective pain management is essential for improving patients' quality of life, particularly for those grappling with chronic conditions like rheumatoid arthritis (RA)

Figure 12.4. In the realm of rheumatology, combination therapy approaches are increasingly recognized for their potential to enhance treatment efficacy beyond that of monotherapy

Figure 12.5. Effective physical therapy and rehabilitation play a pivotal role in the management of rheumatologic conditions, particularly in enhancing patient outcomes and improving quality of life

Figure 12.6. Dietary modifications have emerged as critical components in the management of rheumatological conditions, particularly concerning gout and rheumatoid arthritis (RA)

Figure 12.7. The integration of Complementary and Alternative Medicine (CAM) in the management of rheumatological conditions has gained significant attention

Figure 12.8. The provision of psychological support and counseling is an essential component of therapeutics in rheumatology, particularly for patients navigating chronic conditions such as rheumatoid arthritis (RA)

Figure 12.9. The integration of diverse therapeutic strategies in rheumatology is becoming increasingly vital for enhancing patient outcomes

Figure 12.10. The exploration of genetic research in rheumatology is pivotal in advancing therapeutic strategies for conditions such as rheumatoid arthritis (RA)

Figure 12.11. Precision imaging modalities, including magnetic resonance imaging (MRI) and ultrasound, allow for the early detection of joint inflammation and damage, which is crucial given that timely intervention can prevent long-term disability

Figure 12.12. The integration of Artificial Intelligence (AI) and Machine Learning (ML) into rheumatology represents a transformative approach to enhancing therapeutic strategies for patients with systemic autoimmune rheumatic diseases (SARDs)

Figure 12.13. Personalized medicine approaches in rheumatology represent a significant advancement in tailoring treatments to individual patient profiles, particularly in complex diseases like rheumatoid arthritis (RA) and systemic sclerosis (SSc)

Figure 12.14. As the field of rheumatology continues to evolve, future research directions must emphasize the exploration of novel therapeutic targets that address the complexities of autoimmune diseases

PREFACE

The diagnosis and management of systemic and inflammatory musculoskeletal diseases have been profoundly altered over the past few decades. Disabilities that were previously poorly described are now improved in diagnosis and treated more effectively because of advances in immunology, molecular biology, and therapeutic investigation. Despite such advancement, rheumatologic disease continues to be a major diagnostic challenge and clinical heterogeneity and requires that professionals remain abreast of evolving clinical patterns and management options.

These disorders affect millions of individuals and often mandate chronic care. They are a wide spectrum of presentations from confined joint complaints to multi-organ systemic disease and can manifest at any age, affecting quality of life and productivity. Most of these disorders also have overlapping features, necessitating careful differentiation by clinical judgment, laboratory support, and imaging. Continuous updates in disease terminology, biologics, and disease-modifying drugs mandate that practitioners and students employ general and updated references that integrate the state-of-the-art of science and clinical practice.

Textbook of Rheumatology Volume 2 builds on the fundamental principles established in Volume 1, presenting an extensive discussion of selected rheumatologic diseases and therapeutic methods. Volume 2 integrates detailed descriptions of the pathology of disease, diagnostic features, clinical manifestations, and evidence-based treatment regimens. Every chapter is written to include a scientific basis as well as practical tips, making the textbook of rheumatology Volume 2 a must-have book for those committed to delivering quality care in rheumatology.

Chapter 1 outlines *Rheumatoid Arthritis*, the most common and best-characterized of the autoimmune diseases to symmetrically afflict the joints. It outlines its pathogenesis -- synovial hyperplasia, pannus, and joint destruction -- as well as classification criteria, extra-articular disease, and long-term consequences. It supplies an overview of historic synthetic and biologic disease-modifying antirheumatic drugs, along with how to initiate treatment, follow, and evaluate response.

Chapter 2 is on *Systemic Lupus Erythematosus,* a prototypic systemic autoimmune disorder with diverse clinical features ranging from mucocutaneous lesions and arthritis to nephritis, hematologic abnormalities, and neuropsychiatric features. The chapter covers its immunopathogenesis, including loss of tolerance, autoantibody production, and immune complex deposition. Special emphasis is laid on disease flare, organ-based classification, laboratory monitoring, and management based on disease activity and organ involvement.

Chapter 3 addresses *Spondyloarthritides*, which are inflammatory rheumatic conditions that include ankylosing spondylitis, psoriatic arthritis, reactive arthritis, and inflammatory bowel disease-associated arthritis. They all have common aspects like axial disease, enthesitis, and HLA-B27 association, and differ from each other on the basis of their characteristic disease patterns. Imaging modalities, classification criteria, and treatment with NSAIDs, biologics, and targeted synthetic drugs are discussed in depth.

Chapter 4 discusses *Sjogren's Syndrome*, an autoimmune disorder that mainly affects exocrine glands to produce dry eyes and dry mouth. Besides the sicca manifestations, the chapter proceeds with systemic manifestations like fatigue, arthritis, vasculitis, and lymphoma risk. Diagnosis with tests like antibody assays and salivary gland biopsy is discussed along with current treatment modalities focused on symptom treatment and management of systemic complications.

Chapter 5 discusses *Systemic Sclerosis (Scleroderma),* a complex autoimmune connective tissue disorder characterized by vasculopathy, fibrosis, and immune dysregulation. The chapter describes its two primary forms, limited and diffuse cutaneous, and internal organ complications such as pulmonary hypertension, interstitial lung disease, renal crisis, and gastrointestinal dysmotility. Treatment options, including immunosuppressants, antifibrotic therapy, and vascular-targeted therapies, are discussed with organ-specific treatment in focus.

Chapter 6 outlines *Idiopathic Inflammatory Myopathies,* which are a group of disorders including polymyositis, dermatomyositis, inclusion body myositis, and immune-mediated necrotizing myopathy. The clinical spectrum is from muscle weakness proximally to skin rash, lung disease, and malignancy association.

Chapter 7 addresses *Vasculitides,* a group of diseases characterized by inflammation of blood vessels causing ischemia, hemorrhage, and organ injury. Large-, medium-, and small-vessel vasculitides are addressed, including giant cell arteritis, polyarteritis nodosa, granulomatosis with polyangiitis, and IgA vasculitis. Classification criteria, biopsy findings, imaging procedures such as PET-CT and angiography, and the treatment regimens with corticosteroids, cytotoxic agents, and biologic drugs are accorded significance.

Chapter 8 covers *Gout and Pseudogout,* the most common crystal-induced arthropathies. The chapter covers the pathophysiology of monosodium urate and calcium pyrophosphate crystal deposition, clinical presentation of acute monoarthritis and tophaceous disease, and the diagnostic use of synovial fluid analysis. Acute flare treatment and chronic urate-lowering therapy are covered in depth, with comorbidity and chronic kidney disease in mind.

Chapter 9 describes *Osteoarthritis,* the most prevalent arthritis. It focuses on the degenerative process with cartilage loss, subchondral bone remodeling, and osteophyte formation. Risk factors such as age, obesity, and joint injury are described, alongside the clinical presentation of joint pain, stiffness, and functional limitation. Nonpharmacologic therapy, analgesics, intra-articular interventions, and surgery are outlined in a patient-centered model.

Chapter 10 covers *Calcium and Bone Metabolism Disorders,* including osteoporosis, osteomalacia, Paget's disease, and parathyroid-hormone-related bone changes. The chapter outlines calcium and phosphate homeostasis, hormonal regulation by PTH and vitamins, as well as markers for bone remodeling.

Chapter 11 discusses *Juvenile Idiopathic Arthritis,* the most common chronic rheumatologic disease of children. The chapter describes the subtypes of classification, including oligoarticular, polyarticular, systemic, and enthesitis-related arthritis. Clinical presentation, uveitis risk, and diagnostic strategy are discussed. Treatment is tailored to severity and type of disease, with a discussion of NSAIDs, methotrexate, biologics, and long-term follow-up to prevent growth disturbances and joint damage.

Chapter 12 is put together in a perspective of synthesizing pharmacologic strategies by disease group. The chapter compares drug classes like NSAIDs, corticosteroids, csDMARDs, biologic medications, and Janus kinase inhibitors. It gives recommendations on drug choice, safety monitoring, immunization practice, and resistant disease management.

The book is addressed to a broad-based audience of rheumatologists, internists, pediatricians, orthopedic surgeons, and allied health providers who have shared responsibilities in the treatment of patients with autoimmune and inflammatory conditions. It is also a required book for postgraduate trainees and medical students appearing for board exams or clinical practice exams in their postgraduate or final exams. Owing to its emphasis on theory and practice, the book promotes academic education, clinical decision making, and interprofessional practice in rheumatologic care.

RHEUMATOID ARTHRITIS (RA)

1

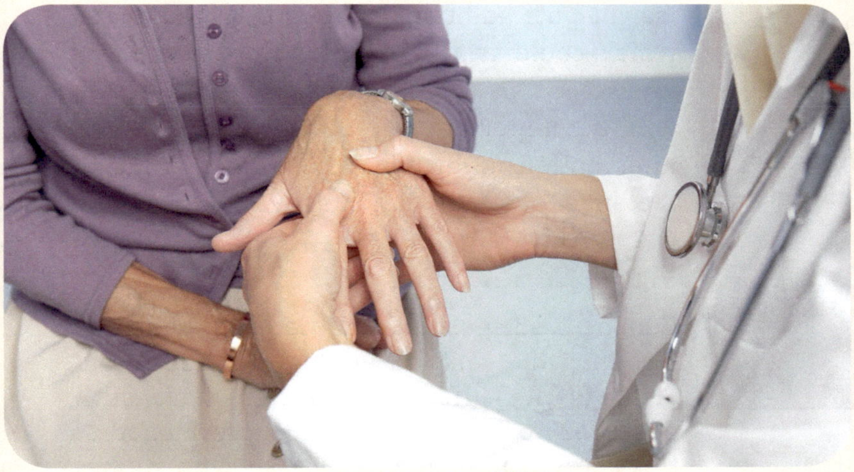

LEARNING OBJECTIVES

After studying this chapter, you will be able to:

1. Identify causes and risk factors of rheumatoid arthritis.
2. Know the symptoms and diagnosis of rheumatoid arthritis.
3. Consider treatment options for rheumatoid arthritis.
4. Focus on living with rheumatoid arthritis.

Introduction

Rheumatoid Arthritis (RA) is not only a severe health issue but also a complex interplay of bodily and psychological factors that collectively impact the suffering. Being a chronic autoimmune disorder, RA triggers constant inflammation, primarily of the joints, and is marked by debilitating pain and functional loss. The prevalence of arthritis is staggering, with approximately 3 million Australians experiencing it, making it a major cause of chronic pain and disability in Australia (Bates et al., 2014). It is essential to know the extensive lived experience of RA patients since there are many individuals with symptoms extending beyond the physical realm, such as emotional distress, social isolation, and increased healthcare needs. This multifactorial nature is usually compounded by comorbid illnesses, such as sleep disorders, that can have additional effects on patient outcomes and overall life quality (Gaspar et al., 2016). Therefore, thorough studies of its multifaceted effects are critical to the improvement of support structures and treatment protocols (Figure 1.1).

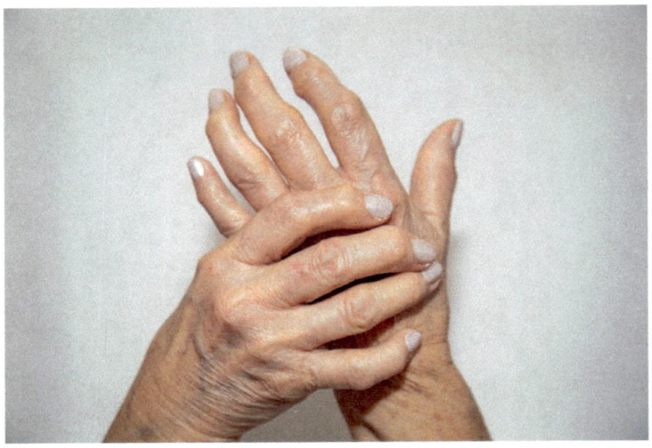

Figure 1.1. Rheumatoid arthritis (RA).

Source: https://www.verywellhealth.com/thmb/i0lfbNRPtQ7Kh3MrQgEAPTBabWE=/1500x0/filters:no_upscale():max_bytes(150000):strip_icc()/GettyImages-1390310510-2c62d564d3e648ccbdddb6921a50ae68.jpg

1.1. Causes and Risk Factors of Rheumatoid Arthritis

Learning Outcome

1. Understand genetic predisposition;
2. Explain environmental triggers;
3. Focus on hormonal influences;
4. Discuss age-related factors;
5. Focus on gender differences;
6. List lifestyle factors (e.g., smoking, diet);
7. Identify infections and autoimmune responses;
8. Describe family history of autoimmune diseases;
9. Identify socioeconomic factors.

Rheumatoid Arthritis (RA) is a multifactorial autoimmune disease characterized by intermittent swelling of the joints, with a host of causes and risk factors for its onset. Of specific interest here is the contribution of genetic susceptibility, in patients who have a first-degree relative with RA, being many times more likely to contract the disease, there being some suggestion that up to 70% of victims accept such family links. In addition to genetic factors, demographic aspects such as gender and age play a contributing role; women, particularly women over the age of 50, have a higher incidence of RA compared to men (Yanusman, 2023).

Additionally, lifestyle factors, including obesity and a history of joint trauma, also contribute to the risk because greater body weight puts additional pressure on the joints, which could trigger inflammatory pathways. Knowledge of these causes and risk factors will be important for early detection and intervention, ultimately with a goal of reducing the effect of RA on patients' lives.

1.1.1. Genetic Predisposition

Genetic predisposition knowledge is critical in unveiling the complex etiology of rheumatoid arthritis (RA). Hereditary factors have been observed to be central to the prevalence of this chronic autoimmune disease, with studies determining that approximately 41.6% of the patients diagnosed with RA present a family history for the disease. This genetic predisposition is compounded by environmental factors, such as smoking and disruption of microbiota, that may trigger immunological responses which put individuals at risk for developing RA (Conti et al., 2019).

In addition, the presence of some genetic markers, such as the HLA-DRB1 gene, has been associated with higher susceptibility to the disease. Therefore, knowledge of genetic predisposition not only helps identify vulnerable populations but also highlights the need for preventive and early interventions to reduce disease onset and severity (Figure 1.2).

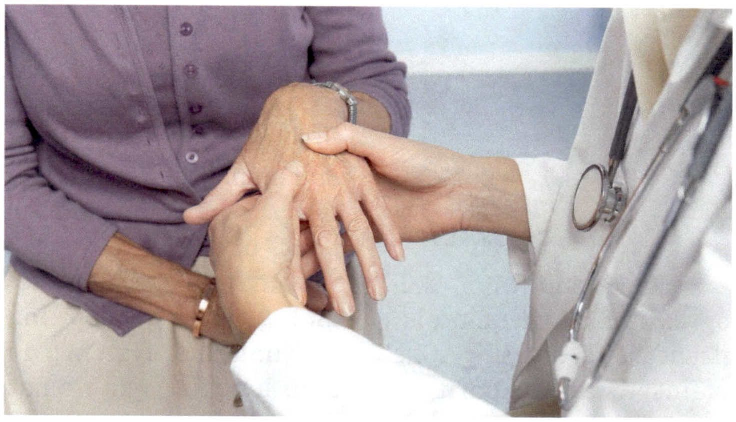

Figure 1.2. Understanding genetic predisposition plays a crucial role in unraveling the complex etiology of rheumatoid arthritis (RA).

Source: https://cdn.pfizer.com/pfizercom/2023-09/banner_section/GettyImages-91559463_1600X900_opt.jpg.

1.1.2. Environmental Triggers

RA pathogenesis is largely influenced by many environmental stimuli, which synergize with genetic predisposition to promote the onset of disease. Recent evidence suggests that dysbiosis of the gut, an imbalance in intestinal microbiota, can be a critical environmental factor for the development of RA. Alterations in gut microbiota play a role in inflammatory responses and increased intestinal permeability, both of which have been shown to occur prior to RA manifestations. In addition, immune dysfunctions caused by these microbial alterations add another layer of complexity to the disease onset. The complexity of such interactions underscores the need for an intimate knowledge of the way environmental factors become intertwined with genetic susceptibility. A systems perspective on RA pathophysiology necessitates further investigation of these environmental triggers, as characterized in the literature, for their potential contribution to disease progression and patient outcome (Horta-Baas et al., 2023; Talele et al., 2024).

1.1.3. Hormonal Influences

The function of hormones in the etiology and progression of rheumatoid arthritis (RA) is a significant area of investigation, particularly in terms of differences between the sexes. Research indicates that hormonal fluctuations, especially at menopause, play an important role in disease onset; women are at greater risk of developing RA than men, with more severe disease and loss of function usually occurring in involved women. Decline in estrogen levels and ovarian activity during menopause has been associated with high proinflammatory cytokines that increase inflammatory responses in the body (Sobek et al., 2024). Additionally, the relationship between genetic, environmental, and sex hormones underscores the complexity of autoimmune diseases like RA, and evidence indicates that personalized management approaches are required (Sobek et al., 2024). Identification of these hormonal actions not only illuminates disease mechanisms but also provides a basis for targeted therapies (Figure 1.3).

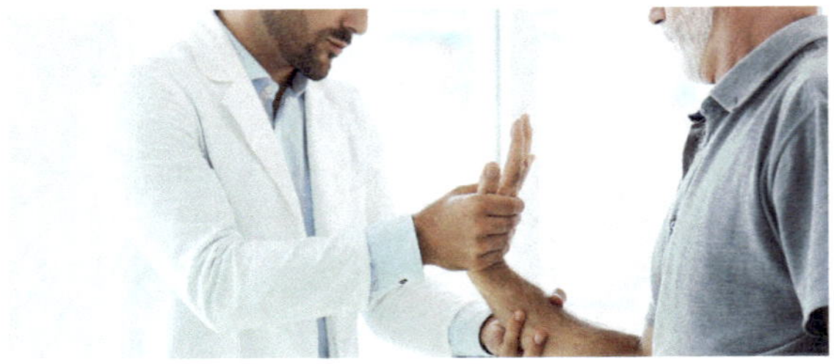

Figure 1.3. The influence of hormones on the development and progression of rheumatoid arthritis (RA) is a significant area of investigation, particularly as it pertains to the disparities observed between genders.

Source: https://medizinonline.com/wp-content/uploads/2024/05/iStock-855557166-1920x814.jpg.

1.1.4. Age-Related Factors

With advancing age, the onset and course of rheumatoid arthritis (RA) can be decided in large measure by age-influenced factors. Frequent in older individuals is a higher frequency of RA, which correlates with physiological alterations and comorbid conditions that often exaggerate the disease with increasing age.

Particularly relevant is the onset age of RA, as the literature has established older RA onset age as predictive of increased risk for the development of such conditions as interstitial lung disease (RA-ILD) (Busby et al., 2019).

Even the aging process might affect the efficacy of treatment, for example, disease-modifying antirheumatic drugs (DMARDs). A paper applying the International Classification of Functioning, Disability and Health (ICF) Core Set for RA underscores how varying responsiveness to treatment in older patients reflects the complex interplay of age, treatment responsiveness, and overall health status (Cieza et al., 2009). Knowledge about these is important so as to tailor efficacious management strategies to older patients with RA.

1.1.5. Gender Differences

Gender variance in rheumatoid arthritis (RA) is a significant consideration in understanding the prevalence and experience of RA among women and men. Research finds women are much more likely to be diagnosed with RA than men, with a rate of some 2-3 times higher among women. This may be attributed to hormonal differences and genetic susceptibility, which influence the immune system's reactions to them. In addition, the symptomatology and course of RA vary with gender; women have more pain and fatigue, whereas men may have a more aggressive disease course. Additionally, gender-adjusted response to treatment is observed, as demonstrated by differences in drug response to disease-modifying drugs. These gender differences are an indication of individualized treatment. Examining these factors is critical to enhancing patient care and following ACR/EULAR guidelines that stress reaching remission rather than just maintaining low disease activity (Hansell et al., 2013; Carpenter et al., 2019) (Figure 1.4).

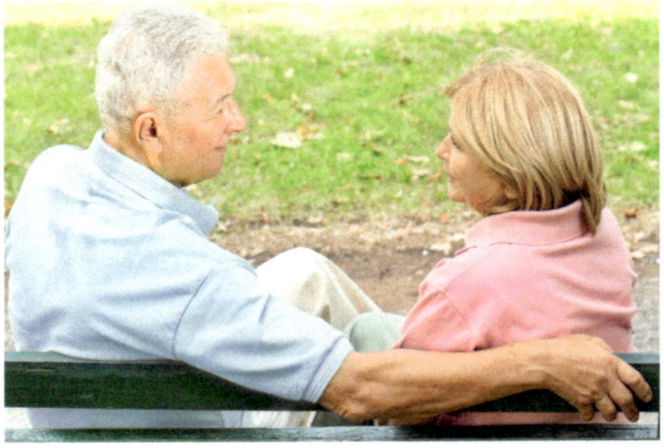

Figure 1.4. The progression and symptomatology of RA often manifest differently across genders; women frequently report greater pain and fatigue, while men may experience a more aggressive disease course.

Source: https://images.ctfassets.net/222znibi5gto/ppm_wysiwyg_fid6820_asset/1e91cc8fab23532a32cbba9922598c99/10612996_XL.jpg.

1.1.6. Lifestyle Factors (e.g., Smoking, Diet)

Lifestyle factors are significant in the development and progression of rheumatoid arthritis (RA), particularly smoking and diet. Available evidence indicates that smoking is a potent risk factor for RA, aggravating the severity of the disease and facilitating adverse treatment effects. Smoking tends to create a state of dysbiosis in the microbiome of the gut, which is observed in RA patients, pointing towards the lifestyle-disease pathology interlink (Picchianti-Diamanti et al., 2018). Dietary intervention plays a significant role as well; some foods are either pro-inflammatory or anti-inflammatory in their effects on clinical manifestations. Future studies suggest that gut microbiota alterations correlate with dietary metabolites, which may also modulate inflammatory processes in RA patients (Coras et al., 2020). Thus, integrating healthier lifestyle regimens, like cessation of smoking and a balanced diet, may not only ameliorate clinical symptoms but also improve control of the disease in RA patients.

1.1.7. Infections and Autoimmune Responses

The intricate interplay between infections and autoimmune responses lies at the heart of rheumatoid arthritis (RA) pathogenesis. The microbiota of the hosts, which via co-evolution takes up a symbiotic relationship with the immune system, can modulate RA chronic inflammation. Alterations in gut bacterial composition can disrupt the equilibrium between inflammation and tolerance, precipitating the onset of autoimmune activity. Most notably, recent data have implicated RA with dysbiosis of oral and gut microbiota and suggested that mucosal infections may be the initiators of autoimmune reactions that extend to joints and other organs (Picchianti-Diamanti et al., 2018). Apart from this, understanding the microbiota mechanisms in this regard and how various drug therapies affect them requires an integrative treatment modality that is not only genetic and environmental in nature but also infection (Chaplain et al., 2019). This understanding has the potential to lead to targeted therapeutic intervention to combat RA successfully (Figure 1.5).

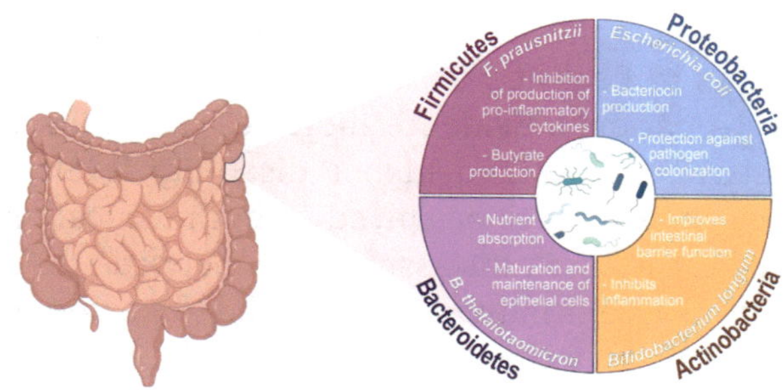

Figure 1.5. Chronic inflammation in RA can be influenced by the host's microbiota, which, through a process of co-evolution, forms a symbiotic relationship with the immune system.

Source: https://www.frontiersin.org/files/Articles/1098386/fmicb-14-1098386-HTML/image_m/fmicb-14-1098386-g001.jpg.

1.1.8. Family History of Autoimmune Diseases

The contribution of family history to the etiology of autoimmune diseases, including rheumatoid arthritis (RA), underscores a critical study area in the investigation of genetic susceptibility. From evidence, it seems that having a positive first-degree family history of autoimmune diseases significantly increases people's risk of acquiring autoimmune illnesses like RA, and studies have established that familial inheritance may enhance susceptibility to autoimmune reaction (Annibale et al., 2018). In addition, the dialogue between genetics and the environment, such as infection and intestinal microbiota, plays a key role in both the onset and progression of the diseases. Mucosal sites, for instance, can be responsible for initiating autoimmune responses centrally, particularly in genetically predisposed individuals, and lead to manifestations in the whole body typical of diseases like RA (Picchianti-Diamanti et al., 2018). Therefore, recognition of the importance of family history might prove to be essential when making early intervention and preventive policies accessible to risk groups.

1.1.9. Socioeconomic Factors

The impact of socioeconomic determinants on rheumatoid arthritis (RA) patients is multidimensional and extensive, and plays a significant role in the incidence as well as management of the disease. Socioeconomic status, such as income level, education, and occupation, has the ability to regulate access to healthcare resources and thereby change the outcome of treatment and the well-being of RA patients. Evidence indicates that a lower socioeconomic status is associated with increased disease activity and higher disability levels in individuals with RA and emphasizes a need for these problems to be solved by both clinical practice and public health interventions. Furthermore, studies highlight the associations between the lower occupational class and moderate-to-severe foot pain, wherein individuals with RA reported lower scores of quality of life and foot health, which also indicates the strong impact of broader social determinants in the expression and control of disease (Finney et al., 2018). Therefore, overcoming these socioeconomic barriers is essential to improve the overall treatment efficacy and status of the patients' health in RA (Callahan et al., 2014) (Figure 1.6).

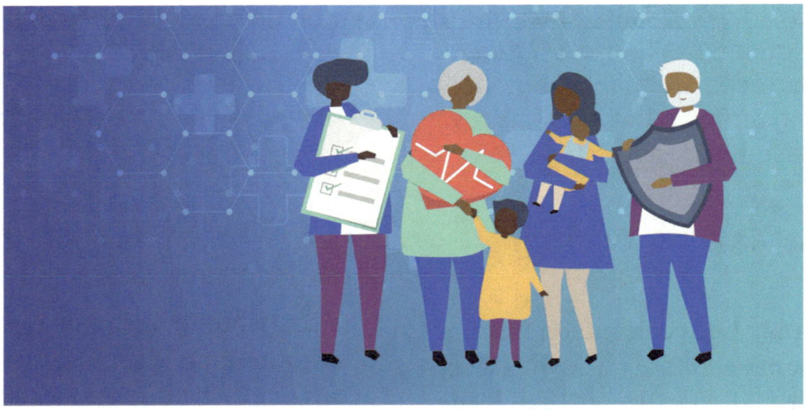

Figure 1.6. Socioeconomic status, which encompasses income, education, and occupation, can affect access to healthcare resources, thereby altering treatment outcomes and quality of life for RA patients.

Source: https://production-tcf.imgix.net/app/uploads/2019/12/18171821/taylor_header-01.png?auto=format%2Ccompress&q=80&fit=crop&w=1200&h=600.

Test Your Knowledge

1. How does smoking influence the risk of developing RA?
2. What is the role of environmental factors (e.g., infections, pollutants) in triggering RA?

1.2. Symptoms and Diagnosis of Rheumatoid Arthritis

Learning Outcome

1. Identify common physical symptoms;
2. Explain joint-specific symptoms;
3. Understand systemic symptoms;
4. Know the early signs of RA;
5. Explain diagnostic criteria;
6. Describe laboratory tests;
7. Define imaging techniques;
8. Focus on differential diagnosis;
9. Learn the importance of early diagnosis.

In the clinical environment of rheumatology, the diagnosis of rheumatoid arthritis (RA) is heavily based on the identification of specific symptoms and laboratory tests.

Patients typically present with classic symptoms, such as stiffness in the morning, swelling of the joints, most commonly of the hands and wrists, accompanied by systemic manifestations like fatigue and fever that are characteristic of this autoimmune disease. Diagnosis is also confirmed by serological evidence, with rheumatoid factor and anti-cyclic citrullinated peptide antibodies playing crucial roles in diagnosing RA.

In addition to the traditional application of radiographs, the newer imaging techniques like MRI and ultrasound have been found to be even more sensitive for detecting early erosive disease characteristic of RA. Of particular importance, RA differentiation from other arthritis is complicated by overlapping symptoms in conditions like osteoarthritis and septic arthritis and must be obtained with close observation for accurate diagnosis. Early diagnosis remains paramount to improving patient outcomes via timely therapeutic intervention.

1.2.1. Common Physical Symptoms

Rheumatoid arthritis (RA) represents a range of common physical symptoms that have significant effects on quality of life for the afflicted. Arthritis pain, often accompanied by swelling and stiffness, primarily in the morning or after periods of inactivity, is one of the symptomatic indicators. Over time, ongoing inflammation will result in joint damage and deformities, needing extensive medical intervention. In addition, systemic manifestations of fatigue, fever, and weight loss can occur as well, causing overall loss of well-being. Notably, atypical but severe complications such as rheumatoid meningitis, with neurological manifestations of seizures and psychosis, in the absence of a prior diagnosis of RA (Berk et al., 2018). The interplay between such symptoms highlights the chronic and multifaceted nature of the disease, indicating the need for ongoing research into the effectiveness of care practices and the identification of potential predictive markers for associated degrees of fatigue (Assassi et al., 2011) (Figure 1.7).

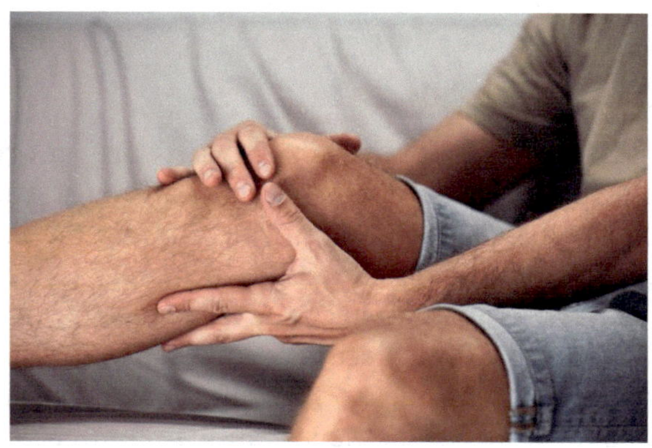

Figure 1.7. The hallmark symptoms are joint pain, often accompanied by swelling and stiffness, particularly in the mornings or after periods of inactivity.

Source: https://docsmedicalgroup.com/docsurgentcare/wp-content/uploads/sites/2/elementor/thumbs/5-common-causes-of-kneecap-pain-min-qict7l5kwt4wtgmqgmzmrpp5nuzqx7hi26vdmir7qy.jpg.

1.2.2. Joint-Specific Symptoms

The signs specific to a joint are pivotal to the early detection and diagnosis of rheumatoid arthritis (RA), since they are likely to present before the official coding of the condition in clinical documentation. Presentations of pain, stiffness, and swelling in a joint may significantly predict future development of RA, so clinicians need to remain vigilant to such presentations. It has been shown by study that a great number of patients are already presenting with these symptoms well before an absolute RA diagnosis, and research has indicated that 44% of patients presented with either one or more joint symptoms at least six months prior to their recorded diagnosis (Hansell et al., 2013). This highlights the importance of why these early signs need to be recognized, as treatment would have a significant impact on disease progression. As highlighted in studies, understanding the nuances of joint-specific symptoms is crucial and provides a pathway for preemptive treatment that may alleviate long-term joint damage as well as improve overall patient outcomes (Aletaha et al., 2013).

1.2.3. Systemic Symptoms

Systemic manifestations in RA are more widespread than local inflammation of the joints, which have a significant impact on the patient's general well-being and quality of life. These symptoms can occur as fatigue, fever, and malaise, most often secondary to the underlying autoimmune process that characterizes the disease. In this case, the systemic inflammation not only affects the synovial joints but can potentially affect other organ systems, causing comorbidities that complicate treatment. Note should be taken of these systemic manifestations, as they demonstrate the importance of early diagnosis and comprehensive treatment modalities that inhibit damage to the joints while also tackling these more systemic symptoms. New findings on the role of diet and intestinal microbiota establish their potential to influence inflammation, suggesting that nutritional therapy may be a complementary approach to conventional treatment in managing RA systemic symptoms (Diaconu et al., 2018; Agustín-Perez et al., 2020). Such an integrative approach emphasizes the need for a multilevel management in addressing RA's multirotational character (Figure 1.8).

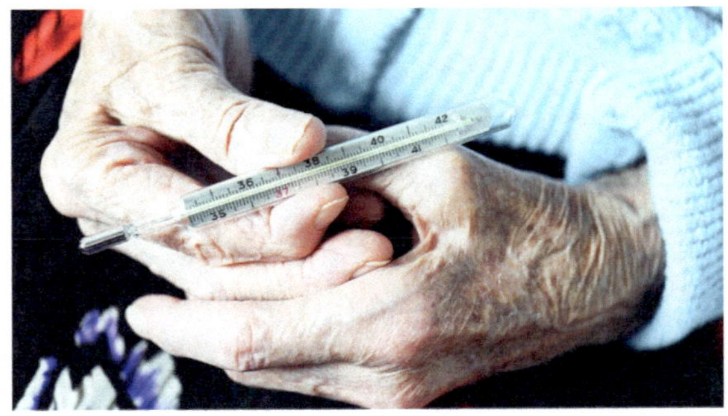

Figure 1.8. Systemic symptoms can manifest as fatigue, fever, and malaise, often resulting from the underlying autoimmune process that characterizes the disease.

Source: https://i0.wp.com/post.medicalnewstoday.com/wp-content/uploads/sites/3/2022/05/arthritis_fevers_GettyImages1296449470_Header-1024x575.jpg?w=1155&h=1528.

1.2.4. Early Signs of RA

Early signs of rheumatoid arthritis (RA) are typically subtle but significant, and are a harbinger of important signs that should be given urgent attention for effective management. Electronic health records (EHRs) studies show high levels of indicator markers, with 83.5% of the patients having two or more markers before diagnosis. In particular, 44% of such patients had joint symptoms or signs at presentation at least six months before coded diagnosis, an indicator of the delay in official recognition (Hansell et al., 2013). In addition, new NICE guidelines place greater importance on early recognition and referral for inflammatory arthritis patients. This emphasis on timely intervention is critical, particularly in the large number of patients seen with musculoskeletal complaints, which makes it difficult to diagnose RA within diverse clinical presentations (Cassell et al., 2011). Prompt intervention has the potential to significantly influence disease course and patient outcomes.

1.2.5. Diagnostic Criteria (e.g., ACR/EULAR)

The diagnostic criteria of rheumatoid arthritis (RA), particularly the American College of Rheumatology/European League Against Rheumatism (ACR/EULAR) criteria, are pivotal tools to achieve early and accurate diagnosis. The criteria emphasize the importance of recognizing typical clinical, laboratory, and imaging features of RA in an effort to intervene as early as possible. Notably, composite index inclusion to measure the activity of disease is most critical in guiding treatment strategies to aim at endpoints such as remission or low disease activity. Further, novel diagnostic testing by the application of B-cell gene expression and MRI offers potential enhancement of conventional paradigms, where recent studies indicate these tests are cost-effectiveness for diagnosing RA in early stages (Buisman et al., 2016). While there has been progress, challenges remain regarding the application of these diagnostic guidelines to all patients, emphasizing the necessity of continuous investigation into innovative methods to maximize RA diagnosis and improve patient outcomes (Aletaha et al., 2016) (Figure 1.9).

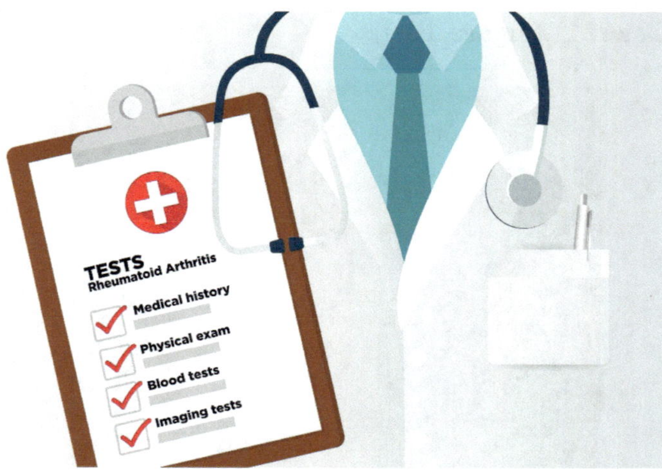

Figure 1.9. The integration of composite indices to measure disease activity is critical in steering treatment strategies toward target outcomes, such as remission or low disease activity.

Source: https://creakyjoints.org/wp-content/uploads/2018/11/0918_RA-Tests.jpg.

1.2.6. Laboratory Tests (e.g., RF, anti-CCP)

Diagnostic and monitoring laboratory investigations are essential for RA diagnosis and treatment, enabling identification of specific autoantibodies associated with RA. The anti-CCP and RF are frequently used among such tests; they are associated with disease severity and progression if identified. Recent research underscores the role of anti-CarP antibodies, which are now significant diagnostic markers for RA, providing a substitute to anti-CCP and RF for enhanced diagnostic sensitivity (Alessandri et al., 2016). Identification of immune complexes in the circulation in RA patients has additionally given us better insight into the pathogenesis of the disease. Strikingly, citrullinated antigens such as fibrinogen and vimentin are also found in these complexes, more with anti-CCP positivity, which underscores the probable role in inflammation and joint damage (Ceuleneer et al., 2010). Therefore, these tests not only help to diagnose RA but also direct therapeutic intervention.

1.2.7. Imaging Techniques (e.g., X-Rays, MRI)

Imaging modalities are an integral component of RA diagnosis and therapy and offer information not easily accessible to standard sources. X-rays have been used for years to image erosions and damage of joints characteristic of RA, but are not well-suited to detect early changes and thus must be developed beyond their current status. Magnetic Resonance Imaging (MRI) has emerged as a valuable tool, enabling the detection of soft tissue lesions and bone edema, hence facilitating early disease detection and monitoring disease progression. Certain recent studies have examined complementary methods, such as ultrasound and dual energy computed tomography (DECT), which were more sensitive for detecting crystalline deposits in relation to the conditions mentioned above. For instance, although conventional radiography remains a reference standard, the integration of newer imaging technologies has the ability to enhance diagnostic assurance, to lead to improved patient outcomes and potential cost savings in treatment, as illustrated by their application in cost-efficient diagnostic models for conditions like Seronegative rheumatoid arthritis (Wu et al., 2016; Alvis-Zakzuk et al., 2021) (Figure 1.10).

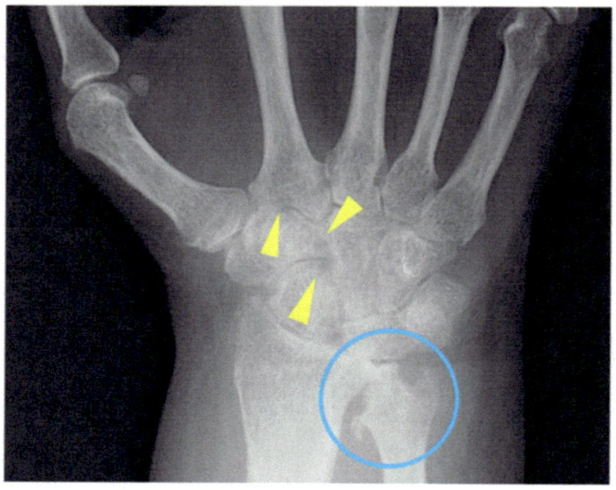

Figure 1.10. X-rays have long been utilized to visualize joint damage and erosions characteristic of RA.

Source: https://www.mdpi.com/diagnostics/diagnostics-12-02134/article_deploy/html/images/diagnostics-12-02134-g002-550.jpg

1.2.8. Differential Diagnosis

Differential diagnosis is a critical component of the diagnostic evaluation of patients suspected to have rheumatoid arthritis (RA), involving the differentiation of RA from other conditions that present overlapping clinical features. The conditions include osteoarthritis, psoriatic arthritis, and systemic lupus erythematosus, all of which have distinct clinical features as well as prognosis. Differential diagnosis not only plays a crucial role in the proper treatment of the patient but also in order to prevent unnecessary treatments that may complicate the clinical course. Autoantibody presence, disease activity levels, and patients' medical histories are determinants of differential diagnosis. Besides, as elaborated in recent studies, early and correct diagnosis influences patient outcome and therapeutic treatment by enabling early intervention with disease-modifying antirheumatic drugs, hence enhancing the long-term prognosis in RA patients (Aletaha et al., 2016; FitzGerald et al., 2013).

1.2.9. Importance of Early Diagnosis

Early diagnosis and detection of rheumatoid arthritis (RA) are crucial in an effort to avert the potentially disabling consequences of the disease. Early diagnosis allows one to initiate disease-modifying therapy early enough, and this can significantly influence clinical outcomes and enhance the quality of life for patients. NICE guidance currently emphasizes early identification of inflammatory arthritis to enable timely treatment and referral, which is a key issue given the large volume of patients presenting with musculoskeletal complaints (Cassell et al., 2011). In addition, technological improvements in imaging diagnosis, such as MRI and ultrasound, have provided meaningful information about the initial pathophysiology of RA, allowing subclinical inflammation that otherwise would go undiagnosed to be identified (Jans et al., 2017). Therefore, stressing the importance of early diagnosis is not only crucial for the management of RA but also for better, longer-term outcomes in sufferers (Figure 1.11).

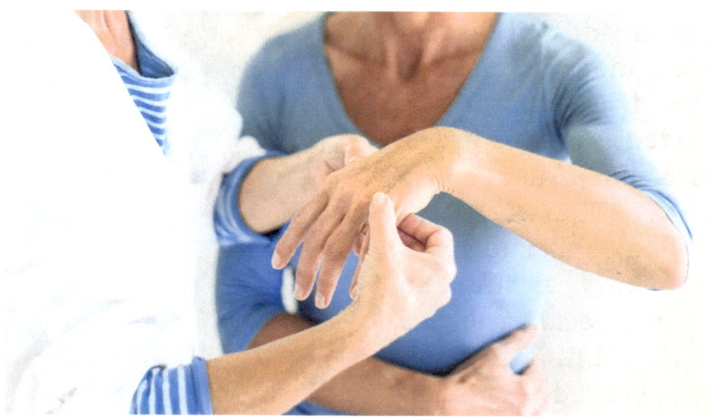

Figure 1.11. Early diagnosis allows for the prompt initiation of disease-modifying treatments, which can significantly improve clinical outcomes and enhance the quality of life for patients.

Source: https://images.everydayhealth.com/images/arthritis/rheumatoid-arthritis/things-a-rheumatologist-wants-you-to-know-about-ra-alt-1440x810.jpg.

Test Your Knowledge

1. What is the significance of morning stiffness in RA diagnosis?
2. Which joints are typically affected first in RA?

1.3. Treatment Options for Rheumatoid Arthritis

Learning Outcome

1. Understand pharmacological treatments;
2. Identify non-steroidal anti-inflammatory drugs;
3. Define disease-modifying antirheumatic drugs (DMARDs);
4. Focus on biologic therapies;
5. Discuss corticosteroids;
6. Explain physical therapy and rehabilitation;
7. Describe lifestyle modifications;
8. Learn complementary and alternative therapies;
9. Know importance of a multidisciplinary approach.

The treatment of rheumatoid arthritis (RA) has been revolutionized, with numerous options available for the patient's individual needs and presentation. Among these options are disease-modifying antirheumatic drugs (DMARDs), biologic agents, and targeted synthetic drugs, all aimed at the control of inflammation and prevention of joint destruction. A recent report emphasized that both rheumatologists and patients consider quality of life and treatment effectiveness while deciding on the most appropriate therapy, pointing towards a common interest in shared decision-making (SDM) during the treatment course (Comellas et al., 2020). Additionally, disability impairment due to arthritis is important to maximize therapeutic strategies since arthritis negatively impacts day-to-day functioning and productivity in most individuals (Bates et al., 2014). These findings emphasize the need for individualized treatment programs that take into account both medical effectiveness and patients' quality of life, ultimately enhancing overall treatment outcomes for patients with this chronic condition.

1.3.1. Pharmacological Treatments

Pharmacological treatment of rheumatoid arthritis (RA) plays a central role in managing symptoms and arresting disease progression. Disease-modifying antirheumatic drugs (DMARDs) are one of the primary agents used to attempt to alter the course of the disease and prevent long-term joint damage.

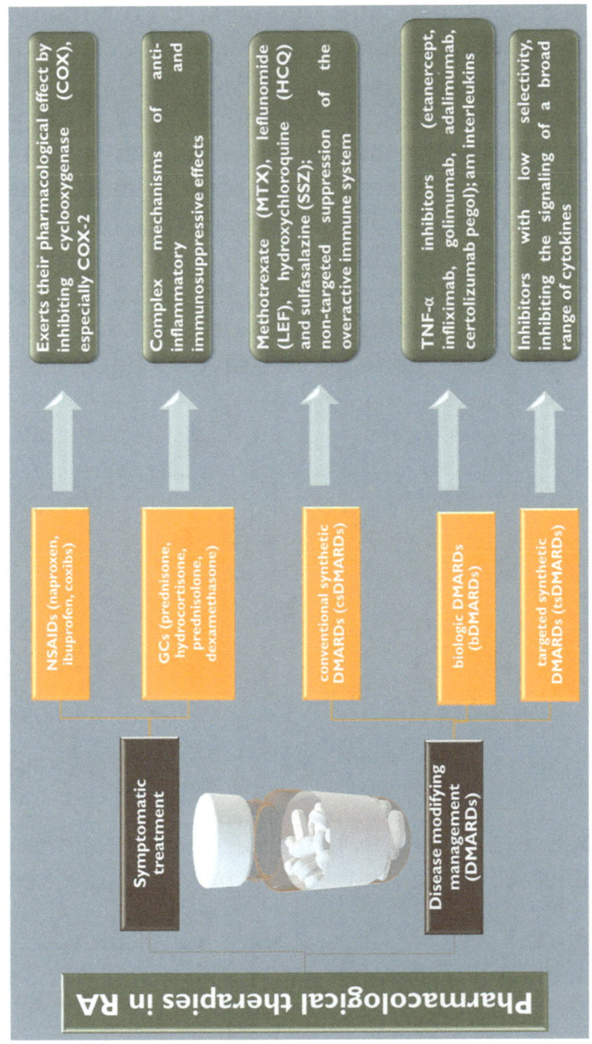

Figure 1.12. The pharmacological treatment of rheumatoid arthritis (RA) is critical in managing symptoms and slowing disease progression.

Source: https://pub.mdpi-res.com/cells/cells-10-02857/article_deploy/html/images/cells-10-02857-ag.png?1635236038.

Tumor necrosis factor inhibitors (TNFi) have also been useful in maximizing clinical benefit for patients by effectively inhibiting inflammatory pathways responsible for joint destruction. While successful, some percentage of patients will not respond adequately to TNFi, and so the value of secondary treatment strategies and ongoing research into new drugs and biosimilars (Kraft et al., 2017). Additionally, knowledge from studies into concomitant conditions, i.e., juvenile primary fibromyalgia syndrome, is that serial monitoring and tailored pharmacologic management are required to manage pain and optimize functioning effectively (Boneparth et al., 2019). By combining these insights, clinicians can make well-rounded treatment plans that put patient outcomes first (Figure 1.12).

1.3.2. Non-Steroidal Anti-Inflammatory Drugs (NSAIDs)

Non-steroidal anti-inflammatory drugs (NSAIDs) are an integral part of the management of inflammatory diseases such as rheumatoid arthritis (RA), primarily due to their analgesic and anti-inflammatory action. Such medications, amongst others that are frequently utilized , such as ibuprofen and naproxen, alleviate pain and inflammation symptoms and thereby improve the quality of life of RA patients. Despite their utility, NSAIDs are not risk-free, particularly concerning cardiovascular outcomes. Scientific studies have indicated that cyclo-oxygenase 2 selective NSAIDs are strongly associated with an increased risk of acute myocardial infarction (AMI) (Langhorne et al., 2006). Additionally, although nonselective NSAIDs do tend to have similar anti-inflammatory benefits, they do appear to raise the risk of AMI, with some medications like diclofenac demonstrating a frighteningly elevated relative risk (Langhorne et al., 2006). Thus, though NSAIDs continue to play a vital role in RA therapy, cautious consideration of their possible side effects is important for best patient management.

1.3.3. Disease-Modifying Antirheumatic Drugs (DMARDs)

The management of rheumatoid arthritis (RA) primarily involves the use of disease-modifying antirheumatic drugs (DMARDs), and these are required for slowing down disease activity and alleviating joint damage. Such drugs, both the conventional synthetic DMARDs and the newer biological agents, are aimed at reducing inflammation, as well as improving patients' quality of life. Current data indicate that some DMARDs, such as denosumab, are effective in controlling joint damage and improving bone mineral density in patients with RA if added to conventional therapies (Genant et al., 2019). There is some evidence to indicate that early treatment with DMARDs is linked with better outcomes in the long term, so early diagnosis and low disease activity or remission orientation of treatment protocols are warranted (Aletaha et al., 2016). As the studies keep on discovering new treatments, the significance of DMARDs will continue to be basic in tackling the complicated requirements of RA patients and mitigating the long-term effects of the disease (Figure 1.13).

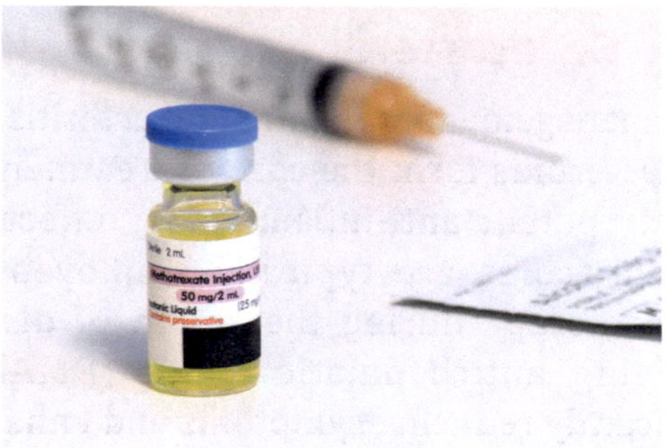

Figure 1.13. The management of rheumatoid arthritis (RA) primarily involves the use of disease-modifying antirheumatic drugs (DMARDs), which are essential for slowing disease progression and alleviating joint damage.

Source: https://images.ctfassets.net/yixw23k2v6vo/1KUU6U2kXeYbJOyucfbWQZ/6d2558d586d681be9dc73ef6a59c9d2e/large-GettyImages-1430136500-3000x2000.jpg.

1.3.4. Biologic Therapies

Biologic treatments are a paradigm change in the management of rheumatoid arthritis (RA) with targeted actions to control the immune system and reduce inflammation. Compared to traditional systemic treatment, biologics specifically target pro-inflammatory cytokines or immune cells involved in RA pathology, leading to increased disease control and potentially an improvement in the quality of life for patients. According to one study examining patient experience with intravenous (IV) biologic therapy, an overwhelming percentage of patients reported extensive satisfaction with their treatment, which reflects the shift in attitude in favor of newer modalities over more traditional subcutaneous regimens (Black et al., 2017). Besides, clinical guideline adherence, such as performing the Disease Activity Score in 28 joints (DAS 28), remains highly relevant for treatment efficacy assessment and the realization of optimal patient outcomes (Borg et al., 2013). This reflects the role of patient attitudes and clinical guideline adherence in the transition to biologic medications for RA.

1.3.5. Corticosteroids

In the management of rheumatoid arthritis (RA), corticosteroids form the core of treatment due to their potent anti-inflammatory effect. The glucocorticoids are typically employed as a bridge therapy during the action of disease-modifying antirheumatic drugs (DMARDs), significantly reducing symptoms and enhancing the quality of life in patients. Current studies emphasize the effectiveness of corticosteroid treatment with high doses, demonstrating a higher probability of clinical remission in comparison to low doses, particularly in acute conditions involving inflammatory arthropathies like adult-onset Still's disease (Berardicurti et al., 2019). This indicates that corticosteroids can not only control pain but also enable the tapering off of systemic inflammation. Apart from that, fresh guidelines emphasize the addition of corticosteroids with other non-corticosteroid immunomodulatory medications for optimizing the treatment of RA, hence enhancing patient safety and minimizing long-term corticosteroid use (Dick et al., 2018). Hence, corticosteroids remain a cornerstone in the therapy against rheumatoid arthritis (Figure 1.14).

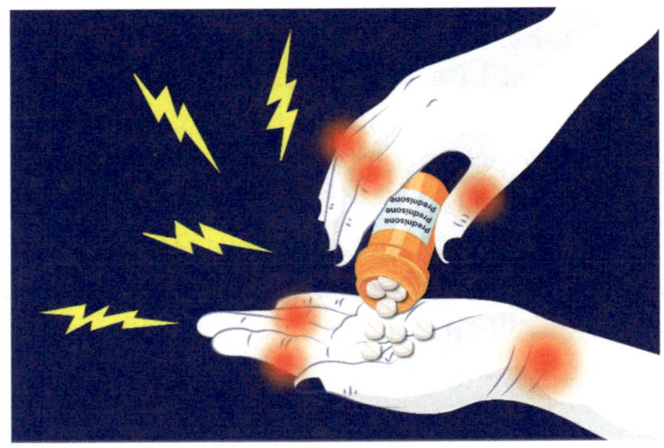

Figure 1.14. In the management of rheumatoid arthritis (RA), corticosteroids play a pivotal role due to their potent anti-inflammatory properties.

Source: https://creakyjoints.org/wp-content/uploads/2019/01/0119_Prednisone.jpg.

1.3.6. Physical Therapy and Rehabilitation

The role that physical therapy and rehabilitation have in the treatment of rheumatoid arthritis (RA) is essential, as it directly impacts improving patient functional status and quality of life. An interdisciplinary approach, tailored to individual patient needs, has to incorporate strategies dealing with biological, social, and individual influences on recovery. The development of tailored rehabilitation programs is significant in reducing pain, increasing joint mobility, and preventing deformities, which significantly contributes to global patient function (Grygus & Nogas, 2020). Furthermore, as clinical resources for health care continue to evolve, having an understanding of the effectiveness of these programs becomes increasingly important in justifying clinical practice and determining cost-effectiveness (Stucki & Liang, 1994). By incorporating rehabilitation interventions into the overall framework of RA management, clinicians can foster improved health results in conjunction with improved patient experience, recognizing the value of personalized care in this challenging field.

1.3.7. Lifestyle Modifications

Lifestyle modification is a crucial component of rheumatoid arthritis (RA) management, both for reducing symptoms and for improving quality of life. Lifestyle modification may involve diet with an abundance of anti-inflammatory foods, such as omega-3 fatty acids, to minimize inflammation and pain within the joints.

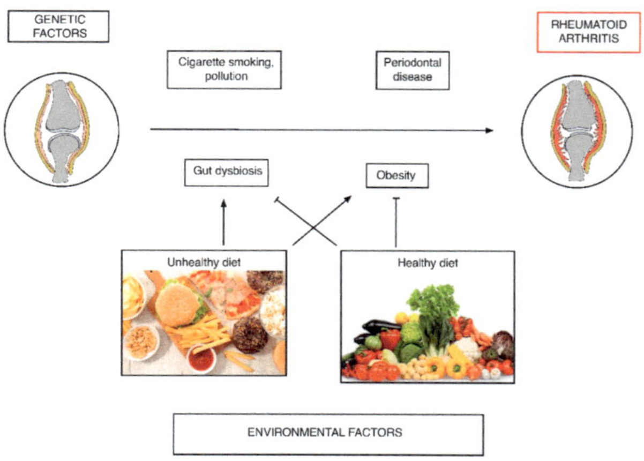

Figure 1.15. Lifestyle modifications play a crucial role in the management of rheumatoid arthritis (RA), influencing both symptom relief and overall quality of life.

Source: https://pub.mdpi-res.com/nutrients/nutrients-12-01456/article_deploy/html/images/nutrients-12-01456-g001.png?1591385304.

Exercise is also beneficial in preserving joint function and reducing stiffness; low-impact exercises, such as swimming or cycling are useful. Furthermore, research points towards monitoring and potential alteration of lifestyle factors, including smoking and stress levels, which were discovered to be related to disease severity and progression.

In a study, the RA patients were observed to have dysbiosis of the gut related to lifestyle choices, which emphasizes the relationship between diet, microbial well-being, and the activity of the disease (Picchianti-Diamanti et al., 2018). Moreover, a perspective of the emotional and social dimensions of rheumatoid arthritis can reinforce coping strategies and optimize patient support interventions (Bates et al., 2014) (Figure 1.15).

1.3.8. Complementary and Alternative Therapies

In the management of rheumatoid arthritis (RA), complementary and alternative treatments have been reported to increase in popularity as adjunctive therapy to traditional treatment. Techniques like acupuncture, herbal remedies, and mind-body interventions like meditation have been investigated for their potential symptom-relieving properties as well as to promote overall well-being. Research has indicated that patients with chronic illnesses, including RA, are more likely to seek mind-body therapies to improve the quality of life, reflecting a trend towards greater emphasis on overall care (Contreras, 2019).

Tai Chi, a mind-body exercise, has also been identified to be particularly beneficial not only for stress reduction but also for improving physical function and pain mitigation across various conditions, including arthritis (Beroes et al., 2016). This convergence of interest in non-pharmacological treatments highlights the importance of incorporating complementary therapies into RA treatment plans to encourage an overall approach that addresses physical and psychological health.

1.3.9. Importance of a Multidisciplinary Approach

Multidisciplinary treatment is important in the management of rheumatoid arthritis (RA) since it involves a multiplicity of healthcare providers who address the various factors of the disease. RA's nature necessitates not only medication but also treatment from professionals , such as physical therapists, occupational therapists, and nutritionists. This cooperative process enhances patient education, which has been one of the main explanations for the improvement of clinical outcomes, particularly in aspects of taking care of foot health, as cited by (Graham et al. (2012). Furthermore, it is important to learn the broader implications of arthritis beyond physical disabilities, particularly in light of its strong association with disability and chronic pain, as indicated by a study by Bates et al. (2014). By applying various disciplines, medical teams can offer patients highly comprehensive care tailored to their unique requirements, ultimately resulting in more efficient self-management strategies and overall enhanced quality of life for RA patients (Figure 1.16).

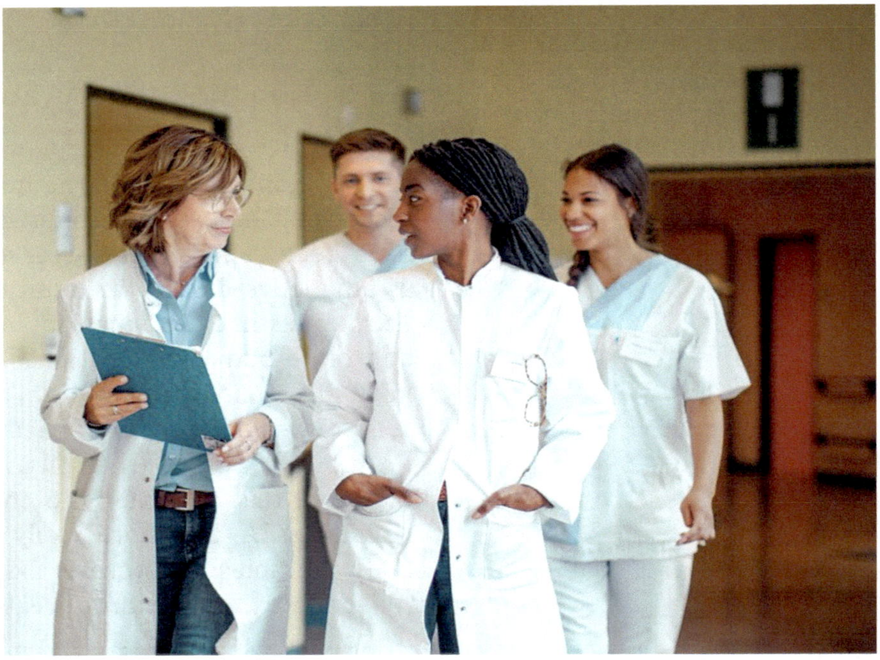

Figure 1.16. The complexity of RA necessitates not only pharmacological interventions but also support from specialists , such as physical therapists, occupational therapists, and dietitians.

Source: https://media.post.rvohealth.io/wp-content/uploads/sites/5/2021/06/healthcare-workers-walking-together-1296x728-header.jpg.

Test Your Knowledge

1. What are the first-line DMARDs for RA?
2. How do biologic DMARDs differ from conventional synthetic DMARDs?

1.4. Living with Rheumatoid Arthritis

Learning Outcome

1. Understand coping strategies;
2. Discuss impact on daily activities;
3. Focus on psychological effects;
4. Describe support systems and resources;
5. Know the role of patient education;
6. Managing flares and remission;
7. Focus on nutrition and dietary considerations;
8. Understand exercise and physical activity;
9. Explain long-term outlook and prognosis.

Living with rheumatoid arthritis (RA) is a complicated matter beyond physical pain, and it is more or less affecting patients' psychological and social lives. Although individuals are coping with living with continuous chronic pain and fatigue, they attempt to adjust and discover ways of coping that allow survival as well as a sense of control. Involvement in activities , such as the making of art has been a successful avenue to expression and release of feelings, allowing the patients to employ creativity as a means of pain control and for rebirth of self-knowledge (Atchley et al., 2011). Moreover, the psychological impact of RA typically comes with fatigue and low mood, further validating the need for effective self-management through the incorporation of physical exercise and mental health interventions (Calin et al., 2013). Through these coping strategies, patients with RA are able to attain normalcy and empowerment in their lives, eventually enhancing their quality of life despite RA.

1.4.1. Coping Strategies

Coping strategies play a significant role in managing the emotional and physical distress of rheumatoid arthritis (RA). Psychological distress, as is common to the majority of RA patients, significantly diminishes the likelihood of keeping them adherent to treatment protocols and navigating everyday lives, thereby exacerbating their conditions. Proper coping strategies, such as acceptance and optimism, were discovered to be effective in impacting therapeutic outcomes and disease management (Santiago et al., 2015). Second, engaging in creative activities like visual art-making has been an effective coping strategy, offering psychological benefits in self-expression and catharsis. Members often describe these activities as a relief they need to have from pain and as a way of reclaiming their sense of self, more easily navigating the complex emotional landscape of dealing with chronic illness (Atchley et al., 2011). Thus, multiplicity of coping mechanisms is critical to the development of quality of life in RA patients (Figure 1.17).

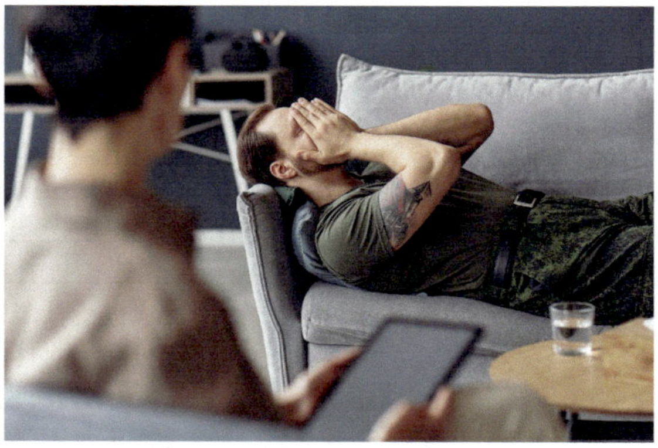

Figure 1.17. Coping strategies play a crucial role in managing the emotional and physical challenges associated with rheumatoid arthritis (RA).

Source: https://altusbiologics.com/wp-content/uploads/2024/08/022.jpg.

1.4.2. Impact on Daily Activities

The impact of RA on activities of daily living is staggering, causing a significant impairment to the quality of patients' lives. Studies show that nearly 51.9% of RA patients have a moderate-to-extensive impact on their daily life, including significant areas , such as work and emotional state (Arteaga et al., 2017). This disability is not just physical but personal and social too, where individuals often struggle to maintain interpersonal relationships and personal responsibilities.

Despite high overall satisfaction with treatment outcomes, with over 80% of patients expressing satisfaction with their current therapies, there remains a notable gap in addressing their everyday challenges, as many patients feel their rheumatologists seldom inquire about the personal difficulties they face (Arteaga et al., 2017). In addition, arthritis is also identified as a major cause of disability in Australia, with an estimated occurrence in 15% of the population, and there is a demand for increased understanding and better support mechanisms.

1.4.3. Psychological Effects

The psychological impacts of rheumatoid arthritis (RA) are a significant aspect of the patient's presentation with the condition. Successful therapy of chronic pain and disability often leads to disabling psychological distress, with heightened states of depression and anxiety, that can significantly inhibit patients from recovering effectively to treatment. Santiago et al., (2015) highlights that patients with RA tend to have mental health problems, and this interferes with coping and compliance with therapy. Furthermore, research indicates that patients who have increased levels of disease activity are more likely to worsen psychologicalally, and there is a study that has evidence with which it was noted that such patients had higher anxiety and depression levels following education programs when compared to patients with lower disease activity (Brus et al., 1997). This underscores the importance of the inclusion of psychological support in treatment protocols because mental health treatment can be critical in encouraging overall disease management as well as improving the quality of patients' lives (Figure 1.18).

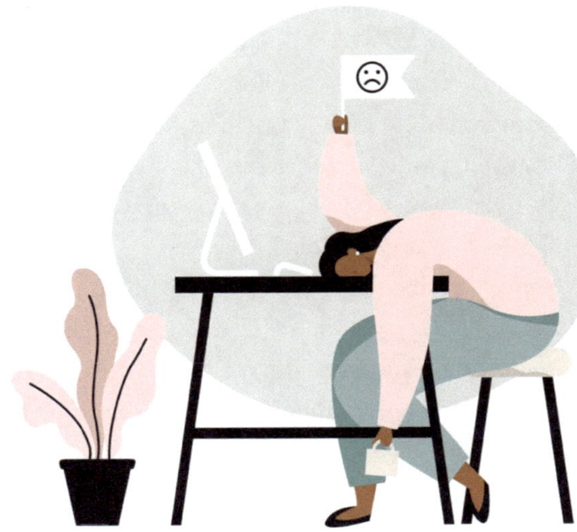

Figure 1.18. Managing chronic pain and disability often leads to debilitating psychological distress, including heightened levels of anxiety and depression, which can significantly impede patients ability to respond to treatment effectively.

Source: https://ysm-res.cloudinary.com/image/upload/ar_16:9,c_fill,dpr_3.0,f_auto,g_faces:auto,q_auto:eco,w_500/v1/yms/prod/3e4a41d0-17fb-4dbf-ba9e-c0b94abef3c8.

1.4.4. Support Systems and Resources

The management of rheumatoid arthritis (RA) challenges involves profound support systems and resources that have a direct bearing on the quality of life of the person affected. The intricacies involved in managing RA involve more than physical symptoms to encompass emotional and social elements, which call for extensive support systems. Evidence shows that understanding lived experiences of the arthritic population may enlighten regarding the type of resources needed for coping strategies, as well as community support systems for enhancing daily functioning (Bates et al., 2014). Furthermore, whereas RA is not taken into account in certain regions, such as Africa, these inequities should be addressed in planning interventions and targeted resource allocation (Abdel-Nasser et al., 2012). While individuals grapple with RA's long-term disability and pain, service delivery that addresses their needs can empower them, foster resilience, and improve health status among heterogeneous populations.

1.4.5. Role of Patient Education

Effective patient education plays a crucial role in the treatment of rheumatoid arthritis (RA), with great influence on clinical results and patients' capacity for active involvement in their own management. Studies reveal that a well-planned educational program has the capacity to enhance patients' understanding of their disease, such as total disease behavior, specific foot health information, and self-management skills important in maintaining mobility and quality of life (Graham et al., 2012). Furthermore, patient education facilitates an interactive treatment relationship between patients and health care professionals, which is essential for tailoring treatment techniques to individual patient needs (Graham et al., 2012). Despite the presumed benefits, challenges in the form of financial constraints and challenges in creating effective relations hinder offering the best possible education, and the need for specific interventions is emphasized (Graham et al., 2012). Eliminating such barriers is important as timely education enables early diagnosis and proper utilization of treatment strategies, eventually resulting in improved patient outcomes in the management of RA (Figure 1.19).

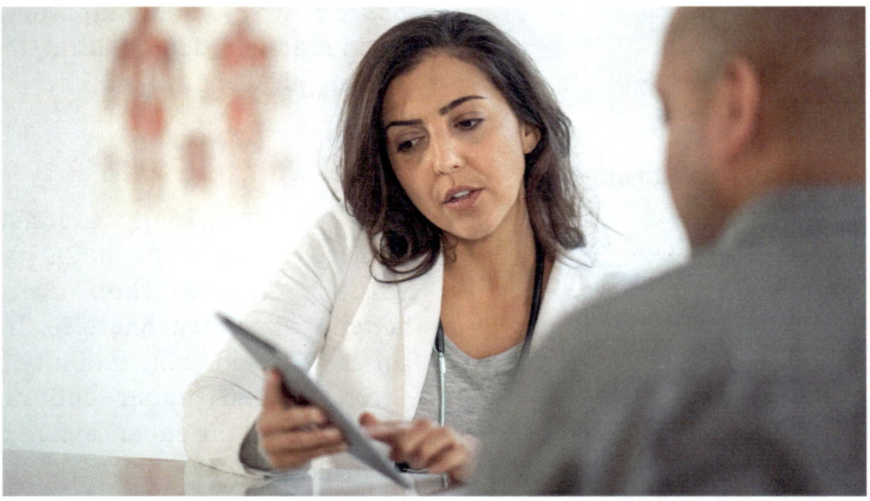

Figure 1.19. Effective patient education plays a crucial role in the management of rheumatoid arthritis (RA), significantly influencing clinical outcomes and empowering patients to take an active role in their treatment.

Source: https://post.healthline.com/wp-content/uploads/2020/02/nurse-doctor-office-1296x728-header-1296x728.jpg.

1.4.6. Managing Flares and Remission

Appropriate management of RA flares and remission is essential in maintaining the quality of life of the patients as well as avoiding damage to the joints. Strategies , such as careful monitoring of the disease activity through frequent evaluation, timely use of ultrasound scans, can lead to early intervention during flares and possibly prevent escalation to more severe stages of the disease (Chowdhury et al., 2020). According to recent reviews, patient education in recognizing signs and symptoms of flare and adherence to treatment regimens has a strong impact on the rate of remission (Talele et al., 2024). The pharmacological treatment of RA, including the administration of disease-modifying antirheumatic drugs (DMARDs) and biologics, is also equally critical in decelerating the rate and severity of flares. With the synergy of medical treatment and lifestyle modification, including exercise and dietary changes, overall management strategies can be optimized, resulting in a more stable disease state and improved long-term outcomes for patients with RA.

1.4.7. Nutrition and Dietary Considerations

Understanding the dietary management of RA is increasingly becoming well known as a key way to promote patient outcomes. Current knowledge indicates that the choice of foods has the power to radically modulate inflammation and influence immune effects in patients with this autoimmune disease. For instance, anti-inflammatory diets , such as the Mediterranean diet rich in omega-3 fatty acids have been effective in reducing the activity of the disease and systemic inflammation characteristic of RA. In addition, interaction between the gut microbiota and diet further complicates the progression and management of the disease. Alterations in gut microbiota composition have been linked to RA severity, suggesting that dietary management, in combination with probiotics and prebiotics, can provide benefits in therapy. By adding personalized nutritional interventions, medical professionals can better support RA patients in managing symptoms and improving general quality of life, further underlining the applicability of whole-patient management strategies for the treatment of autoimmune illnesses (Antczak et al., 2024; Sobek et al., 2024) (Figure 1.20).

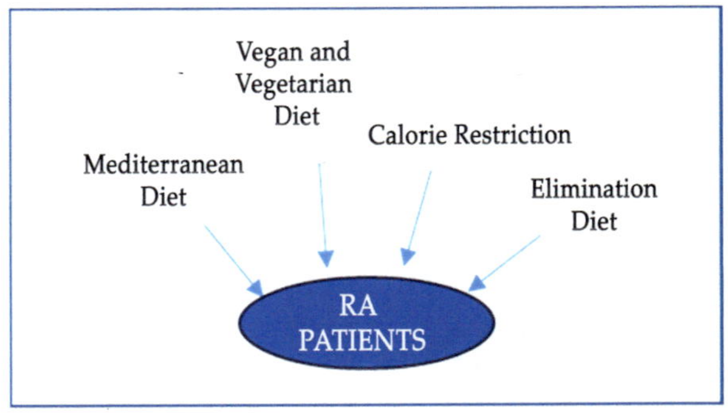

Figure 1.20. Understanding the role of nutrition in managing rheumatoid arthritis (RA) is increasingly recognized as vital for improving patient outcomes.

Source: https://www.mdpi.com/cimb/cimb-45-00341/article_deploy/html/images/cimb-45-00341-g001.png.

1.4.8. Exercise and Physical Activity

Engagement in daily exercise and physical activity is important in RA patients as it can actually enhance their overall health and functional ability. Exercise, in return, offers an increase in joint mobility, greater muscle strength, and higher endurance, which all contribute to the enhancement of a good quality of life. Evidence indicates that the majority of RA patients experience challenges in adhering to health recommendations due mainly to dependency, pain, and disability feelings, which could undermine their self-efficacy in living with their condition (Rasker et al., 1993). Surprisingly, integration of activity regimens specifically tailored might induce empowerment among the patients, which will enhance self-management resilience. In addition, combining exercise with psychological therapy has the potential to alleviate complex conditions , such as fatigue, a common complaint of chronic disease , such as RA (Calin et al., 2013). By promoting a total exercise strategy, health professionals can assist patients in overcoming exercise barriers and maximizing their health benefits.

1.4.9. Long-Term Outlook and Prognosis

The long-term course and prognosis for RA patients can be extremely unpredictable based on a wide array of variables, including timing of diagnosis and the success of early intervention strategies. In most cases, the chronic nature of RA provides the potential for persistence of symptoms over a lifetime, with attendant potential disability and compromised quality of life. Studies have shown that approximately one quarter of patients experience unrelenting disease activity, which, without treatment, will result in severe functional impairment (Ballan, 1996). However, improvements in treatment regimens, especially the development of biologic agents and disease-modifying anti-rheumatic drugs (DMARDs), have significantly improved patient outcomes. Registries like Pharma Child indicate that the monitoring and management of adverse events, including infections, remain critical for long-term care, and highlight the need for comprehensive treatment plans taking into consideration disease and associated risks alike (Giancane, 2019). In turn, active control could enhance long-term prognosis, allowing for better functional outcomes in RA patients (Figure 1.21).

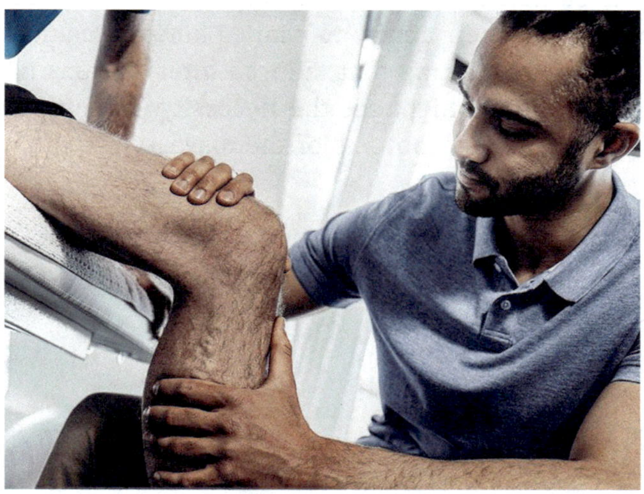

Figure 1.21. The chronic nature of RA means that symptoms can persist over time, leading to potential disability and reduced quality of life.

Source: https://media.post.rvohealth.io/wp-content/uploads/sites/3/2022/02/Rheumatoid_arthritis_GettyImages1318050809_Thumb_new-732x549.jpg.

Test Your Knowledge

1. What types of exercise are beneficial for patients with RA?
2. How can diet and nutrition influence inflammation in RA?

Summary

The complex interaction between RA and comorbidities highlights the intricacy of managing it as a chronic condition. The findings show that certain immunological components, such as undetectable mannose-binding lectin, are linked with poorer survival among RA patients, particularly with bronchiectasis, so there is a requirement for global patient assessments (Bulsara et al., 2019). Besides, methotrexate's contribution in lowering the risk for interstitial lung disease among RA patients aims to highlight the importance of tailored treatment strategies (Busby et al., 2019). This suggests that RA management should not only consider the direct consequences of the disease but also its potential complications, in support of a multidimensional treatment approach involving ongoing surveillance, if any, for comorbid diseases. Continuing research and clinical surveillance are necessary to enhance outcomes for patients and quality of life in individuals with RA.

RA significantly affects the lives of those affected, with persistent pain and disability rendering it one of the major chronic conditions, impacting almost 3 million individuals in Australia alone, accounting for 15 percent of the population (Bates et al., 2014). It has been discovered in research that despite the established cost of RA on health, it has been necessary to know about the experiences of the patients, i.e., how their lifestyle is influenced by symptoms and whether the available support system is sufficient or not (Bates et al., 2014). In addition, studies examining tailored foot orthoses have shown their ability to change kinematic and kinetic parameters in RA patients with foot impairments, suggesting that tailored interventions may improve mobility and reduce pain. Together, these findings highlight the necessity to improve care strategies for RA, addressing physical and psychosocial symptoms of the disease.

KEY TERMS FROM THIS CHAPTER

- Acute myocardial infarction (AMI)
- Antidiuretic hormone (ADH)
- Arthritis
- Arthropathies
- Biologic treatments
- Cardiovascular
- Chronic autoimmune disease
- Chronic pain
- Complex interplay
- Demographic aspects
- Diagnosis
- Diagnostic
- Diagnostic assurance
- Effective management
- Electronic health records (EHRs)
- Emotional distress
- Genetic predisposition
- Hormones
- Immunological
- Joint trauma

Critical Thinking Questions

1. **Which of the following is the most common joint involvement in early rheumatoid arthritis?**
   a. Distal interphalangeal joints
   b. Metacarpophalangeal joints
   c. Hip joints
   d. Sacroiliac joints
2. **Rheumatoid arthritis is primarily characterized by:**
   a. Non-inflammatory joint degeneration
   b. Asymmetric joint involvement
   c. Autoimmune-mediated synovial inflammation
   d. Septic arthritis
3. **Which autoantibody is most specific for diagnosing RA?**
   a. Antinuclear antibody (ANA)
   b. Anti-cyclic citrullinated peptide (anti-CCP) antibody
   c. Rheumatoid factor (RF)
   d. Anti-dsDNA
4. **Morning stiffness in RA typically lasts for:**
   a. Less than 15 minutes
   b. About an hour or more
   c. Only at night
   d. Occurs after exercise
5. **Which of the following is NOT a common extra-articular manifestation of RA?**
   a. Rheumatoid nodules
   b. Interstitial lung disease
   c. Uveitis
   d. Vasculitis

Answers to Critical Thinking Questions

1. (b); 2. (c); 3. (b); 4. (b); 5. (c).

Short Answer Questions

1. What is the role of genetics in the development of RA?
2. Which HLA allele is most strongly associated with RA
3. What are the most common presenting symptoms of RA?
4. How does RA differ from osteoarthritis in terms of joint involvement?
5. What is the role of NSAIDs in RA management?
6. When should DMARDs be initiated in RA treatment?
7. How does RA impact daily life and physical function?
8. What lifestyle changes can help manage RA symptoms?

References

1. Abdel-Nasser, A., Adebajo, A., Arnett, F., Beaglehole, R., Beaglehole, R., Beighton, P., et al. (2012). Estimating the burden of rheumatoid arthritis in Africa: A systematic analysis. https://core.ac.uk/download/28973477.pdf (accessed on 17th June 2025).
2. Dick, A. D., Rosenbaum, J. T., Al-Dhibi, H. A., Belfort, R., Jr, Brézin, A. P., Chee, S. P., Davis, J. L., Ramanan, A. V., Sonoda, K. H., Carreño, E., Nascimento, H., Salah, S., Salek, S., Siak, J., Steeples, L., & Fundamentals of Care for Uveitis International Consensus Group (2018). Guidance on Noncorticosteroid Systemic Immunomodulatory Therapy in Noninfectious Uveitis: Fundamentals Of Care for UveitiS (FOCUS) Initiative. *Ophthalmology*, *125*(5), 757–773. https://doi.org/10.1016/j.ophtha.2017.11.017 (accessed on 17th June 2025).
3. Agustín-Perez, M., Bustamante, M. F., Cedola, F., Coras, R., et al. (2020). Design of an anti-inflammatory diet (*ITIS diet*) for patients with rheumatoid arthritis. https://core.ac.uk/download/323064574.pdf (accessed on 17th June 2025).
4. Alessandri, C., Barbati, C., Ceccarelli, F., Colasanti, T., et al. (2016). Prevalence, sensitivity and specificity of antibodies against carbamylated proteins in a monocentric cohort of patients with rheumatoid arthritis and other autoimmune rheumatic diseases. https://core.ac.uk/download/74321024.pdf (accessed on 17th June 2025).
5. Aletaha, D., Anderson, J., Arnett, F. C., Backman, J. T., Bartlett, S. J., Bernatsky, S., et al. (2013). Symptom complexes at the earliest phases of rheumatoid arthritis: A synthesis of the qualitative literature. https://core.ac.uk/download/30625453.pdf (accessed on 17th June 2025).
6. Aletaha, D., McInnes, I. B., & Smolen, J. S. (2016). *Rheumatoid Arthritis*. https://core.ac.uk/download/77600864.pdf (accessed on 17th June 2025).
7. Alvis-Zakzuk, N. J., Castillo, E., Pineda, C., Sandoval, H., et al. (2021). Quantifying potential cost-savings through an alternative imaging-based diagnostic process in presumptive seronegative rheumatoid arthritis. https://core.ac.uk/download/481668853.pdf (accessed on 17th June 2025).
8. Annibale, B., Carabotti, M., Conti, L., Esposito, G., et al. (2018). Risk factors associated with the occurrence of autoimmune diseases in adult coeliac patients. https://core.ac.uk/download/188824534.pdf (accessed on 17th June 2025).
9. Antczak, J., Bocianiak, B., Fenrych, U., Hamerska, M., et al. (2024). The importance of diet, intestinal microbiome and physical activity in rheumatoid arthritis (RA)–Review. https://core.ac.uk/download/613694736.pdf (accessed on 17th June 2025).
10. Arteaga, M. J., Batlle-Gualda, E., Carmona, L., Cea-Calvo, L., et al. (2017). Perceptions of patients with rheumatic diseases on the impact on daily life and satisfaction with their medications: RHEU-LIFE, a survey to patients treated with subcutaneous biological products. https://core.ac.uk/download/199450378.pdf (accessed on 17th June 2025).
11. Assassi, S., Fischbach, M., GENISOS Study Group, Gonzalez, E. B., et al. (2011). Predictors of fatigue severity in early systemic sclerosis: A prospective longitudinal study of the GENISOS cohort. https://core.ac.uk/download/323073807.pdf (accessed on 17th June 2025).
12. Atchley, S., Axford, J., Vivat, B., Bury, M., Charmaz, K., Fisher, P., Reynolds, F., et al. (2011). Visual art-making as a resource for living positively with arthritis: An interpretative phenomenological

analysis of older women's accounts. https://core.ac.uk/download/20665876.pdf (accessed on 17th June 2025).

13. Ballan, J. C. (1996). *A Review of Juvenile Rheumatoid Arthritis*. https://core.ac.uk/download/235074323.pdf (accessed on 17th June 2025).

14. Barn, R., Brandon, M., Rafferty, D., Steultjens, M., et al. (2013). Kinematic, kinetic and electromyographic response to customized foot orthoses in patients with tibialis posterior tenosynovitis, *pes plano valgus* and rheumatoid arthritis. https://core.ac.uk/download/16458497.pdf (accessed on 17th June 2025).

15. Beral, V., Berkel, J., Bullard, J., Coleman, M., Gulliford, M., Møller, H., Phekoo, K., et al. (2013). Cancer recording and mortality in the General Practice Research Database and linked cancer registries.

16. Berardicurti, O., Carubbi, F., Ciccia, F., Cipriani, P., Giacomelli, R., Guggino, G., Liakouli, V., et al. (2019). Managing adult-onset Still's disease: The effectiveness of high-dosage of corticosteroids as first-line treatment in inducing the clinical remission. Results from an observational study. https://core.ac.uk/download/287858909.pdf (accessed on 17th June 2025).

17. Berk, M., Kenyon, L. C., Lee-Ching, C., Park, E. J., et al. (2018). Rheumatoid meningitis *sine arthritis*. https://core.ac.uk/download/213444660.pdf (accessed on 17th June 2025).

18. Beroes, J. M., Hempel, S., Miake-Lye, I. M., Shanman, R., et al. (2016). An evidence map of the effect of Tai Chi on health outcomes. https://core.ac.uk/download/323076047.pdf (accessed on 17th June 2025).

19. Black, S., DeHoratius, R. J., Gaylis, N. B., Kafka, J., et al. (2017). Patient-reported outcome assessment of inflammatory arthritis patient experience with intravenously administered biologic therapy. https://core.ac.uk/download/129192309.pdf (accessed on 17th June 2025).

20. Boneparth, A. D., CARRA Registry Investigators, Connelly, M., Schikler, K. N., et al. (2019). Demographic, clinical, and treatment characteristics of the juvenile primary fibromyalgia syndrome cohort enrolled in the Childhood Arthritis and Rheumatology Research Alliance Legacy Registry. https://core.ac.uk/download/323073272.pdf (accessed on 17th June 2025).

21. Borah, R., Reddibathina, L. H., Mudagal, M. P., Ramachandran, S., et al. (2023). Menopausal transition and the development of rheumatoid arthritis: An overview. https://core.ac.uk/download/588487544.pdf (accessed on 17th June 2025).

22. Borg, A. A., Caruana Galizia, J. P., & Frendo, M. (2013). Concordance with the British Society of Rheumatology (BSR) 2010 recommendations on eligibility criteria for the first biologic agent. https://core.ac.uk/download/46602399.pdf (accessed on 17th June 2025).

23. Brus, H. L. M., Rasker, J. J., Taal, E., et al. (1997). Patient education and disease activity: A study among rheumatoid arthritis patients. https://core.ac.uk/download/pdf/11474797.pdf (accessed on 17th June 2025).

24. Buisman, L. R., Hazes, J. M. W., Luime, J. J., Oppe, M., et al. (2016). A five-year model to assess the early cost-effectiveness of new diagnostic tests in the early diagnosis of rheumatoid arthritis. https://core.ac.uk/download/43291966.pdf (accessed on 17th June 2025).

25. Bulsara, M., Carroll, G. J., Coleman, S., Easter, J., et al. (2019). Undetectable mannose binding lectin is associated with HRCT proven bronchiectasis in rheumatoid arthritis (RA). https://core.ac.uk/download/213608148.pdf (accessed on 17th June 2025).

26. Busby, A., Creamer, P., Dixey, J., Kiely, P., et al. (2019). Is incident rheumatoid arthritis interstitial lung disease associated with methotrexate treatment? Results from a multivariate analysis in the ERAS and ERAN inception cohorts. https://core.ac.uk/download/287581915.pdf (accessed on 17th June 2025).

27. Calin, A., van Tubergen, A., Belza, B., Cote-Arsenault, D., Dernis-Labous, E., Irvine, E., Dagfinrud, H., et al. (2013). Patient perspectives of managing fatigue in ankylosing spondylitis, and views on potential interventions: A qualitative study. https://core.ac.uk/download/16460591.pdf (accessed on 17th June 2025).

28. Callahan, L. F., Martin, K. R., Mingo, C. A., Schoster, B., et al. (2014). Individual and community socioeconomic status: Impact on mental health in individuals with arthritis. https://core.ac.uk/download/29150971.pdf (accessed on 17th June 2025).

29. Carpenter, L., Creamer, P., Dixey, J., for ERAS and ERAN, et al. (2019). Remission vs low disease activity: Function, quality of life and structural outcomes in the Early Rheumatoid Arthritis Study and Network. https://core.ac.uk/download/287582096.pdf (accessed on 17th June 2025).

30. Cassell, J., Davies, K., Nicholson, A., Rait, G., et al. (2011). The early presentation and management of rheumatoid arthritis cases in primary care. https://core.ac.uk/download/9127596.pdf (accessed on 17th June 2025).

31. Chaplain, M. A. J., Eftimie, R., & Macfarlane, F. R. (2019). Quantitative predictive modelling approaches to understanding rheumatoid arthritis: A brief review. https://core.ac.uk/download/286356117.pdf (accessed on 17th June 2025).

32. Wu, Y., Chen, K., & Terkeltaub, R. (2016). Systematic review and quality analysis of emerging diagnostic measures for calcium pyrophosphate crystal deposition disease. *RMD open*, *2*(2), e000339. https://doi.org/10.1136/rmdopen-2016-000339(accessed on 17th June 2025).

33. Chowdhury, R., Duquenne, L., Emery, P., Mankia, K., et al. (2020). The role of ultrasound across the inflammatory arthritis continuum: Focus on "at-risk" individuals. https://core.ac.uk/download/341797736.pdf (accessed on 17th June 2025).

34. Sobek, K. Łucja, Mazur, M., Waz, D., Szarłowicz, J., Goliszek, Z., Tabin-Barczak, W., ... Samuła, S. (2024). The Impact of Diet and Lifestyle on the Course of Autoimmune Diseases. *Quality in Sport*, *36*, 56879. https://doi.org/10.12775/QS.2024.36.56879(accessed on 17th June 2025).

35. Cieza, A., Kvien, T. K., Moe, R., Reinsberg, J., et al. (2009). Responsiveness of the International Classification of Functioning, Disability and Health (ICF) Core Set for rheumatoid arthritis. https://core.ac.uk/download/12175841.pdf (accessed on 17th June 2025).

36. Comellas, M., Dilla, T., Díaz Torne, C., Díaz, S., et al. (2020). What matters most to patients and rheumatologists? A discrete choice experiment in rheumatoid arthritis. https://core.ac.uk/download/304372039.pdf (accessed on 17th June 2025).

37. Conti, F., Di Franco, M., Guzzo, M. P., Iannuccelli, C., et al. (2019). Mucosa-environment interactions in the pathogenesis of rheumatoid arthritis. https://core.ac.uk/download/231748449.pdf (accessed on 17th June 2025).

38. Contreras, J. (2019). *Utilization of Mind-Body Practices for Adults with Fibromyalgia: 2017 National Health Interview Survey*. https://core.ac.uk/download/231832574.pdf (accessed on 17th June 2025).

39. Coras, R., Guma, M., & Murillo-Saich, J. D. (2020). Circulating pro- and anti-inflammatory metabolites and its potential role in rheumatoid arthritis pathogenesis. https://core.ac.uk/download/323308678.pdf (accessed on 17th June 2025).

40. Picchianti-Diamanti, A., Panebianco, C., Salemi, S., Sorgi, M. L., Di Rosa, R., Tropea, A., Sgrulletti, M., Salerno, G., Terracciano, F., D'Amelio, R., Laganà, B., & Pazienza, V. (2018). Analysis of Gut Microbiota in Rheumatoid Arthritis Patients: Disease-Related Dysbiosis and Modifications Induced by Etanercept. *International journal of molecular sciences, 19*(10), 2938. https://doi.org/10.3390/ijms19102938(accessed on 17th June 2025).

41. D'Amelio, R., Picchianti-Diamanti, A., & Rosado, M. M. (2018). Infectious agents and inflammation: The role of microbiota in autoimmune arthritis. https://core.ac.uk/download/153366739.pdf (accessed on 17th June 2025).

42. De Ceuleneer, M., De Keyser, F., Deforce, D., Elewaut, D., et al. (2010). Citrullinated vimentin as an important antigen in immune complexes from synovial fluid of rheumatoid arthritis patients with antibodies against citrullinated proteins. https://core.ac.uk/download/55843039.pdf (accessed on 17th June 2025).

43. Diaconu, C. C., Hainarosie, R., Iancu, M. A., Iftimie, G., et al. (2018). The importance of early arthritis in patients with rheumatoid arthritis. https://core.ac.uk/download/216809651.pdf (accessed on 17th June 2025).

44. Finney, A., Katsambas, A., Sav, A., Dufour, A. B., Keenan, A. M., Garrow, A. P., van der Zwaard, B. C., et al. (2018). Foot pain and foot health in an educated population of adults: Results from the Glasgow Caledonian University Alumni Foot Health Survey. https://core.ac.uk/download/293885566.pdf (accessed on 17th June 2025).

45. FitzGerald, O. R., Stephen, S., Opeyemi, S., Staunton, B., et al. (2013). Biomarkers of inflammatory arthritis and proteomics. https://core.ac.uk/download/288637789.pdf (accessed on 17th June 2025).

46. Gaspar, M. P., Gaspar, P. S., Jacoby, S. M., Kane, P. M., et al. (2016). Evaluation and management of sleep disorders in the hand surgery patient. https://core.ac.uk/download/83049675.pdf (accessed on 17th June 2025).

47. Santiago, T., Geenen, R., Jacobs, J. W., & Da Silva, J. A. (2015). Psychological factors associated with response to treatment in rheumatoid arthritis. *Current pharmaceutical design, 21*(2), 257–269. https://doi.org/10.2174/1381612820666140825124755(accessed on 17th June 2025).

48. Genant, H. K., Nitta, T., Okubo, N., Soen, S., et al. (2019). Effects of the anti-RANKL antibody denosumab on joint structural damage in patients with rheumatoid arthritis treated with conventional synthetic disease-modifying antirheumatic drugs (*DESIRABLE study*): A randomized, double-blind, placebo-controlled phase 3 trial. https://core.ac.uk/download/323072454.pdf (accessed on 17th June 2025).

49. Giancane, G. (2019). Pharmacovigilance in juvenile idiopathic arthritis patients (*PharmaChild*) treated with biologic agents and/or methotrexate. A Pediatric Rheumatology International Trials Organization (PRINTO)/Pediatric Rheumatology European Society (PRES) registry. https://core.ac.uk/download/201719507.pdf (accessed on 17th June 2025).

50. Graham, A. S., Hammond, A., & Williams, A. E. (2012). Foot health education for people with

rheumatoid arthritis: the practitioner's perspective. *Journal of foot and ankle research*, *5*(1), 2. https://doi.org/10.1186/1757-1146-5-2 (accessed on 17th June 2025).

51. Grygus, I., & Nogas, A. (2020). Main provisions of the concept of physical therapy for patients with rheumatoid arthritis. *Journal of Education, Health and Sport*, *10*(3), 340–351. https://doi.org/10.12775/JEHS.2020.10.03.037(accessed on 17th June 2025).
52. Hansell, A., Tate, A. R., Nicholson, A., Tate, A. R., Tate, A. R., Lovis, C., Edwards, C. J., et al. (2013). Optimising use of electronic health records to describe the presentation of rheumatoid arthritis in primary care: A strategy for developing code lists. https://core.ac.uk/download/9837008.pdf (accessed on 17th June 2025).
53. Horta-Baas, G., et al. (2023). Gut-joint axis: Gut dysbiosis can contribute to the onset of rheumatoid arthritis via multiple pathways. https://core.ac.uk/download/635719447.pdf (accessed on 17th June 2025).
54. Jans, L., Sudol-Szopińska, I., & Teh, J. (2017). *Rheumatoid Arthritis: What do MRI and Ultrasound Show*. https://core.ac.uk/download/160734620.pdf (accessed on 17th June 2025).
55. Kraft, W. K., Mantravadi, S., & Ogdie, A. (2017). Tumor necrosis factor inhibitors in psoriatic arthritis. https://core.ac.uk/download/83049994.pdf (accessed on 17th June 2025).
56. Langhorne, P., Madhok, R., Singh, G., Wu, O., et al. (2006). Risk of acute myocardial infarction with nonselective non-steroidal anti-inflammatory drugs: A meta-analysis. https://core.ac.uk/download/1394549.pdf (accessed on 17th June 2025).
57. Rasker, J. J., Seydel, E., Taal, E., Wiegman, O., et al. (1993). Health status, adherence with health recommendations, self-efficacy and social support in patients with rheumatoid arthritis. https://core.ac.uk/download/pdf/11456304.pdf (accessed on 17th June 2025).
58. Bates, S. et al (2014). *Arthritis and Disability*. https://core.ac.uk/download/pdf/30673486.pdf (accessed on 17th June 2025).
59. Talele, C., Gohil, D., Kumari, M., Shah, N., & Sadhu, P. (2024). Comprehensive review of rheumatoid arthritis: Insights, challenges, and prospects. https://core.ac.uk/download/603897628.pdf (accessed on 17th June 2025).
60. Yanusman, A. (2023). The effect of physical activity on elderly woman with rheumatoid arthritis symptoms. https://core.ac.uk/download/614371065.pdf (accessed on 17th June 2025).

SYSTEMIC LUPUS ERYTHEMATOSUS (SLE)

2

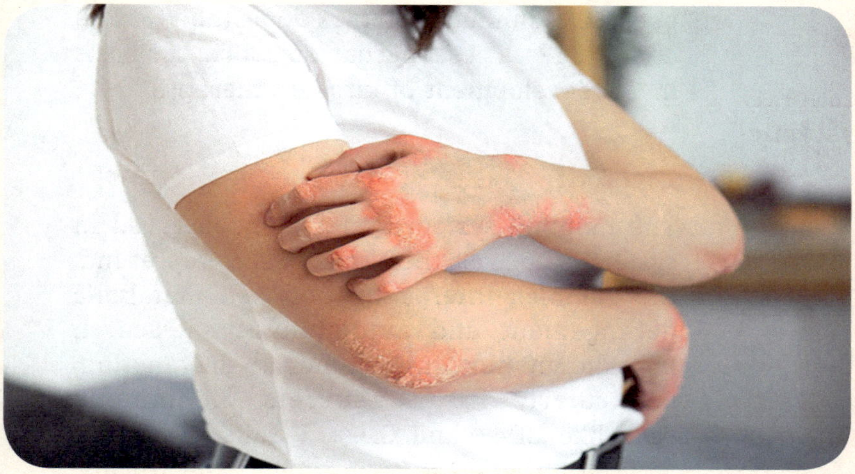

LEARNING OBJECTIVES

After studying this chapter, you will be able to:

1. Understand the pathophysiology of SLE.
2. Explain the clinical manifestations of SLE.
3. Focus on the diagnosis of SLE.
4. Learn the treatment and management of SLE.

Introduction

Systemic Lupus Erythematosus (SLE) is a complex autoimmune illness where the immune system's inability to distinguish self from non-self-cells leads to diffuse inflammation and tissue damage. SLE pathogenesis remains multifactorial with contributions from genetic, environmental, and hormonal factors that interact to promote its etiology and course. It is critical to understand the sophisticated immune mechanisms, most notably the role of T regulatory lymphocytes (Tregs), which are tasked with promoting immune tolerance and controlling inflammation. An observed decrease in FoxP3+ Tregs in renal tissue among lupus nephritis patients would be in support of a mechanism of disease aggravation (Afeltra et al., 2015). Besides, SLE can affect the lower limbs significantly, causing joint and muscular discomfort, together with vascular impairment that degrades the quality of life (Cherry et al., 2014). Therefore, it is critical to enhance our knowledge about SLE to develop holistic management plans and improve patient outcomes (Figure 2.1).

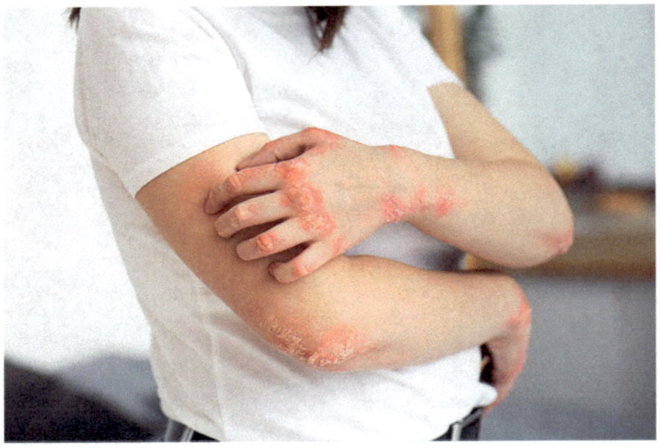

Figure 2.1. Systemic lupus erythematosus.

Source: https://jsshospital.in/wp-content/uploads/2024/05/Suffering-with-Systemic-Lupus-Erythematosus-Lupus.jpg.

2.1. Pathophysiology of SLE

Learning Outcome

1. Understand immune system dysfunction;
2. Identify genetic factors contributing to SLE;
3. Focus on environmental triggers;
4. Discuss the role of hormones in SLE;
5. Learn mechanisms of autoimmunity;
6. Focus on the inflammatory processes involved;
7. Describe organ systems affected by SLE;
8. Focus on differences between SLE and other autoimmune diseases;
9. Know current research on pathophysiology.

Systemic lupus erythematosus (SLE) pathophysiology is traditionally explained as a complex interaction of genetic, environmental, and immunologic components that combine in a dysregulated immune response. The hallmark of the illness is the hyperactivation of B cells that produce autoantibodies against a wide variety of self-antigens and form immune complexes. These immune complexes can deposit in tissues, causing inflammation and tissue damage, a process crucial to SLE clinical manifestations. Moreover, the autoimmune phenomenon entails the participation of different forms of immune cells, including T cells, which play critical functions in the perpetuation of inflammation (Agarwal et al., 2019). Among audio vestibular SLE complications, studies cite abnormality of inner ear structures as a consequence of the autoimmune response and vascular injury because of immune complex deposition (Stadio et al., 2017). These mechanisms form the basis in the development of targeted therapy.

2.1.1. Immune System Dysfunction

The immune system dysfunction observed in systemic lupus erythematosus (SLE) represents the complex interaction between metabolic derangement and autoimmunity. Research has shown how mitochondrial dysfunction, particularly in the subsets of immune cells like CD4+ and CD8+ T cells, results in worsening disease symptoms. Specifically, oxygen consumption rate, spare respiratory capacity, and maximal respiration testing reflect compromised mitochondrial function in these cells, reflecting an extreme metabolic reprogramming with SLE (Yennemadi et al., 2023). Furthermore, recent clinical trials for KZR-616, an immunoproteasome inhibitor, reflect promising immunomodulatory effects, which are key to treating the dysregulated immune responses inherent in SLE patients (Fan et al., 2022). Such an identification not only increases our understanding of immune pathophysiology but also holds promise for the development of targeted therapy directed towards correcting metabolic imbalance, which can lead to improved patient outcomes in SLE treatment (Figure 2.2).

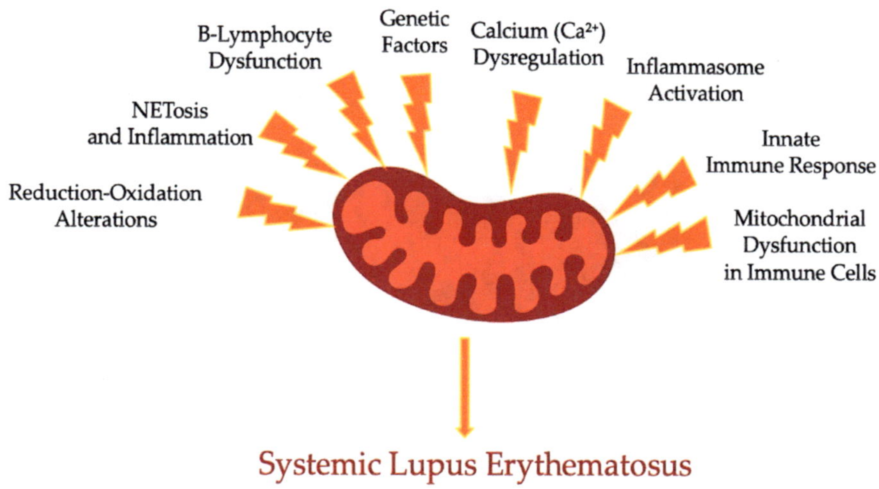

Figure 2.2. The immune system dysfunction observed in systemic lupus erythematosus (SLE) underscores the complex interplay between metabolic disturbances and autoimmunity.

Source: https://www.mdpi.com/diseases/diseases-12-00226/article_deploy/html/images/diseases-12-00226-g001.png.

2.1.2. Genetic Factors Contributing to SLE

Genetic factors play a central role in the etiology and pathogenesis of Systemic Lupus Erythematosus (SLE), controlling the onset and severity of the disease. The polygenic disorder has a strong inherited component, with certain genetic loci, such as those implicated in the regulation of the immune system, which are highly linked with SLE susceptibility. For instance, the existence of antibodies, such as anti-Carp has been linked with erosive disease in SLE-associated arthritis and has highlighted specific genetic pathways that predispose to this phenotype (Alessandri et al., 2018). Furthermore, studies have indicated that environmental factors, as well as genetic dispositions, can lead to malignancies in SLE patients, as mentioned in a long-term cohort study comparing pertinent clinical factors and cancer prognosis (Dey et al., 2013). Therefore, understanding these genetic foundations is crucial in order to develop targeted therapies and improve diagnostic methods in individuals suffering from SLE.

2.1.3. Environmental Triggers

Information on the contribution of environmental stimuli to Systemic Lupus Erythematosus (SLE) pathogenesis is needed to develop effective targeted therapies. Some studies have established that some environmental stimuli, such as exposure to UV light, infection, and certain drugs, can enhance SLE activity and cause disease flares. For instance, UV radiation has been identified as one of the major determinants, triggering cutaneous and systemic involvement through action on the immune system. Moreover, viral and bacterial infections could trigger the immune system and cause the dysregulation characteristic of SLE. Moreover, some drug exposures have been implicated in drug-induced lupus, emphasizing the importance of a well-taken patient history in trying to determine inciting stimuli. As seen with recent studies, knowledge of these environmental interactions is critical, as they guide both clinical care and prevention measures for those who are at risk of developing SLE (Mohamad et al., 2009; Smith et al., 2018) (Figure 2.3).

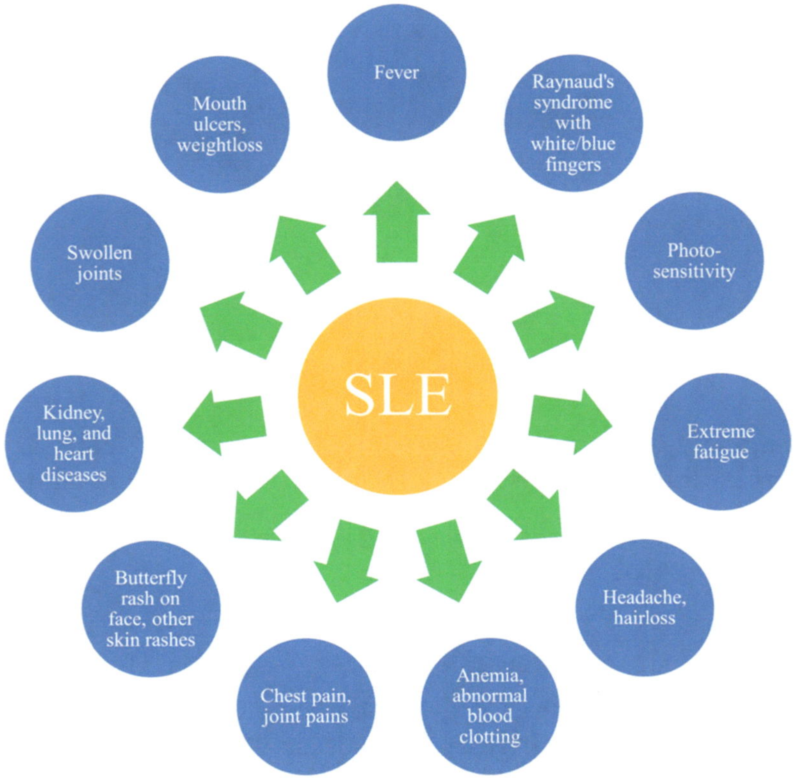

Figure 2.3. Understanding the role of environmental triggers in the pathogenesis of Systemic Lupus Erythematosus (SLE) is critical for developing targeted therapeutic strategies.

Source: Kaye A D, Tassin J P, Upshaw W C, et al. (December 03, 2024) Evolving Treatment Strategies for Systemic Lupus Erythematosus in Clinical Practice: A Narrative Review . Cureus 16(12): e75062. doi:10.7759/cureus.75062

2.1.4. Role of Hormones in SLE

Systemic Lupus Erythematosus (SLE) pathogenesis and presentation are a critical field of research, especially given the disease's high female prevalence. Sex steroid hormones, and notably estrogen, have been invoked as having the ability to modulate immune function and potentially exacerbate autoimmune diseases like SLE. There is evidence that hormonal variations can influence gene expression patterns, which can increase genetic susceptibility to autoimmune disorders in women. Moreover, microRNAs, which are regulated by sex hormones, have emerged as key players in SLE pathophysiology because they regulate immune and inflammatory processes (Sharma & Eghbali, 2014). In addition, the interface between these hormones and immune-mediated disease suggests the intricate role of hormonal status in disease and emphasizes the importance of a subtle understanding of how therapeutic approaches will assist SLE patients (Adelchi et al., 2018). This intricacy suggests gender-specific treatment in managing SLE.

2.1.5. Mechanisms of Autoimmunity

Autoimmunity mechanisms are crucial to decipher in explaining the pathogenesis of systemic lupus erythematosus (SLE). Among these mechanisms of autoimmunity are crucial genetically predisposed defects in tolerance, leading to autoreactive lymphocyte activation. Environmental factors , such as microbial infection, also play a key role in triggering these autoimmune responses.

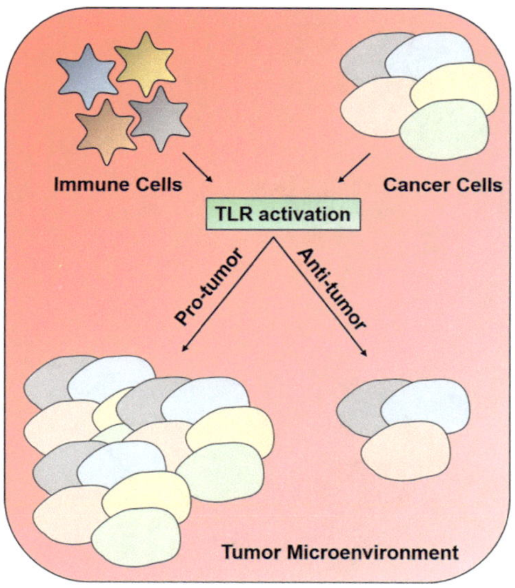

Figure 2.4. The discovery of Toll-like receptors (TLRs) significantly enhances our understanding of this phenomenon, as TLRs can initiate innate and adaptive immune responses upon encountering pathogen-associated molecules.

Source: https://pub.mdpi-res.com/cancers/cancers-12-00297/article_deploy/html/images/cancers-12-00297-ag.png?1583586818.

Recognition of Toll-like receptors (TLRs) enhances our understanding of this process considerably, as TLRs are able to induce innate and adaptive immunity when stimulated by pathogen-associated molecules. But this same pathway can also inadvertently induce autoimmunity, providing a mechanism whereby infection may precipitate subsequent autoimmune disease like SLE. The information gained from recent conferences, such as the 6th European Lupus Meeting, is reflective of new studies and the necessity for new therapeutic strategies aimed at these pathological mechanisms of autoimmunity in SLE (Anders et al., 2005; Ioannou et al., 2005) (Figure 2.4).

2.1.6. Inflammatory Processes Involved

The underlying inflammatory mechanisms of Systemic Lupus Erythematosus (SLE) are complex and multifactorial and in turn usually lead to dysregulation of immune cells, resulting in tissue damage. Central to SLE is the activity of T regulatory lymphocytes (Tregs), which are important for immune tolerance. Studies have shown that Foxp3, a Treg marker, is significantly lower in renal biopsies of lupus nephritis patients, particularly for class IV cases with the worst inflammation (Afeltra et al., 2015). Such a reduction indicates an inappropriate immune-regulatory response, which results in unregulated inflammatory processes. Moreover, SLE may have different symptoms, including audiovestibular complications, where sensorineural hearing loss may be associated with systemic inflammation. These results corroborate the systemic nature of SLE's involvement in more than one organ system, which in turn reinforces the necessity of diagnosing and treating the inflammatory mechanisms inherent within this autoimmune disease (Adelchi et al., 2018).

2.1.7. Organ Systems Affected by SLE

Systemic lupus erythematosus (SLE) is a multifaceted autoimmune disease that impacts numerous organ systems, significantly complicating its clinical picture. Arguably, the most commonly affected system is the musculoskeletal system, with patients experiencing inflammation and pain in the joints, often leading to significant mobility impairment. In addition, renal manifestation is widespread and lupus nephritis is a severe expression that will lead to end-stage renal disease if left untreated (Anand et al., 2023). Even the central nervous system can be involved with seizures and encephalopathy occurring later in the disease course (Anand et al., 2023). Besides, the auditory and vestibular systems are not spared; SLE can lead to hearing impairment and balance abnormalities, as a result of immune-mediated damage to inner ear structures, suggesting an even broader array of neurological effects. Thus, SLE's extensive influence on multiple organ systems points to the complexity of this autoimmune disease (Figure 2.5).

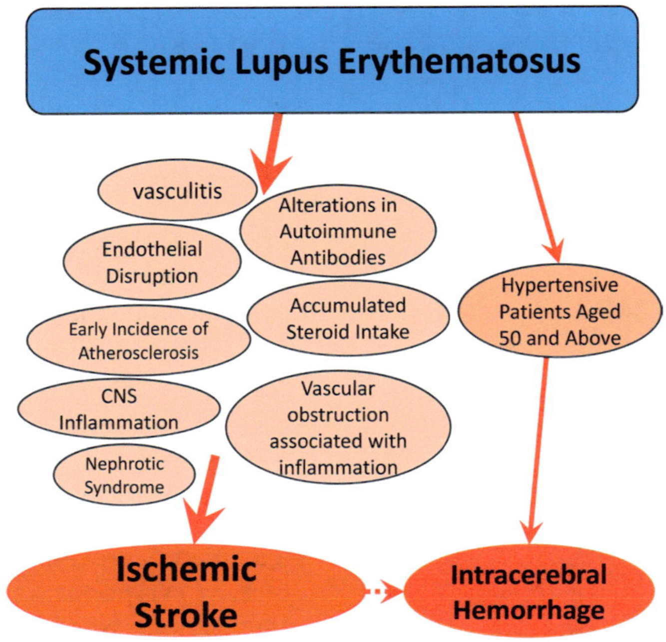

Figure 2.5. Systemic lupus erythematosus (SLE) is a multifaceted autoimmune disorder that impacts various organ systems, significantly complicating its clinical presentation.

Source: https://pub.mdpi-res.com/medicines/medicines-11-00015/article_deploy/html/images/medicines-11-00015-g001.png?1722420272.

2.1.8. Differences Between SLE and Other Autoimmune Diseases

It is critical to understand the differences between systemic lupus erythematosus (SLE) and other autoimmune diseases to make the correct diagnosis and treatment. SLE is distinguished by its systemic impact, affecting multiple organ systems, as opposed to the more focal autoimmune illnesses , such as rheumatoid arthritis or Sjögrens syndrome. Of special mention is the fact that SLE manifests a unique constellation of symptoms, including cutaneous and neuropsychiatric symptoms, which can potentially make its diagnosis harder than in diseases like scleroderma or vasculitis. Evidence indicates that patients with SLE are frequently observed to have diverse responses to therapy, as reflected by variability in cerebral perfusion among patient groups with SLE compared to other forms of autoimmune vasculitis (Maffione et al., 2015). In addition, racial and ethnic differences in disease impact further complicate the disease picture, making it critical to have individually appropriate strategies in clinical practice (Anderson et al., 2012).

2.1.9. Current Research on Pathophysiology

Recent studies in the pathophysiology of systemic lupus erythematosus (SLE) have shown significant progress toward the comprehension of its complex mechanisms, the need for new treatment approaches. SLE is characterized by its diverse manifestations, and in the majority of instances, this results in multi-organ damage, with difficulty in providing management strategies for patients. More recent studies have also pointed to the promise of biological agents, such as potential use of belimumab and anifrolumab that target specific pathways of SLE pathogenesis (Saegusa et al., 2025). Additionally, novel animal models, particularly humanized mouse models, provide a more accurate representation of disease mechanisms through direct exploration of human immune responses within an orchestrated environment (Chilmi et al., 2024). These developments not only improve understanding of its pathophysiology but also pave the way for personalized therapeutic approaches, enabling researchers to better stratify patients and improve therapeutic impact in this difficult autoimmune illness (Figure 2.6).

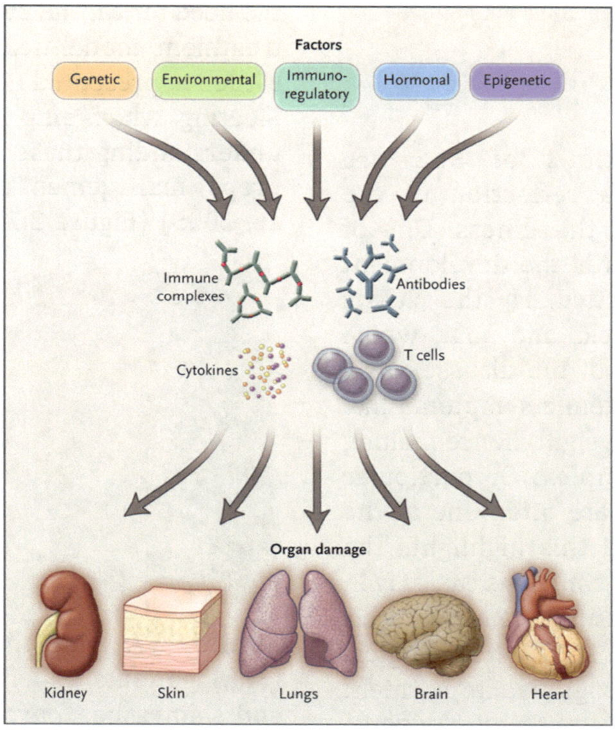

Figure 2.6. SLE is characterized by diverse clinical manifestations, often resulting in multi-organ damage, which complicates management options for affected individuals.

Source: https://www.nejm.org/cms/10.1056/NEJMra1100359/asset/2825f5eb-c31b-4562-81d2-351d3ad42f8b/assets/images/large/nejmra1100359_f1.jpg.

Test Your Knowledge

1. What is the role of B cells and plasma cells in the pathogenesis of lupus?
2. How does defective clearance of apoptotic cells lead to autoimmunity in SLE?

2.2. Clinical Manifestations of SLE

Learning Outcome

1. Identify common symptoms of SLE;
2. Explain cutaneous manifestations;
3. Discuss musculoskeletal symptoms;
4. Focus on renal involvement in SLE;
5. Identify neurological symptoms;
6. Discuss hematological abnormalities;
7. Describe cardiovascular complications;
8. Focus on gastrointestinal manifestations;
9. Learn the variability of symptoms among patients.

The clinical presentations of SLE are extraordinarily varied, a reflection of the multi-systemic nature of the illness. One of the characteristic features is the development of cutaneous lesions, particularly the classic butterfly rash on the cheeks and nose, which presents as an early sign of the disease. Also, patients present with systemic symptoms like fatigue, fever, and loss of weight, hence making the diagnosis rather complex. Of particular note, oral manifestations are often one of the earliest signs of SLE, and this highlights the significant role that dental clinicians can play in early diagnosis of autoimmune diseases in their development (Bossù et al., 2018). Neurological manifestations, including cognitive impairment and vasculitis, present an additional challenge to SLE, and the need for close monitoring and personalized therapeutic intervention (Maffione et al., 2015). It is important to understand these manifestations to enhance patient outcomes and quality of life through early intervention.

2.2.1. Common Symptoms of SLE

Systemic Lupus Erythematosus (SLE) has a vast array of symptoms that are quite variable among the individuals affected and, hence, diagnosis and treatment are challenging. Patients usually complain of fatigue, arthritis, and skin rashes and often the characteristic butterfly rash over the cheeks and nose. SLE can also have hematologic involvement with anemia and thrombocytopenia and affect other organ systems and cause complications like nephritis and neurological conditions. One of the most often overlooked SLE-related symptoms is sensorineural hearing loss, which can be insidious or acute and suggestive of inner ear participation in systemic autoimmune disorders (Adelchi et al., 2018). This broad spectrum of clinical presentations underscores the need for careful evaluation and personalized treatment modalities, as indicated in current evidence presented at the 6th European Lupus Meeting, which emphasized the significance of understanding these diverse symptoms in the proper management of the disease (Ioannou et al., 2005) (Figure 2.7).

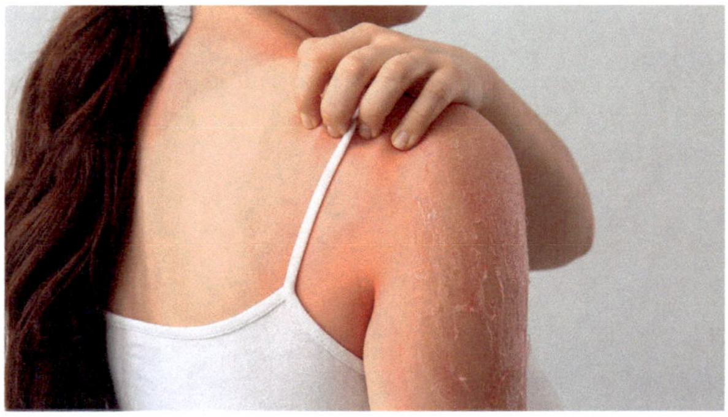

Figure 2.7. Systemic Lupus Erythematosus (SLE) patients experience fatigue, joint pain, and skin rashes, particularly the characteristic butterfly rash across the cheeks and nose.

Source: https://images.healthshots.com/healthshots/en/uploads/2024/03/14150531/lupus.jpg.

2.2.2. Cutaneous Manifestations

Skin manifestations of Systemic Lupus Erythematosus (SLE) reflect the complex interplay between cutaneous pathology and autoimmune process. The disease typically begins with classical skin lesions, including the widespread butterfly rash across the cheeks and nose, most commonly triggered by sunlight. Cutaneous findings are not just for show; they can precede or follow systemic disease and therefore need vigilant follow-up and treatment. As reported in recent studies, the identification of oral and cutaneous manifestations early is essential to optimize the treatment outcome, with clinicians pointing out the requirement for meticulous clinical examinations to produce an accurate diagnostic construct (Bossù et al., 2018). Additionally, studies have also recognized the increased susceptibility of SLE patients to infections , such as periodontal disease and fungal infection, mostly due to the inflammatory milieu and effect of immunosuppressive treatment (Smith et al., 2018). Cumulatively, detection and control of these manifestations become part and parcel of providing the best care for patients with SLE and improving the overall quality of life for such patients.

2.2.3. Musculoskeletal Symptoms

As one of the traditional presentations of systemic lupus erythematosus (SLE), musculoskeletal manifestations significantly influence disease activity and quality of life in patients. Patients most commonly present with several musculoskeletal complaints, including arthralgias, myalgias, and even inflammatory arthritis, which contribute significantly to morbidity. Despite the overall appreciation of these manifestations, they are inadequately treated due to a lack of overall evidence and guidelines to address them. Recent studies have shown that the inclusion of patient-reported outcomes in treatment can lead to improvement in health-related quality of life in accordance with subjective patient experience (Parodis et al., 2025). Furthermore, glucocorticoid (GC) pulse therapy, also applied in the treatment of SLE flare-ups, negatively affects musculoskeletal health, leading to detrimental effects , such as loss of bone density (Esteves et al., 2024). Managing these complications by interventions like exercise training can improve management results and patient satisfaction (Figure 2.8).

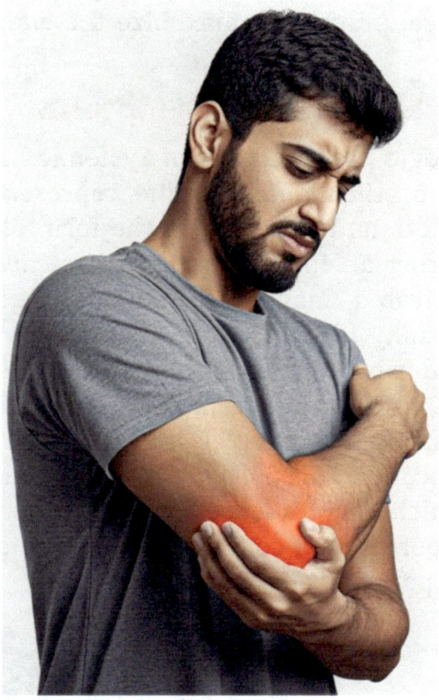

Figure 2.8. Patients report a range of musculoskeletal issues, including arthralgia, myalgia, and even inflammatory arthritis, which contribute to substantial morbidity.

Source: https://www.sghshospitals.com/images/rheumatology.webp.

2.2.4. Renal Involvement in SLE

The renal presentation in systemic lupus erythematosus (SLE), most often in the form of lupus nephritis (LN) significantly enhances the disease morbidity and clinical care. LN has the ability to result in severe renal damage if not treated and when diagnosed late, and, therefore, early biomarkers are important for guiding interventions. Recent studies have defined urinary peptidomic biomarkers that help in the early diagnosis of SLE and LN, helping to stratify patients for focused therapy

(Burkly et al., 2018). Following the identification of these biomarkers, a number of guidelines have been developed, defining regimens of treatment for lupus nephritis in terms of induction and maintenance therapies based on different histological classes of the condition (Bajema et al., 2015). This systemic approach is centered on the critical role of early intervention in the management of renal complications, emphasizing the importance of the integration of early detection strategies in clinical practice to maximize the effectiveness of treatment and recovery of patients with SLE.

2.2.5. Neurological Symptoms

Neurologic presentations in Systemic Lupus Erythematosus (SLE) patients can have a significant impact on their quality of life, representing a formidable diagnosis and management issue. Such presentations tend to be in the form of headache, cognitive impairment, and psychiatric illness, presenting an image of the central nervous system's multifaceted involvement by SLEs. More sophisticated imaging technologies, such as perfusion brain single photon emission computed tomography (SPECT), have also proven the ability to differentiate between responder and non-responder patients to therapeutic interventions through tracking alterations in cerebral perfusion in individuals with autoimmune vasculitis secondary to SLE (Maffione et al., 2015). Also, magnetic resonance spectroscopy (MRS) has helped to define the metabolic changes in the brain, particularly with uncontrolled spells of headache, demonstrating a greater choline/creatine ratio during the spell, and which may be associated with disease activity (Caramia et al., 2018). These tests underscore the importance of controlling neurological symptoms in order to maximize response to treatment in SLE patients (Figure 2.9).

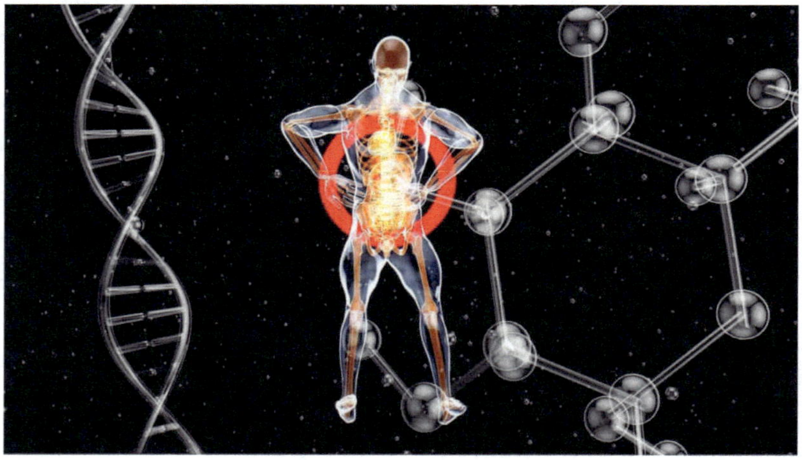

Figure 2.9. Neurological symptoms in patients with Systemic Lupus Erythematosus (SLE) can significantly impact their quality of life, presenting a complex challenge for diagnosis and management.

Source: https://s3.amazonaws.com/production.scholastica/article/82228/medium/photo-1650897492422-1a939d83e4e6?1688054312.

2.2.6. Hematological Abnormalities

Hematologic conditions are among the most frequent manifestations of systemic lupus erythematosus (SLE) with a significant influence on patient prognosis and management. Various studies illustrate that almost 72% of SLE patients present with anemia, typically due to autoimmune hemolytic causes, while a significant percentage also present with leukopenia (32%), lymphopenia (54%), and thrombocytopenia (23%) (Chawla et al., 2023). Further, SLE children also exhibit similar patterns, with hematologic presentations in over 83% of the patients, highlighting the need for prompt identification of these manifestations by the clinician (Ghrahani et al., 2021). Anemia, in particular, also occurs not only as the common initial presentation but also as a multi-factorial complication throughout the course of the development of the diseases. Recognition of the broad spectrum of hematologic abnormalities is essential to properly diagnose and treat SLE, as these disorders offer valuable indices of disease activity and severity.

2.2.7. Cardiovascular Complications

Cardiovascular disease is the greatest concern in patients with systemic lupus erythematosus (SLE), as it is highly responsible for causing morbidity and mortality in them. Pathogenesis usually is immune-mediated vascular damage and increased atherosclerosis due to the underlying chronic inflammation of the condition. The additional risk of thrombotic events like stroke and myocardial infarction is also enhanced by the presence of anti-phospholipid antibodies. There have also been recent developments in the role of biomarkers in early diagnosis prediction, with studies indicating urinary peptides linked to cardiovascular complications in SLE patients (Burkly et al., 2018). Treatments , such as belimumab have also been indicated in treating cardiovascular complications related to SLE, reporting improved clinical outcomes as observed in randomized controlled trials (Kandala et al., 2013). Hence, an effective approach to surveillance and cardiovascular well-being management in SLE patients is required to maximize patient outcomes across the board (Figure 2.10).

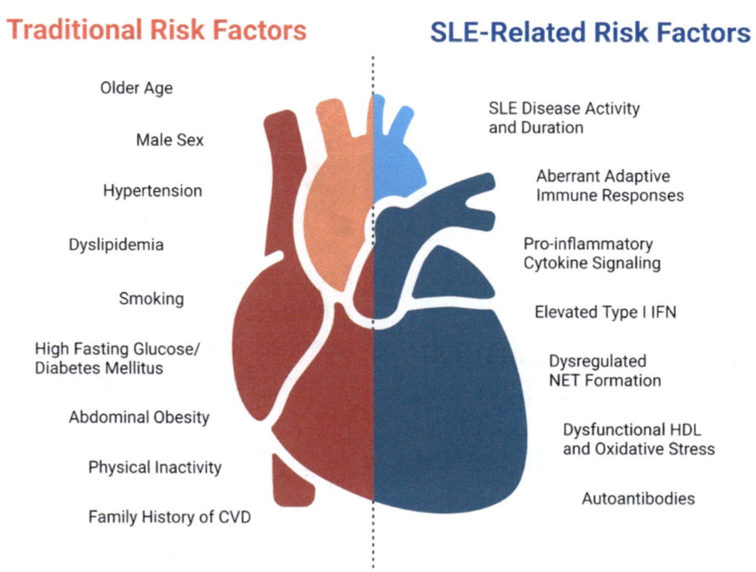

Figure 2.10. Cardiovascular complications are a significant concern for patients with systemic lupus erythematosus (SLE), as they contribute markedly to morbidity and mortality within this population.

Source: https://media.springernature.com/lw1200/springer-static/image/art%3A10.1007%2Fs00281-022-00922-y/MediaObjects/281_2022_922_Fig1_HTML.png.

2.2.8. Gastrointestinal Manifestations

Gastrointestinal manifestations are significant Systemic Lupus Erythematosus (SLE) complications in patients and affect nearly 9.7% of patients who present in the early phase of the disease. Enteritis, pancreatitis, ascites, and hepatitis are the most frequent manifestations, and they have more than just simple symptomatology implications since these manifestations are associated with more active disease and mortality. Interestingly, gastrointestinal disturbances are patients who have comorbidities, i.e., pleural effusion and thrombocytopenia, which also complicate their clinical management (Mehta et al., 2023). Additionally, literature shows that functional gastrointestinal disorders (FGIDs) are prevalent in SLE patients, and their incidence is much higher among them compared to age-matched controls. These conditions manifest as anorectal pain, nausea, and vomiting with potential correlations to drugs , such as non-steroidal anti-inflammatory drugs and glucocorticoids (Realpozo et al., 2019). In general, these gastrointestinal complications emphasize the multifaceted impact of SLE on patient quality of life and well-being.

2.2.9. Variability of Symptoms Among Patients

The variability in symptoms of patients with Systemic Lupus Erythematosus (SLE) is the primary diagnostic and treatment challenge. Heterogeneity can be described in terms of the extremely variable manifestations that affect virtually every organ system, which give rise to a wide range of clinical presentations to confuse healthcare providers. Symptoms, for instance, can vary from musculoskeletal pain and fatigue to more severe sequelae like nephropathy and neuropsychiatric syndromes. Also, some patients may develop audio vestibular symptoms like sensorineural hearing loss, which may occur either in a fluctuating or progressive manner, complicating the patient's clinical presentation and treatment plan, as seen in immune-mediated inner ear disorders in systemic autoimmune diseases (Adelchi et al., 2018). Individualized pharmacological strategies are essential, since psychosocial variables like coping and perceived pain similarly contribute to symptom severity and patient quality of life (Assassi et al., 2011) (Figure 2.11).

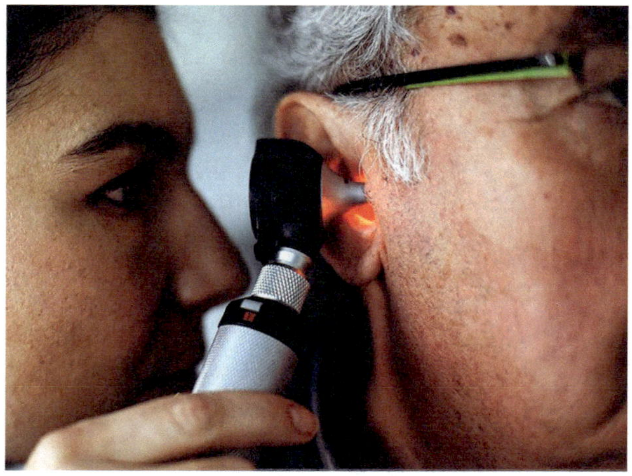

Figure 2.11. Some patients may experience audiovestibular symptoms like sensorineural hearing loss, which can occur in a fluctuating or progressive manner.

Source: https://media.post.rvohealth.io/wp-content/uploads/sites/3/2022/08/sensorineural_hearing_GettyImages1217809756_Thumb-732x549.jpg.

Test Your Knowledge

1. What are the musculoskeletal symptoms of SLE?
2. How is lupus nephritis classified, and what are its clinical signs?

2.3. Diagnosis of SLE

Learning Outcome

1. Learn criteria for SLE diagnosis;
2. Discuss the role of laboratory tests;
3. Focus on the importance of clinical history;
4. Understand differential diagnosis considerations;
5. Explain the use of imaging studies;
6. Identify challenges in diagnosing SLE;
7. Explain the role of biomarkers in diagnosis;
8. Know the importance of multidisciplinary approach;
9. Learn advances in diagnostic techniques.

Diagnosis of systemic lupus erythematosus (SLE) calls for a multi-faceted approach given the heterogeneity of presentation of the disease. Clinicians utilize endorsed criteria by the American College of Rheumatology (ACR) to characterize SLE, which can involve the identification of characteristic symptoms , such as joint pain, weakness, and rashes through laboratory investigations. Existing research puts importance on assessing new biomarkers, such as cell-bound complement activation products (CB-CAPs) and multianalyte assay panels (MAPs), identified as more sensitive than standard serum complement levels in detecting complement activation in potential SLE patients. In fact, it is shown that higher MAP scores also predict the eventual fulfillment of ACR criteria in one and a half years (Alexander et al., 2020). Besides, long-term follow-up of SLE patients emphasizes careful surveillance of serological parameters as they may be linked with increased risks of associated disorders, including cancers (Dey et al., 2013).

2.3.1. Criteria for SLE Diagnosis

Diagnosis of systemic lupus erythematosus (SLE) calls for a multi-faceted approach given the heterogeneity of presentation of the disease. Clinicians utilize endorsed criteria by the American College of Rheumatology (ACR) to characterize SLE, which can involve the identification of characteristic symptoms , such as joint pain, weakness, and rashes through laboratory investigations. Existing research puts importance on assessing new biomarkers, such as cell-bound complement activation products (CB-CAPs) and multianalyte assay panels (MAPs), identified as more sensitive than standard serum complement levels in detecting complement activation in potential SLE patients. In fact, it is shown that higher MAP scores also predict the eventual fulfillment of ACR criteria in one and a half years (Alexander et al., 2020). Besides, long-term follow-up of SLE patients emphasizes careful surveillance of serological parameters as they may be linked with increased risks of associated disorders, including cancers (Dey et al., 2013) (Figure 2.12).

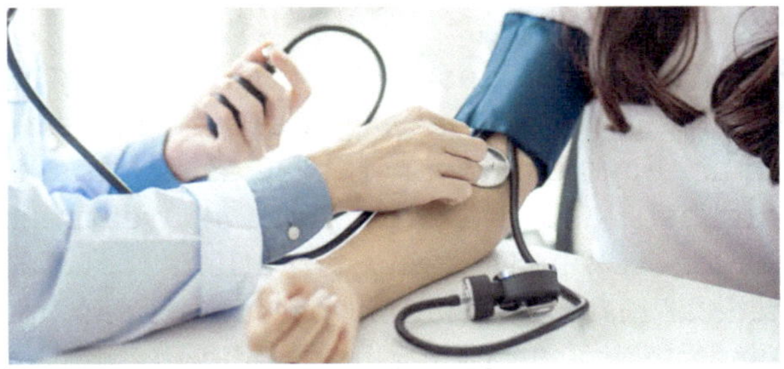

Figure 2.12. Accurate identification of these criteria is crucial, given that early diagnosis can significantly influence patient outcomes and treatment efficacy.

Source: https://images.apollo247.in/pd-cms/cms/2023-04/Shutterstock_1180800871.jpg?tr=q-80,f-webp,w-350,dpr-2.5,c-at_max%20875w.

2.3.2. Role of Laboratory Tests

The laboratory test during the diagnosis and management of Systemic Lupus Erythematosus (SLE) is critical because the tests provide very valuable information about the activity and progress of the disease. For instance, complement activation can be determined using cell-bound complement activation products (CB-CAPs), which were found more often positive in patients with suspected SLE compared to standard serum complement levels (C3 and C4) (Alexander et al., 2020).

Another instance of the utility of lab tests is the measurement of interleukin-2 (IL-2) levels; a high level of serum IL-2 has been strongly correlated with SLE disease activity, and this may be used as a clinical marker for the assessment of disease activity (Sedighi et al., 2014). Not only do these lab tests enhance diagnostic specificity, but they also allow for the prediction of SLE course, thereby impacting treatment planning to better improve patient outcomes. Lastly, the convergence of lab results is essential in the total management of SLE.

2.3.3. Importance of Clinical History

A patient's extensive medical history is important in the management of Systemic Lupus Erythematosus (SLE), as it aids in diagnosis and the selection of treatment options. Understanding a patient's overall medical history, including past infections and hematological status, can help clinicians develop therapeutic interventions suitably. For instance, leukopenia is a frequent complication among patients with SLE, and the treatment of such patients with immunosuppressive therapy can aggravate this condition, making them more vulnerable to infections (Magder et al., 2015).

The second link is that SLE also has an association with oral conditions, which requires a comprehensive patient assessment; oral conditions like periodontitis and fungal infections are more frequent among such patients, complicating their clinical management even further (Smith et al., 2018). Hence, meticulous documentation and monitoring of clinical histories not only enable identification of potential drug interactions and side effects but also enhance the quality of care provided to SLE patients (Figure 2.13).

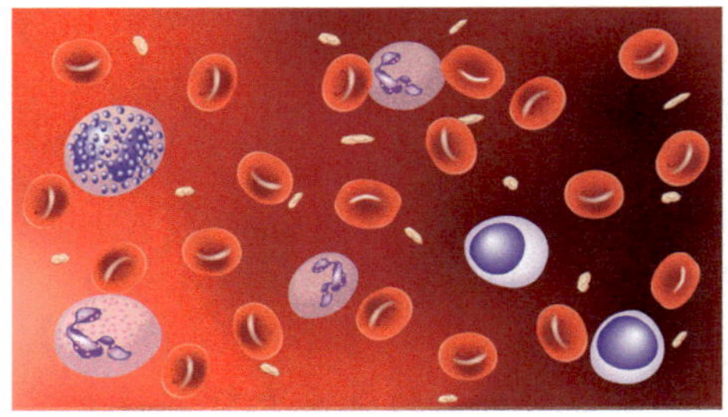

Figure 2.13. Understanding a patient's complete medical background, including prior infections and hematological status, can guide clinicians in tailoring therapeutic interventions effectively.

Source: https://myhematology.com/wp-content/uploads/2024/01/Blood.jpg.

2.3.4. Differential Diagnosis Considerations

Differential diagnosis in SLE is particularly difficult since the symptomatology in SLE is similar to that of most other autoimmune disorders, e.g., rheumatoid arthritis and Sjögrens syndrome. Clinicians should perform careful assessments that include clinical, laboratory, and immunologic data in order to rule out SLE from these conditions. For instance, anti-dsDNA antibodies are a very specific SLE marker, and the rate of positivity in patients is 70–98% (Alessandri et al., 2015).

These types of biomarkers can be of great value to this diagnostic conundrum, where renal findings and serositis further restrict the differential approach. In rare cases, SLE-like acute presentations may be due to other diseases that include epidermolysis bullosa, with the need for careful examination and accurate classification of clinical manifestations (Abiri et al., 2017). Lastly, a differential approach is essential to facilitate proper management and treatment of patients.

2.3.5. Use of Imaging Studies

Imaging studies play a crucial role in the assessment and management of Systemic Lupus Erythematosus (SLE), particularly in evaluating cardiovascular disease and other systemic manifestations. Newer modalities , such as echocardiography, or speckle tracking echocardiography (STE), as it is commonly referred to, have proven more sensitive for detecting small changes within the myocardium than the traditional diagnostic modalities. For instance, studies have established that SLE patients exhibit significantly reduced left ventricular global longitudinal strain (LV GLS) levels, indicating compromised myocardial function with normal ventricular systolic function (Gegenava & Gegenava, 2023).

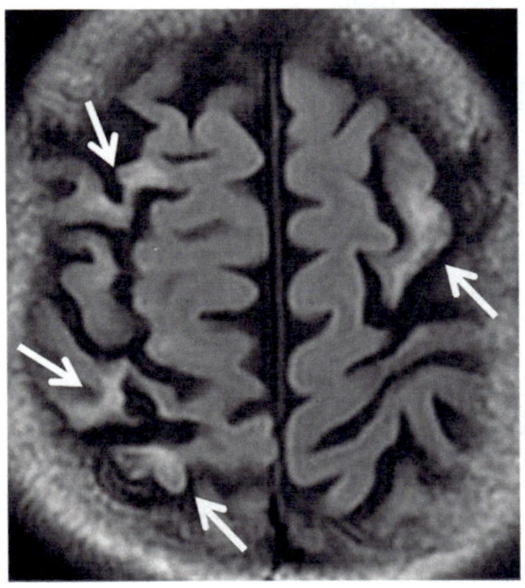

Figure 2.14. Imaging studies play a crucial role in the assessment and management of Systemic Lupus Erythematosus (SLE).

Source: https://www.academicradiology.org/cms/10.1016/j.acra.2014.02.002/asset/c512c39a-e584-479c-ac3f-18a82cc28d87/main.assets/gr3_lrg.jpg.

Further, imaging studies are useful to enhance diagnostic sensitivity in syndromes that overlap, like in the case of pediatric patients with juvenile idiopathic arthritis and SLE manifestations (Velez-Arteaga et al., 2024). By unifying these imaging modalities, clinicians can better stratify risks and tailor treatment strategies, resulting in improved patient outcomes in those patients suffering from this complex autoimmune disease (Figure 2.14).

2.3.6. Challenges in Diagnosing SLE

The diagnosis of systemic lupus erythematosus (SLE) is plagued by challenges due to its inconsistent clinical presentation and overlap with other autoimmune conditions. It is not rare for practitioners to have patients whose clinical presentations overlap with those of other conditions, thus endangering misdiagnosis or delay in therapy. For instance, experience has been such that it has demonstrated the intricacy of differentiating SLE from other illnesses like Wilson's disease, whereby the neuropsychiatric presentation blurs the actual autoimmune process (Bhagoowani et al., 2025). Similarly, SLE may be presented in the form of cerebral vasculitis, which complicates the clinical picture and poses gigantic management challenges (Dudhe et al., 2024). Serological marker-dependent diagnostic criteria can also have their share of inaccuracies, as the markers may be positive in other illnesses or not present in some SLE cases. This multifaceted presentation of SLE needs enhanced clinical expertise and a comprehensive approach to assessment to achieve timely and proper diagnoses and hence improve patient outcomes.

2.3.7. Role of Biomarkers in Diagnosis

Identification and utilization of biomarkers are crucial in the diagnosis and treatment of Systemic Lupus Erythematosus (SLE), a complex autoimmune disorder. Although recent studies have indicated that urinary peptidomic biomarkers have potential for non-invasive preclinical diagnosis, significantly enhancing patients' outcomes through targeted treatment strategies (Burkly et al., 2018). For instance, in 2018, a biomarker panel of 65 urinary peptides discriminated between SLE patients and healthy controls with good effectiveness, with a whopping area under the receiver operating characteristic (ROC) curve of 0.80 (Burkly et al., 2018). Furthermore, CB-CAPs were found to be pertinent in suspected SLE patients, predictive of disease activity. Thus, integrating these biomarkers into the clinical arena may transform the diagnostic environment for SLE, with resulting improved patient risk stratification and improved treatment efficacy (Figure 2.15).

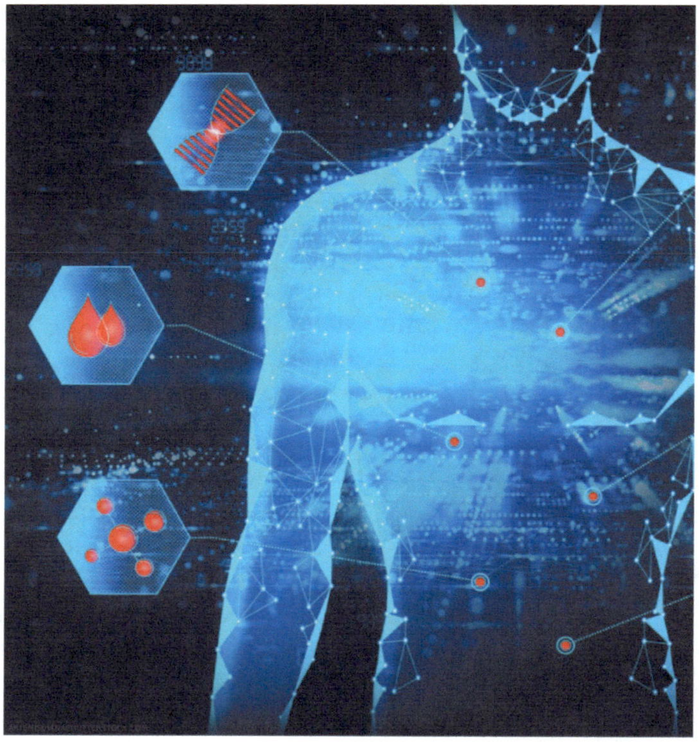

Figure 2.15. The identification and utilization of biomarkers play a crucial role in the diagnosis and management of Systemic Lupus Erythematosus (SLE), a complex autoimmune disorder.

Source: https://www.the-rheumatologist.org/wp-content/uploads/2023/10/shutterstock_2197072529.png.

2.3.8. Importance of Multidisciplinary Approach

The management and interpretation of Systemic Lupus Erythematosus (SLE) must be taken care of in a holistic and multidisciplinary approach due to its complexity as well as multi-organ involvement. Rheumatologists, ophthalmologists, dentists, and immunologists must collaborate in providing holistic patient care because SLE can manifest in numerous ways, with the involvement not just of joints and skin but also eyes and mouth. For instance, eye manifestations range from being mild, such as dry eye syndrome, to severe complications , such as retinal vasculitis, needing subspecialty care (Chukwuyem et al., 2024). Furthermore, oral manifestations of autoimmune diseases, such as those occurring in dental clinics, can affect treatment modalities and patient prognosis equally significantly on early recognition (Bossù et al., 2018). Such a cooperative strategy enables therapeutic regimens, including corticosteroid and biologic use, to be custom fit, ultimately contributing to disease management, monitoring, and quality of life in patients. Thus, multidisciplinary management is essential for effective SLE management.

2.3.9. Advances in Diagnostic Techniques

Recent advances in SLE diagnostic techniques have significantly enhanced clinical results and patient management protocols. Some of the advancements include the utilization of newer magnetic resonance imaging technology, which enables more precise evaluation of SLE neuropsychiatric presentation. These new imaging methods help clinicians diagnose and differentiate SLE-associated neurological complications from other pathologies, and therefore improve the accuracy of treatment and patient prognosis (Alabart et al., 2017). New methods have also been established in the field of immunological testing, that is, the detection of T helper 17 (Th17) cells responsible for SLE pathogenesis. By researching the immunomodulatory effect of drugs like 1α, 25-dihydroxyvitamin D3 on Th17 cell function, scientists are opening the door to specific therapeutic interventions that could improve patient prognosis (Abdollahi et al., 2015). Taken as a whole, these advances represent a paradigm shift in SLE diagnostic practice, emphasizing the importance of early diagnosis and tailoring of management regimens (Figure 2.16).

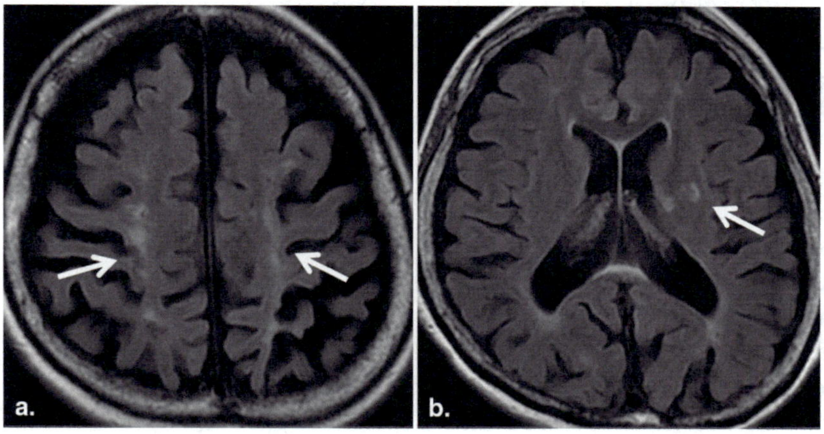

Figure 2.16. The utilization of advanced magnetic resonance imaging (MRI) technologies, which facilitate more precise evaluations of neuropsychiatric manifestations in SLE patients.

Source: https://www.academicradiology.org/cms/10.1016/j.acra.2014.02.002/asset/19e0bcfd-992c-4790-b745-9d54e164b968/main.assets/gr4_lrg.jpg.

Test Your Knowledge

1. What laboratory findings support a diagnosis of lupus nephritis?
2. What are the hematologic criteria in the classification of SLE?

2.4. Treatment and Management of SLE

Learning Outcome

1. Give an overview of treatment goals;
2. Understand pharmacological treatments and non-pharmacological interventions;
3. Discuss the role of lifestyle modifications;
4. Explain management of flares;
5. Know the importance of patient education;
6. Monitoring disease progression;
7. Give psychological support to patients;
8. Discuss future directions in SLE treatment.

Optimal management and treatment of systemic lupus erythematosus (SLE) require an integrated approach to the physical as well as psychosocial aspects of the disease. Increasing evidence supports attention to retention in care, particularly in high-risk groups , such as individuals living in socioeconomically deprived areas, where levels of retention might be significantly lower than in more prosperous communities. It has been identified that 51% of Black SLE patients resided in the most deprived quartile and this was linked to a significant decrease in retention of care and corresponding health outcomes (Ahmad et al., 2020). Aside from monitoring, pharmacologic interventions, including belimumab utilization, have been shown to substantially improve patient responses, particularly in those with typical autoantibody profiles (Kandala et al., 2013). This double emphasis on care continuity and specific pharmacotherapy is essential in mitigating the disparities and complexities involved in the management of SLE optimally.

2.4.1. Overview of Treatment Goals

Management of Systemic Lupus Erythematosus (SLE) involves comprehensive consideration of treatment goals directed toward optimizing patient outcome and minimizing morbidity from the disease. Key objectives are to achieve and sustain remission or low disease activity with sparing use of glucocorticoids due to long-term side effects. In addition to treatment effectiveness, application of the treat-to-target (T2T) strategy based on regular monitoring, such that pre-agreed therapeutic objectives may be achieved, is recommended. This approach, although subtle due to the complex clinical presentation of SLE, has been promising to improve quality of life and disease control in the patient, replicating achievements that have been observed in other chronic illnesses. In addition, attention to the particular requirements of adolescents and young adults with SLE is required, as they also have an inclination to perceive limitations in social opportunities and physical abilities, which points towards the need for psychosocial intervention to promote self-management and coping (Chaitow et al., 2016; Nikolopoulos et al., 2024) (Figure 2.17).

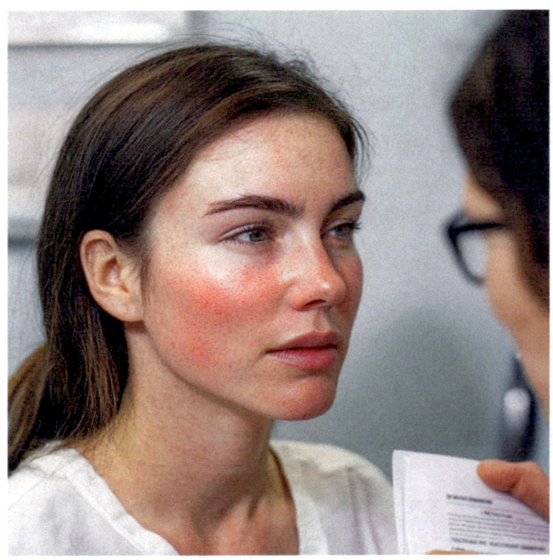

Figure 2.17. The management of Systemic Lupus Erythematosus (SLE) necessitates a comprehensive overview of treatment goals aimed at optimizing patient outcomes and minimizing disease-related morbidity.

Source: https://mdsearchlight.com/wp-content/uploads/2024/11/24526-1731379117185.png.

2.4.2. Pharmacological Treatments

Best management of Systemic Lupus Erythematosus (SLE) relies heavily on a variety of pharmacologic treatments modified to fit the needs of individual patients. Contemporary practice guidelines emphasize first-line use of hydroxychloroquine (HCQ), which is recommended for all patients to avert flares of the disease with vigilant screening for retinal toxicity. During exacerbation, glucocorticoids (GCs) are a valuable bridging treatment, though care should be taken to maintain their use to a bare minimum to minimize maintenance doses in an effort to avoid long-term side effects. Furthermore, early treatment with immunosuppressive drugs (ISDs) , such as methotrexate, mycophenolate, and biologics , such as anifrolumab can significantly enhance disease control and facilitate tapering GCs (Jeanette et al., 2023). For manifestations threatening organs, intravenous cyclophosphamide and rituximab can be employed, emphasizing the importance of patient-centered therapy according to disease severity and response to therapy. This variability reflects the evolving dynamic in the treatment of SLE with a focus on safety in patients and quality of life (Glennon, 2019).

2.4.3. Non-Pharmacological Interventions

In the management of Systemic Lupus Erythematosus (SLE), non-pharmacologic interventions also play a critical role in enhancing the quality of life of patients. Informational and educational assistance, particularly organized exercise, has been shown to be an invaluable resource of adjunct therapy, with impressive efficacy in reducing fatigue and improving functional ability. Research has established that exercise, in addition to enhancing pharmacologic treatment, such as antimalarials and glucocorticoids, also facilitates reduced disease activity and enhanced well-being in SLE patients (Cameron et al., 2023).

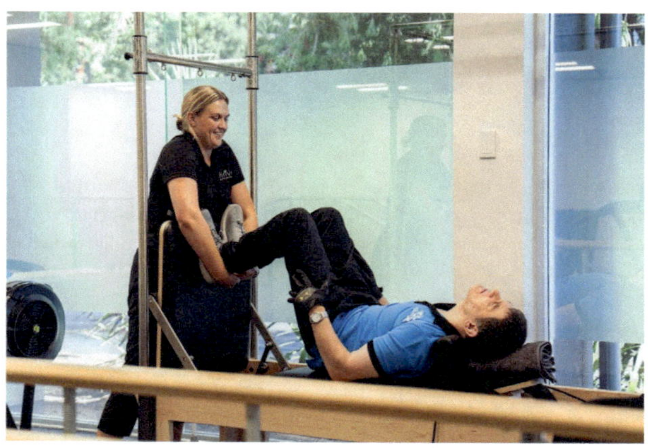

Figure 2.18. Structured exercise has emerged as a particularly effective adjunctive therapy, showing significant benefits in reducing fatigue and improving functional capacity.

Source: https://images.squarespace-cdn.com/content/v1/64e165f66aa02055bda772bb/6c104656-a804-46c7-92d0-f0c890be1405/physiotherapy-pilates-rehabilitation.jpg.

Furthermore, psychoeducative treatments have also been found effective, with results differing by cohort, particularly in altering fatigue levels (Dures et al., 2023). Through the inclusion of such non-pharmacological measures, healthcare workers are able to offer a more holistic model of therapy, stimulating more active patient participation and hopefully reducing overreliance on medication alone. Non-pharmacological approaches thus form part of the holistic management of SLE (Figure 2.18).

2.4.4. Role of Lifestyle Modifications

Lifestyle changes are a major part of treating systemic lupus erythematosus (SLE) and improving the quality of life of the patient. Maintenance of body weight through regular exercise is beneficial for SLE patients, besides promoting improved mental health and reduced fatigue. Exercise has been found to alleviate chronic pain, a common symptom of SLE and other connective tissue diseases, such as systemic sclerosis (Atzeni et al., 2015). In addition, lifestyle changes, particularly diet with anti-inflammatory components, can be added to medical therapies and contribute to symptom management as well (Staniszewska & Baran, 2024). These lifestyle changes are advantageous not only for the overall health condition but also make the patients self-assured with a sense of control over the disease. Thus, embracing an integrative strategy that combines lifestyle modification along with medical treatment is crucial to optimizing the management of patients with SLE.

2.4.5. Management of Flares

Effective management of SLE flares is crucial to avoid complications and enhance the quality of life among patients. By applying the treat-to-target (T2T) strategy, healthcare providers can adjust therapy in order to reach predetermined targets aimed at achieving low disease activity or remission and thus reduce the frequency and severity of flares.

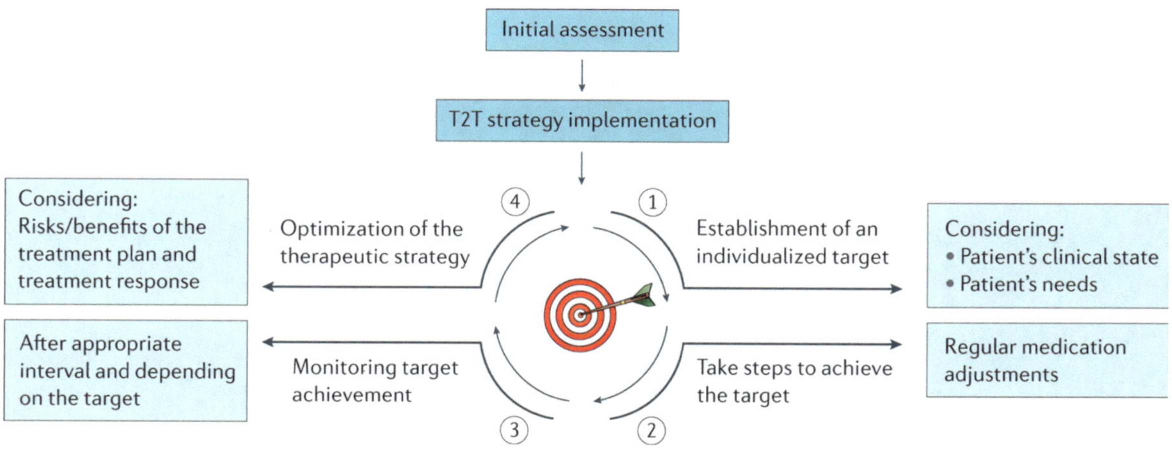

Figure 2.19. Employing a treat-to-target (T2T) strategy, clinicians can adjust therapies to meet predefined objectives that aim for low disease activity or remission, thus reducing the frequency and severity of flares.

Source: https://media.springernature.com/full/springer-static/image/art%3A10.1038%2Fs41584-021-00739-3/MediaObjects/41584_2021_739_Fig1_HTML.png.

This method of management is bolstered by evidence in chronic diseases, where outcomes with target-based therapies have been shown to be superior. Flare management involves a combination of pharmacologic treatments, such as glucocorticoids and immunosuppressants, tailored to individual patient profiles, and lifestyle modifications to minimize triggers. In addition, regular monitoring of disease activity indices, such as described in reports of variations in cognitive impairment associated with SLE, confirms the merit of longitudinal management (Alessandri et al., 2018). Through focusing on effective management strategies, health workers can significantly improve SLE patients' prognosis over the long term and overall improve their well-being (Nikolopoulos et al., 2024) (Figure 2.19).

2.4.6. Importance of Patient Education

Effective education of the patient is essential in managing systemic lupus erythematosus (SLE) since it allows the patient to be actively involved in care and in decision-making regarding treatment. That SLE is long-term and can have complications serves to alert the patient to detect their symptoms early and seek medical attention when necessary. According to the interaction between the treatment regimens, i.e., mycophenolate mofetil, and side effects risks, e.g., susceptibility to leukopenia and infection, there is an imperative for education to ensure that patients adhere to their drugs as prescribed while being vigilant about their health (Magder et al., 2015). Moreover, familiarity with the disease's socioeconomic impact, such as its influence on quality of life and health spending, further supports the need for comprehensive educational interventions (Mak et al., 2009). Ultimately, well-educated patients are better positioned to cope with their illness, adhere to treatment protocols, and improve overall health outcomes in SLE.

2.4.7. Monitoring Disease Progression

Monitoring of disease in systemic lupus erythematosus (SLE) is critical to successful management and treatment, as this condition can lead to significant organ damage and complications. New breakthroughs in identifying biomarkers have enhanced our capacity to quantify disease activity and forecast flares. For instance, a research that utilized urinary peptidomic biomarkers identified a panel of 65 peptides that can distinguish between SLE and healthy controls with an area under the receiver operating characteristic curve of 0.80, as it exhibits the potential of non-invasive testing for early diagnosis and risk stratification (Burkly et al., 2018). Further, cell-bound complement activation products (CB-CAPs) measurement has revealed a higher prevalence of complement activation among patients with probable SLE than in those with typical biomarkers, thereby serving as a reliable predictor for disease progression (Alexander et al., 2020). Such forms of emerging techniques outline the importance of continuous monitoring with the aim of improving patient outcomes for SLE treatment (Figure 2.20).

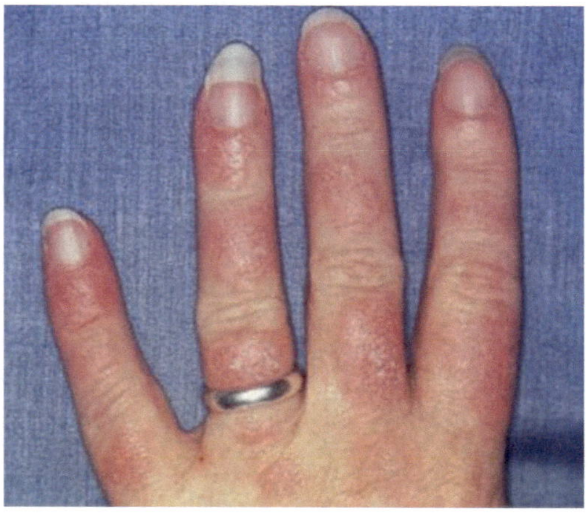

Figure 2.20. Monitoring disease progression in systemic lupus erythematosus (SLE) is critical for effective management and treatment outcomes, as the condition can lead to severe organ damage and complications.

Source: https://img.medscapestatic.com/pi/meds/ckb/24/39224tn.jpg.

2.4.8. Psychological Support for Patients

The psychological impact of Systemic Lupus Erythematosus (SLE) is significant, with patients frequently facing chronic pain and emotional distress that can significantly erode their quality of life. Studies have depicted that fatigue, pain, and musculoskeletal pain are among the most distressing symptoms faced by SLE patients, all of which result in higher rates of depression and anxiety (Aggarwal et al., 2012). The implications of chronic pain in these patients show the importance of specialized psychological treatment, as it is very influential in their mental condition and social activity (Atzeni et al., 2015). Effective pain management strategies not only contribute to relieving physical conditions but also to enhancing the emotional well-being of the patients. Thus, clinicians must optimize psychological treatments that address the intricacies of SLE, fostering resilience and health-related quality of life in individuals struggling with this complex and debilitating disease.

2.4.9. Future Directions in SLE Treatment

As knowledge of systemic lupus erythematosus (SLE) expands, treatment in the future will have greater emphasis on individualized medicine and minimizing differences in care. Because SLE disproportionately affects patients of color and residents of socioeconomically disadvantaged communities, directed initiatives are warranted to maximize retention in care as well as general outcomes. Evidence indicates Black patients retain much lower proportions, and this suggests geo-targeted interventions are needed that more effectively engage these vulnerable groups (Ahmad et al., 2020). Further, the economic burden of SLE indicates an integrated model of care that deals with the psychosocial issues of patients, i.e., employment and education, as well as clinical treatment (Mak et al., 2009). By developing both personalized and fair care approaches, future studies can focus on improving the quality of life of SLE patients and eventually promote improved health outcomes and less discrepancy in treatment access and effectiveness.

Test Your Knowledge

1. What immunosuppressive drugs are used in moderate to severe SLE?
2. How is lupus nephritis managed differently based on the class of disease?

Summary

The management of systemic lupus erythematosus (SLE) requires a comprehensive understanding of its multifaceted nature, including its clinical presentation and response to therapy. The recent research illustrates the effectiveness of belimumab, which is a therapeutic drug that significantly enhances patient responses for up to 52 weeks, as evidenced by SLE Responder Index (SRI) outcomes in BLISS-52 and BLISS-76 studies, where there was an appreciable advantage over placebo or standard treatment (Kandala et al., 2013). Furthermore, the crossover between SLE and auditory manifestations places emphasis on the need for a multidisciplinary approach to managing this complex autoimmune disease. As increasing evidence suggests multiple mechanisms of pathogenesis , including autoimmune attack and immune complex deposition within inner ear structures, further research remains necessary in order to maximize treatment modalities and strategies in patient management (Stadio et al., 2017). Lastly, clinicians and patients grappling with its dilemma should have a good grasp of SLE's implications.

Systematic scrutiny of systemic lupus erythematosus (SLE) instructs us in several valuable lessons about the multidimensional nature of this autoimmune disease. Not the least significant is the positive clinical effectiveness of belimumab, assessed by systematic review and meta-analysis, for SLE patients with antinuclear and/or anti-double-stranded DNA (dsDNA) autoantibodies. In trials , such as BLISS-52 and BLISS-76, belimumab significantly improved results according to the SLE Responder Index (SRI) at 52 weeks, with results demonstrating an odds ratio of 1.63, reflecting considerable therapeutic gain (Kandala et al., 2013). By week 76, however, efficacy was observed to diminish, which suggests variable long-term responses in patients (Kandala et al., 2013). Secondly, the study's identification of diverse participant backgrounds highlights the imperative for a specific treatment approach, in that ethnic and geographical variation may be the determining factor for treatment efficacy. These findings illuminate the multifaceted basis of management plans to ensure optimal care in SLE.

KEY TERMS FROM THIS CHAPTER

- Abnormalities
- Antibodies
- Cause disease flares
- Diffuse inflammation
- Environmental stimuli
- Estrogen
- Genetic loci
- Hyperactivation
- Immune system
- Metabolic imbalance
- Anifrolumab
- Autoantibodies
- Cerebral perfusion
- Dysregulation
- Erythematosus
- Genetic dispositions
- human immune responses
- Immune cells
- Immune-mediated disease
- Metabolic reprogramming

CRITICAL THINKING QUESTIONS

1. **Which of the following antibodies is most specific for SLE?**
   a. Rheumatoid factor
   b. Anti-nuclear antibody (ANA)
   c. Anti-dsDNA antibody
   d. Anti-centromere antibody
2. **The classic malar rash in SLE:**
   a. Spares the nasolabial folds
   b. Involves the palms and soles
   c. Is pruritic and scaly
   d. Worsens in cold temperatures
3. **Which of the following systems is most commonly affected in SLE?**
   a. Endocrine system
   b. Musculoskeletal system
   c. Gastrointestinal system
   d. Respiratory system
4. **A positive ANA test is found in approximately what percentage of SLE patients?**
   a. 25%
   b. 50%
   c. 75%
   d. >95%
5. **Which hematologic abnormality is commonly seen in SLE?**
   a. Polycythemia
   b. Thrombocytosis
   c. Leukopenia
   d. Eosinophilia

Answers to Critical Thinking Questions

1. (c); 2. (a); 3. (b); 4. (d); 5. (c).

Short Answer Questions

1. What immune system dysfunctions are central to the development of SLE?
2. How do autoantibodies contribute to tissue damage in SLE?
3. What are the most common initial symptoms of SLE?
4. How does the classic malar (butterfly) rash present in lupus patients?
5. What is the sensitivity and specificity of ANA in diagnosing SLE?
6. How do anti-dsDNA and anti-Smith antibodies aid in diagnosis?
7. What is the role of hydroxychloroquine in long-term lupus management?
8. When are corticosteroids indicated in lupus treatment?

References

1. Abdollahi, N., Ghoryani, M., Mahmoudi, M., Rastin, M., et al. (2015). Influence of 1 alpha, 25-dihydroxyvitamin D3 on T helper 17 cells and related cytokines in systemic lupus erythematosus. https://core.ac.uk/download/52205683.pdf (accessed on 17th June 2025).
2. Abiri, M., Aghazadeh, N., Bagherian, H., Barzegar, M., et al. (2017). Multigene next-generation sequencing panel identifies pathogenic variants in patients with unknown subtype of epidermolysis bullosa: Subclassification with prognostic implications. https://core.ac.uk/download/188826600.pdf (accessed on 17th June 2025).
3. Afeltra, A., Gigante, A., Margiotta, D. P., Taffon, C., Cianci, R., Barbano, B., Liberatori, M., Amoroso, A., & Rossi Fanelli, F. (2015). The involvement of T regulatory lymphocytes in a cohort of lupus nephritis patients: a pilot study. *Internal and emergency medicine, 10*(6), 677–683. https://doi.org/10.1007/s11739-015-1212-x(accessed on 17th June 2025).
4. Agarwal, A., Al-Mousawi, F., Allen, J., Almawi, W., Anderson, L., Andreae, M., & Annunziato, R. (2019). Glucocorticoids—All-rounders tackling the versatile players of the immune system. https://core.ac.uk/download/227044178.pdf (accessed on 17th June 2025).
5. Aggarwal, R., Almehed, K., Bauernfeind, B., Bjelland, I., Bombardier, C., Brennan, P., & Moberg, C. (2012). An exploration of patient-reported symptoms in systemic lupus erythematosus and the relationship to health-related quality of life. https://core.ac.uk/download/29017094.pdf (accessed on 17th June 2025).
6. Ahmad, U., Bartels, C. M., Chang, I., Ezeh, A., et al. (2020). Investigating lupus retention in care to inform interventions for disparities reduction: An observational cohort study. https://core.ac.uk/download/288432759.pdf (accessed on 17th June 2025).
7. Alessandri, C., Ceccarelli, F., Cipriano, E., Colasanti, T., et al. (2018). Anti-carbamylated protein antibodies as a new biomarker of erosive joint damage in systemic lupus erythematosus. https://core.ac.uk/download/159269169.pdf (accessed on 17th June 2025).
8. Alessandri, C., Ceccarelli, F., Conti, F., Marocchi, E., et al. (2015). Systemic lupus erythematosus with and without anti-dsDNA antibodies: Analysis from a large monocentric cohort. https://core.ac.uk/download/54520771.pdf (accessed on 17th June 2025).
9. Alexander, R. V., Arriens, C., Collins, C. E., Dervieux, T., et al. (2020). Complement activation in patients with probable systemic lupus erythematosus and ability to predict progression to American College of Rheumatology-classified systemic lupus erythematosus. https://core.ac.uk/download/323065797.pdf (accessed on 17th June 2025).
10. Anand, A., Basera, P., Siddiqui, A. S., Singh, A., et al. (2023). Neuropsychiatric systemic lupus erythematosus: A rare case of acute polyneuropathy. https://core.ac.uk/download/553557928.pdf (accessed on 17th June 2025).
11. Anders, H. J., Patole, P. S., Pawar, R. D., Zecher, D., et al. (2005). Molecular mechanisms of autoimmunity triggered by microbial infection. https://core.ac.uk/download/pdf/3779125.pdf (accessed on 17th June 2025).
12. Andersen, J., Aringer, M., Arnaud, L., Bae, S. C., Boletis, J., Bruce, I. N., Cervera, R., et al. (2023). EULAR recommendations for the management of systemic lupus erythematosus: 2023 update. https://core.ac.uk/download/590358195.pdf (accessed on 17th June 2025).
13. Anderson, J., Purdy, C., Ransom, A., Tumiel-Berhalter, L., et al. (2012). Racial disparities in

cancer screening among women with chronic joint pain. https://digitalscholarship.unlv.edu/cgi/viewcontent.cgi?article=1031&context=jhdrp (accessed on 17th June 2025).

14. Assassi, S., Fischbach, M., GENISOS Study Group, Gonzalez, E. B., et al. (2011). Predictors of fatigue severity in early systemic sclerosis: A prospective longitudinal study of the GENISOS cohort. https://core.ac.uk/download/323073807.pdf (accessed on 17th June 2025).

15. Atzeni, F., Bazzichi, L., Casale, R., DI FRANCO, M., et al. (2015). Pain in systemic connective tissue diseases. https://core.ac.uk/download/54524187.pdf (accessed on 17th June 2025).

16. Bajema, I. M., Bertsias, G. K., Boumpas, D. T., Gordon, C., et al. (2015). Lupus nephritis management guidelines compared. https://core.ac.uk/download/77009956.pdf (accessed on 17th June 2025).

17. Staniszewska, I., & Baran, M. (2024). A Role of Physical Activity in Patients with Systemic Lupus Erythematosus – A Literature Review. *Quality in Sport, 15*, 52338. https://doi.org/10.12775/QS.2024.15.52338 (accessed on 17th June 2025).

18. Bargalló Alabart, N., Cervera I Segura, R., & Sarbu, N. (2017). Advanced and conventional magnetic resonance imaging in neuropsychiatric lupus. https://core.ac.uk/download/83829243.pdf (accessed on 17th June 2025).

19. Barker, R. N., Basu, N., Dahal, L. N., Erwig, L. P., et al. (2016). Immunoregulatory soluble CTLA-4 modifies effector T cell responses in systemic lupus erythematosus. https://core.ac.uk/download/77614568.pdf (accessed on 17th June 2025).

20. Bhagoowani, S., Devi, U., Munir, A., Hasnain, U., Khan, S., Iqbal, J., & Akhtar, T. (2025). When copper meets autoimmunity: A rare coexistence of Wilson's disease and systemic lupus erythematosus. *Clinical Case Reports, 13*. https://www.semanticscholar.org/paper/3b1ee6c55da52c215b508316ade3fcf7e17e2938 (accessed on 17th June 2025).

21. Bossù, M., Di Carlo, G., Giovarruscio, F., Polimeni, A., et al. (2018). Autoimmune diseases and their manifestations on oral cavity: Diagnosis and clinical management. https://core.ac.uk/download/159635803.pdf (accessed on 17th June 2025).

22. Ioannou, Y., Bowman, S. J., Rahman, A., & Giles, I. P. (2005). Review of presentations at the 6th European Lupus Meeting 3-5 March 2005. *Lupus, 14*(6), 467–478. https://doi.org/10.1191/0961203305lu2172xx(accessed on 17th June 2025).

23. Burkly, L. C., Mischak, H., Mullen, W., Pejchinovski, M., et al. (2018). Urine peptidome biomarkers for diagnosis of patients with systematic lupus erythematosus. https://core.ac.uk/download/82958552.pdf (accessed on 17th June 2025).

24. Cameron, M., Frade, S., Greene, D., Nutter, J., et al. (2023). Exercise as adjunctive therapy for systemic lupus erythematosus (Review). https://core.ac.uk/download/654326150.pdf (accessed on 17th June 2025).

25. Caramia, F., Francia, A., Morreale, M., Pontecorvo, C., et al. (2018). H-magnetic resonance spectroscopy: Diagnostic tool in recurrent headache in systemic lupus erythematosus. A case report. https://core.ac.uk/download/188832576.pdf (accessed on 17th June 2025).

26. Chaitow, J., Craig, J., Lin, M. W., Mackie, F., et al. (2016). "Lupus means sacrifices" –The perspectives of adolescents and young adults with systemic lupus erythematosus. https://core.ac.uk/download/212686546.pdf (accessed on 17th June 2025).

27. Chawla, K., Dessai, R., Gulati, S., Jain, R., et al. (2023). Study of hematological profile of systemic lupus erythematosus. https://core.ac.uk/download/588568144.pdf (accessed on 17th June 2025).

28. Cherry, L., Edwards, C. J., Teh, L., Williams, B., et al. (2014). An investigation into self-reported foot and lower limb problems associated with systemic lupus erythematosus (SLE): A research proposal.

29. Chilmi, S., Airlangga, D. I., Susianti, H., & Handono, K. (2024). Serological profiles of systemic lupus erythematosus in humanized mice and pristane-induced lupus models. *Folia Medica Indonesian*. https://www.semanticscholar.org/paper/79f5ea192f9a6c97ec45489f59ee28dfac425123 (accessed on 17th June 2025).

30. Chukwuyem, E., Gagliano, C., Musa, M., Ojo, B., et al. (2024). Unveiling ocular manifestations in systemic lupus erythematosus. https://core.ac.uk/download/614041614.pdf (accessed on 17th June 2025).

31. Kandala, N. B., Connock, M., Grove, A., Sutcliffe, P., Mohiuddin, S., Hartley, L., Court, R., Cummins, E., Gordon, C., & Clarke, A. (2013). Belimumab: a technological advance for systemic lupus erythematosus patients? Report of a systematic review and meta-analysis. *BMJ open*, *3*(7), e002852. https://doi.org/10.1136/bmjopen-2013-002852 (accessed on 17th June 2025).

32. Croce, A., D'Aguanno, V., De Vincentiis, M., De Virgilio, A., et al. (2018). Audio-vestibular symptoms in systemic autoimmune diseases. https://core.ac.uk/download/188823057.pdf (accessed on 17th June 2025).

33. Nikolopoulos, D., Lourenço, M. H., Depascale, R., Triantafyllias, K., & Parodis, I. (2024). Evolving Concepts in Treat-to-Target Strategies for Systemic Lupus Erythematosus. *Mediterranean journal of rheumatology*, *35*(Suppl 2), 328–341. https://doi.org/10.31138/mjr.290424.eci(accessed on 17th June 2025).

34. Dey, D., Isenberg, D. A., & Kenu, E. (2013). Cancer complicating systemic lupus erythematosus—A dichotomy emerging from a nested case-control study. https://core.ac.uk/download/29416246.pdf (accessed on 17th June 2025).

35. Di Stadio, A., & Ralli, M. (2017). Systemic lupus erythematosus and hearing disorders: Literature review and meta-analysis of clinical and temporal bone findings. https://core.ac.uk/download/98349075.pdf (accessed on 17th June 2025).

36. Didona, D., Feola, A., Granata, G., Granata, M., et al. (2015). Macrophage activation syndrome as onset of systemic lupus erythematosus: A case report and a review of the literature. https://core.ac.uk/download/153366215.pdf (accessed on 17th June 2025).

37. Dudhe, S., Mishra, G., Parihar, P., Nimodia, D., Shinde, D., & Kumari, A. (2024). Case report: A case report on an 18-year-old female with cerebral vasculitis in systemic lupus erythematosus (SLE). *F1000Research, 13*. https://www.semanticscholar.org/paper/9807715cc47c5a00136550d0618073fe99f9363e (accessed on 17th June 2025).

38. Dures, E., Farisogullari, B., Geenen, R., Machado, P., et al. (2023). Efficacy of non-pharmacological interventions: A systematic review informing the 2023 EULAR recommendations for the management of fatigue in people with inflammatory rheumatic and musculoskeletal diseases. https://core.ac.uk/download/586147649.pdf (accessed on 17th June 2025).

39. Sharma, S., & Eghbali, M. (2014). Influence of sex differences on microRNA gene regulation in

disease. *Biology of sex differences*, *5*(1), 3. https://doi.org/10.1186/2042-6410-5-3 (accessed on 17th June 2025).

40. Esteves, G. P., Barboza, J. M., Ribeiro, W. J. D., Fickert, V. R., Mendes, E. S., Seguro, L., Franco, A. S., et al. (2024). Can a 6-month exercise training program improve musculoskeletal health in individuals with systemic lupus erythematosus post glucocorticoid pulse therapy? Protocol for a randomized controlled trial. *Journal of Clinical Exercise Physiology*. https://www.semanticscholar.org/paper/1407589eadcdaf8d23888ef0aaf3cd6f3e1d89de (accessed on 17th June 2025).

41. Fan, A., Tuch, B., Muchamuel, T., Anderl, J., Leff, R., Henig, N., & Kirk, C. (2022). POS0715 treatment of SLE patients with zetomipzomib (KZR-616), a selective inhibitor of the immunoproteasome, results in circulating gene expression, protein level, and immune cell phenotypic changes with potential correlations to clinical response. *Annals of the Rheumatic Diseases*. https://www.semanticscholar.org/paper/b5b9a0603a32a1bd05a9500469c213bfd0f4d874 (accessed on 17th June 2025).

42. Gegenava, T., & Gegenava, M. (2023). Speckle tracking echocardiography in the assessment of left ventricular systolic function in patients with autoimmune disorders: Review and meta-analysis. *European Heart Journal–Cardiovascular Imaging*. https://www.semanticscholar.org/paper/d5c9fb5d14109f83054bf07ea7d25aa59e3c2d16 (accessed on 17th June 2025).

43. Ghrahani, R., Sugianli, A. K., & Yudiana, H. S. (2021). Clinical manifestation and hematologic interpretation of pediatric systematic lupus erythematosus at initial presentation: 2-years observation. https://core.ac.uk/download/478924048.pdf (accessed on 17th June 2025).

44. Glennon, M. K. (2019). *Today's Fibromyalgia*. https://core.ac.uk/download/286697650.pdf (accessed on 17th June 2025).

45. Maffione, A. M., Anagnostou, C., Civitelli, L., Collorone, S., et al. (2015). Role of brain perfusion SPECT with 99mTc HMPAO in the assessment of response to drug therapy in patients with autoimmune vasculitis: A prospective study. https://core.ac.uk/download/54523723.pdf (accessed on 17th June 2025).

46. Magder, L. S., Petri, M., & Subedi, A. (2015). Effect of mycophenolate mofetil on the white blood cell count and the frequency of infection in systemic lupus erythematosus. https://core.ac.uk/download/155271769.pdf (accessed on 17th June 2025).

47. Mak, A., Clarke, A. E., Bertoli, A. M., et al. (2009). The socioeconomic burden of SLE. https://core.ac.uk/download/37962189.pdf (accessed on 17th June 2025).

48. Mehta, P., Aggarwal, A., Rajasekhar, L., Shobha, V., Mathew, A. J., Kavadichanda, C., Ghosh, P., et al. (2023). Gastrointestinal manifestations in systemic lupus erythematosus: Data from an Indian multi-institutional inception (INSPIRE) cohort. *Rheumatology*. https://www.semanticscholar.org/paper/21a0bb68cf4ee0eabad160eff6b46083e098a4c7 (accessed on 17th June 2025).

49. Mohamad, W. M. (2009). Effects of adjuvant honey therapy on disease activity, lymphocyte function and lymphocyte subsets in patients with systemic lupus erythematosus. https://core.ac.uk/download/32600194.pdf (accessed on 17th June 2025).

50. Munguía Realpozo, P., Pinto, C. M., Carrasco, M. G., Carrasco, M. G., Martínez, S. M., Mogollan

Delfín, T., et al. (2019). THU0272 functional gastrointestinal disorders in women with systemic lupus erythematosus. *Annals of the Rheumatic Diseases, 78*, 414–414. https://www.semanticscholar.org/paper/b75306e2c212590067d2091c226843b215714653 (accessed on 17th June 2025).

51. Parodis, I., Wincup, C., Touma, Z., Andersen, J., Strand, V., & Sjöwall, C. (2025). Holistic approaches in systemic lupus erythematosus: Do physicians avoid addressing difficult-to-treat but highly relevant symptoms? *RMD Open, 11*. https://www.semanticscholar.org/paper/616cdc8a552c3fcbb8dbdfaa164fb487ae4bdd21 (accessed on 17th June 2025).
52. Saegusa, K., Tsuchida, Y., Komai, T., Tsuchiya, H., & Fujio, K. (2025). Advances in targeted therapy for systemic lupus erythematosus: Current treatments and novel approaches. *International Journal of Molecular Sciences, 26*. https://www.semanticscholar.org/paper/fc644ff3148f35c77236b9f02f48ee0a803f46ad (accessed on 17th June 2025).
53. Sedighi, S., Aghaei, M., Musavi, S., Nomali, M., et al. (2014). Relationship between serum level of interleukin-2 in patients with systemic lupus erythematosus and disease activity in comparison with control group. https://core.ac.uk/download/52204560.pdf (accessed on 17th June 2025).
54. Velez-Arteaga, M., Carrera-Barriga, G. C., Moreno-Montenegro, K., Gallegos, C., Nicolalde, B. I., Leon, B., & Guijarro, K. (2024). Rhupus syndrome in the pediatric population: A comprehensive systematic literature review. *Medicine, 103*. https://www.semanticscholar.org/paper/31d465208592b6015ed45cca2e5f4b9b262cc15d (accessed on 17th June 2025).
55. Yennemadi, A. S., Keane, J., & Leisching, G. (2023). Mitochondrial bioenergetic changes in systemic lupus erythematosus immune cell subsets: Contributions to pathogenesis and clinical applications. *Lupus, 32*, 603–611. https://www.semanticscholar.org/paper/c9c1cccea10ebf055c3905d08618009d55b85a35 (accessed on 17th June 2025).

SPONDYLOARTHRITIDES

3

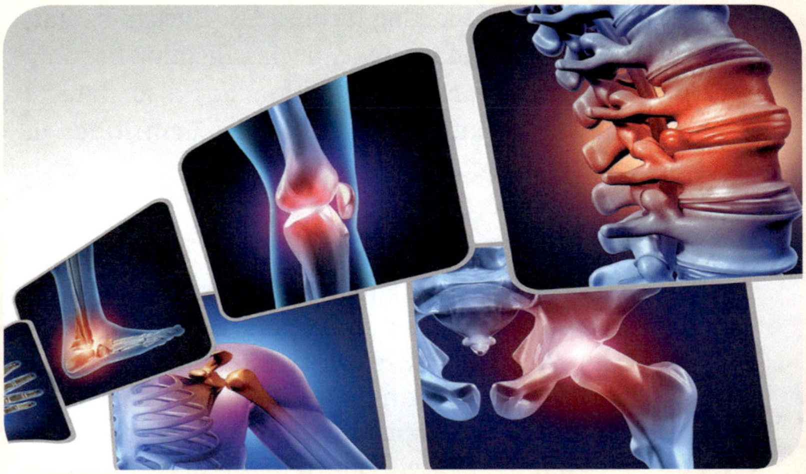

LEARNING OBJECTIVES

After studying this chapter, you will be able to:

1. Identify types of spondyloarthritides.
2. Focus on pathophysiology.
3. Discuss diagnosis.
4. Explain treatment and management.

Introduction

Spondyloarthritides represent a heterogeneous group of inflammatory rheumatic illnesses that share the link with the HLA-B27 antigen and a spectrum of musculoskeletal and extra-musculoskeletal manifestations. Presentation can be extremely variable among subjects, often involving axial symptoms in the form of sacroiliitis and non-radiographic forms and extra-articular symptoms like uveitis and psoriasis. New treatments, particularly the development of biologic drugs against such cytokines as tumor necrosis factor-alpha (TNFα), have significantly altered treatment and encouraged patient outcomes. TNF blockade therapy is a prime example of the remarkable progress made in treating this condition, with strong success in symptom abatement and better quality of life (Barr & Keat, 2010). Further, the management of ocular complications, a characteristic of HLA-B27-related spondyloarthritides, also experienced significant improvement, with biologic drugs proving beneficial in refractory cases

(Gueudry et al., 2017). These intricacies need to be realized to intervene effectively and look after the patient (Figure 3.1).

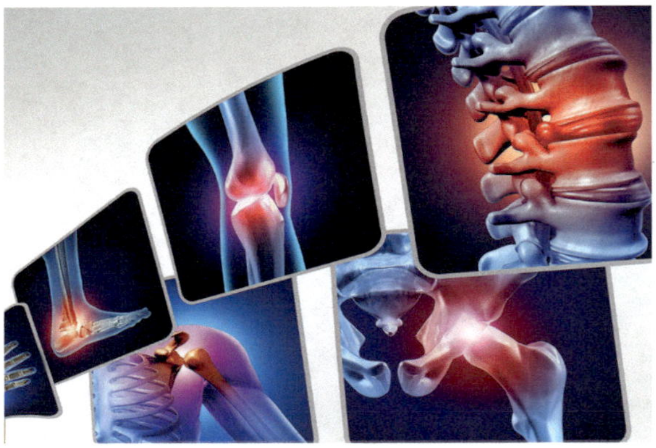

Figure 3.1. Spondyloarthritides.

Source: https://www.the-rheumatologist.org/wp-content/uploads/2022/05/ASPsA-stock-art.png.

3.1. Types of Spondyloarthritides

Learning Outcome

1. Understand ankylosing spondylitis;
2. Explain psoriatic arthritis;
3. Discuss reactive arthritis;
4. Focus on enteropathic arthritis;
5. Define undifferentiated spondyloarthritis;
6. Focus on juvenile spondyloarthritis;
7. Identify non-radiographic axial spondyloarthritis.

Spondyloarthritides are a heterogeneous series of inflammatory rheumatic diseases characterized by overlapping manifestations, including axial and peripheral arthritis, enthesitis, and sometimes extra-articular features. Some such well-established ones among them are ankylosing spondylitis, psoriatic arthritis, reactive arthritis, and juvenile *spondyloarthritis*. In particular, with juvenile *spondyloarthritis*, how intriguing that the disease would manifest differently from adults, with peripheral joint inflammation more frequently than the spine or sacroiliac joints, potentially leading to difficulties in diagnosis and classification (Eshed et al., 2018).

The Spondyloarthritis International Society (ASAS) has established criteria for facilitating early diagnosis of these conditions and instituted the significance of the diagnosis of inflammatory back pain and sacroiliitis through the utilization of advanced imaging techniques (Burgos-Vargas, 2012). Such adaptability in classification not only facilitates early intervention but also detects the complexities of the spondyloarthritides in clinical practice.

3.1.1. Ankylosing Spondylitis

Ankylosing spondylitis (AS) forms a significant component of the spondyloarthritides (SpA), representing a disease of inflammation most commonly affecting the spine and sacroiliac joints. It leads to persistent inflammation, more commonly evolving into pain and stiffness, particularly in the lumbar area, and can ultimately lead to a fusion of the vertebrae, affecting mobility and quality of life.

The diagnosis of AS relies on a combination of imaging studies and clinical examination, through well-documented criteria , such as the modified New York criteria for diagnosis (Glasnović et al., 2011). Recent advances in the pathophysiologic mechanisms of AS, more specifically the role of the HLA-B27 antigen, have been important in enhancing diagnostic and therapeutic potential. Moreover, the development of tumor necrosis factor (TNF) blockers has revolutionized the treatment of patients, which has drastically diminished symptoms and avoided structural damage, thereby highlighting the importance of proper and early diagnosis (Sieper, 2009) (Figure 3.2).

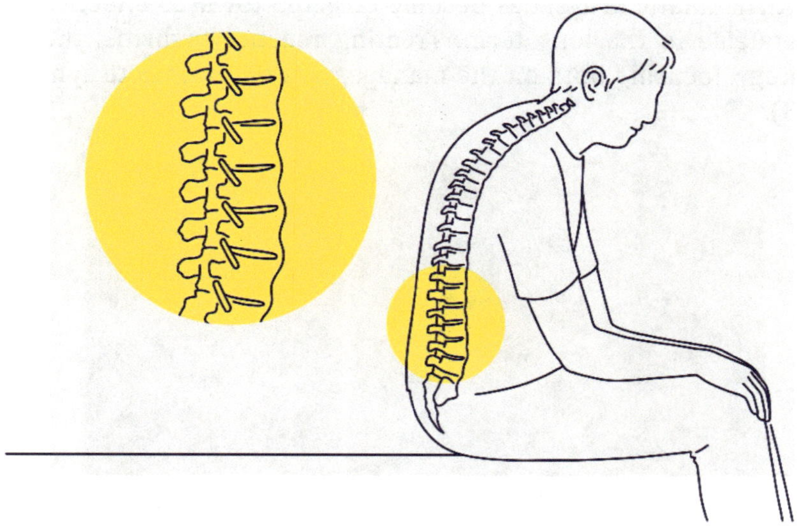

Figure 3.2. Ankylosing spondylitis (AS).

Source: https://www.health.com/thmb/5RBOmqHvlrzPYxKVUhb9aMAQACg=/4000x0/filters:no_upscale():max_bytes(150000):strip_icc()/Health-ankylosing-spondylitis-overview-MiraNorian-7099547-final-e9885ae0972d4d5685e283301ec3f3cc.jpg.

3.1.2. Psoriatic Arthritis

Psoriatic arthritis (PsA) is a heterogeneous form of inflammatory arthritis that commonly occurs in patients with psoriasis, a chronic inflammatory skin disorder. Peripheral joint and axial symptoms characterize PsA, as a subtype of *spondyloarthritis*, and it is clinically challenging to treat. Recent advances in the pathophysiology of PsA, in particular regarding immune mechanisms underlying inflammation and joint destruction, have pinpointed significant progress in therapy. The introduction of biologic agents, anti-tumor necrosis factor (anti-TNF), has transformed PsA treatment, facilitating efficient control of both arthritic and extra-articular presentations, such as uveitis and skin lesions. These have been particularly beneficial in resistant cases, illustrating the need for ongoing studies to further develop therapeutic strategies and optimize long-term results in affected patients (Sieper, 2009; Gueudry et al., 2017).

3.1.3. Reactive Arthritis

Reactive arthritis, a type of *spondyloarthritis*, usually occurs after an infection, most commonly in the genitourinary or intestinal tract. It is defined by a triad of symptoms: arthritis, urethritis, and conjunctivitis, frequently resulting in crippling joint pain that may be confused with other rheumatic diseases. The condition is highly linked with the HLA-B27 antigen, which suggests a genetic predisposition that increases one's susceptibility to inflammatory reactions (Glasnović et al., 2011). Over the past years, enhancements in the understanding of spondyloarthritides have enlightened us on the immune system mechanisms of reactive arthritis, specifically interaction between the immune system and inflammation that initiates joint destruction (Sieper, 2009).

As a result, proactively using medicine, including non-steroidal anti-inflammatory drugs and disease-modifying antirheumatic drugs, has become targeted towards effective relief of symptoms and prevention of sequelae in the long term. Treating reactive arthritis, therefore demands an interdisciplinary strategy, focusing both on the management of immediate symptoms and on long-term care (Figure 3.3).

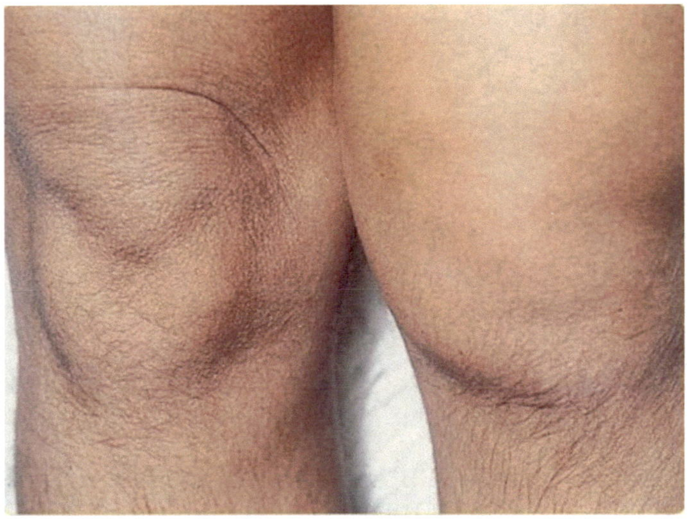

Figure 3.3. Reactive arthritis, a form of *spondyloarthritis*, typically arises following an infection, often in the genitourinary or gastrointestinal tract.

Source: https://upload.wikimedia.org/wikipedia/commons/4/4d/SOA-arthritis.jpg.

3.1.4. Enteropathic Arthritis

Enteropathic arthritis, which is an inflammatory arthritis, occurs most frequently as part of inflammatory bowel diseases (IBD) , such as Crohn's disease and ulcerative colitis. The coincidence highlights the complicated relationship between inflammation elsewhere in the body and gut health, with the demonstration that in some instances, arthritis precedes or coincides with bowel symptoms. Spondyloarthritides manifestations can be present in enteropathic arthritis patients, with peripheral joint inflammation and inflammatory back pain, and leading to severe disability if untreated. Most importantly, it is the pathophysiology underlying that connects IBD intestinal inflammation to the inflammatory mechanisms via genetic and environmental triggers that are comparable. Effective management of enteropathic arthritis can not only enhance musculoskeletal performance but also the quality of life in patients, as therapies targeting intestinal inflammation, such as TNF inhibitors, have been found beneficial not only in enhancing arthritic symptoms but also gastrointestinal symptoms (Elewaut et al., 2009).

3.1.5. Undifferentiated Spondyloarthritis

Undifferentiated *Spondyloarthritis* (uSpA) is an intricate and frequently confusing presentation in the spectrum of the spondyloarthritides, and is defined by inflammatory back pain and a variety of peripheral manifestations that fall short of fulfilling strict criteria for established subtypes. With ongoing research, knowledge regarding uSpA has become ever more critical, including its early recognition and treatment. The development of the Spondyloarthritis International Society (ASAS) classification criteria has made it much easier to identify at-risk patients for ankylosing spondylitis (AS) and other forms of *spondyloarthritis* so that one can intervene early with TNF blockers, which have been shown to improve patient outcomes (Sieper, 2009). In addition, the incorporation of novel concepts , such as inflammatory back pain (IBP) and magnetic resonance imaging for sacroiliitis, has transformed diagnostic processes, further reiterating the necessity for multidimensional approaches to counter the varying presentations of uSpA (Burgos-Vargas, 2012) (Figure 3.4).

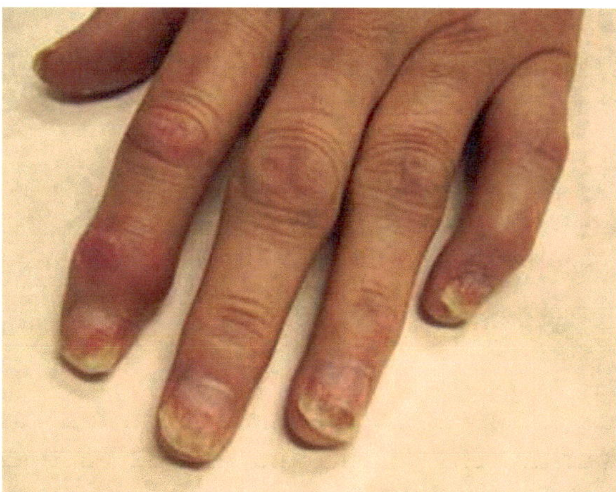

Figure 3.4. Undifferentiated *Spondyloarthritis* (uSpA).

Source: https://media.springernature.com/lw685/springer-static/image/chp%3A10.1007%2F978-3-319-52567-9_150/MediaObjects/339799_1_En_150_Fig1_HTML.jpg.

3.1.6. Juvenile Spondyloarthritis

Juvenile *Spondyloarthritis* (JSpA) is one of the large groups of the spondyloarthritides with a typical childhood onset and particular clinical presentations. It predominantly affects the axial skeleton and may also involve peripheral joints, presenting both diagnostic and therapeutic difficulties. Uveitis is one of the typical complications and is an inflammatory eye disease commonly associated with HLA-B27 positivity. The management of JSpA has changed significantly over the past few years; biologic treatments, especially anti-TNFα drugs, have been found to be the primary treatments of refractory cases, not only managing articular but also extra-articular symptoms , such as uveitis. Such developments highlight the significance of early intervention, since left untreated, symptoms may cause permanent joint destruction and compromised quality of life in affected patients. Therefore, understanding the complexities of JSpA still remains essential to improving patient prognosis through personalized therapeutic measures (; Forte et al., 2010; Gueudry et al., 2017).

3.1.7. Non-Radiographic Axial Spondyloarthritis

The emergence of non-radiographic axial *spondyloarthritis* (nr-axSpA) is a crucial step toward the understanding of spondyloarthritides, particularly in the identification and treatment of early disease. Unlike its radiographic counterpart, nr-axSpA lacks well-defined structural damage on X-rays, hence challenging diagnosis. With the evolution of imaging techniques and clinical assessment, physicians have managed to identify inflammation at an earlier stage, thus precipitating earlier intervention. Educational initiatives , such as those sponsored by the British Society for Rheumatology (BSR), attempt to sensitize and educate clinicians on these conditions with a view to enhancing patient outcomes (Coates et al., 2020).

Notably, there has also been treatment innovation for nr-axSpA, with biologics, specifically anti-TNFα, proving to be effective in symptom control and associated extra-articular manifestations like uveitis, which is prevalent among HLA-B27-positive patients (Gueudry et al., 2017). Thus, the integration of novel treatment modalities is essential in the management of the complexities of non-radiographic axial spondyloarthritis (Figure 3.5).

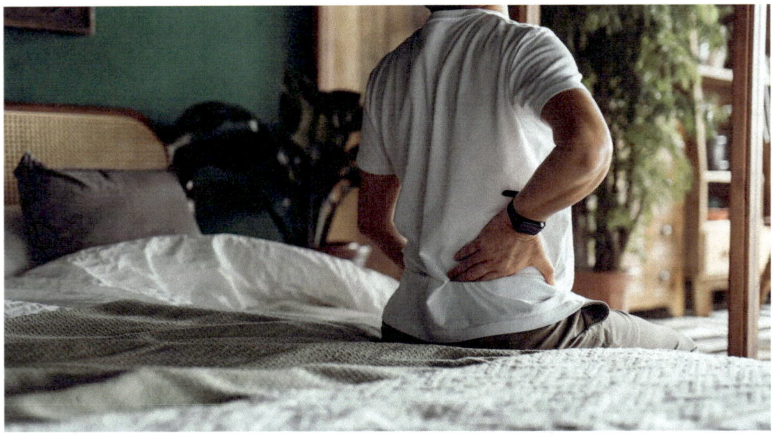

Figure 3.5. Non-radiographic axial *spondyloarthritis.*

Source: https://images.everydayhealth.com/images/arthritis/ankylosing-spondylitis/what-is-nonradiographic-axial-*spondyloarthritis*-1440x810.jpg?sfvrsn=825a92b1_5.

Test Your Knowledge

1. What are the major subtypes of spondyloarthritides?
2. How is ankylosing spondylitis distinguished from non-radiographic axial spondyloarthritis?

3.2. Pathophysiology

Learning Outcome

1. Identify genetic factors and HLA-B27;
2. Discuss immune system involvement;
3. Understand inflammatory processes;
4. Discuss the role of cytokines;
5. Focus on bone remodeling and erosion;
6. Learn extra-articular manifestations;
7. Identify environmental triggers;
8. Know the interaction between genetics and environment;
9. Describe current research on pathophysiology.

The pathophysiologic process of the spondyloarthritides (SpA) is complex, with complex immune mechanisms involved in inflammation and structural disease. The presence of haematopoietic cells, in this case dendritic cells bearing the HLA-B27 antigen, with abnormal misfolding capacities that set off an inflammatory cascade, is one of the main features of SpA. Such misfolding may extend to T helper 17 cell function, which are the cells implicated in mediating inflammation in other autoimmune conditions. Furthermore, stromal cells have become critical components in the sustenance of inflammatory reactions in joints. The occurrence of cytokines, particularly TNF-alpha, further substantiates the immunopathogenesis of the disease by its widespread contribution to conditions like Crohn's disease and SpA (Churg et al., 2015). These cell-cell interactions and cytokine patterns are a necessity to understand to make way for therapeutic interventions to avoid the disabling effect of spondyloarthritides (Elewaut et al., 2009).

3.2.1. Genetic Factors and HLA-B27

Knowledge of the genetic aspect, i.e., the role of the HLA-B27 antigen, is crucial in understanding the pathophysiology of spondyloarthritides (SpA). HLA-B27 is strongly associated with the development of ankylosing spondylitis, a predominant subtype of SpA.

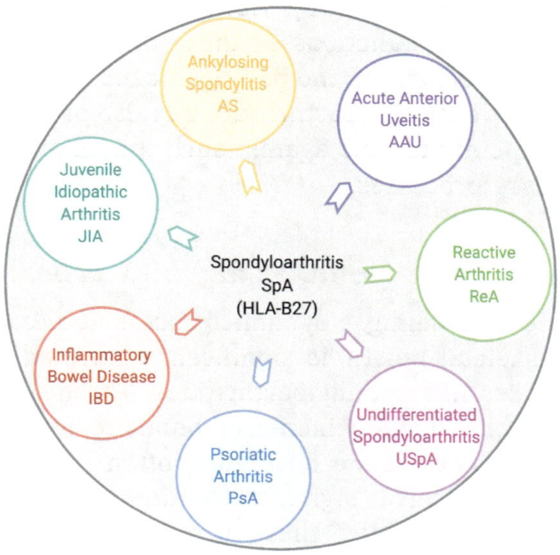

Figure 3.6. An understanding of genetic factors, particularly the role of the HLA-B27 antigen, is crucial for elucidating the pathophysiology of spondyloarthritides (SpA).

Source: https://www.frontiersin.org/files/Articles/586494/fimmu-11-586494-HTML-r1/image_m/fimmu-11-586494-g001.jpg.

Research highlights that HLA-B27 can influence immune system interactions, with findings indicating that dendritic cell disruption and T helper 17 cell function are associated with the misfolding nature to cause inflammation (Elewaut et al., 2009). Furthermore, newer genetic studies have identified additional associations besides HLA-B27, such as interleukin-23 receptor polymorphisms, suggesting a complex pattern of interaction between multiple genetic determinants of susceptibility and disease progression (Sieper, 2009). Thus, these conditions give hints towards potential therapeutic targets, and thorough research into the genetic etiology of such inflammatory disorders must be undertaken (Figure 3.6).

3.2.2. Immune System Involvement

The immune system plays a central role in the pathogenesis of spondyloarthritides, particularly with reference to interaction with bone metabolism and inflammation. New advances in understanding these diseases have highlighted the contribution of immune processes, particularly tumor necrosis factor blockers, that significantly improve the prognosis for patients by minimizing inflammation and structural damage (Sieper, 2009). Also, genetic studies have been successful in detecting associations with some immune-related genes, such as HLA-B27, interleukin-23 receptor, and ARTS1, which emphasize the genetic components of these diseases and their immunological basis (Sieper, 2009). Clinical findings corroborate these findings, showing that recurrent symptoms , such as inflammatory back pain, sacroiliitis, and enthesitis correlate highly with immune dysregulation in patients, thereby emphasizing the need to understand the immune system's role in developing useful diagnostic and therapeutic approaches for spondyloarthritides.

3.2.3. Inflammatory Processes

Inflammatory pathways are key to the pathophysiology of spondyloarthritides, characterized by severe inflammation of the joints with resulting acute and chronic structural damage. The chief issue with these diseases is how inflammatory mediators engage with and produce joint remodeling, something that is most evident in spondyloarthritides. It has been shown by research that joint destruction, though common, co-exists with extensive instances of new bone formation and enthesopathy, resulting in ankylosis and reduced mobility (Lories et al., 2007). Furthermore, spondyloarthritides have overlapping clinical presentations with conditions , such as Behcet's disease, which is also typified by recurrent inflammatory attacks and high pro-inflammatory cytokines , such as IL-1 and TNF-alpha that are implicated in the causation of the disease (Allenspach et al., 2020). This intricate play of inflammatory mechanisms underscores the complexity and heterogeneity in spondyloarthritides and the necessity of a differentiated understanding to facilitate effective management and treatment (Figure 3.7).

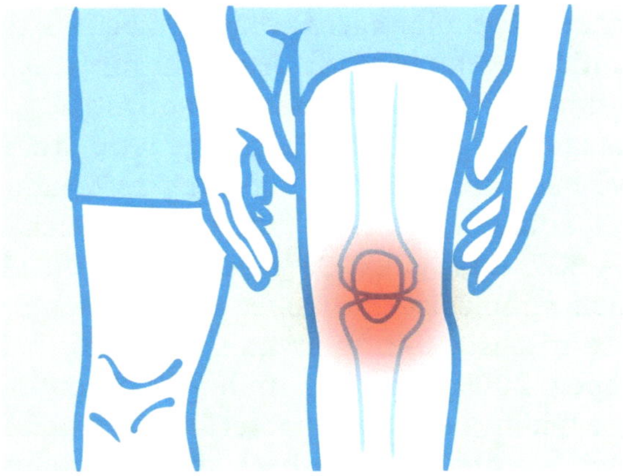

Figure 3.7. Inflammatory processes play a crucial role in the pathophysiology of spondyloarthritides, characterized by significant joint inflammation that leads to both acute symptoms and chronic structural changes.

Source: https://onsen.eu/en/photos/news/spondyloartropatia-kopia.webp.

3.2.4. Role of Cytokines

Cytokines are also pivotal in the pathogenesis of spondyloarthritides (SpA), influencing both the inflammatory disease process and the consequent clinical manifestations. Of the many hundreds of cytokines that have been implicated, TNF-alpha is one of the crucial pro-inflammatory mediators that have been involved in the different forms of SpA, including psoriatic arthritis. Case-control studies also highlighted the deep association of TNF-alpha gene polymorphisms with disease susceptibility, which pointed toward a genetic predisposition in the context of cytokine function (Baraliakos et al., 2011). Other cytokines, particularly interleukin-23, are also involved in the immunopathogenesis of SpA, which was identified as pivotal in T helper 17 cell activation and consequent inflammation (Elewaut et al., 2009). Hence, understanding the intricate functions of these cytokines not only sheds light on the pathogenic mechanisms that drive spondyloarthritides but also provides therapeutic targets against such inflammatory disease processes.

3.2.5. Bone Remodeling and Erosion

Bone remodeling, a dynamic process necessary for skeletal health, is significantly affected by diseases like spondyloarthritides. The disease is characterized by increased bone erosion and aberrant new bone formation, often resulting in ankylosis. It is significant to understand the interplay between these processes because osteoclast activation by inflammation results in bone resorption and mediators like bone morphogenetic proteins and WNTs can promote abnormal osteogenesis. Notably, studies have demonstrated that conventional anti-inflammatory therapy may not be sufficient to stop disease progression toward ankylosis, suggesting a multidimensional connection between inflammation and the processes of bone remodeling (de Vlam et al., 2009). Moreover, in juvenile *spondyloarthritis*, the initial inflammatory reaction is likely to affect peripheral joints prior to the involvement of central structures like the sacroiliac joints, rendering early diagnosis and treatment approaches problematic (Eshed et al., 2018). This underlines the necessity of the use of individually tailored therapeutic methods to cure both bone erosion and bone remodeling in spondyloarthritides (Figure 3.8).

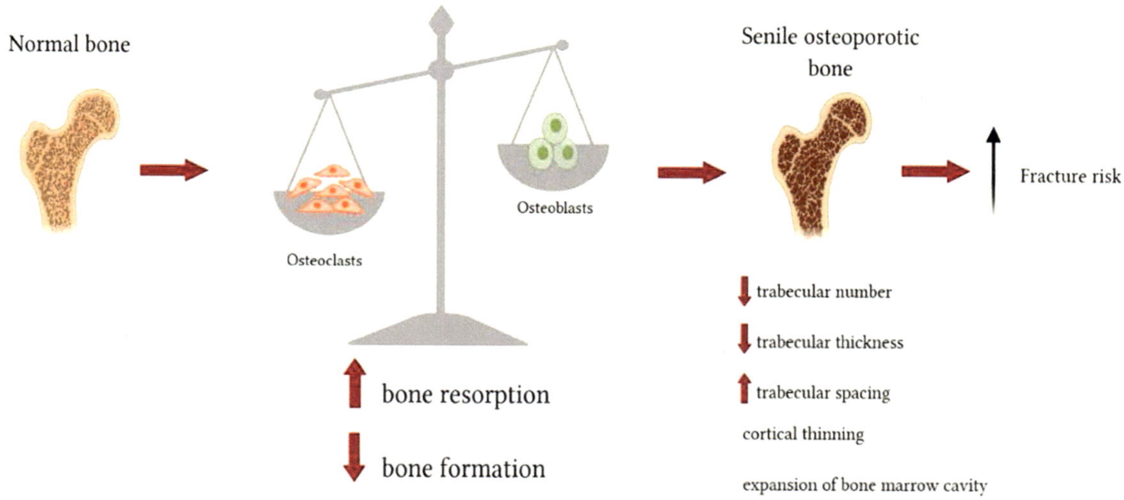

Figure 3.8. Bone remodeling, a dynamic process crucial for maintaining skeletal integrity, is significantly altered in conditions like spondyloarthritides.

Source: https://pub.mdpi-res.com/ijms/ijms-21-03679/article_deploy/html/images/ijms-21-03679-g001.png?1591380300

3.2.6. Extra-Articular Manifestations

Spondyloarthritides' extra-articular manifestations, particularly those of HLA-B27, play an important role in the quality of life of patients and underscore the heterogeneity of the disease. Uveitis, IBD, and psoriasis are frequent extra-articular manifestations of axial *spondyloarthritis* and need careful management due to the higher morbidity of the patients. Of these, uveitis is the most common presentation, which creates clinical challenges with its potential to lead to vision impairment and necessitate emergent treatment with local corticosteroids and cycloplegic agents. Refractory cases, however, may require biologic agents, particularly anti-TNFα therapy, which has proved useful in diminishing repeat uveitis attacks (Gueudry et al., 2017). Other than ocular involvement, anti-TNF therapies also exhibited differential responsiveness in the treatment of skin lesions and gastrointestinal manifestations, stressing the importance of developing individualized treatment regimens based on extra-articular burden of disease (Elewaut et al., 2009). This will be key to optimizing the patient's well-being as well as adequately addressing complications.

3.2.7. Environmental Triggers

The environmental trigger role in spondyloarthritides (SpA) pathogenesis is increasingly known to be crucial to account for the onset and triggering of disease. Numerous factors, including infections, physical trauma, and lifestyle aspects, have been proposed to induce inflammatory responses in the context of SpA. For instance, microbial infections are thought to initiate responses in genetically predisposed individuals with emphasis on the interplay between environmental stimuli and host genetics, with particular focus on the HLA-B27 allele. Interestingly, even though SpA exhibits multiple clinical manifestations, these environmental influences affect disease presentation and response to therapy so that SpA is less sensitive to traditional therapies than many other rheumatic diseases , such as rheumatoid arthritis. Besides, recent studies have also identified overlapping genetic risk variants of other inflammatory disorders, such as Behcet's disease, to enhance the diversity of environmental stimuli in the overall framework of autoinflammatory disorders (Bose et al., 2018; Allenspach et al., 2020) (Figure 3.9).

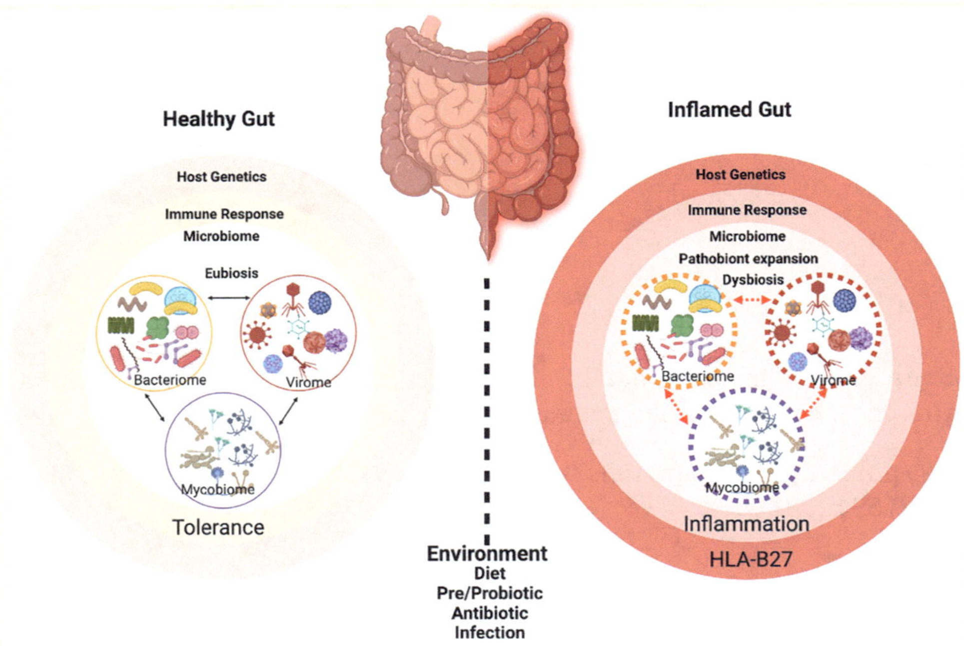

Figure 3.9. Microbial infections are thought to provoke reactions in genetically predisposed individuals, highlighting the interaction between environmental agents and host genetics, particularly concerning the HLA-B27 allele.

Source: https://www.frontiersin.org/files/Articles/586494/fimmu-11-586494-HTML-r1/image_m/fimmu-11-586494-g002.jpg.

3.2.8. Interaction Between Genetics and Environment

The interaction between environmental influences and predisposing genes plays a pivotal role in the establishment and progression of spondyloarthritides (SpA). Genetic determinants, particularly the HLA-B27 allele, have been strongly associated with SpA, which represents an inherited component that predisposes to these inflammatory diseases (Bose et al., 2018). However, individuals who bear this genetic predisposition do not always manifest the disease, proving the significance of environmental elements , such as infections, mechanical pressure, and lifestyle (Andersen et al., 2017). Diet and lifestyle habits, for instance, can precipitate or aggravate chronic inflammatory diseases , such as SpA, which can, in turn, affect reactions to biologics against pro-inflammatory agents (Andersen et al., 2017). This interaction suggests that while genetics provides the initial risk assessment, environmental influences ultimately determine the clinical presentation and response to treatment, and thus a diverse strategy is required for the understanding and management of spondyloarthritides (Figure 3.10).

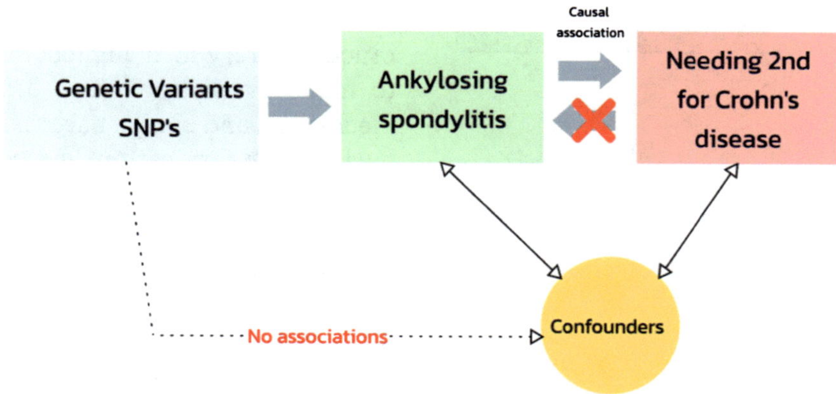

Figure 3.10. A summarized illustration of the Mendelian randomization causal association assessment between Ankylosing Spondylitis (exposure) and the need for a second-line therapy in Crohn's disease (outcome).

Source: https://www.mdpi.com/jcm/jcm-13-07496/article_deploy/html/images/jcm-13-07496-g001-550.jpg.

3.2.9. Current Research on Pathophysiology

Modern developments in the understanding of spondyloarthritides have always highlighted the central role played by genetic factors and inflammatory processes in their pathogenesis. Of particular note, research has determined that TNF-alpha is a significant pro-inflammatory cytokine with which involvement in the aetiopathogenesis of conditions like psoriatic arthritis has been established, with evidence that polymorphisms of some TNF-alpha genes are involved in susceptibility to these conditions in populations like Romanian patients (Baraliakos et al., 2011). Also, a recent study using administrative health care data indicates that various case definitions of rheumatoid arthritis capture varying degrees of accuracy compared to rheumatologist diagnoses, suggesting an interplay of gene, clinical, and diagnostic factors possibly influencing the identification of inflammatory arthritis cases (Hanly et al., 2015). This suggests that there is a need for ongoing research to further elucidate these disorders and maximize patient outcomes.

Test Your Knowledge

1. How do mechanical stress and biomechanical factors contribute to disease progression?
2. How does chronic inflammation lead to new bone formation and ankylosis?

3.3. Diagnosis

Learning Outcome

1. Understand clinical evaluation and history;
2. Explain physical examination techniques;
3. Focus on imaging studies;
4. Discuss laboratory tests ;
5. Learn differential diagnosis;
6. Describe the role of rheumatologists;
7. Understand diagnostic criteria;
8. Identify challenges in diagnosis;
9. Know the importance of early diagnosis.

The diagnosis of spondyloarthritides (SpA) is a multifaceted exercise that entails meticulous consideration of clinical presentation, patient history, and some diagnostic criteria. At the center of this exercise is the identification of sentinel symptoms , such as inflammatory back pain, peripheral arthritis, and enthesitis, which prompts clinicians to classify SpA correctly (Glasnović et al., 2011). ASAS (Assessment in AS Working Group) classification criteria play a vital role in the diagnosis of various forms of SpA, such as ankylosing spondylitis (AS) and psoriatic arthritis (PsA). Of special interest here are the modified New York criteria for AS and the CASPAR criteria for PsA, providing structured methods of diagnosis that are often supplemented with radiologic techniques to determine sacroiliitis (Glasnović et al., 2011). Conversely, research that is coming out suggests that conditions like Behcet Disease may be similar to SpA but with relatively lower sacroiliitis in patients with such diseases and thus influencing diagnostic practice.

3.3.1. Clinical Evaluation and History

Thorough clinical evaluation and full patient history are central in the diagnosis of spondyloarthritides in that they facilitate the differentiation of various forms of back pain. Back pain of the lower back is extremely prevalent in patients reporting to general practitioners, which, in most instances, is bound to make evaluation more difficult due to its mechanical and benign nature. But inflammatory back pain identification, less common but more harmful, is crucial for correct management strategies (Moosajee & Kalla, 2016). Disease activity and functional impairment assessment provide background, especially in diseases like nonpsoriatic peripheral spondyloarthritis, where classification criterion fulfillment is necessary to establish a diagnosis. Current studies have proven the efficacy of adalimumab and other treatments, with special focus on highlighting the importance of initial clinical evaluation leading to better outcomes in care for patients with poor response to conventional treatments (Karunaratne et al., 2015). Clinical evaluation thus serves not only to provide diagnostic data but also to guide therapeutic interventions in spondyloarthritides management (Figure 3.11).

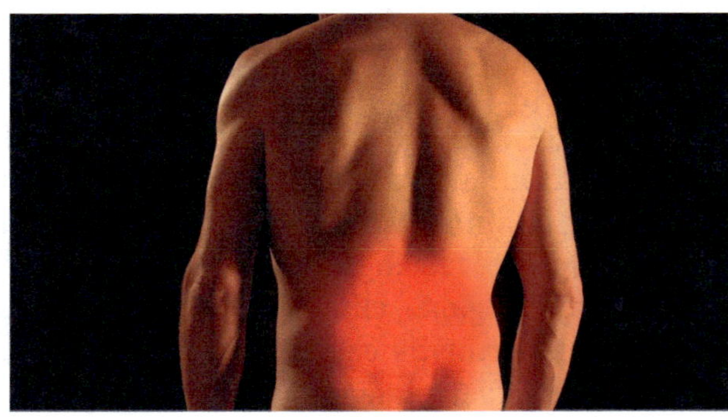

Figure 3.11. Lower back pain is particularly prevalent among patients consulting general practitioners, often complicating the assessment due to its benign and mechanical nature in many cases.

Source: https://alignmotionphysio.com.au/uploads/services/lower-back-pain-guide-image-1.jpg.

3.3.2. Physical Examination Techniques

Accurate diagnosis of spondyloarthritides to a

great extent depends upon the employment of meticulous physical examination techniques that enable clinicians to identify important clinical findings. Traditionally, examination of such conditions, particularly axial *spondyloarthritis*, begins with an appropriate history taking, and is preceded by a systematic physical examination emphasizing measurement of spinal mobility and inflammatory pain. New findings, including refined definitions of inflammatory back pain (IBP) and employment of imaging modalities , such as magnetic resonance imaging, further enhanced the possibility of detecting early features of the disease (Burgos-Vargas, 2012). Furthermore, continuous continuing professional development courses, such as the British Society for Rheumatology, highlight the need to remind healthcare providers of examination skills and diagnostic innovation (Coates et al., 2020). Continuous education focuses on having to master physical examination skills in order to increase the accuracy of diagnostics in various patient populations, particularly children.

3.3.3. Imaging Studies (X-Rays, MRI)

Whereas imaging tests , such as X-rays and magnetic resonance imaging (MRI) in the diagnosis and treatment of spondyloarthritides (SpA) are crucial to offer greater insight into the disease course and enable early intervention. X-rays traditionally are employed to assess structural deformities of the spine and sacroiliac joints, which offer a two-dimensional representation of usual changes observed with spinal fusion and inflammation. But MRIs have come to be a crucial tool in the early diagnosis, particularly in the diagnosis of sacroiliitis, which is long before radiographic changes are evident. Early diagnosis is crucial because evidence indicates that early recognition significantly improves the response to therapy with TNF-alpha blockers (Burgos-Vargas, 2012). Furthermore, technological progress in imaging has helped to elaborate in greater depth the immunological process of bone destruction and new bone formation, thereby informing the most effective treatments (Sieper, 2009). Such imaging modalities are therefore at the heart of the world management and assessment of SpA (Figure 3.12).

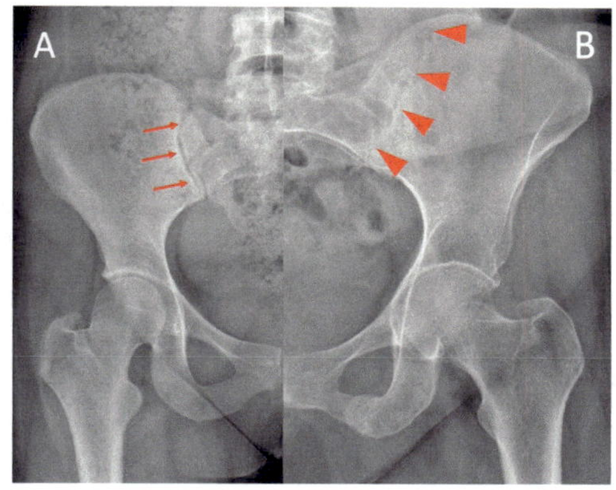

Figure 3.12. X-rays are traditionally utilized to assess structural changes in the spine and sacroiliac joints, offering a visual representation of characteristic alterations associated with spinal fusion and inflammation.

Source: https://www.mdpi.com/medicina/medicina-61-00039/article_deploy/html/images/medicina-61-00039-g001.png.

3.3.4. Laboratory Tests (Blood Tests, Markers)

Laboratory studies, such as some of the blood work and biomarkers, are critical to the diagnosis and management of spondyloarthritides, a group of rheumatic inflammatory disorders. The laboratory studies can identify whether inflammatory markers, such as C-reactive protein and erythrocyte sedimentation rate, are present, which are indicators of systemic inflammation and will guide treatment. Genetic tests for the HLA-B27 antigen are also critical in the diagnosis of some of the spondyloarthritides, particularly ankylosing spondylitis. Recent advances in biobanking, such as the Rheumatology BioBank (RheumaBank), provide valuable tools for pairing genetic and biological samples with clinical data, thereby generating a greater understanding of disease mechanisms and responsiveness to therapy (Assirelli et al., 2023). Furthermore, studies have suggested that marrying lifestyle variables with molecular profiles may be applied to tailor treatment regimens to most benefit patients undergoing TNF inhibitor therapy (Andersen et al., 2017), thereby contributing towards developing a more integrated approach towards the management of such multifactorial illnesses.

3.3.5. Differential Diagnosis

Differential diagnosis between the spondyloarthritides is a complex issue due to the heterogeneity of these inflammatory conditions. Accurate labeling of the *spondyloarthritis* subtype is crucial for optimal treatment and intervention. Standard clinical procedures may not be sufficient because, at an early stage, these share overlapping symptoms with conditions like rheumatoid arthritis and psoriatic arthritis. Therefore, sophisticated imaging methods, especially magnetic resonance imaging (MRI), are more and more used to distinguish faint inflammatory and erosive changes that can be missed with conventional methods.

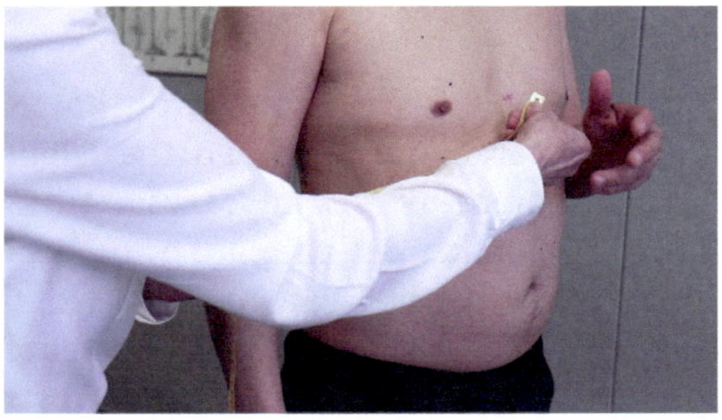

Figure 3.13. Accurate identification of the subtype of *spondyloarthritis* is crucial for effective management and intervention.

Source: https://i.ytimg.com/vi/721_1vxzrb0/maxresdefault.jpg.

High sensitivity of MRI increases the clinician's ability to make well-informed decisions, especially when standard clinical assessments are unrevealing (Duer et al., 2005). Continuing education in medicine is vital in equipping medical practitioners with newer diagnostic tools and techniques, including initiatives by professional organizations like the British Society for Rheumatology (Coates et al., 2020). Continuous learning raises detailed comprehension, which ultimately improves patient outcomes in this diverse disease background (Figure 3.13).

3.3.6. Role of Rheumatologists

Rheumatologists are important in the diagnosis and treatment of spondyloarthritides, some of which are axial *spondyloarthritis* (axSpA) and psoriatic arthritis (PsA). These specialists are important in recognizing the clinical nuances between characteristics common to these conditions, especially because treatment strategies for axial PsA will largely emulate those established in axSpA due to insufficient in-depth studies targeting the former (Bernatschek et al., 2023). Aside from that, rheumatologists apply constantly evolving diagnostic criteria, such as those by the *Spondyloarthritis* International Society (ASAS), to ensure maximum early detection and treatment outcomes of conditions like ankylosing spondylitis, ultimately improving the outcome for patients (Burgos-Vargas, 2012). Rheumatologists treat patients on an individualized basis by solving the complicated nature of spondyloarthritides through their expertise while promoting ongoing research endeavors towards optimizing treatment protocols.

3.3.7. Diagnostic Criteria

The diagnostic criteria for the spondyloarthritides (SpA) have also altered significantly in the last decade, reflecting both clinical developments and scientific breakthroughs. Criteria are valuable for facilitating early diagnosis and efficient management, as certain subtypes, like axial and peripheral SpA, require specialized management approaches. The development of detailed classification criteria has been instrumental in recognizing affected patients, to intervene at an early stage, capable of maximizing outcomes. Current research highlights the central role of inflammatory mediators, such as TNF-alpha, in SpA pathogenesis and thus supports the centrality of genetic determinants in diagnosis and drug responsiveness (Baraliakos et al., 2011). Furthermore, the efficacy of TNF blockers in altering disease course supports the importance of precise diagnostic criteria to guide therapy (Sieper, 2009). Hence, finessing the criteria of diagnosis is not only significant for classification purposes but also for maximizing the treatment approaches to offset structural damage (Figure 3.14).

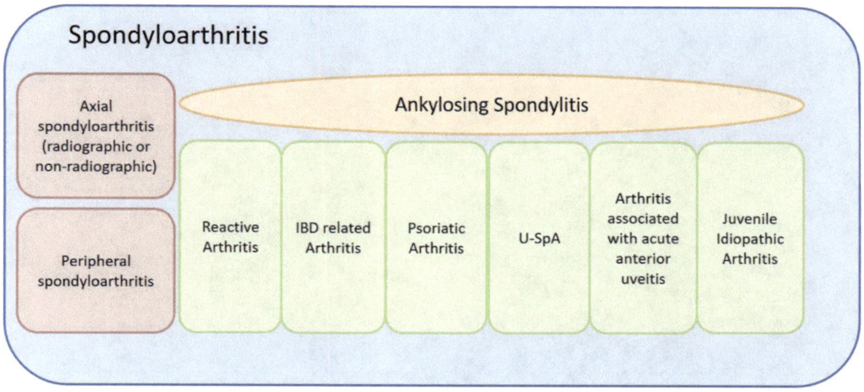

Figure 3.14. The diagnostic criteria for spondyloarthritides (SpA) have evolved significantly in recent years, reflecting advancements in both clinical practice and scientific understanding.

Source: https://www.rheumatic.theclinics.com/cms/10.1016/j.rdc.2020.01.008/asset/4284a47b-4371-4775-a20b-c936297b6f0c/main.assets/gr1_lrg.jpg.

3.3.8. Challenges in Diagnosis

Diagnosis of spondyloarthritides is extremely difficult and relies on overlapping symptomatology and varying presentations of the disease. For instance, juvenile spondyloarthritis tends to begin with peripheral joint inflammation, which may confuse doctors into mixing it with other types of juvenile idiopathic arthritis, thus making the identification process more difficult (Eshed et al., 2018). Similarly, in adult axial spondyloarthritis, there are considerable diagnostic delays of several years (even many years), thus impacting both work productivity and health-related quality of life (Smith, 2020). Furthermore, utilization of standard imaging methods, such as sacroiliac joint radiographs, has potential false negatives with early inflammatory changes, thus further delaying effective treatment. These diagnostic challenges underscore the importance of increased awareness and the application of advanced imaging modalities, such as magnetic resonance imaging, to permit early and accurate diagnosis in both the pediatric and adult patient populations suffering from these disabling conditions.

3.3.9. Importance of Early Diagnosis

Early diagnosis of spondyloarthritides is too important to be overvalued because early detection of these conditions influences the overall management and outcome of the patients afflicted with them. Early management allows one to implement special treatments that can halt the advancement of the disease and improve the quality of life. For instance, a study involving HLA-B27 positive patients identified that the detection of the most important clinical features , such as inflammatory back pain and sacroiliitis, is critical in diagnosing spondyloarthritis appropriately (Glasnović et al., 2011). Moreover, heterogeneity in the diagnosis of rheumatoid arthritis cases proves the necessity to develop proper diagnostic criteria with a need for stringent assessment in clinics (Hanly et al., 2015). Delayed diagnosis poses the risk of permanent joint damage and consequent loss of functional ability. It is, hence, important that awareness and skill in the diagnosis of healthcare professionals are enhanced so that the delivery of early treatment and successful outcomes in spondyloarthritides patients can be guaranteed (Figure 3.15).

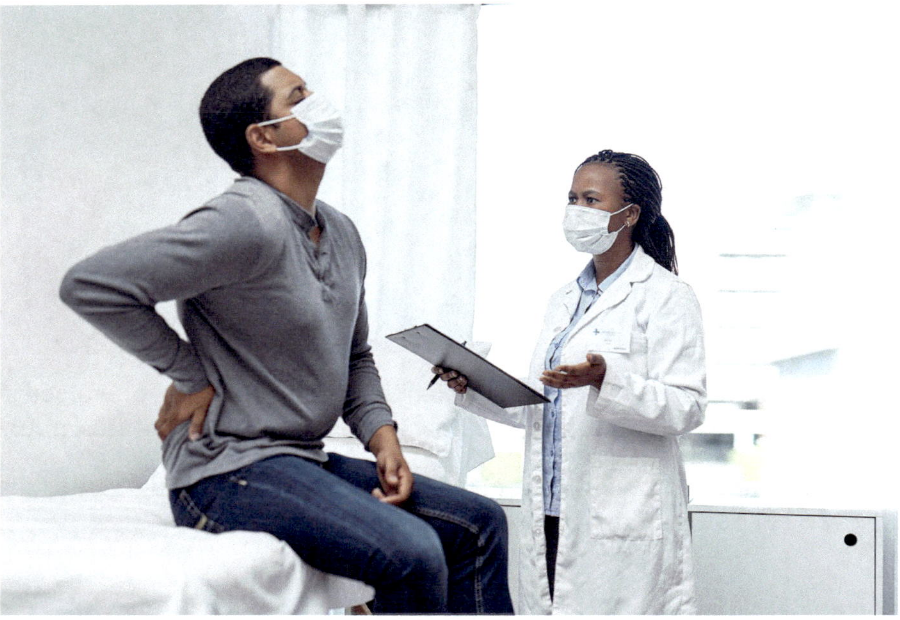

Figure 3.15. The importance of early diagnosis in spondyloarthritides cannot be overstated, as timely identification of these conditions significantly influences the overall management and prognosis of affected patients.

Source: https://www.verywellhealth.com/thmb/H9Pn2RadzlSbOvyLzejv4P9B6OM=/1500x0/filters:no_upscale():max_bytes(150000):strip_icc()/GettyImages-1301555105-6ec1649a53ef4a598b831312d59a4e9a.jpg.

Test Your Knowledge

1. When is MRI preferred over X-ray in evaluating SPA?
2. How is sacroiliitis identified and graded on imaging?

3.4. Treatment and Management

Learning Outcome

1. Understand pharmacological treatments;
2. Explain biologic therapies;
3. Focus on physical therapy and exercise;
4. Discuss lifestyle modifications;
5. Describe surgical options;
6. Know pain management strategies;
7. Discuss the role of patient education;
8. Explain the multidisciplinary approach;
9. know future directions in treatment.

Treatment and management of the spondyloarthritides (SpA) has been transformed, most significantly by therapeutic innovations , such as TNF blockers that dramatically improve patient outcomes. These medications represent a quantum leap, providing options not previously available to patients with this disease. Evidence has been demonstrated that relates the efficacy of TNF blockers to the quality of the underlying immune response and extrarheumatic manifestations, including uveitis and psoriasis, which are crucial considerations in the management (Sieper, 2009). However, management of the spondyloarthritides is not limited to pharmacologic management; management of the low back pain, a ubiquitous symptom and common cause of doctor visits, is a sine qua non to patient quality of life (Moosajee & Kalla, 2016).

Furthermore, a comprehensive treatment plan should also take into account long-term safety and efficacy, with a multidisciplinary treatment strategy to optimize the treatment for this complicated group of disorders.

3.4.1. Pharmacological Treatments (NSAIDs, DMARDs)

The management of spondyloarthritides, particularly ankylosing spondylitis (AS), in the majority of cases involves pharmacologic treatment with nonsteroidal anti-inflammatory drugs (NSAIDs) and disease-modifying antirheumatic drugs (DMARDs). NSAIDs are generally most frequently prescribed as a first line of treatment due to their effectiveness in reducing pain and inflammation, enhancing patients' quality of life. Although DMARDs are employed to modify disease development, they often act with partial success when employed alone for managing the symptoms of AS (Pant et al., 2023).

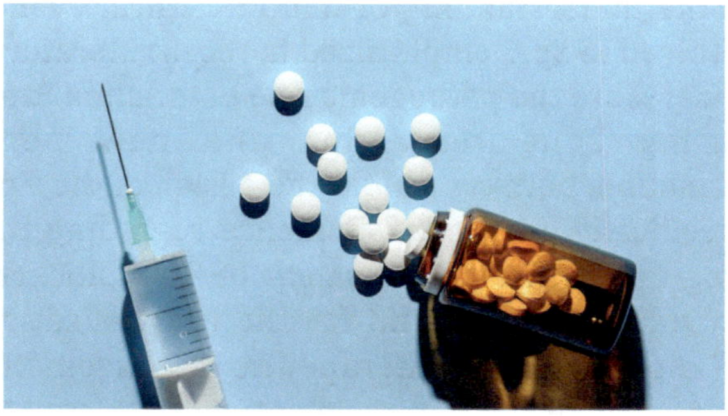

Figure 3.16. The management of spondyloarthritides, particularly ankylosing spondylitis (AS), often involves pharmacological treatments , such as nonsteroidal anti-inflammatory drugs (NSAIDs) and disease-modifying antirheumatic drugs (DMARDs).

Source: https://images.everydayhealth.com/images/arthritis/ankylosing-spondylitis/cs-what-you-need-to-know-about-dmards-for-ankylosing-spondylitis-alt-1440x810.jpg.

A multidisciplinary treatment plan , including physical therapy and the pharmacological drugs has therefore been shown to dramatically improve patient outcomes. Furthermore, where conventional therapy is not yielding adequate response, the presence of biologics, including TNF inhibitors, can be truly valuable with their capacity to engage important inflammatory pathways (Cauli et al., 2008). This entire regimen of treatment is testimony to the benefits of personalized treatment of such long-term illnesses as spondyloarthritides (Figure 3.16).

3.4.2. Biologic Therapies

Biologic agents have revolutionized the treatment of spondyloarthritides (SpA) by specifically addressing individual components of the immune response that contribute to the development of disease. These therapies, particularly TNF blockers, have been highly effective in controlling disease activity and symptoms of SpA, alleviating suffering in those patients who previously had few treatment options. Advances in the understanding of immunological events involved in SpA, emphasized in recent literature, underscore the pathogenic role of inflammation during bone resorption and new bone formation, both critical for the design of therapy specifically addressed. Evidence regarding the long-term efficacy and safety of TNF blockers provides a background for the rationalization of individualized therapeutic management. Moreover, recent genetic discoveries related to ankylosing spondylitis, e.g., with HLA-B27 and novel inflammatory markers—can potentially lay the groundwork for future biologic treatment breakthroughs (Sieper, 2009; Aaltonen et al., 2018).

3.4.3. Physical Therapy and Exercise

Physical therapy and physical exercise are both crucial in the treatment of spondyloarthritides (SpA), providing patients with useful aids in terms of maintaining mobility while minimizing pain. Regular physical exercise is not only vital to enhance flexibility and strength but also general cardiovascular health, which is particularly pertinent considering the cardiovascular complications of pharmacologic treatment for SpA (Corea et al., 2025). Research has indicated that tailored exercise programs are capable of reducing stiffness and enhancing functional capacity, which can result in enhanced quality of life among SpA patients (Sieper, 2009). Furthermore, integration of physical therapy into treatment allows for customized adaptation based on patient-specific symptoms and disease course. Thus, through the promotion of an active life and by making the rehabilitation process easier, exercise and physical therapy become essential components in the overall therapy of spondyloarthritides, complementing pharmacological treatment and addressing the multifaceted problems of this chronic disease (Figure 3.17).

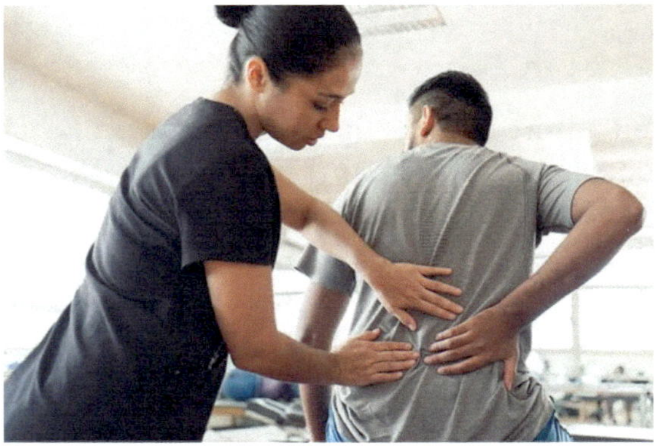

Figure 3.17. Physical therapy and exercise play crucial roles in the management of spondyloarthritides (SpA), providing patients with effective strategies for maintaining mobility and alleviating pain.

Source: https://images.everydayhealth.com/images/arthritis/ankylosing-spondylitis/cs-tips-from-physical-therapists-on-how-to-manage-as-722x406.jpg?sfvrsn=69ecf9a6_1.

3.4.4. Lifestyle Modifications

Within the management of spondyloarthritides, lifestyle modification becomes a necessary component of the process to further enhance outcomes for patients and avoid disease worsening. Exercise, even that which is prescribed on an individual basis, has been shown to enhance functional mobility along with pain reductions, in line with other evidence confirming the role of exercise therapy in the context of juvenile idiopathic arthritis (Kern, 2019). Study participants tend to explain needing to alter their exercise routine due to their shifting disease states as a sign of a proactive self-management style (Porter, 2025). Lifestyle alterations also encompass dietary modifications, stress coping behaviors, and smoking cessation, all of which contribute to overall health and may further boost immune function. Therefore, as these patients become actively engaged in such overall modifications, they can display not only physical gratifications but psychological advantages too, which underscores the requirement for a multi-dimensional treatment process and continuous management of spondyloarthritides.

3.4.5. Surgical Options

In the management of spondyloarthritides, surgical treatment is typically reserved when conservative therapy has not alleviated symptoms or improved quality of life. Surgery in such instances may involve interventions , such as decompression or spinal fusion to address extreme structural deformity or disabling pain that occurs with arthritis and inflammation. It is crucial to differentiate between the basic etiology of the symptoms because some patients would complain of inflammatory manifestations that can lead to progressive impairment if left untreated. Secondly, the complexity of spondyloarthritides necessitates multi-disciplinary management to optimize results, particularly for those who have significant functional impairment. While surgical procedures can bring great relief to non-responsive patients compared to traditional therapies, indications must be carefully assessed because surgery has risks that can impact general health and exacerbate existing conditions (Forss, 2022) (Figure 3.18).

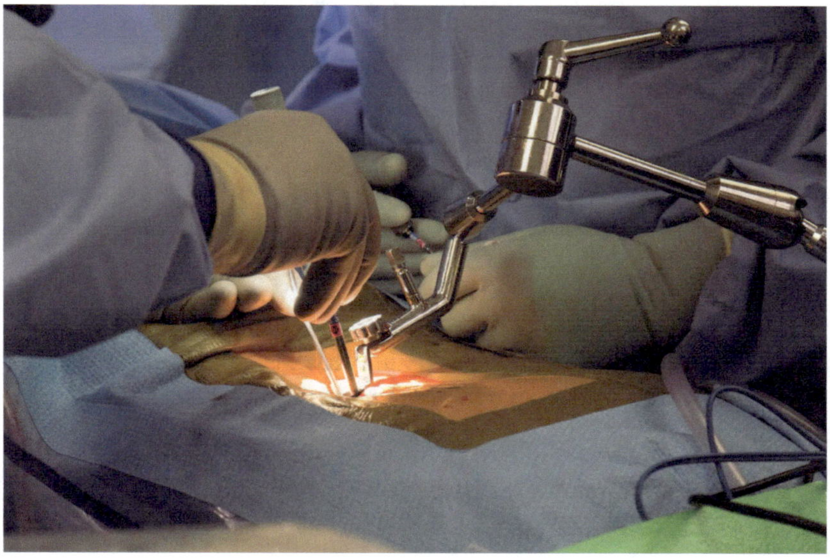

Figure 3.18. Surgical interventions may involve procedures , such as spinal fusion or decompression, aimed at addressing severe structural deformities or debilitating pain linked to inflammation and arthritis.

Source: https://pharmaceutical-journal.com/wp-content/uploads/2021/01/spine-surgery-15-scaled.jpg.

3.4.6. Pain Management Strategies

Effective pain treatment of spondyloarthritides (SpA) is crucial in lowering symptoms and improving the quality of life. As it is a very frequent and annoying symptom that is often encountered in clinical practice, the discrimination between benign mechanical back pain and inflammatory back pain is of utmost significance (Moosajee & Kalla, 2016). Current advances have led to the development of targeted therapies, particularly TNF blockers, which have revolutionized treatment by demonstrating dramatic effectiveness in reducing inflammation and associated pain in SpA patients (Sieper, 2009). Besides pharmacotherapy, a good pain management program should include physical therapy, exercise, and education to foster self-management practices. Incorporating these strategies not only provides relief of immediate pain but also helps in bringing about long-term functional enhancement and enriches the global treatment environment in persons affected by the disabling consequences of spondyloarthritides.

3.4.7. Role of Patient Education

Successful patient education is crucial in spondyloarthritides management since informed patients can engage more actively in their own treatment processes and avoid related complications. Through providing thorough knowledge regarding the disease, its progression, and potential interventions, healthcare professionals enhance patient autonomy.

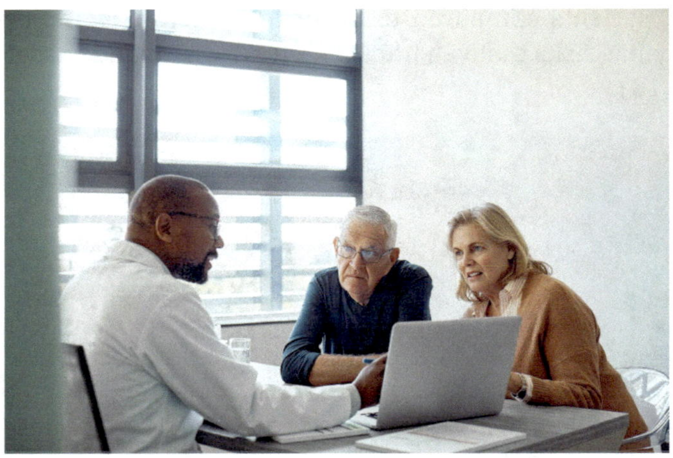

Figure 3.19. Effective patient education plays a crucial role in the management of spondyloarthritides, as informed patients are better equipped to engage in their treatment processes and mitigate associated complications.

Source: https://www.rheumatologyadvisor.com/wp-content/uploads/sites/18/2023/10/Couple.Computer.Doctor_G_1366811808-scaled.jpg.

Such empowerment is particularly critical in the face of the complex nature of spondyloarthritis and its potential co-morbidities, which often necessitate a multidisciplinary treatment strategy by various specialists (Armuzzi et al., 2018). Furthermore, the psychological impact of spondyloarthritis, including anxiety and depression, highlights the need for addressing mental health as much as physical symptoms. Through systematic education interventions, healthcare professionals can facilitate compliance with disease management regimens, enhance coping, and ultimately enhance overall quality of life in patients suffering from these chronic illnesses. In this respect, patient education assumes a focal role in effective disease management and integral care (Figure 3.19).

3.4.8. Multidisciplinary Approach

Multidisciplinary treatment is essential in spondyloarthritides (SpA) due to the complexity and heterogeneity of the disease. Multidisciplinary management in SpA often involves coordination among providers within rheumatology, physical medicine, dermatology, and gastroenterology to address the multifaceted nature of immune-mediated inflammatory diseases (IMIDs). Such coordination is not only necessary to diagnose and manage the underlying inflammatory back pain, but also to manage secondary conditions like psoriasis and inflammatory bowel disease, which frequently co-present with SpA. Integrating multiple forms of expertise ensures that treatments remain patient-specific, hence improving patient outcomes and quality of life. Keeping in mind the financial cost and disability caused by lower back pain, an active, joint management strategy can easily combat these problems (Moosajee & Kalla, 2016; Armuzzi et al., 2018). This multi-step strategy emphasizes the need for consistency between experts in achieving the maximum treatment for sufferers of spondyloarthritides.

3.4.9. Future Directions in Treatment

The future trends in treatment of spondyloarthritides promise to be revolutionary, and the combination of targeted therapies and personalized medicine is the focus.

There is evidence shown by recent studies that Janus kinase inhibitors, such as tofacitinib, not only suppress disease activity but also possess the potential to enhance concomitant metabolic factors like insulin resistance in rheumatoid arthritis and type 2 diabetes patients, representing an important breakthrough in dual-benefit therapy in comorbid patients (Cipriani et al., 2024).

In addition, research biobanking , such as RheumaBank enables systematic collection of the biological specimens and data essential to studying pathogenetic processes and optimizing therapeutic methods on a personalized level (Assirelli et al., 2023). These novel approaches not only further enlighten us about spondyloarthritides but also pave the way for more effective, personalized interventions with the potential to significantly improve patient outcomes and quality of life (Figure 3.20).

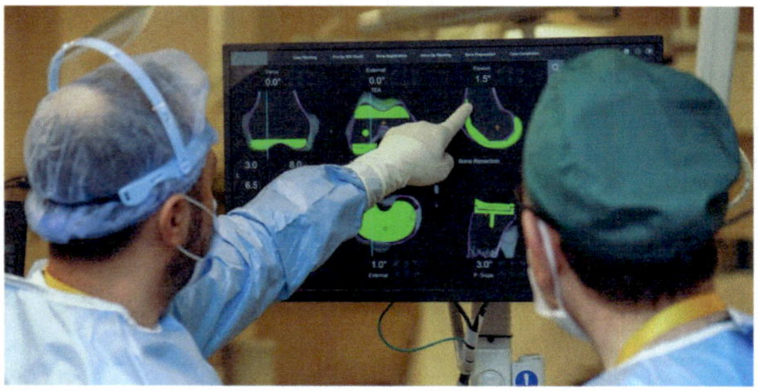

Figure 3.20. The future directions in the treatment of spondyloarthritides promise to be transformative, emphasizing the integration of targeted therapies and personalized medicine.

Source: https://assets.isu.pub/document-structure/241220163851-4e3dfd61db7ee89767cefd5174c2c45a/v1/53154ae479e841235d5451804c056cbd.jpeg.

Test Your Knowledge

1. How is treatment monitored for efficacy and safety in SPA patients?
2. What non-pharmacologic treatments are essential for SPA management?

Summary

The investigation of spondyloarthritides (SpA) ends by acknowledging the immense progress in the comprehension and treatment of these multifactorial illnesses. Given that the past decade has seen considerable growth, the creation of accurate classification criteria and early-diagnosis approaches has played a pivotal role in enhancing patient outcomes. The introduction of TNF blockers is a revolution, with most SpA patients who hitherto had little effective therapy finding relief. Furthermore, the intricate understanding of SpA pathogenesis, particularly the interaction between immune responses and bone destruction, underscores the utility of targeted therapeutic interventions in arresting structural damage (Sieper, 2009). Despite these advances, there still exist challenges, particularly in accurately identifying cases of linked conditions like rheumatoid arthritis within administrative databases that significantly vary in terms of sensitivity and specificity (Hanly et al., 2015). Eventually, further research must be conducted to further refine treatment strategies and improve the quality of life of affected individuals.

Summary of spondyloarthritides points reflects tremendous progress in treatment options and sophistication of disease management. The biologic technology of TNF blockade therapy has transformed the approach to addressing severe ankylosing spondylitis significantly, greatly improving patient symptoms and quality-of-life outcomes. Nevertheless, issues remain, particularly about changes in skeletal disease and cost-effectiveness of these biologic therapies (Barr & Keat, 2010). In addition, non-specific diagnostic criteria of early disease impede timely interventions, and the majority of patients continue to remain susceptible (Barr et al., 2010). Moreover, including the International Classification of Functioning, Disability and Health (ICF) in practice should systematically address functioning and disability in ankylosing spondylitis patients, such that it is easier to deliver individualized healthcare interventions. Therefore, as progress is noted, persistent problems highlight the need for ongoing research and development of treatment protocols.

KEY TERMS FROM THIS CHAPTER

- Aetiopathogenesis
- Ankylosing spondylitis
- Ankylosing spondylitis (AS)
- Anti-inflammatory drugs
- Antirheumatic drugs
- Biologic drugs
- Blockade therapy
- Cycloplegic agents
- Cytokines
- Diagnostic innovation
- Disease
- Efficient management
- Genetic etiology
- Heterogeneous series
- Immune system
- Morphogenetic proteins
- Pathophysiologic mechanisms
- Peripheral arthritis
- Physical therapy
- Polymorphisms

Critical Thinking Questions

1. **Which of the following is a hallmark feature of ankylosing spondylitis?**
   a. Symmetric distal interphalangeal joint involvement
   b. Involvement of the sacroiliac joints
   c. Erosions at the MCP joints
   d. Involvement of the cervical spine only
2. **Which gene is most strongly associated with ankylosing spondylitis?**
   a. HLA-DR4
   b. HLA-DQ2
   c. HLA-B27
   d. HLA-A1
3. **Dactylitis ("sausage digits") is most commonly seen in:**
   a. Rheumatoid arthritis
   b. Osteoarthritis
   c. Psoriatic arthritis
   d. Systemic lupus erythematosus
4. **Reactive arthritis typically occurs after which of the following?**
   a. Viral respiratory infections
   b. Streptococcal throat infections
   c. Gastrointestinal or genitourinary infections
   d. Fungal infections
5. **Which of the following is a typical extra-articular manifestation of ankylosing spondylitis?**
   a. Uveitis
   b. Malar rash
   c. Oral ulcers
   d. Raynaud's phenomenon

Answers to Critical Thinking Questions

1. (b); 2. (c); 3. (c); 4. (c); 5. (a).

Short Answer Questions

1. What are the major subtypes of spondyloarthritides?
2. How is ankylosing spondylitis distinguished from non-radiographic axial spondyloarthritis?
3. What is the role of HLA-B27 in the pathogenesis of spondyloarthritides?
4. How do innate immune pathways contribute to enthesitis in SpA?
5. What are the ASAS classification criteria for axial and peripheral spondyloarthritis?
6. How is HLA-B27 testing used in the diagnostic workup of SpA?
7. What is the first-line treatment for axial spondyloarthritis?
8. How effective are NSAIDs in managing SpA symptoms?

References

1. Aaltonen, K., Askling, J., Chatzidionysiou, K., Di Giuseppe, D., et al. (2018). Opportunities and challenges for real-world studies on chronic inflammatory joint diseases through data enrichment and collaboration between national registers: The Nordic example. https://core.ac.uk/download/157588385.pdf (accessed on 17th June 2025).
2. Allenspach, E. J., Eklund, K. K., Perazzio, S. F., Seppänen, M., et al. (2020). Behcet disease (BD) and BD-like clinical phenotypes: NF-kappa B pathway in mucosal ulcerating diseases. https://core.ac.uk/download/479169561.pdf (accessed on 17th June 2025).
3. Andersen, K. W., Andersen, V., Bek Sørensen, S., Bojesen, B., et al. (2017). A proposal for a study on treatment selection and lifestyle recommendations in chronic inflammatory diseases: A Danish multidisciplinary collaboration on prognostic factors and personalized medicine. https://core.ac.uk/download/269294992.pdf (accessed on 17th June 2025).
4. Armuzzi, A., Ayala, F., Bettoli, V., Bianchi, L., et al. (2018). Multidisciplinary management of spondylarthritis-related immune-mediated inflammatory disease. https://core.ac.uk/download/195754331.pdf (accessed on 17th June 2025).
5. Assirelli, E., Brusi, V., Ciaffi, J., Faldini, C., Lisi, L., Mancarella, L., Naldi, S., et al. (2023). Building a rheumatology biobank for reliable basic/translational research and precision medicine. https://core.ac.uk/download/611909296.pdf (accessed on 17th June 2025).
6. Gueudry, J., Thorne, J. E., Bansie, R., Braun, J., van Hagen, P. M., & Bodaghi, B. (2017). Biologic Therapy for HLA-B27-associated Ocular Disorders. *Ocular immunology and inflammation*, *25*(2), 169–178. https://doi.org/10.1080/09273948.2016.1234625(accessed on 17th June 2025).
7. Baraliakos, C. C., Ciofu, C., Bara, D., Danning, G., Dougados, M., Fitzgerald, O., Garcia-Valladares, M., et al. (2011). A pilot study of the association of tumor necrosis factor alpha polymorphisms with psoriatic arthritis in the Romanian population. https://core.ac.uk/download/pdf/8619927.pdf (accessed on 17th June 2025).
8. Barr, A., & Keat, A. (2010). Spondyloarthritides: evolving therapies. *Arthritis research & therapy*, *12*(6), 221. https://doi.org/10.1186/ar3178(accessed on 17th June 2025).
9. Bernatschek, A., Bürki, K., Ciurea, A., Exer, P., et al. (2023). Characterization of patients with axial psoriatic arthritis and patients with axial spondylarthritis and concomitant psoriasis in the SCQM registry. https://www.zora.uzh.ch/id/eprint/234522/1/e002956.full.pdf (accessed on 17th June 2025).
10. Boonen, A., Braun, J., Cieza, A., Kiltz, U., et al. (2017). Developing and validating an index for measuring health in patients with ankylosing spondylitis. https://core.ac.uk/download/85215567.pdf (accessed on 17th June 2025).
11. Bose, T., Damoiseaux, J. G. M. C., Generali, E., Selmi, C., et al. (2018). Nature versus nurture in the spectrum of rheumatic diseases: Classification of spondylarthritis as autoimmune or autoinflammatory. https://core.ac.uk/download/572842290.pdf (accessed on 17th June 2025).
12. Burgos-Vargas, R. (2012). The assessment of the Spondylarthritis International Society concept and criteria for the classification of axial spondylarthritis and peripheral spondylarthritis: A critical appraisal for the pediatric rheumatologist. https://core.ac.uk/download/pdf/81079348.pdf (accessed on 17th June 2025).

13. Cauli, A., Mathieu, A., Spadaro, A., ALONSO, L., Anderson, M., Apolone, G., Badia, X., et al. (2008). The psoriatic arthritis cost evaluation study: A cost-of-illness study on tumor necrosis factor inhibitors in psoriatic arthritis patients with inadequate response to conventional therapy. https://core.ac.uk/download/pdf/8206126.pdf (accessed on 17th June 2025).

14. Chandrababu, R., Jacob, D., & Lazarus, E. R. (2022). Efficacy of cling film dressing on palmoplantar psoriatic lesions among patients with psoriasis: A randomized controlled trial. https://core.ac.uk/download/571640431.pdf (accessed on 17th June 2025).

15. Churg, A., D'Hulst, A. I., D'Hulst, A. I., Oberholzer, A., Ananthakrishnan, A. N., Chassaing, B., Vuillemenot, B. R., et al. (2015). The effect of cigarette smoke exposure on the development of inflammation in lungs, gut and joints of TNFΔARE mice. https://core.ac.uk/download/55798655.pdf (accessed on 17th June 2025).

16. Cipriani, P., Di Cola, I., Di Muzio, C., Giacomelli, R., Iagnocco, A., Ruscitti, P., Shariat Panahi, A., et al. (2024). The effects of suppressing inflammation by tofacitinib may simultaneously improve glycemic parameters and inflammatory markers in rheumatoid arthritis patients with comorbid type 2 diabetes: A proof-of-concept, open, prospective, clinical study. https://core.ac.uk/download/611902511.pdf (accessed on 17th June 2025).

17. Coates, L. C., Dubash, S., Helliwell, P. S., Marzo-Ortega, H., et al. (2020). BSR Spondylarthritis Course, 27 February 2020. Spondylarthritis: Pathogenesis, diagnosis and management. https://core.ac.uk/download/334600662.pdf (accessed on 17th June 2025).

18. Codacci Pisanelli, M., Costi, U., De Santis, A., Gabriele, L., et al. (2018). The use of x-ray CT and MRI in the study of sacroiliac joints in patients with Behcet disease and acute anterior uveitis. https://core.ac.uk/download/158327793.pdf (accessed on 17th June 2025).

19. Corea, F., Lanari, A., Micheli, S., Silvestrelli, G., et al. (2025). Clinical pharmacology and vascular risk. https://core.ac.uk/download/pdf/8443032.pdf (accessed on 17th June 2025).

20. de Vlam, K., Lories, R. J. U., & Luyten, F. P. (2009). Progress in spondylarthritis: Mechanisms of new bone formation in spondylarthritis. https://core.ac.uk/download/pdf/8291777.pdf (accessed on 17th June 2025).

21. Duer, A., Hørslev-Petersen, K., & Østergaard, M. (2005). Can magnetic resonance imaging differentiate undifferentiated arthritis? https://core.ac.uk/download/pdf/3814081.pdf (accessed on 17th June 2025).

22. Elewaut, D., & Matucci-Cerinic, M. (2009). Treatment of ankylosing spondylitis and extra-articular manifestations in everyday rheumatology practice. https://core.ac.uk/download/55761196.pdf (accessed on 17th June 2025).

23. Elewaut, D., & Melis, L. (2009). Progress in spondylarthritis. Immunopathogenesis of spondylarthritis: Which cells drive disease? https://core.ac.uk/download/pdf/8308904.pdf (accessed on 17th June 2025).

24. Eshed, I., Herregods, N., Jans, L., Sudoł-Szopińska, I., et al. (2018). Classifications and imaging of juvenile spondylarthritis. https://core.ac.uk/download/200225208.pdf (accessed on 17th June 2025).

25. Forss, A. (2022). Medical and surgical treatment of inflammatory bowel disease. https://core.ac.uk/download/516464049.pdf (accessed on 17th June 2025).

26. Forte, G., Galasso, D., & Marigliano, N. (2010). Focus on: Le spondiloartriti. La diagnosi

precoce può modificare il decorso della malattia? https://core.ac.uk/download/604644005.pdf (accessed on 17th June 2025).

27. Hanly, J. G., Skedgel, C., & Thompson, K. (2015). The use of administrative health care databases to identify patients with rheumatoid arthritis. https://core.ac.uk/download/41991036.pdf (accessed on 17th June 2025).
28. Karunaratne, P. M., Mease, P., Pangan, A. L., Rahman, P., et al. (2015). Randomized controlled trial of adalimumab in patients with nonpsoriatic peripheral spondylarthritis. https://core.ac.uk/download/55847961.pdf (accessed on 17th June 2025).
29. Kern, M. (2019). Exercise therapy for juvenile idiopathic arthritis. https://open.bu.edu/bitstream/2144/38663/7/Kern_bu_0017N_14858.pdf (accessed on 17th June 2025).
30. Lories, R. J. U., & Luyten, F. P. (2007). Bone morphogenetic proteins in destructive and remodeling arthritis. https://core.ac.uk/download/pdf/7636126.pdf (accessed on 17th June 2025).
31. Pant, S., Raj, S., Sharma, A. C., Srivastava, N., et al. (2023). Treatment modalities of ankylosing spondylitis. https://core.ac.uk/download/553310165.pdf (accessed on 17th June 2025).
32. Porter, S. B. (2025). Exercise behavior in ankylosing spondylitis. https://core.ac.uk/download/17182800.pdf (accessed on 17th June 2025).
33. Sieper J. (2009). Developments in the scientific and clinical understanding of the spondyloarthritides. *Arthritis research & therapy*, *11*(1), 208. https://doi.org/10.1186/ar2562(accessed on 17th June 2025).
34. Smith, R. (2020). Axial spondyloarthropathies in the Western Cape. https://core.ac.uk/download/288496305.pdf (accessed on 17th June 2025).
35. Glasnović, M., Bosnjak, I., Sram, M., Vranjes, Z., Vcev, A., Dobrosević, B., Petricević, J. S., Horvatić, E., Orkić, Z., Tadzić, R., Soldo, A., Sisljagić, D., & Dinjar, K. (2011). Clinical characteristics of patients with spondyloarthritides and HLA-B27 positive antigen. *Collegium antropologicum*, *35*(2), 397–402. (accessed on 17th June 2025).

SJOGREN'S SYNDROME

4

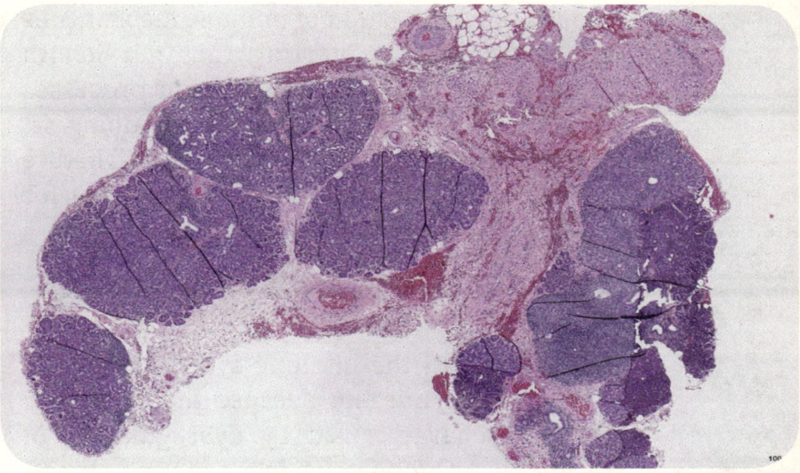

LEARNING OBJECTIVES

After studying this chapter, you will be able to:

1. pathophysiology of Sjogren's syndrome.
2. symptoms and diagnosis.
3. treatment and management.
4. complications and comorbidities.

Introduction

Sjogren's Syndrome is a complex autoimmune disease predominantly characterized by dry mouth and dry eyes due to the invasion of immune cells into exocrine glands, i.e., salivary and lacrimal glands. The condition not only destroys the quality of life but also leads to systemic complications in other organs. The pathogenesis of Sjogren's Syndrome is not entirely clear, with both genetic predispositions and environmental factors playing significant roles in disease development. As highlighted by current research, the diagnosis process can be particularly daunting, considering that there are no definitive tests for Sjogren's; therefore, biopsy, clinical assessment, and serologic testing are all commonly utilized to make the diagnosis. Understanding the multifactorial etiology of Sjogren's syndrome is important in the implementation of optimal treatment regimens and the improvement of outcomes in patients. Also, associated autoimmune diseases, including burning mouth syndrome, further complicate the clinical picture, requiring extensive studies of common pathophysiological mechanisms (Löwhagen, 1999; Ji et al., 2017) (Figure 4.1).

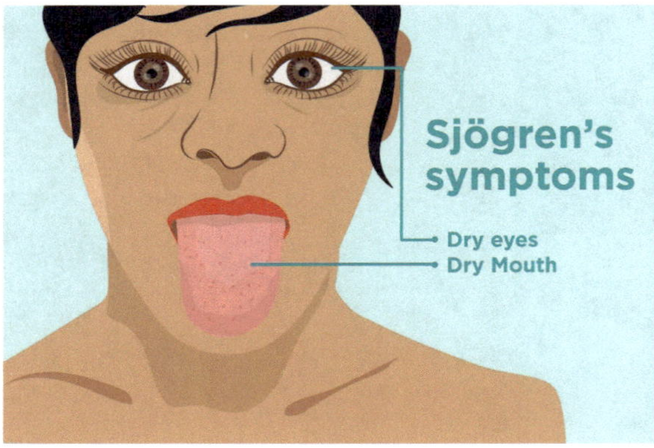

Figure 4.1. Sjogren's syndrome.

Source: https://www.cyprusdermaclinic.com/wp-content/uploads/2022/09/308351691_595617705369550_8819631735619909492_n.jpg.

4.1. Pathophysiology of Sjogren's Syndrome

Learning Outcome

1. Understand immune system involvement;
2. Discuss the role of exocrine glands;
3. Explain mechanisms of glandular dysfunction;
4. Identify genetic factors contributing to the disease;
5. Focus on environmental triggers;
6. Learn inflammatory processes;
7. Know the differences between primary and secondary Sjogren's;
8. Discuss the impact on salivary and lacrimal glands.

The pathophysiology of Sjögren's Syndrome (SS) is supported by a complex interplay between immune dysregulation and genetic predisposition. At the very core of the disease is the overexpression of interferon (IFN) signatures, which are elevated in patients and play an important role in disease progression. Type I IFN signaling has been shown to be implicated in many features of SS, such as the lymphocytic infiltration of exocrine glands, autoantibody production, and apoptosis of glandular cells (Lessard et al., 2013). Further, recent evidence suggests that the gut microbiome may also play a potential role in the immune modulation in autoimmune conditions , such as SS. For instance, probiotic treatment has been promising in the relief of dry eye syndrome through the modulation of immune mechanisms and microbiota, suggesting that gut health can influence the pathophysiologic processes underlying SS (Choi et al., 2020). In doing so, these findings highlight the multifactorial nature of Sjögren's Syndrome and pave the way for novel therapeutic interventions.

4.1.1. Immune System Involvement

The function of the immune system is pivotal to Sjögren's Syndrome because the disease is primarily characterized by dysregulation of the immune reactions against exocrine glands. The autoimmune disorder, which is especially characterized by its effects on salivary and lacrimal glands, displays a complex interaction between innate and adaptive immunity. Research highlights the role of invariant natural killer T cells (iNKT) that control immune activity and cause inflammation in the affected tissues, with potential as biomarkers of disease progression (Ji et al., 2017). Furthermore, the autoimmune response in Sjögren's Syndrome is often provided by T-helper lymphocytes actively attacking glandular tissue, with severe damage and inflammation followed (Gallo et al., 2017). This immune dysregulation not only explains Sjögren's pathogenesis but also emphasizes the requirement for specifically targeted therapeutics aimed at controlling the underlying immune mechanisms that sustain the syndrome's chronic manifestations (Figure 4.2).

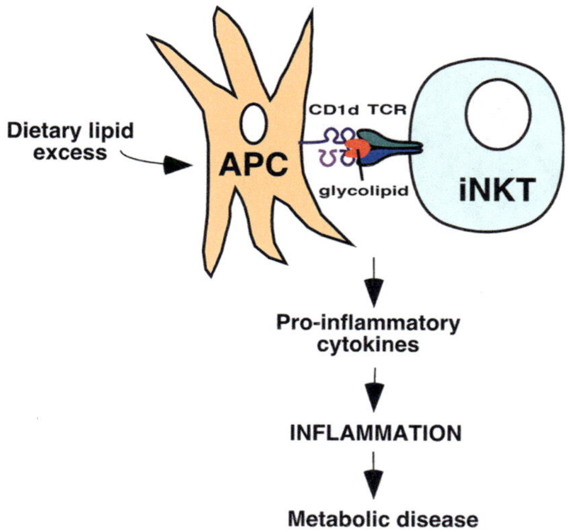

Figure 4.2. The role of invariant natural killer T cells (iNKT), which modulate immune activity and contribute to inflammation within the affected tissues, suggesting their potential as biomarkers for disease progression.

Source: https://www.pnas.org/cms/10.1073/pnas.1200498109/asset/9191c2ce-2c25-4c06-9b53-2a77b2071f5f/assets/graphic/pnas.1200498s109fig01.jpeg.

4.1.2. Role of Exocrine Glands

The role of human exocrine glands is diverse, particularly with reference to the way they operate in autoimmune diseases , such as Sjögren's Syndrome (pSS). Salivary and lacrimal glands are the primary exocrine glands that secrete aqueous fluids essential to provide moisture to the oral cavity and the eyes. In pSS patients, the immune system attacks these exocrine glands by mistake, leading to inflammatory destruction and the characteristic dryness features.

Lymphocytic infiltration of the glands is responsible for pSS pathogenesis, which focuses on them being vulnerable to autoimmune attack (Bhattacharya et al., 2017). Pointedly, dysregulation of immunity also indicates a potential association between activity in exocrine glands and systemic inflammation because correlations between pSS disease activity and autophagy in T lymphocytes have been proven in research, which emphasizes the function of such organs in both local and systemic disease expression (Gallo et al., 2017).

Thus, knowledge of the exocrine gland function not only helps in the diagnosis of pSS but also provides avenues for specific therapeutic interventions.

4.1.3. Mechanisms of Glandular Dysfunction

The pathophysiology of glandular dysfunction in Sjögren's syndrome is multifactorial and entails intricate mechanisms of both autoimmune-mediated damage and perturbed neurovascular interactions. Central to the pathophysiology is lymphocytic infiltration of exocrine glands with attendant severe architectural alterations and impaired glandular function.

Especially, studies have demonstrated that dysfunctional vascular response to parasympathetic stimulation in salivary glands leads to hyposalivation, a widespread symptom of the condition, on the basis of much weaker blood flow responses in nonobese diabetic mice compared to controls (Berggreen et al., 2013). Besides, the association of hearing impairment with Sjögren's syndrome highlights an overall systemic impact whereby autoimmune responses also affect sensory mechanisms, suggesting the intricate relationship between glandular dysfunction and sensory mechanisms (Thanooja, 2012).

Thus, it is crucial to understand these mechanisms fully to devise pinpoint therapeutic interventions against the severity of this disabling autoimmune disorder (Figure 4.3).

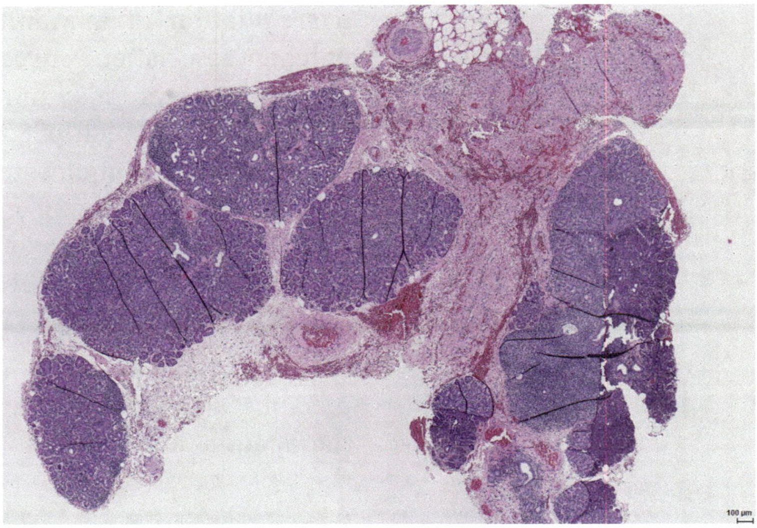

Figure 4.3. Infiltration of lymphocytes into exocrine glands, leading to significant architectural changes and impaired glandular function.

Source: https://www.surveyophthalmol.com/cms/10.1016/j.survophthal.2019.10.004/asset/d15f9e61-9e9b-4b7d-b14f-eb01f2504662/main.assets/gr3_lrg.jpg.

4.1.4. Genetic Factors Contributing to the Disease

The genetic basis of Sjogren's Syndrome (SS) is important in the understanding of the disease's etiology and pathogenesis. Several genetic markers have been identified through research to contribute to the potential predisposition of individuals to autoimmune disorders, such as SS. An example of this includes the polymorphism of genes involved in immune function that can increase susceptibility to out-of-control immune responses, which are typical in SS. Also, the interaction of environmental stimuli and predispositions of a genetic nature, such as infections by viruses, can increase the likelihood of disease development. Association evidence with other autoimmune diseases, such as systemic lupus erythematosus, and the development of type 1 interferon (T1 IFN) pathways has also been observed, suggesting the sharing of a common genetic origin of autoimmune dysregulation in predisposed individuals (Allanore et al., 2022). Furthermore, research has indicated the significance of metabolic factors, i.e., the impact of diabetes mellitus on ocular health, and that genetic factors might also interact with metabolic disorders to influence symptom severity in SS (Priya et al., 2015).

4.1.5. Environmental Triggers

In the multifactorial etiology of Sjogren's Syndrome, environmental determinants play an increasingly important role in disease causation and exacerbation. Chemical exposures, infection, and climatic influences can act to trigger autoimmune activity in affected individuals. Data have shown that some autoimmune disorders, including Sjogren's Syndrome, are female-dominated, suggesting that interactions between environmental and hormonal factors might lead to pathogenesis (Chandrasekaran et al., 2024). Furthermore, studies show that some biologic treatments can influence the immune reaction to environmental antigens and complicate treatment (Lin et al., 2023). The ability to differentiate these environmental determinants is significant in that it can potentially lead to improved preventative measures and personalized treatment approaches for patients. Awareness of the interaction among genetic susceptibilities and environmental exposures thus has the potential to improve the care and prognosis of individuals afflicted with Sjogren's Syndrome (Figure 4.4).

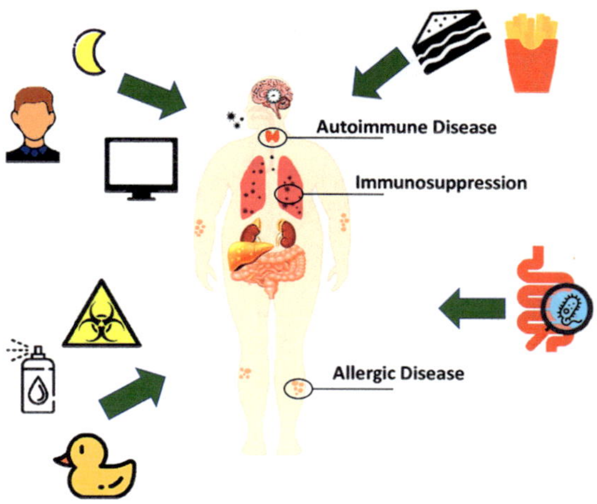

Figure 4.4. Factors , such as exposure to certain chemicals, infections, and even climate conditions can exacerbate the autoimmune responses seen in affected individuals.

Source: https://media.springernature.com/lw685/springer-static/image/chp%3A10.1007%2F978-3-030-38366-4_13-1/MediaObjects/471956_0_En_13-1_Fig1_HTML.png.

4.1.6. Inflammatory Processes

Inflammatory processes are central to Sjogren's Syndrome pathophysiology, an autoimmune-mediated disorder involving primary exocrine gland damage. Pathologic immune response in the syndrome leads to lymphocytic infiltration of salivary and lacrimal glands, tissue injury, and functional impairment. An inflammatory environment can amplify symptoms and lead to dryness and discomfort in patients with this condition. Interestingly, the response to conventional immunomodulatory therapy is typically poor, and other treatments are under consideration. For instance, the use of rituximab, a CD20-positive B-cell antibody, has proved to be advantageous in the management of treatment-refractory cases, improving pulmonary function in patients with associated interstitial lung disease as seen in more recent research (Adamali et al., 2016). Besides, understanding molecular mechanisms of inflammation enhances the development of personalized therapy, ultimately leading to better patient outcomes for autoimmune disorders like Sjogren's Syndrome (Lin et al., 2023).

4.1.7. Differences Between Primary and Secondary Sjogren's

These distinctions between primary and secondary Sjögren's syndrome are significant in understanding the broader implications of the autoimmune disease. Primary Sjögren's syndrome occurs independently, with the autoimmune mechanism primarily targeting the exocrine glands to create dry eyes and dry mouth without any associated other underlying autoimmune disease. On the other hand, secondary Sjögren's is associated with other autoimmune disorders, such as rheumatoid arthritis or lupus, thus the clinical picture and management are complicated due to the interference of greater than one autoimmune mechanism. Primary Sjögren's syndrome has been discovered by research to be mediated by mechanisms , such as disrupted cell polarity and lymphocytic invasion that compromise normal gland function (Langara, 2017). Secondly, with further research, the efficacy of non-pharmacological interventions remains questionable in terms of symptom treatment of primary Sjögren's (Cockshott et al., 2015). The identification of these differences is crucial to designing specific therapies and improving patient outcomes in both syndromes (Figure 4.5).

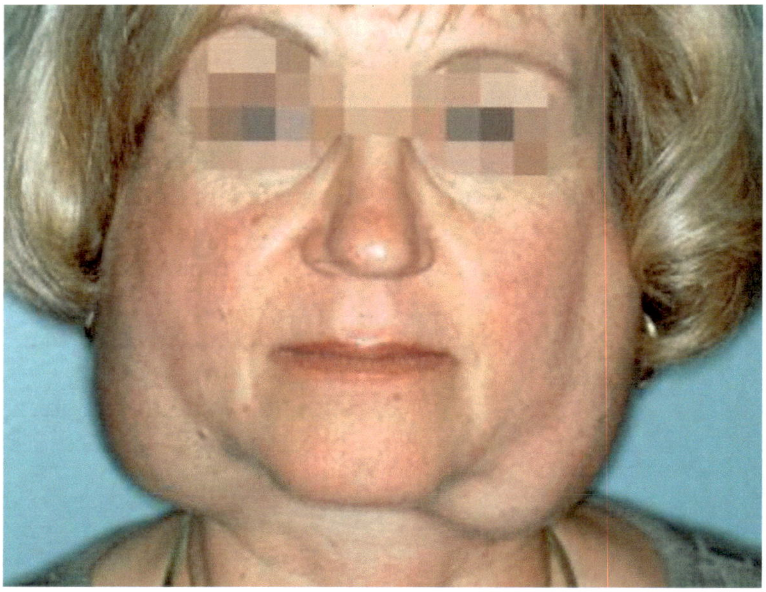

Figure 4.5. Secondary Sjögren's is associated with other autoimmune conditions, such as rheumatoid arthritis or lupus, complicating the clinical presentation and management due to the interplay of multiple autoimmune processes.

Source: https://img.medscapestatic.com/pi/meds/ckb/16/39216tn.jpg.

4.1.8. Impact on Salivary and Lacrimal Glands

Its impact on the salivary and lacrimal glands is widespread, leading to debilitating dryness that has a profoundly adverse impact on patients' quality of life. The disease mainly targets these exocrine glands, generating hyposalivation and decreased tear secretion, characteristic features of the disorder. The most common complaints from the patients are persistent dry eyes and mouth in the form of dysphagia, altered taste, and burning or gritty eye symptoms. Most importantly, clinical markers , such as the Schirmer I test and Tear Break-Up Time that are pivotal for follow-up and diagnosis of disease progression can be correlated with the severity of dry eyes (Roma, 2015). Moreover, the systemic complications of Sjogren's syndrome, including a risk of developing lymphoma, serve to emphasize the need for early diagnosis and treatment of affected glands (Caffery, 2009). Thus, the understanding of glandular involvement is significant in developing overall treatment strategies.

Test Your Knowledge

1. How does chronic inflammation lead to the destruction of salivary and lacrimal glands?
2. What genetic predispositions are associated with Sjögren's syndrome?

4.2. Symptoms and Diagnosis

Learning Outcome

1. Identify common symptoms of Sjogren's syndrome;
2. Focus on ocular manifestations;
3. Explain oral manifestations;
4. Discuss fatigue and systemic symptoms;
5. Learn diagnostic criteria;
6. Explain laboratory tests for diagnosis;
7. Describe imaging studies and their relevance;
8. Learn differential diagnosis;
9. Identify challenges in diagnosing Sjogren's syndrome.

The manifestations of Sjögren's Syndrome are predominantly seen as mucous membrane dryness, and the eyes and mouth are involved to a great degree, leading to conditions , such as keratoconjunctivitis and xerostomia. Joint pain, fatigue, and other systemic symptoms are also shown by patients, making it difficult to diagnose.

Proper assessment is required as the disease can be misinterpreted as other autoimmune diseases. Specific laboratory tests, such as the presence of anti-Ro/SSA and anti-La/SSB antibodies, can enhance the diagnostic yield, alongside salivary gland biopsies that show lymphocytic infiltrate typical of gland damage. Studies indicate that underlying immune mechanisms, in this case, the role of innate immunity and invariant natural killer T cells, can contribute to the pathophysiology of the disease and also serve as potential biomarkers for the activity of the disease (Barbera et al., 2019). Moreover, accurate differentiation from immunoglobulin G4-related diseases is of primary importance because these conditions may mimic overlapping features (Gallo et al., 2017).

4.2.1. Common Symptoms of Sjogren's Syndrome

Sjogren's Syndrome, an autoimmune disorder with exocrine gland dysfunction, is clinically manifested by a particular set of symptoms. The most frequent symptoms are xerostomia and keratoconjunctivitis sicca, which often disable the patients and may drastically change their quality of life. In addition to these typical symptoms, fatigue and arthralgia may occur, contributing to their compromised daily activity. The condition also usually occurs alongside other autoimmune diseases, as suggested by evidence that connective tissue disorders tend to present with overlapping signs and complications during pregnancy, thereby emphasizing the complexity and systemic nature (Caramia et al., 2018). The occurrence of other related comorbidities may also exacerbate challenges for patients, necessitating holistic treatment protocols (Jha & Chaudhari, 2020). A complicated symptomatology as such emphasizes early diagnosis and specially focused interventions to effectively treat Sjogren's Syndrome (Figure 4.6).

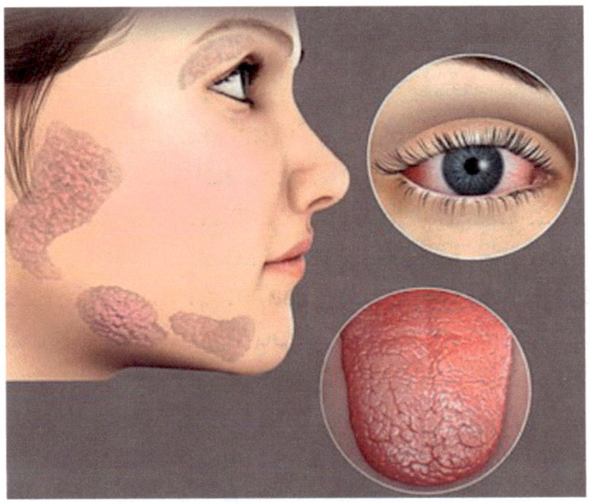

Figure 4.6. Sjogren's Syndrome, an autoimmune disorder characterized by the dysfunction of exocrine glands, primarily manifests through a distinctive set of symptoms.

Source: https://upload.wikimedia.org/wikipedia/commons/thumb/5/54/Sjogrens_Syndrome.jpg/330px-Sjogrens_Syndrome.jpg.

4.2.2. Ocular Manifestations

The ophthalmic presentation of Sjögren's Syndrome is a significant issue as this autoimmune disease affects secretory function from exocrine glands to the largest degree, producing common symptoms , such as dry eye syndrome. The prevalence of dry eye syndrome in patients with Sjögren's has been well documented and reported to a large degree by studies, referring to a high rate of patients reporting various severity levels, from mild to severe dry eyes (Chandrasekaran et al., 2024). Decreased tear production not only compromises comfort but can also lead to more serious complications, including corneal damage and compromise of vision. Contributing to the complicated clinical scenario, ocular involvement commonly accompanies other systemic manifestations of the disease, demonstrating the interrelation character of autoimmune disorders (Thanooja, 2012). Hence, management of these eye symptoms is very important as it is a significant factor in determining the quality of life of individuals suffering from Sjögrens Syndrome.

4.2.3. Oral Manifestations

The oral features of Sjögren's syndrome are significant and complex and are primarily a result of the disease's impact on exocrine glands, particularly the salivary glands. The patient is predisposed to xerostomia, or dry mouth, caused by diminished saliva production, and leads to discomfort during chewing, swallowing, and talking. Dryness also enhances dental issues, like increased caries and periodontal disease, indicating the need for scrupulous oral hygiene and regular dental care. Moreover, Sjögren's syndrome's inflammatory process may also contribute to sialadenitis, the inflammation of salivary glands themselves, further complicating oral health. Studies show a correlation between inflammatory activity as reflected by some autoantibodies and severity of oral symptoms and implicate the possibility of a pathophysiological relationship between systemic and oral manifestations of Sjögren's syndrome (Gallo et al., 2017; Yakimenko et al., 2019). Therefore, recognition of such oral manifestations is important in the overall management of such patients (Figure 4.7).

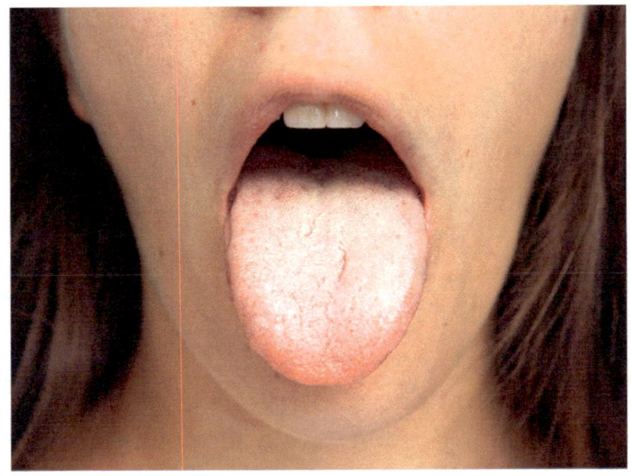

Figure 4.7. Patients often experience xerostomia, or dry mouth, which arises from decreased saliva production, leading to difficulties in chewing, swallowing, and speaking.

Source: https://www.riverwalkdentalorthodontics.com/wp-content/uploads/2023/08/Xerostomia-1200x900.jpg.

4.2.4. Fatigue and Systemic Symptoms

Among the many systemic manifestations of Sjogren's Syndrome, one of the most common and disabling ones is chronic fatigue. This is frequently associated with the autoimmune features of the disease, where the immune system of the body attacks its own tissues in error, resulting in a host of systemic issues like joint pain and dryness of the mucous membranes. It has been observed that nearly half of patients with primary Sjogren's Syndrome (pSS) have extensive sensorineural hearing loss, which is also possibly correlated with the degree of fatigue and other systemic features. Surprisingly, psychological symptoms , such as depression can also enhance fatigue, thus contributing to poor patient prognosis. The relationship between immunological factors, such as the presence of anti-SS antibodies and tiredness, suggests a deeper association between autoimmune processes and the overall symptomology of Sjogren's. These systemic symptoms significantly impair the quality of life of patients, as an indicator of the significance of overall management plans in pSS (Thanooja, 2012; Ranjitham et al., 2018).

4.2.5. Diagnostic Criteria

Accurate diagnosis of Sjögren's Syndrome (SS) is dependent on clearly defined criteria that include both clinical presentation and laboratory findings. Commonly, symptoms are present in the presentation of dry eyes and mouth, necessitating accurate evaluation using objective parameters like the Schirmer test and salivary flow measurement. Furthermore, serologic tests can reveal the occurrence of autoantibodies, particularly anti-Ro/La markers, as good predictors of SS. Studies have pointed out the significance of such immunological markers as major diagnostic features, and that their detection helps in differentiating SS from other autoimmune diseases , such as systemic lupus erythematosus, which can have overlapping symptoms (Caramia et al., 2018). More advanced techniques , such as high-resolution mass spectrometry, have also proved crucial in identifying individual autoantibody profiles, including those against LaA, thus enhancing diagnostic specificity for SS (Arentz et al., 2013). The multi-faceted approach is crucial for early and accurate diagnosis, influencing, in turn, patient management strategies (Figure 4.8).

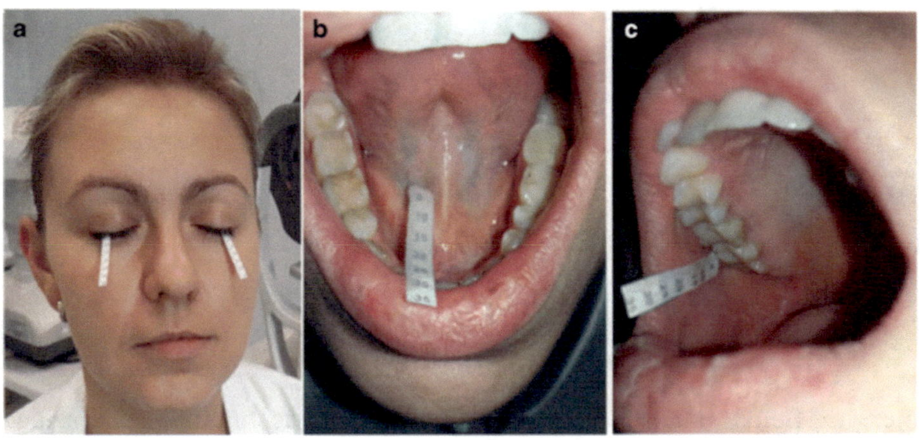

Figure 4.8. a Lacrimal Schirmer test, b Salivary Schirmer test 1. c Salivary Schirmer test 2.

Source: https://media.springernature.com/lw685/springer-static/image/art%3A10.1007%2Fs00784-020-03741-3/MediaObjects/784_2020_3741_Fig1_HTML.png.

4.2.6. Laboratory Tests for Diagnosis

Diagnosis of Sjögren's syndrome is often preceded by a battery of laboratory tests that examine numerous diverse functions of the immune system and salivary gland function. These may frequently include autoantibody profiles, i.e., quantitation of anti-Ro/SSA and anti-La/SSB antibodies, most commonly associated with the syndrome. Additionally, sialometry and sialography can be employed to assess salivary gland flow rates and morphology, respectively, providing evidence of gland involvement. Recent studies also suggest that ocular surface testing, such as tear film stability and ocular staining, could be highly beneficial for in-depth evaluation, especially in patients with concomitant dry eye symptoms. Moreover, studies are indicating that air quality could further aggravate ocular surface compromise in patients with Sjögrens syndrome, which would suggest the need for a multidimensional approach in diagnostic strategies (Gallo et al., 2017). Hence, the combination of laboratory exams and careful clinical observation is significant in proving the presence of Sjögren's syndrome and in managing its diverse implications.

4.2.7. Imaging Studies and Their Relevance

Imaging studies are at the center of Sjögren's Syndrome diagnosis and treatment, and they keep broadening our understanding of this highly complex autoimmune disease. Of the various imaging methods, salivary gland imaging has been of prime interest because it has been extensively utilized and has been instrumental in determining glandular dysfunction, along with disease activity follow-up. With the aid of advanced imaging, clinicians not only can confirm the diagnosis of primary Sjögren's syndrome but are also able to evaluate the course of the disease and its accompanying lymphoproliferative complications, all of which are paramount in patient management (Bootsma et al., 2020). Emerging frontiers , such as oculomics, have also begun to highlight the role of ocular imaging in identifying systemic disease markers of Sjögren's Syndrome. This novel approach highlights the potential of imaging studies to facilitate early diagnosis and disease progression monitoring on ocular health, hence opening new avenues for translational medicine. (Figure 4.9)

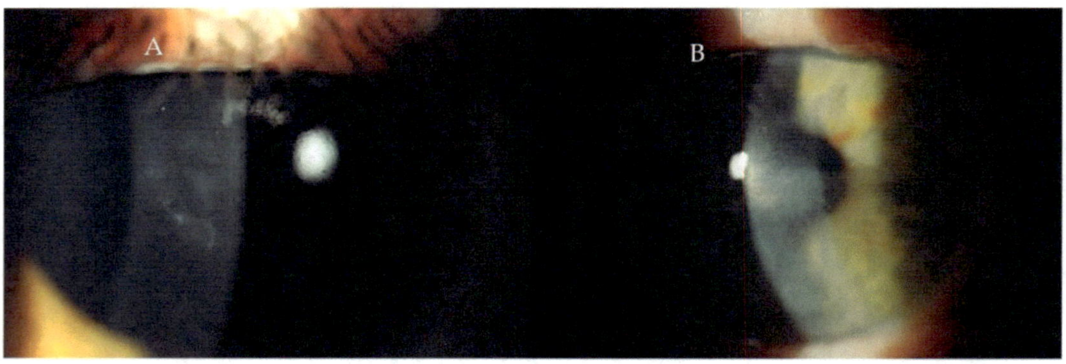

Figure 4.9. Emerging fields , such as oculomics have begun to highlight the relevance of ocular imaging in identifying systemic disease markers associated with Sjögren's Syndrome.

Source: https://www.mdpi.com/diagnostics/diagnostics-15-00643/article_deploy/html/images/diagnostics-15-00643-g003.png.

4.2.8. Differential Diagnosis

In the context of autoimmune diseases, the differential diagnosis of Sjögren's syndrome is rather challenging owing to its imitative presentation in other conditions. Of greatest importance in this exercise is differentiation of Sjögren's from immunoglobulin G4-related disease, systemic lupus erythematosus, and rheumatoid arthritis, since these have similar symptoms, particularly salivary gland involvement and the systemic effect. For instance, immunoglobulin G4-related diseases have emerged as multifactorial multi-organ diseases with an autoimmune attack on salivary glands, and identification is necessary since these diseases were previously thought to be just a variant of Sjögrens syndrome (Gallo et al., 2017). Additionally, advancements in the glycomic techniques suggest that incorrect glycosylation can serve as biomarkers for distinguishing autoimmune conditions, highlighting the significance of glyco-biomarkers for developing diagnostic and prognostic methods under differential diagnosis frameworks (Alavi & Axford, 2008). Hence, meticulous evaluation is essential for accurate determination and treatment of Sjögren's syndrome in the context of such uncertain diseases (Figure 4.10).

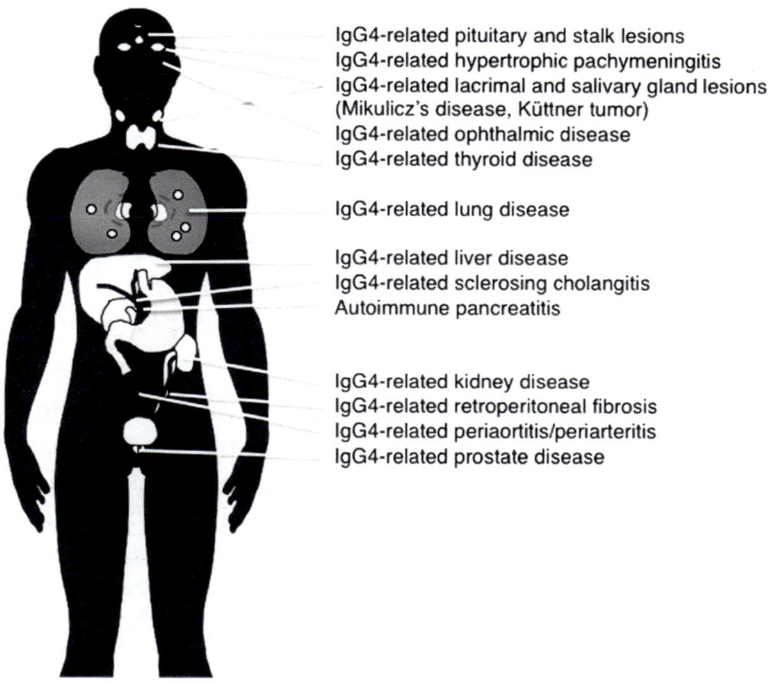

Figure 4.1.0. Immunoglobulin G4-related diseases have emerged as complex multi-organ conditions characterized by an autoimmune reaction that targets salivary glands, making identification crucial since these disorders were previously regarded as mere variants of Sjögrens syndrome.

Source: https://www.jmaj.jp/assets/10.31662_jmaj.2018-0017/JMAJF0017-01-.jpg.

4.2.9. Challenges in Diagnosing Sjogren's Syndrome

Diagnosis of Sjögren's Syndrome is extremely difficult, primarily due to its heterogeneous clinical presentation and its similarity with other autoimmune conditions. This is more difficult to diagnose or delay diagnosing because some of its clinical manifestations, such as mouth and eye dryness, are easily confused with other conditions. Moreover, variability in the symptoms may hide the presence of the syndrome, making it even harder to diagnose (Mahroum et al., 2022). Recent literature has focused on symptom management and patient empowerment, and it has been suggested that patients' concerns need to be attended to by healthcare professionals in order to navigate successfully diagnostic uncertainties (Abourazzak et al., 2018). Additionally, the lack of absolute serological markers for Sjögren's makes it difficult to differentiate it from diseases with overlapping clinical presentations, hence necessitating a multidisciplinary diagnostic process. All these illustrate that understanding the clinical nuances and etiologic rationale is critical for early and accurate diagnosis of Sjögren's Syndrome.

Test Your Knowledge

1. What oral complications are commonly associated with xerostomia?
2. Which diagnostic tests are used to assess tear and saliva production?

4.3. Treatment and Management

Learning Outcome

1. Understand the overview of treatment options;
2. Explain symptomatic relief for dry eyes;
3. Learn management of dry mouth;
4. Focus on pharmacological treatments;
5. Discuss the role of lifestyle modifications;
6. Know the importance of regular monitoring;
7. Focus on a multidisciplinary approach to care;
8. Know emerging therapies and research;
9. Focus on patient education and support.

Effective treatment and management of Sjogren's Syndrome demand an overall approach, owing to its complex nature as well as the variety of symptoms involved. Relief from symptoms , such as dry mouth and eyes is primarily the target of management, as they significantly impair the quality of life of the patient. Salivary substitutes and stimulants are usually prescribed to control xerostomia, while ocular lubricants and anti-inflammatory agents can help remove ocular dryness, indicating the relative importance of local treatment in relieving symptoms. Moreover, it is essential to monitor for systemic involvement since Sjogren's has the potential to affect other organs and cause non-Hodgkin lymphoma (Bogacz et al., 2023). Therefore, a standard diagnostic protocol is required to detect and treat it in an early stage. Ongoing research into more novel therapeutic agents, including immune-modulating therapies, has the potential to further refine the management strategy, further highlighting the importance of a unified approach both to relief of symptoms and regard for the disease's systemic expression.

4.3.1. Overview of Treatment Options

The treatment for Sjögren's syndrome is multidisciplinary and encompasses symptomatic relief as well as management of systemic manifestations. Symptomatic relief of xerostomia and dry eyes primarily includes over-the-counter saliva substitutes and prescription medications , such as pilocarpine, which stimulate the secretion of saliva. For individuals with extreme pain or inflammation, corticosteroids and NSAIDs are the most effective anti-inflammatory medications. Also, disease-modifying antirheumatic drugs (DMARDs) , such as hydroxychloroquine are employed to manage autoimmune manifestations, offering dual benefit in managing joint symptoms as well as the immune disorder. Biologic agents are being explored as therapeutic options, with evidence of effectiveness in decreasing severe manifestations of the syndrome, although closely monitored due to potential side effects and heightened risk of infection (Lin et al., 2023). The heterogeneity of the treatment context emphasizes the requirement for individualized therapy based on patient needs and symptom-specific, aimed at optimizing quality of life (Greenstein, 2017) (Figure 4.11).

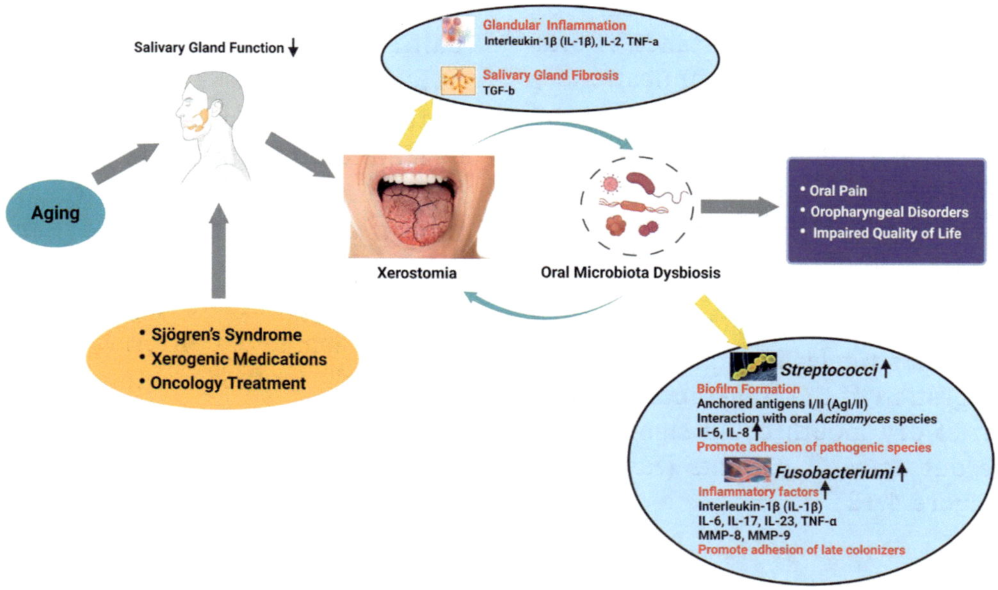

Figure 4.11. Symptomatic relief for xerostomia and dry eye involves the use of over-the-counter artificial saliva substitutes and prescription medications , such as pilocarpine, which stimulate saliva production.

Source: https://www.mdpi.com/ijms/ijms-25-12815/article_deploy/html/images/ijms-25-12815-g003.png.

4.3.2. Symptomatic Relief for Dry Eyes

Dry eye patients, particularly those with Sjögren's Syndrome, may develop significant discomfort that is debilitating in regard to daily function. Symptom control is desirable in the treatment of this disorder, and several forms of treatment exist. Artificial tears remain a cornerstone of treatment, providing lubrication and hydration and symptom relief. However, more recent advances highlight the role of immunomodulatory agents , such as cyclosporine A (CsA), which are increasingly recognized for their therapeutic potential in managing underlying inflammation of dry eye syndrome. Clinical evidence suggests that CsA not only enhances tear secretion but also patient-reported symptom scores, and thus it has great promise as a treatment option (Bouzoukis et al., 2008). Moreover, understanding the multifactorial etiology of xerostomia ; an Sjögren's Syndrome comorbidity often seen in patients, would be key in the decision-making process for treatment modalities. As technology advances, inclusion of symptomatic and disease-modifying therapies will be essential in optimizing patient outcomes.

4.3.3. Management of Dry Mouth

Dry mouth management, particularly for Sjögren's Syndrome, should include a holistic approach based on symptomatic relief and enhancing the quality of life in patients suffering from this condition. This autoimmune dysfunction syndrome of decreased salivary gland activity requires interventions that reverse levels of moisture and minimize pain. One of the primary measures involves the use of saliva substitutes and stimulants, which may provide temporary relief from xerostomia. Additionally, it is necessary to educate patients about the importance of oral hygiene to prevent further complications , such as dental caries and infections. Current research has shown the possible benefits of interprofessional education (IPE) programs that allow for increased awareness among healthcare providers regarding oral signs of systemic illnesses like Sjögren's Syndrome, thereby translating to improved care practices and team management strategies (Rothmund, 2016). With the integration of these methods, holistic management of dry mouth could significantly enhance the outcomes of patients (Renner et al., 1997) (Figure 4.12).

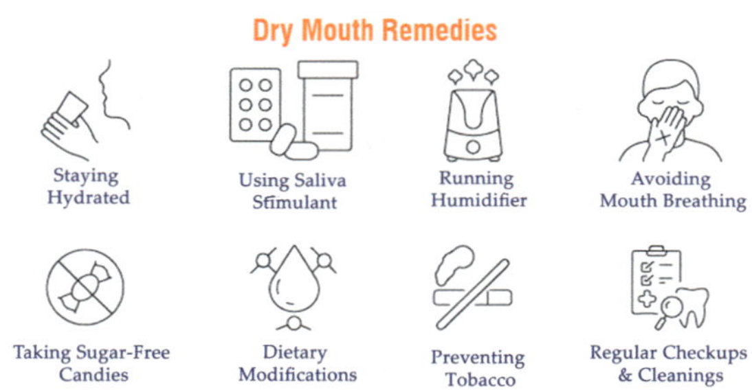
Dry Mouth Remedies
Staying Hydrated
Using Saliva Stimulant
Running Humidifier
Avoiding Mouth Breathing
Taking Sugar-Free Candies
Dietary Modifications
Preventing Tobacco
Regular Checkups & Cleanings

Figure 4.12. Dry mouth remedies.

Source: https://www.yashodahospitals.com/wp-content/uploads/2025/03/Dry-Mouth-Understanding-the-Symptoms_Body-2-1.png.

4.3.4. Pharmacological Treatments

Management of the polymeric symptoms of Sjögren's Syndrome (SD) often necessitates a multidisciplinary approach to pharmacologic treatments, aimed at alleviating individualized symptoms while improving patients' quality of life in general.

Initial treatment often addresses dryness symptoms and includes, for instance, local lubrication of the eyes and mouth. Systemic treatments, including anti-inflammatory drugs, can decrease autoimmune responses and manage systemic manifestations. The response emphasizes the individualized treatment, reaffirming the importance of facilitating individuals to be actively engaged in the control and management of their condition by maintaining, promoting, and stimulating secretions and protecting them from the damaging effects of the disease (Benjamin et al., 2025). Furthermore, ongoing pharmacological research continues to explore new therapies that are capable of delivering additional relief, particularly in those with more established symptoms, thereby being an integral part of overall management strategies for SD (Benjamin et al., 2024). Overall, a well-coordinated pharmacological approach is crucial to optimize patient outcomes for Sjögren's Syndrome.

4.3.5. Role of Lifestyle Modifications

Lifestyle modification is a key element in the management of Sjögren's Syndrome, which is a systemic autoimmune disorder characterized by dry eyes and mouth. Patients can benefit from the introduction of interventions that enhance their overall state as well as alleviate symptoms. For instance, the use of humidifiers and hydration can enhance the pain associated with dry mucous membranes, and the frequent application of artificial tears can provide symptomatic relief. Also, dietary modifications that include nutrient-dense foods can support immunity and overall health, thereby offering a natural way to treat this chronic disease. Furthermore, routine exercise can improve circulation and minimize fatigue, which are common complaints of Sjögren's Syndrome patients.

As dry eye disease is increasing with many systemic medications, including anti-psychotic medications that have been found to have a prevalence of 32% in patients (Jena et al., 2017), it becomes necessary to conduct routine eye checks to monitor and follow up accordingly on patient care (Lin et al., 2023) (Figure 4.13).

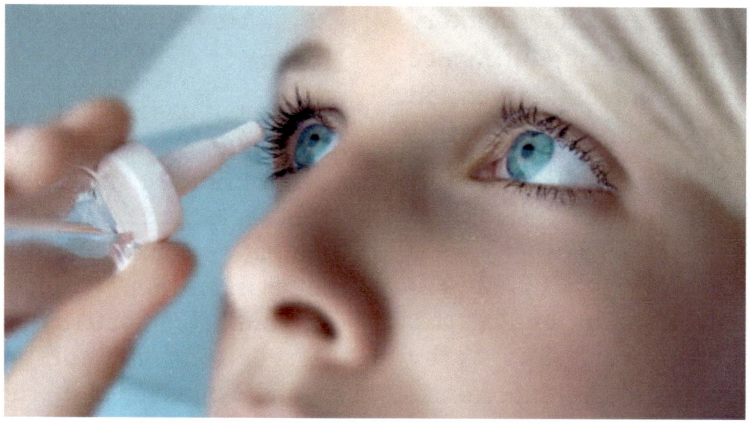

Figure 4.13. Maintaining hydration and utilizing humidifiers can alleviate the discomfort associated with dry mucous membranes, while regular use of artificial tears can provide symptomatic relief.

Source: https://lh3.googleusercontent.com/proxy/hyP7KM9zw2Unlez OMW4f99pCyEjN8zuxCaM6VG4LzFSM2l2XQDMRzipizKCblxy6Nk1KIrM gKn2cnbK95e4b1rh jWDENbYxo2LKvR8qC34vtO3MZFw.

4.3.6. Importance of Regular Monitoring

Close follow-up is critical to the management of Sjogren's Syndrome because it allows doctors to keep track of the progression of the disease and intervene early in the event of looming complications. Without frequent check-ups, patients risk encountering underdiagnosed symptoms , such as sensorineural hearing loss, which is discovered to affect a high number of patients with primary Sjogren's Syndrome, and indicates the vulnerability to severe impairment of hearing (Thanooja, 2012).

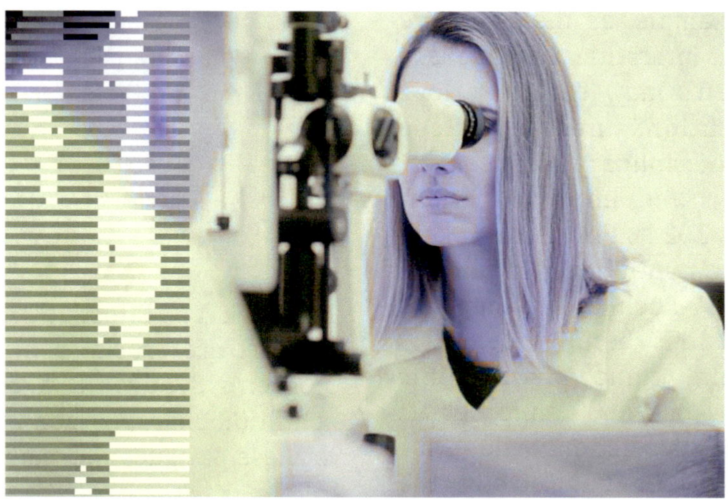

Figure 4.14. Regular monitoring is crucial for managing Sjogren's Syndrome, as it allows healthcare providers to track the progression of the disease and promptly address emerging complications.

Source: https://juniceyecare.com.au/wp-content/uploads/2023/12/sjogren-syndrome-treatment.jpg.

This emphasizes the need to follow auditory function as well as traditional symptoms since early detection can lead to timely intervention that minimizes disease impacts. Further, measuring the association between major immunological markers and symptom onset can enhance personalized treatment regimens (Soyza et al., 2018). Regular check-ups do not just guarantee active management of Sjogren's Syndrome but also empower patients by involving them in their healthcare experience, generating more understanding of their disease and the necessity to be cautious in protecting their quality of life (Figure 4.14).

4.3.7. Multidisciplinary Approach to Care

An interdisciplinary management of care is essential in the management of Sjögren's Syndrome, a multi-factorial autoimmune condition with symptoms of dry mouth and eyes, among other systemic signs. The strategy is through care coordination by multi-disciplinary healthcare providers like rheumatologists, ophthalmologists, dentists, and pulmonologists in an attempt to address the numerous aspects of the disease. For example, as the literature on autoimmune-linked interstitial lung disease (ILD) suggests, Sjögren's may lead to serious pulmonary complications needing close observation and interdisciplinary management to avert exacerbation and improve patient outcomes (Good et al., 2024). Furthermore, the comorbidity of Sjögren's with other conditions leads to misdiagnosis, such as in the case of lacrimal gland lesions being incorrectly attributed to lacrimal gland pleomorphic adenoma rather than Sjögren's (Cannon et al., 2010). Thus, combined care not only allows for enhanced diagnostic efficiency but also plots the treatment modalities according to individualized patient needs, ultimately enhancing their quality of life.

4.3.8. Patient Education and Support

Patient education and care success is critical in Sjögren's Syndrome management, a complex autoimmune condition characterized by dryness, fatigue, and pain. Research indicates that patients have intense sleep disturbances that worsen their general health and function (Carvajal et al., 2018). Tailored educational interventions, including methods , such as cognitive behavioral therapy for insomnia, may allow patients to better control their symptoms and improve sleep. Furthermore, evidence shows that patient empowerment and enhancing access to educational resources are crucial in facilitating engagement with activities of daily living (Abourazzak et al., 2018). By treating the unique challenges posed by Sjögren's Syndrome with whole-person support systems, physicians can inform patients more about their illness and improve the overall quality of life. In addition to assisting patients in alleviating their symptoms, such multifaceted treatments also enhance patient and family resilience and social support (Figure 4.15).

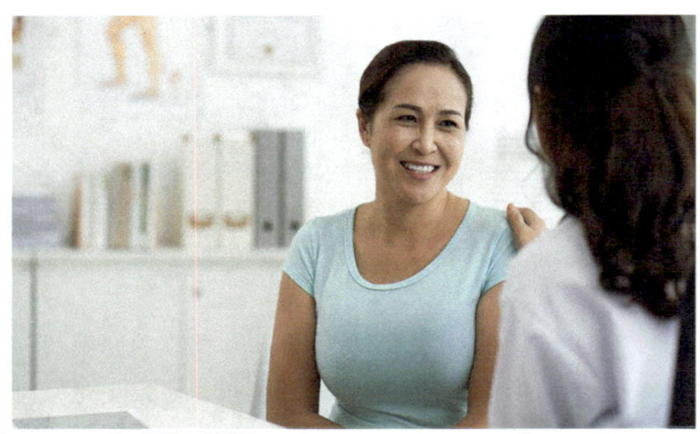

Figure 4.15. Effective patient education and support are crucial components in managing Sjögren's Syndrome, a complex autoimmune condition characterized by symptoms , such as dryness, fatigue, and pain.

Source: https://magazine.medlineplus.gov/images/uploads/main_images/sjogrens-what-you-need-to-know.jpg.

4.3.9. Emerging Therapies and Research

In recent years, novel therapies and research have made significant advances in the diagnosis and management of Sjögren's Syndrome, a systemic autoimmune disease that almost exclusively affects exocrine glands. Researchers are exploring new biologic treatments targeting novel pathways in the autoimmune mechanism. As an example, innovations in mitogen-activated kinase pathway blockade have produced promising early results, enhancing symptom control and reducing the activity of the disease in affected individuals (Blake et al., 2022). In addition, genomic approaches utilized in similar inflammatory conditions, such as inflammatory bowel disease, provide insights into potential mechanisms of treatment challenges and response variability, paving the way for personalized treatment in Sjögren's Syndrome as well (Lin et al., 2023). These advances not only promise better patient outcomes but also elevate our general understanding of the pathogenesis and systemic effects of the disease, paving the way for more optimal treatment patterns in the future.

Test Your Knowledge

1. How is fatigue managed in patients with Sjögren's syndrome?
2. What role does corticosteroid therapy play in systemic involvement?

4.4. Complications and Comorbidities

Learning Outcome

1. Understand potential complications of Sjogren's syndrome;
2. Focus on the increased risk of lymphoma;
3. Learn association with other autoimmune diseases;
4. Know the impact on quality of life;
5. Explain psychological effects of the disease;
6. Describe oral health complications;
7. Focus on musculoskeletal manifestations;
8. Identify neurological complications;
9. Discuss long-term prognosis.

Understanding the complications and comorbidities associated with Sjögren's syndrome is vital to improving patient outcomes and management. The patients with this autoimmune disorder are usually afflicted by secondary medical conditions, for instance, increased susceptibility to infection and risk of glandular-associated complications, including lymphoma. Research has also established that Sjögren's syndrome patients experience a greater prevalence of various comorbidities, including hypertension and complicated infections, worsened by immunosuppressive therapy commonly used against autoimmune disorders (Greenstein, 2017). Furthermore, as shown in experience with other connective tissue diseases, such as in pregnancy, interdependence of the complications leads to a complex clinical condition that necessitates a worldwide approach strategies (Jha & Chaudhari, 2020). The interaction among the factors underscores the necessity for ongoing monitoring and tailor-made interventions in an attempt to avoid injury and enhance the quality of life for those involved.

4.4.1. Potential Complications of Sjogren's Syndrome

Sjögren's Syndrome, which is most widely recognized to induce dry mouth and eyes, has multifaceted implications that affect numerous body systems. The chronic inflammation associated with the syndrome can lead to increased incidence of eye surface disorders, including keratoconjunctivitis sicca, which can significantly impair vision and decrease quality of life (Chandrasekaran et al., 2024). Patients also typically have systemic complications , such as fatigue, arthralgias, and predisposition to other autoimmune diseases. A more recent study underlines the potential involvement of CD4+ T lymphocyte autophagy in disease progression, in correlation with the intensity of Sjögren's complications (Bhattacharya et al., 2017). This increased awareness of complications supports the necessity of a holistic approach to treatment, addressing both symptoms and immune dysregulation at its core in order to enhance patient outcomes in those with this chronic condition (Figure 4.16).

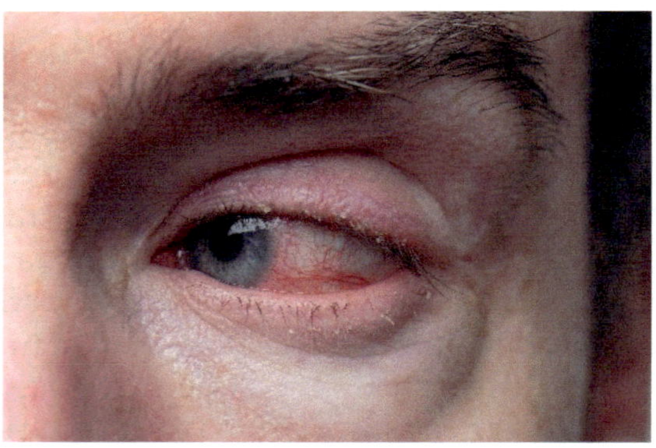

Figure 4.16. The chronic inflammation associated with the syndrome may lead to increased risks of ocular surface diseases, including keratoconjunctivitis sicca, which can significantly impair vision and diminish quality of life

Source: https://www.nyclasik.com/wp-content/uploads/2022/07/blepharitis.jpg.

4.4.2. Increased Risk of Lymphoma

Sjogren's syndrome, a condition that is autoimmune in nature and mostly affects exocrine glands, has in more recent times been discovered to be associated with an extremely high risk for lymphoproliferative disorders, particularly lymphoma. This explains why doctors must use utmost care in following Sjogren's patients for signs of malignant transformation, a very common occurrence in early Non-Hodgkin Lymphoma. A study indicates that primary malignant lymphomas, particularly those that arise in the salivary glands , such as the parotid, remain undiagnosed until surgery is needed, leading to delays in treatment (Cicero et al., 2011). Moreover, patients diagnosed with Sjogren's syndrome usually come with a multitude of comorbidities, which may enhance their risk of developing cancerous diseases, including lymphoma (Greenstein, 2017). Therefore, management based on a comprehensive approach that includes periodic screening and patient activation on symptoms of lymphoma is necessary to maximize outcomes in this high-risk group.

4.4.3. Association with Other Autoimmune Diseases

The association with other conditions of autoimmune nature augments evidence for the intricate nature of immune network interactions within autoimmune pathology. Sjögren's patients frequently present with comorbidities , such as rheumatoid arthritis, systemic lupus erythematosus, and thyroid diseases, suggesting a shared immunological mechanism. The autoimmune process of Sjögren's, which is mediated primarily by T-helper lymphocytes targeted to exocrine glands, also copies the pathogenesis of other autoimmune conditions, including those immunoglobulin G4-related conditions that involve salivary and other glandular organs as well (Gallo et al., 2017). In addition, it has been shown in recent research that the disrupted gut microbiota can profoundly affect immune modulation in various autoimmune diseases, including the dry eye symptoms that occur in many Sjögren's patients (Choi et al., 2020). This interconnectivity of autoimmune diseases not only highlights the clinical challenge posed by diagnosis as well as management but also emphasizes the necessity of adopting a holistic approach in intervention for management (Figure 4.17).

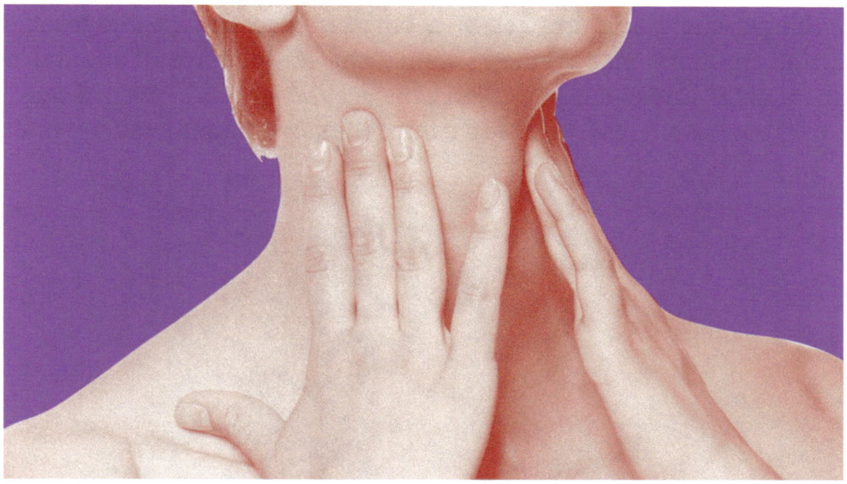

Figure 4.17. Patients with Sjögren's frequently exhibit comorbid conditions , such as rheumatoid arthritis, systemic lupus erythematosus, and thyroid disorders, suggesting a shared underlying immunological mechanism.

Source: https://jnj-content-lab2.brightspotcdn.com/dims4/default/5e0ee3b/2147483647/strip/true/crop/1920x1080+0+0/resize/1440x810!/quality/90/?url=https%3A%2F%2Fjnj-production-jnj.s3.us-east-1.amazonaws.com%2Fbrightspot%2F07%2F4e%2F73c278334ac5ae4ce708a90f9645%2F0924-sjogrens-disease-tone-1.png.

4.4.4. Impact on Quality of Life

The quality of life is significantly impaired by Sjogren's syndrome, predominantly due to its disabling features , such as chronic dryness of the mouth and eyes, which have a profound impact on daily living activity functioning and emotional well-being. It frustrates individuals and makes them socially withdrawn since they may not be able to communicate and socialize effectively. Studies indicate a highly significant proportion of patients with moderate to severe dry eyes, with significant evidence of corneal surface damage and discomfort, emphasizing the need for correct management procedures (Chandrasekaran et al., 2024). In addition, comorbidities that are related, such as musculoskeletal aches and fatigue, also play a role in enhancing the overall decrease in quality of life among patients and hence in requiring integrated care approaches that tackle both the physical and mental aspects of disease (Lin et al., 2023). It is thus essential to determine and tackle such multifaceted effects to enhance patient care and treatments.

4.4.5. Psychological Effects of the Disease

The psychiatric manifestations of Sjogren's Syndrome extend beyond its somatic presentations and significantly affect the patient's mental status and quality of life. Depression and anxiety also occur among patients, primarily due to the chronic pain owing to symptoms , such as xerostomia and xerophthalmia, resulting in withdrawal from society and isolation. The unpredictability of flare-ups aggravates stress levels, and it becomes difficult for people to manage daily activities. According to research, patients may feel overwhelmed as they struggle with the challenges of this autoimmune disease, which can deteriorate their coping ability and resilience (Basu et al., 2018). Moreover, the psychological impact of a chronic disease like Sjogren's Syndrome tends to necessitate multidisciplinary management, hence the importance of mental health care along with conventional medical interventions (Choudhary et al., 2023). Accordingly, management of the psychological components is essential for comprehensive patient management (Figure 4.18).

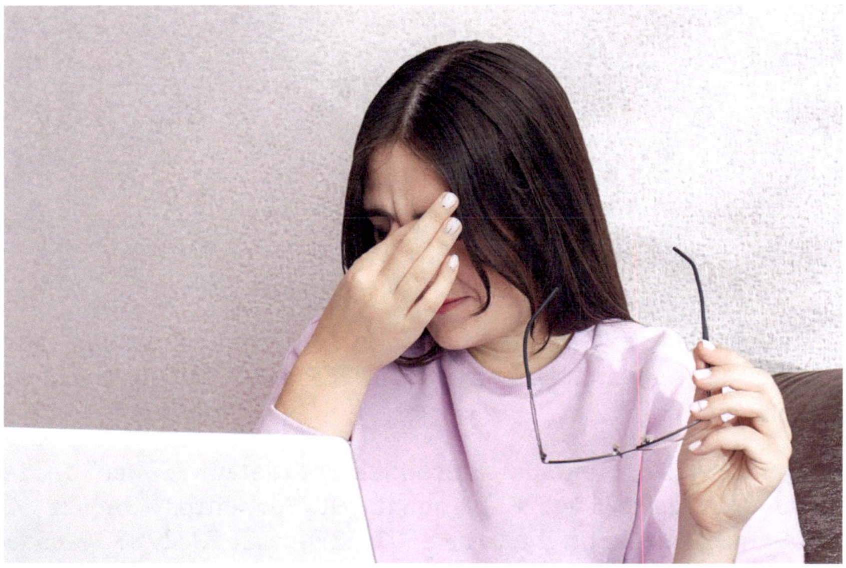

Figure 4.18. Patients often experience anxiety and depression, primarily due to the chronic discomfort caused by symptoms , such as xerostomia and xerophthalmia, which can lead to social withdrawal and a sense of isolation.

Source: https://mydr.com.au/wp-content/uploads/2013/02/sjogrens_syndrome_orig-e1559717501632.jpeg.

4.4.6. Oral Health Complications

Sjogren's Syndrome is characterized by serious oral complications of health, primarily due to its effect on exocrine glands that leads to xerostomia or dryness of the mouth. The syndrome not only damages the salivary function but also makes the patient more susceptible to dental caries, periodontal disease, and fungal infections. Research has shown that systemic autoimmune patients, to which Sjogren's is a case, have a considerably higher prevalence of periodontal disease; 99.2% of autoimmune patients presented with gingivitis versus 85.5% in non-autoimmune patients (Kumar et al., 2011). Further, xerostomia impacts the oral microflora as well, further increasing the likelihood of bacterial infection and dental caries. Furthermore, studies have also shown that sensorineural hearing loss, which is a common finding among Sjogren's patients, is also commonly accompanied by the presence of specific autoantibodies, which indicate the relationship between oral health status and the general manifestations of the condition (Thanooja, 2012). Hence, thorough dental care and follow-up are recommended for these patients.

4.4.7. Musculoskeletal Manifestations

The musculoskeletal manifestations of Sjögrens syndrome are notable in frequency and impact on the patients' quality of life. Joint pain, stiffness, and inflammation are common complaints, affecting approximately 30-50% of patients with autoimmune disease.

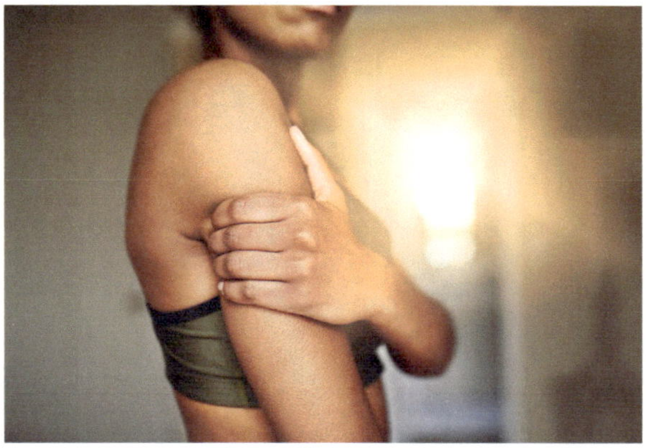

Figure 4.19. Joint pain, stiffness, and inflammation are commonly reported symptoms, affecting approximately 30-50% of individuals with this autoimmune condition.

Source: https://www.health.com/thmb/PKwZTXvF-HV_8PWgkRpSSdlhbOw=/1500x0/filters:no_upscale():max_bytes(150000):strip_icc()/GettyImages-636083506-2000-385caefb6262485683605763ab537f2b.jpg.

They can also mimic rheumatoid arthritis, making diagnosis and treatment more difficult. Of notable interest, musculoskeletal findings may even comprise weakness and fatigue of the muscles, further complicating the clinical picture. Research indicates that patterns of antibodies, as reflected by the presence of anti-SS-A and anti-SS-B antibodies, can correlate with such findings, suggesting a causative immunological link. Also, the interaction between the severity of musculoskeletal symptoms and systemic inflammation has been documented and proves the importance of careful clinical assessment in their identification in the case of Sjögrens syndrome patients (Archimandritis et al., 2002; Thanooja, 2012). The knowledge of these manifestations is necessary for the creation of individualized therapeutic regimens aiming at alleviation of patient discomfort and maximization of functional status (Figure 4.19).

4.4.8. Neurological Complications

Neurological Sjögren's Syndrome complications may significantly impact the quality of life, which may manifest in various forms as cognitive dysfunction, neuropathies, or central nervous system involvement. These are frequently a result of the autoimmune pathology of the disease, with resultant nervous system inflammation and damage. For instance, studies show the changes that can be experienced by the patients can be detected by top-level imaging techniques like MR-spectroscopy that capture metabolic changes during exacerbation of neurological symptoms. The imaging has also been used with success to follow related autoimmune diseases, thus reinforcing its potential in Sjögren's Syndrome treatment (Caramia et al., 2018). Additionally, the prevalence of comorbidity, particularly infections and immunologic complications, contributes to the neurological load in these patients, as observed in some populations studied on systemic lupus erythematosus (Greenstein, 2017). This calls for rigorous neurological assessment and multidisciplinary care in treating Sjögren's Syndrome patients.

4.4.9. Long-Term Prognosis

The long-term prognosis for patients with Sjogren's Syndrome is influenced by various factors, including the disease's systemic involvement and potential complications, such as the development of lymphoproliferative disorders. While many individuals experience manageable symptoms primarily affecting exocrine glands, there is a notable risk of primary malignant lymphoma, particularly involving the salivary glands. As highlighted in studies, early-stage Non-Hodgkin Lymphoma of the parotid gland often exhibits an excellent prognosis, achieving a loco-regional control rate of 87.5% following appropriate management strategies (Cicero et al., 2011). Additionally, understanding the autoimmune mechanisms underlying Sjogren's can illuminate long-term outcomes and therapeutic approaches, particularly as the interplay between autoimmune processes and chronic conditions like COVID-19 has garnered attention in recent discussions (Mahroum et al., 2022). Thus, continuous monitoring and interdisciplinary management are vital for optimizing long-term health in individuals with Sjogren's Syndrome.

Test Your Knowledge

1. How does the disease affect renal function (e.g., interstitial nephritis)?
2. What are the cardiovascular risks associated with chronic inflammation in Sjögren's?

Summary

Sjogren's syndrome is a multifaceted autoimmune condition with extensive quality of life compromise for the majority of individuals through its signature clinical manifestations of dry eyes and dry mouth. The complexity of the involvement of its etiology, particularly the role of innate immunity and invariant natural killer T cells, underscores the need for ongoing studies to demystify the precise mechanisms of the disease process (L et al., 2019). Furthermore, demarcation of Sjogren's syndrome from overlapping syndromes , such as burning mouth syndrome, highlights the importance of accurate diagnostic markers that can aid in early intervention (Ji et al., 2017). With growing knowledge on underlying pathophysiology and exploration of potential biomarkers, the medical community will be able to refine diagnostic accuracy and outcomes in patients. Future research should be directed in these fields for enhancing therapy and relief for patients of this disabling syndrome, eventually culminating in a more comprehensive approach to autoimmune disease treatment.

A complete realization of Sjogren's Syndrome recognizes several critical aspects highlighting its complexity and the impact on the patients. The autoimmune condition affects predominantly exocrine glands, leading to dry mouth and dry eyes and seriously deforms the quality of life. Recent advances in genome-based approaches have recognized some of the molecular pathways behind Sjogren's, which have enhanced our understanding of the treatment challenges and the therapy available. For example, therapeutic interventions, typically the same as for other autoimmune conditions, are to prevent inflammatory responses and treat complications , such as risk of infection, just like with inflammatory bowel disease therapy, where failure can occur (Lin et al., 2023). Additionally, the search for immunological dynamics of Sjogren's recalls the study of parasite-host dynamics in diseases , such as human African trypanosomiasis, with potential for cross-disciplinary understanding regarding immune modulation and outcome of treatments (Beverley et al., 2013).

KEY TERMS FROM THIS CHAPTER

- Cognitive behavioral therapy
- Cyclosporine A (CsA)
- Dryness
- Dysregulation
- Erythematosus
- Etiologic rationale
- Gland pleomorphic adenoma
- Glandular dysfunction
- Glandular tissue
- Guarantee active management
- Holistic management
- Human exocrine glands
- Immunomodulatory agents
- Immunomodulatory therapy
- Inflammation
- Interprofessional education (IPE)
- Interstitial lung disease (ILD)

Critical Thinking Questions

1. **Sjögren's syndrome is primarily characterized by dysfunction of which glands?**
   a. Endocrine glands
   b. Exocrine glands
   c. Lymph nodes
   d. Sweat glands
2. **The two hallmark symptoms of Sjögren's syndrome are:**
   a. Arthralgia and fatigue
   b. Xerostomia and xerophthalmia
   c. Myalgia and weight loss
   d. Fever and photosensitivity
3. **Which autoantibodies are most commonly associated with Sjögren's syndrome?**
   a. Anti-dsDNA and anti-Sm
   b. Anti-SSA (Ro) and anti-SSB (La)
   c. Anti-centromere and anti-Scl-70
   d. Rheumatoid factor and anti-MPO
4. **What test is used to evaluate tear production in suspected Sjögren's syndrome?**
   a. Slit-lamp exam
   b. Schirmer's test
   c. Fluorescein staining
   d. Fundoscopy
5. **Which of the following is considered a definitive diagnostic test for Sjögren's syndrome?**
   a. ANA test
   b. Salivary gland biopsy
   c. Chest X-ray
   d. ESR

Answers to Critical Thinking Questions

1. (b); 2. (b); 3. (b); 4. (b); 5. (b).

Short Answer Questions

1. What autoimmune mechanisms lead to glandular dysfunction in Sjögren's syndrome?
2. How do T and B lymphocytes contribute to tissue damage in Sjögren's?
3. What are the hallmark symptoms of primary Sjögren's syndrome?
4. How does secondary Sjögren's syndrome differ in clinical presentation?
5. What are the main goals of treatment in Sjögren's syndrome?
6. Which topical therapies are commonly used for dry eyes and dry mouth?
7. What is the most serious long-term complication of Sjögren's syndrome?
8. How does Sjögren's increase the risk of non-Hodgkin lymphoma?

References

1. Mahroum, N., Elsalti, A., Alwani, A., Seida, I., Alrais, M., Seida, R., Esirgun, S. N., Abali, T., Kiyak, Z., Zoubi, M., & Shoenfeld, Y. (2022). The mosaic of autoimmunity - Finally discussing in person. The 13th international congress on autoimmunity 2022 (AUTO13) Athens. *Autoimmunity reviews*, *21*(10), 103166. https://doi.org/10.1016/j.autrev.2022.103166 (accessed on 17th June 2025).
2. Abourazzak, H., Anderson, J., Bowman, S., Bravo, F., Brito-Zeron, P., Broadbent, J., Choi, J., et al. (2018). Mixed-methods study identifying key intervention targets to improve participation in daily living activities in primary Sjögren's syndrome patients. https://core.ac.uk/download/151208350.pdf (accessed on 17th June 2025).
3. Adamali, H., Dodds, N., Edey, A., Gunawardena, H., et al. (2016). Rituximab in autoimmune connective tissue disease-associated interstitial lung disease. https://core.ac.uk/download/83929026.pdf (accessed on 17th June 2025).
4. Alavi, A., & Axford, J. S. (2008). Glyco-biomarkers: potential determinants of cellular physiology and pathology. *Disease markers*, *25*(4-5), 193–205. https://doi.org/10.1155/2008/863032(accessed on 17th June 2025).
5. Allanore, Y., Allanore, Y., Assassi, S., del Galdo, F., et al. (2022). Type 1 interferon activation in systemic sclerosis: A biomarker, a target or the culprit. https://core.ac.uk/download/541347915.pdf (accessed on 17th June 2025).
6. Archimandritis, A., Czaja, A. J., Hansen, B. U., Jorgensen, C., Vitali, C., Vitali, C., Vogel, C., et al. (2002). The liver is a common non-exocrine target in primary Sjögren's syndrome: A retrospective review. https://core.ac.uk/download/pdf/3226420.pdf (accessed on 17th June 2025).
7. Arentz, G., Chataway, T. K., Colella, A., Gordon, T. P., et al. (2013). An immunodominant La/SSB autoantibody proteome derives from public clonotypes. https://core.ac.uk/download/43326799.pdf (accessed on 17th June 2025).
8. Barbera, L. L., Ciccia, F., Guggino, G., Pizzo, M. L., Rizzo, C., & Sireci, G. (2019). Invariant NKT cells and rheumatic disease: Focus on primary Sjögren syndrome. https://core.ac.uk/download/287859163.pdf (accessed on 17th June 2025).
9. Basu, N., Goni, M., Murray, A. D., Waiter, G., et al. (2018). Neural indicators of fatigue in chronic diseases: A systematic review of MRI studies. https://core.ac.uk/download/159067075.pdf (accessed on 17th June 2025).
10. Benjamin, S., Bombardieri, M., Bowman, S., Carty, S., Ciurtin, C., Crampton, B., Dawson, A., et al. (2025). British Society for Rheumatology guideline on management of adult and juvenile onset Sjögren disease. https://core.ac.uk/download/644552182.pdf (accessed on 17th June 2025).
11. Benjamin, S., Bombardieri, M., Bowman, S., Carty, S., et al. (2024). British Society for Rheumatology guideline on management of adult and juvenile onset Sjögren disease. https://core.ac.uk/download/603470350.pdf (accessed on 17th June 2025).
12. Berggreen, E., Delaleu, N. H., Hajdaragic-Ibricevic, H., Jonsson, R., et al. (2013). Impaired vascular responses to parasympathetic nerve stimulation and muscarinic receptor activation in the

submandibular gland in non-obese diabetic mice. https://core.ac.uk/download/479085814.pdf (accessed on 17th June 2025).

13. Beverley, S. M., Hoare, C. A., Jennings, F. W., Johnson, R. T., Poltera, A. A., & WHO. (2013). Imaging African trypanosomes. https://core.ac.uk/download/17049882.pdf (accessed on 17th June 2025).

14. Bhattacharya, A., Tzioufas, A. G., Finucci, A., Minniti, A., Rizzo, A., Alessandri, C., Li, C., et al. (2017). CD4 T lymphocyte autophagy is upregulated in the salivary glands of primary Sjögren's syndrome patients and correlates with focus score and disease activity. https://core.ac.uk/download/98348664.pdf (accessed on 17th June 2025).

15. Blake, J., Bremner, F. D., Carroll, A. S., D'Sa, S., et al. (2022). Neurology and the histiocytosis: A case of Rosai-Dorfman-Destombes disease. https://core.ac.uk/download/533458307.pdf (accessed on 17th June 2025).

16. Bogacz, R., Gaik, M., Magda, I., Osuch, K., et al. (2023). A focus on Sjögren's dry eye disease – Pathogenesis, patient management, and new advancements in therapy. https://core.ac.uk/download/587246699.pdf (accessed on 17th June 2025).

17. Bootsma, H., Glaudemans, A. W. J. M., Kroese, F. G. M., Mossel, E., et al. (2020). Imaging in primary Sjögren's syndrome. https://core.ac.uk/download/518766465.pdf (accessed on 17th June 2025).

18. Börjesson, O., Elvin, K., Fei, G. Z., Gunnarsson, I., et al. (2009). Predictors of the first cardiovascular event in patients with systemic lupus erythematosus–A prospective cohort study. https://core.ac.uk/download/pdf/8500115.pdf (accessed on 17th June 2025).

19. Bouzoukis, D. I., Diakonis, V. F., Kymionis, G. D., Siganos, D., et al. (2008). Treatment of chronic dry eye: Focus on cyclosporine. https://core.ac.uk/download/pdf/8299294.pdf (accessed on 17th June 2025).

20. Caffery, B. (2009). *Sjögren's Syndrome: A Clinical and Biochemical Analysis.* https://core.ac.uk/download/144143384.pdf (accessed on 17th June 2025).

21. Cannon, P., Davis, G., Dolman, P., Ghabrial, R., et al. (2010). Lesions mimicking lacrimal gland pleomorphic adenoma. https://core.ac.uk/download/12783642.pdf (accessed on 17th June 2025).

22. Caramia, F., Francia, A., Morreale, M., Pontecorvo, C., et al. (2018). H-magnetic resonance spectroscopy: Diagnostic tool in recurrent headache in systemic lupus erythematosus. A case report. https://core.ac.uk/download/188832576.pdf (accessed on 17th June 2025).

23. Carvajal, C. P., Goodchild, C. E., Hackett, K. L., Hackett, K. L., Hackett, K. L., Hackett, K. L., et al. (2018). Experience of sleep disruption in primary Sjögren's syndrome: A focus group study. https://core.ac.uk/download/146501626.pdf (accessed on 17th June 2025).

24. Chandrasekaran, B., Divya, D., Sri, D., Priya, R., & Kokila, D. (2024). A study on the prevalence of dry eye disease in newly diagnosed autoimmune disorders in a tertiary eye care hospital. https://core.ac.uk/download/640069956.pdf (accessed on 17th June 2025).

25. Jha, N., & Chaudhari, H. K. (2020). Connective tissue disorders in pregnancy: maternal and fetal perspective. *International Journal of Reproduction, Contraception, Obstetrics and Gynecology*, *9*(3), 1124–1131. https://doi.org/10.18203/2320-1770.ijrcog20200887(accessed on 17th June 2025).

26. Choi, S. H., IM, S. H., Kim, H. M., Kim, J., et al. (2020). IRT5 probiotics changes immune modulatory protein expression in the extra orbital lacrimal glands of an autoimmune dry eye mouse model. https://core.ac.uk/download/299810317.pdf (accessed on 17th June 2025).

27. Choudhary, R., Nagaraju, R., Nagi, R., Rathore, M., et al. (2023). Effectiveness of pharmacological interventions for Sjogren syndrome–A systematic review. https://core.ac.uk/download/570979994.pdf (accessed on 17th June 2025).

28. Cicero, G., Dispenza, C., Dispenza, F., Kulamarva, R., et al. (2011). Primary non-Hodgkin's lymphoma of the parotid gland. https://core.ac.uk/download/53270437.pdf (accessed on 17th June 2025).

29. Cockshott, E., Fox, P., Goodchild, C. E., Higgins, J. L., Newton, J. L., Deane, K. H. O., et al. (2015). A systematic review of non-pharmacological interventions for primary Sjögren's syndrome. https://core.ac.uk/download/41990342.pdf (accessed on 17th June 2025).

30. De Soyza, A., Strauss, A., Barker, A. F., Quittner, A. L., Wong, C., Wilson, C. B., Apfelbacher, C. J., et al. (2018). "The missing ingredient": The patient perspective of health-related quality of life in bronchiectasis: A qualitative study. https://core.ac.uk/download/195287509.pdf (accessed on 17th June 2025).

31. Gallo, A., Martellucci, S., Fusconi, M., Pagliuca, G., Greco, A., De Virgilio, A., & De Vincentiis, M. (2017). Sialendoscopic management of autoimmune sialadenitis: a review of literature. Trattamento scialendoscopico delle scialoadeniti autoimmuni: revisione della letteratura. *Acta otorhinolaryngologica Italica : organo ufficiale della Societa italiana di otorinolaringologia e chirurgia cervico-facciale, 37*(2), 148–154. https://doi.org/10.14639/0392-100X-1605(accessed on 17th June 2025).

32. Ji, E. H., Diep, C., Liu, T., Li, H., Merrill, R., Messadi, D., & Hu, S. (2017). Potential protein biomarkers for burning mouth syndrome discovered by quantitative proteomics. *Molecular pain, 13*, 1744806916686796. https://doi.org/10.1177/1744806916686796(accessed on 17th June 2025).

33. Good, S., Sparks, J., & Volkmann, E. (2024). Screening, diagnosis, and monitoring of interstitial lung disease in autoimmune rheumatic diseases: A narrative review. https://core.ac.uk/download/618291919.pdf (accessed on 17th June 2025).

34. Greenstein, L. S. (2017). Comorbidities in South Africans with systemic lupus erythematosus. https://core.ac.uk/download/188772450.pdf (accessed on 17th June 2025).

35. Langara, H. A. (2017). Insights into the molecular mechanism of Sjogren's syndrome. https://open.bu.edu/bitstream/2144/26241/5/Langara_bu_0017N_13150.pdf (accessed on 17th June 2025).

36. Lessard, C. J., Li, H., Ice, J. A., & Sivils, K. L. (2013). Interferons in Sjögren's syndrome: Genes, mechanisms, and effects. https://core.ac.uk/download/pdf/82852371.pdf (accessed on 17th June 2025).

37. Lin, S. (2023). Using genomic approaches to characterize the immune response to biologicals. https://core.ac.uk/download/590000217.pdf (accessed on 17th June 2025).

38. Löwhagen, O. (1999). Asthma and asthma-like disorders. https://core.ac.uk/download/pdf/82066054.pdf (accessed on 17th June 2025).

39. Mohana Priya, P. (2015). Study the prevalence of diabetic retinopathy and dry eye in diabetes

mellitus patients and comparing with duration and urea, creatinine level. https://core.ac.uk/download/235669308.pdf (accessed on 17th June 2025).

40. Punitha Ranjitham, S. (2018). Detection of antibodies to extractable nuclear antigens by ELISA for the diagnosis of connective tissue disorders in ANA positive patients. https://core.ac.uk/download/235668332.pdf (accessed on 17th June 2025).

41. Ramesh Kumar, S. G. (2011). A case-control study to compare the prevalence of periodontal disease in patients with and without systemic autoimmune diseases. https://core.ac.uk/download/235667294.pdf (accessed on 17th June 2025).

42. Renner, R. P., Shay, K., & Truhlar, M. R. (1997). Oropharyngeal candidiasis in the older patient. https://deepblue.lib.umich.edu/bitstream/2027.42/111172/1/j.1532-5415.1997.tb01517.x.pdf (accessed on 17th June 2025).

43. Roma, J. (2015). Diagnostic performance of dry eye tests in primary Sjogren's syndrome patients in Indian setting. https://core.ac.uk/download/235669314.pdf (accessed on 17th June 2025).

44. Rothmund, W. L. (2016). Oral manifestations of menopause: An interprofessional intervention for dental hygiene and physician assistant students. https://core.ac.uk/download/230656501.pdf (accessed on 17th June 2025).

45. Soumya Jena. (2017). Tear film analysis in patients on chronic anti-psychotic therapy. https://core.ac.uk/download/288215953.pdf (accessed on 17th June 2025).

46. Thanooja, C. V. (2012). Audiological profile in primary Sjogren's syndrome in an Indian setting. https://core.ac.uk/download/235655074.pdf (accessed on 17th June 2025).

47. Yakimenko, D. (2019). The role of autoimmune reactions in formation and progressing of Sjogren's syndrome as systemic damage of organism. https://core.ac.uk/download/287359025.pdf (accessed on 17th June 2025).

SYSTEMIC SCLEROSIS (SCLERODERMA)

5

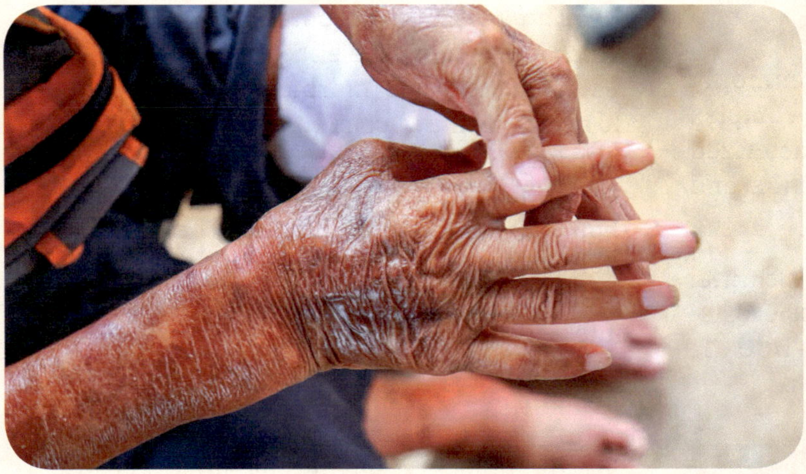

LEARNING OBJECTIVES

After studying this chapter, you will be able to:

1. Understand pathophysiology of systemic sclerosis
2. Focus on clinical manifestations
3. Learn diagnosis and assessment
4. Explain treatment and management

Introduction

Systemic sclerosis, or scleroderma, is a profound and complex autoimmune disease with pathological connective tissue growth and extensive fibrosis. Systemic sclerosis is one of the most dangerous expressions in the spectrum of the scleroderma disease and poses a significant clinical problem because of its high mortality and morbidity. The interrelationship between immune-inflammatory reactions and vascular damage leading to tissue fibrosis underscores the complex nature of the diseases. Researchers continue to want to understand the etiology and precipitating factors, which remain unknown, and therefore, it remains difficult to manage effectively. Although the management of many of the disease's complications has treatments, they are largely palliative rather than curative. Innovative approaches, such as immunosuppressive methodologies like autologous stem cell transplantation, have some benefit; however, consideration must be given for risk versus benefit, keeping in mind the complexities (Denton, 2016; Allanore et al., 2021). Systemic sclerosis insights are necessary to develop better therapeutic interventions (Figure 5.1).

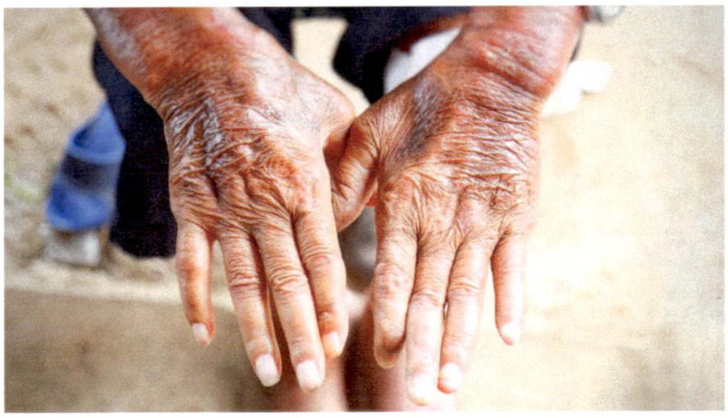

Figure 5.1. Systemic sclerosis, commonly known as scleroderma, represents a complex and severe autoimmune disorder characterized by aberrant connective tissue production and extensive fibrosis.

Source: https://i0.wp.com/post.healthline.com/wp-content/uploads/2022/03/sclerosis-scleroderma-systemic-sclerosis-body1.jpg?w=1155&h=1528.

5.1. Pathophysiology of Systemic Sclerosis

Learning Outcome

1. Understand immune system dysfunction
2. Discuss the role of fibrosis in scleroderma
3. Identify vascular changes and endothelial damage
4. Focus on genetic factors and susceptibility
5. Describe environmental triggers
6. Learn pathways of collagen production
7. Know the impact of inflammation
8. Discuss organ involvement mechanisms
9. Explain current research on pathophysiology

The pathophysiology of systemic sclerosis is a complex interaction of dysregulation of the immune system, vascular alterations, and generalized fibrosis with resultant severe organ dysfunction. The most important part of the process is myofibroblast function, which involves the laying down of the extracellular matrix and causing fibrosis in the affected tissue. Research has come to identify oxidative stress as the key factor in the pathogenesis of systemic sclerosis and has suggested that excessive production of reactive oxygen species can induce cellular senescence and hence also promote tissue damage and fibrosis (Piera-Velazquez & Jimenez, 2015). The disease is also associated with fibroproliferative vasculopathy, which exerts immense effects on circulation and results in extreme morbidity (Jimenez et al., 2013). It is the recent work that stresses the necessity of defining the molecular mechanisms of myofibroblast activation and the pathways they take, as this will ultimately result in new therapeutic avenues to preclude the disabling effects of the disease and improve patient outcomes.

5.1.1. Immune System Dysfunction

The immune system derangement observed in systemic sclerosis (scleroderma) is a key feature in the pathological process and course of the disease. Characterized as an autoimmune disease, it is an inappropriate immunological response that will end up in diffuse fibrosis and damage to most organ systems. Research pins down the combination of stressors in early life and subsequent hyper-arousal responses, these having been linked to immune dysfunction and thus show psychological stress can exacerbate scleroderma symptoms and management in general (Kearney & Hicks, 2016). Further, gastrointestinal tract involvement is a frequent complication, and this presents in up to 90% of patients, resulting in the generation of dysmotility that exacerbates malnutrition and quality of life deterioration (Tomcik & Oreska, 2019). These reviews illustrate the central role of immune dysfunction in systemic sclerosis, as immune dysregulation not only leads to tissue damage but also severe comorbidities that have a crucial impact on patient morbidity and mortality (Figure 5.2).

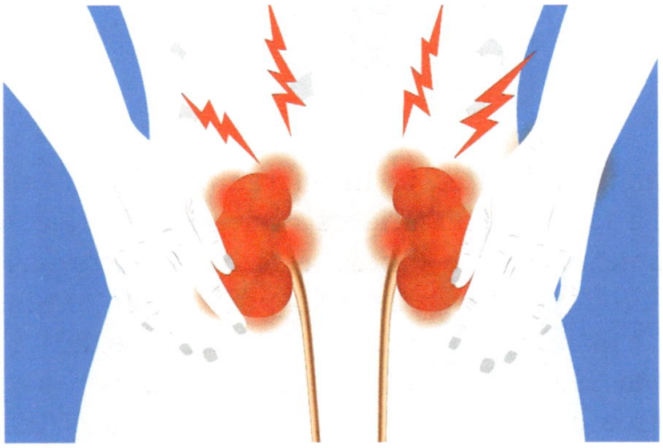

Figure 5.2. The immune system dysfunction observed in systemic sclerosis (scleroderma) significantly contributes to the disease's pathological progression and severity.

Source: https://creakyjoints.org/wp-content/uploads/0719_Gout-and-Kidney-Disease.jpg.

5.1.2. Role of Fibrosis in Scleroderma

Scleroderma fibrosis is a central process in which there is a complex interplay of cellular events leading to the excess production of collagen and extracellular matrix molecules. The resultant abnormal fibrotic response leads to thickening of the tissue and dysfunction of organs, a primary reason for morbidity and mortality in the disease. Critical factors implicated in the fibrotic process include oxidative stress, which initiates cellular senescence, and dysregulation of cytokines, inducing collagen synthesis. For instance, studies have demonstrated that oxidative stress has been established as an important mechanism that initiates the fibroproliferative vasculopathy observed in scleroderma, and that therapeutic intervention may be pivotal in treating oxidative damage. Moreover, the molecular basis of fibrosis, particularly the associations with interferon regulatory factor 5, indicates that genetic susceptibility to pathological fibrotic behavior plays a crucial role in disease susceptibility and phenotypic heterogeneity in scleroderma (; Gabrielli et al., 2013; Piera-Velazquez & Jimenez, 2015).

5.1.3. Vascular Changes and Endothelial Damage

The vasculopathy in systemic sclerosis (scleroderma) is a significant component of the disease's multifaceted pathophysiology, particularly secondary to endothelial damage. The damage is a key factor in precipitating a cascade of inflammatory processes and resultant fibrosis, causing impaired circulation and tissue ischemia. Endothelial cells have been thought to become stimulated through various stimuli, leading to the production of reactive oxidizing species (ROS), which are responsible for the vascular damage characteristic of both lc-SSc and dc-SSc (Gambardella et al., 2018).

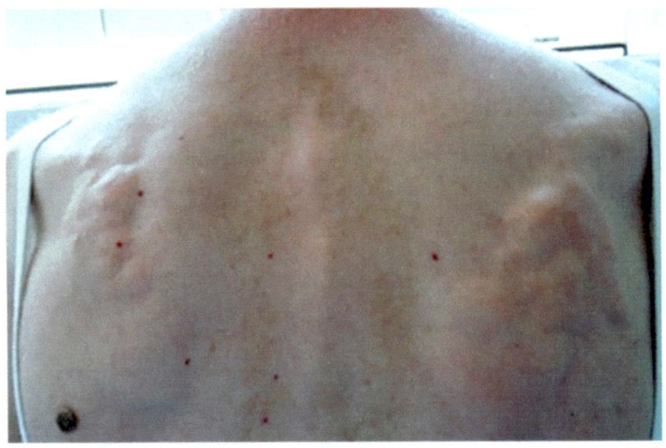

Figure 5.3. The vascular changes observed in systemic sclerosis (scleroderma) significantly contribute to the disease's complex pathophysiology, particularly through endothelial damage.

Source: https://reu.termedia.pl/f/fulltexts/190576/RU-62-190576-g002.jpg.

Further, gastrointestinal involvement is frequent in SSc, contributing to vascular impairment and establishing the key interaction between endothelial impairment and gastrointestinal manifestations (Abraham et al., 2017). The multiformality of such vascular alterations also demands ongoing study into the specific mechanisms of these alterations as a potential avenue for new therapies in minimizing endothelial injury and improving patient outcomes in systemic sclerosis (Figure 5.3).

5.1.4. Genetic Factors and Susceptibility

The genetic map of scleroderma shows important findings related to the hereditary factors for disease susceptibility. Various genetic loci responsible for systemic sclerosis have been detected based on recent studies, marking the etiologic complexity of the illness. Notably, a large-scale study with over 1,800 cases and 3,400 controls of scleroderma recognized six polymorphic amino acid positions and seven single nucleotide polymorphisms (SNPs) in the human leukocyte antigen (HLA) region to establish significant associations with SSc risk. Furthermore, the common path the genetic risk factors for different autoimmune diseases follow shows a shared pathway that would enhance our knowledge regarding systemic sclerosis when understood in autoimmunity (Richard-Miceli & Criswell, 2012). These findings not only outline previously mentioned genetic associations but also underscore the necessity of future investigation into the interaction of these genes in order to provide improved diagnostic and therapeutic strategies in the management of systemic sclerosis (Figure 5.4).

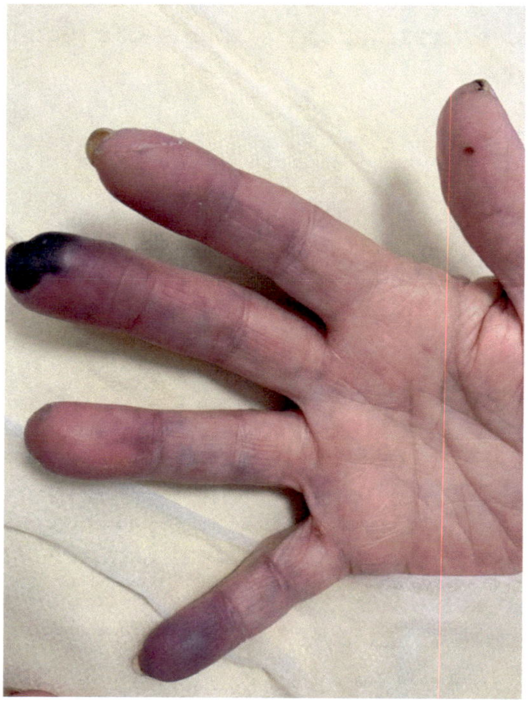

Figure 5.4. The genetic landscape of systemic sclerosis (scleroderma) reveals significant insights into the hereditary factors contributing to disease susceptibility.

Source: https://www.bjaed.org/cms/10.1016/j.bjae.2022.10.004/asset/1cceca41-ab64-412b-97a1-1938b24e350e/main.assets/gr2_lrg.jpg.

5.1.5. Environmental Triggers

The intricate interaction between environmental stimuli and systemic sclerosis (scleroderma) is currently recognized as a primary determinant of the disease's etiology. Environmental exposures, including chemical agents, viral infections, and certain foods, have been implicated in triggering and perpetuating scleroderma symptoms. For instance, the presence of transposable elements in the genome might be triggered by such environmental factors, potentially as a causative agent of the autoimmune mechanisms that characterize this disease (Macia et al., 2019). The reduced vitamin D status, which is characterized as an ordinary environmental factor, has also been revealed to be implicated in the severity and development of scleroderma. Vitamin D status has also been shown to be linked with inflammatory markers, suggesting a potential modulating effect on immune dysregulation (Cortese et al., 2015). Understanding these environmental interactions is critical for the application of targeted therapeutic strategies and patient care in systemic sclerosis.

5.1.6. Pathways of Collagen Production

The pathways of collagen production are crucially altered in systemic sclerosis (scleroderma), leading to fibrosis in excess characteristic of this complex disease. The target for such fibrosis is a variety of growth factors, such as transforming growth factor beta (TGF-β), connective tissue growth factor (CTGF), and platelet-derived growth factor (PDGF), that lead to the differentiation of myofibroblasts from fibroblasts. This event is central to collagen deposition; however, in systemic sclerosis, it is deranged, and there is overproduction of collagen and other extracellular matrix proteins. These pathologic changes ultimately compromise tissue structure and organ function, resulting in the multisystemic disease manifestations. These excessive fibrotic responses are also amplified by chronic inflammation, further obscuring the therapeutic rationale. Understanding the molecular mechanisms governing collagen production and the activity of myofibroblasts is important as it can pave the way for novel anti-fibrotic treatments aimed at this central feature of systemic sclerosis (Castro et al., 2010; Jimenez et al., 2013) (Figure 5.5).

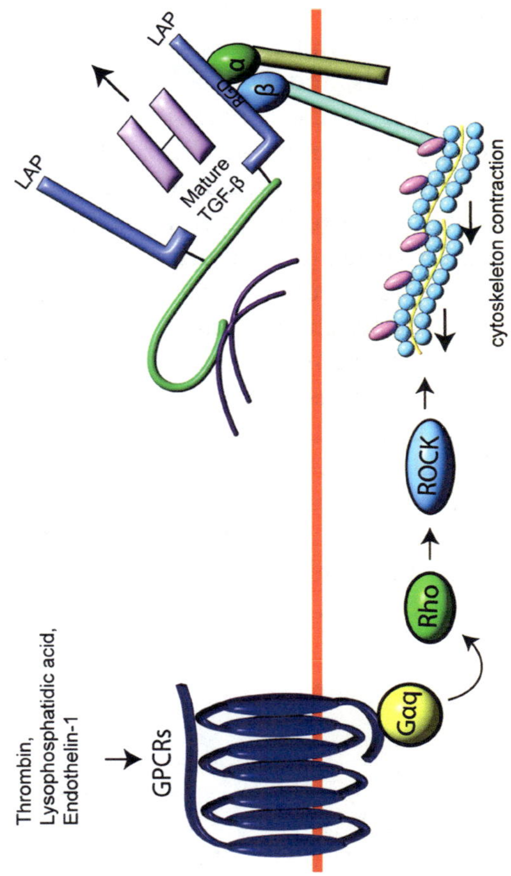

Figure 5.5. Central to this fibrotic process are various growth factors, notably transforming growth factor beta (TGF-β), connective tissue growth factor (CTGF), and platelet-derived growth factor (PDGF), which promote the differentiation of fibroblasts into myofibroblasts.

Source: https://media.springernature.com/lw1200/springer-static/image/art%3A10.1038%2Fs41401-024-01235-6/MediaObjects/41401_2024_1235_Fig4_HTML.png.

5.1.7. Impact of Inflammation

The complex role of inflammation in systemic sclerosis (scleroderma) has a significant influence on the severity and progression of the disease. The autoimmune disease is characterized by vasculopathy, along with fibrosis, pathways that are intrinsically linked to inflammatory pathways. Persistent inflammation has been implicated as part of the pathophysiology of interstitial lung disease, one of the most lethal threats to life in systemic sclerosis, and clinical phenotypes are associated with distinct inflammatory markers. Intriguingly, interleukin-6 (IL-6) has been considered the primary mediator of progression from inflammation to fibrosis, highlighting the connection between the two processes (Denton et al., 2020). Moreover, the presence of specific immune mediators and inflammatory cells, such as alternatively activated macrophages, also indicates that not just inflammation facilitates the process of fibrosis development but might also define the course of the disease (Bernstein et al., 2021). Understanding these inflammatory pathways is imperative in developing targeted therapeutic strategies, ultimately serving the patient's outcome in systemic sclerosis.

5.1.8. Organ Involvement Mechanisms

An understanding of the mechanisms of involvement of organs in systemic sclerosis (scleroderma) is necessary for optimal patient outcomes, as the complex illness has a predisposition to affect many internal organs, the most common of which is the gastrointestinal tract. Research has proven that gastrointestinal symptomatology is predominantly due to dysmotility, which may be dissociated from skin disease. It occurs in as many as 8% of patients, predominantly with disastrous gastrointestinal complications directly proportional to their mortality rates, with a survival rate of only 15%. Functional anti-muscarinic receptor autoantibodies have been recently identified as a new pathogenic pathway for this dysmotility in recent studies, with potential lines of focused therapies (Abraham et al., 2017). Apart from this, autoimmune systemic illness, like systemic sclerosis, also tends to be associated with audiovestibular manifestations like sensorineural hearing loss, making the clinical picture even more complex and underscoring the need for heightened scrutiny and appropriate treatment strategies (Adelchi et al., 2018). These observations enhance global insight into disease pathology and reinforce the search for effective therapies (Figure 5.6).

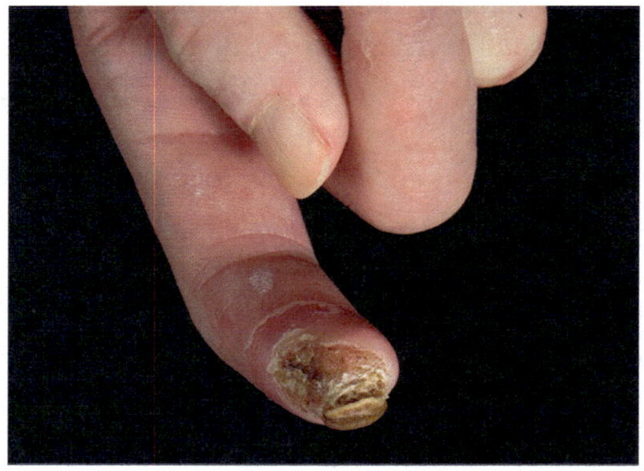

Figure 5.6. Understanding the mechanisms underlying organ involvement in systemic sclerosis (scleroderma) is crucial for improving patient outcomes, as this multifaceted disease often affects various internal organs, with the gastrointestinal tract being the most commonly involved.

Source: https://www.jaad.org/cms/10.1016/j.jaad.2021.10.065/asset/6295596c-b018-4e83-b0db-151bc23a6192/main.assets/gr5_lrg.jpg.

5.1.9. Current Research on Pathophysiology

Understanding the pathophysiology of systemic sclerosis (SSc) is crucial, as it is a combined result of genetic, environmental, and immunological factors. Recent studies have also highlighted the role of oxidative stress as a key contributor to the fibrotic process of the diseases. Evidence shows that an excess of reactive oxygen species may lead to cellular senescence, inducing a cascade of molecular reactions that promote the disability and death of SSc (Piera-Velazquez & Jimenez, 2015). Furthermore, socioeconomic factors, like exposure to tobacco, are also increasingly known to contribute to negative effects on disease severity and progression, although evidence is limited in this regard. Specifically, data on smoking's impact on pulmonary and cutaneous manifestations of SSc offer facts that can guide more effective therapies (Airó et al., 2018). Altogether, the evidence collectively indicates that lifestyle factors and oxidative stress need to be top priorities for future studies on the confusing pathophysiology of systemic sclerosis.

Test Your Knowledge

1. What is the role of fibroblast activation in systemic sclerosis?
2. How does excessive collagen deposition affect skin and organ function?

5.2. Clinical Manifestations

Learning Outcome

1. Understand skin changes and symptoms
2. Know gastrointestinal complications
3. Focus on pulmonary involvement
4. Discuss cardiac manifestations
5. Describe renal implications
6. Identify musculoskeletal symptoms
7. Focus on neurological effects
8. Define Raynaud's phenomenon
9. Describe quality of life considerations

Clinical presentation of systemic sclerosis (scleroderma) is heterogeneous and has the ability to significantly influence the quality of life of patients. Most impressively, gastrointestinal tract (GIT) involvement is a frequent complication, with symptoms secondary to dysmotility of any area of the GIT, resulting in a diverse range of disabling conditions , such as dysphagia and abdominal pain. Astoundingly, these GIT symptoms can occur independently of cutaneous involvement, complicating diagnosis and plans for management (Abraham et al., 2017). Also, sensorineural hearing loss can occur as one of the systemic autoimmune disorders in patients, which can present variably as sudden or fluctuant auditory loss, often accompanied by vestibular findings and tinnitus (Adelchi et al., 2018). The multisystem nature of such clinical presentations is an impetus for holistic treatment strategies with emphasis on symptomatic therapy, but highlighting the importance of detection and treatment of the diverse manifestations of this condition.

5.2.1. Skin Changes and Symptoms

Systemic sclerosis or scleroderma is very apparent through a number of cutaneous changes that are very visible and distressing to patients. Initial changes are thickening and tightening of the skin, or sclerodactyly, which affects the fingers and severely limits movement. At the same time , alterations like telangiectasia—dilatation of blood vessels visible on the skin's surface—are common, with cosmetic complaints. Also, sequelae like sicca syndrome can develop, which impair oral function and quality of life as mouth width and openings are reduced, generating eating and speech difficulties (Onesti et al., 2016). There is evidence that environmental factors, such as tobacco exposure, may increase skin and pulmonary involvement of the disease and therefore have an effect on the overall evolution of systemic sclerosis (Airó et al., 2018). This interplay of the symptoms portrays the complexity of managing systemic sclerosis and highlights the need for multidimensional management approaches (Figure 5.7).

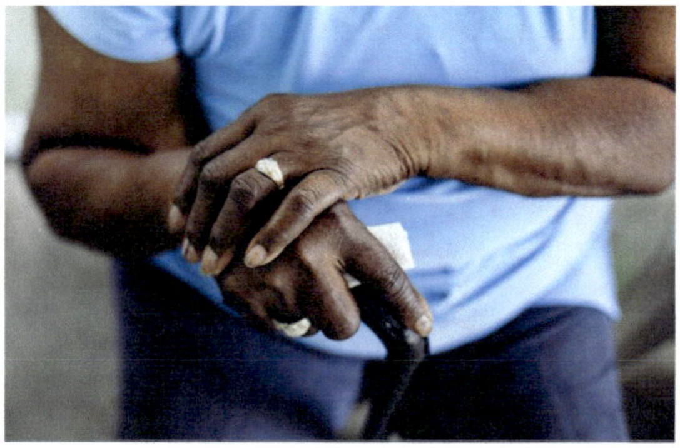

Figure 5.7. Patients may experience skin thickening and tightness, often referred to as sclerodactyly, which affects the fingers and can severely limit mobility.

Source: https://dims.healthgrades.com/dims3/MMH/bb6e16f/2147483647/strip/true/crop/883x575+70+0/resize/768x500!/quality/75/?url=https%3A%2F%2Fucmscdn.healthgrades.com%2Fb0%2F64%2F8340f55c087abb974b20022f469a%2Fhg-hands-on-cane-1296x728-header-1024x575.jpg.

5.2.2. Gastrointestinal Complications

The gastro-intestinal manifestations of systemic sclerosis (scleroderma) present serious challenges that can severely compromise the quality of life of patients. They are a consequence of progressive atrophy and fibrosis of the gastro-intestinal tract, leading to symptoms of dysphagia, gastroesophageal reflux, and constipation. The most prevalent is esophageal dysmotility and it occurs in over 90% of patients and complicate food ingestion and digestion. Additionally, studies have indicated a higher risk of more intense symptoms in specific groups, such as African Americans, who can experience pulmonary fibrosis and renal crises with gastroesophageal complications, demonstrating the multifaceted impact of the disease (Boin et al., 2017). Systemic symptoms could also be exacerbated with gastrointestinal participation, making treatment protocols more complex and requiring special interventions. Identifying these concerns is critical to effective management and improved patient outcomes, emphasizing the need for ongoing research into diverse modes of managing affected persons (Akin et al., 2018).

5.2.3. Pulmonary Involvement

Pulmonary disease is a major systemic sclerosis (SSc) problem, significantly affecting patient morbidity and mortality. The disorder often leads to complications , such as pulmonary fibrosis and pulmonary arterial hypertension, both of which may be insidious in onset and significantly compromise lung function. Most surprisingly, pulmonary fibrosis in SSc patients is quite common, with studies indicating that 43% of them are affected by this condition, often being related to specific serological features , such as positivity for anti-topoisomerase I (Boin et al., 2017).

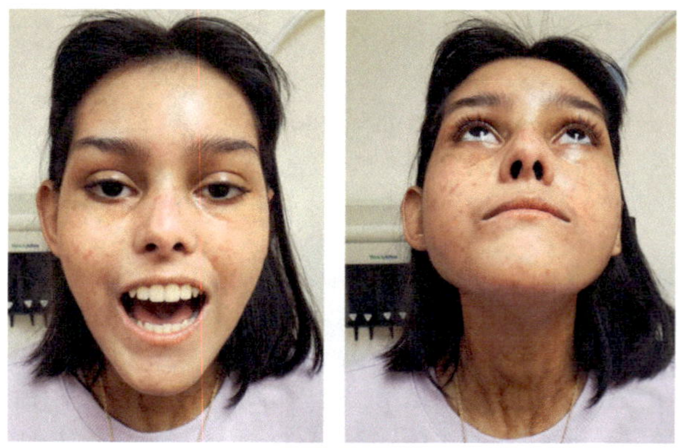

Figure 5.8. Pulmonary involvement is a critical concern in systemic sclerosis (SSc), significantly impacting patient morbidity and mortality.

Source: https://www.rheumatic.theclinics.com/cms/10.1016/j.rdc.2021.07.004/asset/fb921b10-f8dc-439f-9cf3-bf049f38302f/main.assets/gr3_lrg.jpg.

Moreover, restrictive ventilatory defect, expressed as FVC <50% predicted, demonstrates the severity of pulmonary disease in a proportion of patients. The challenge to diagnose and manage pulmonary involvement necessitates early detection for improved outcome, particularly since pulmonary complications can occur within the first few years of SSc development (Alabrudziński et al., 2025). Vigilance and early action are, therefore, essential in managing these potentially life-threatening manifestations of the disease (Figure 5.8).

5.2.4. Cardiac Manifestations

The cardiac involvement of systemic sclerosis (scleroderma) presents specific clinical challenges and adds to exacerbating patient morbidity and mortality. Among the cardiac sequelae, diastolic dysfunction is especially prevalent, followed by conduction blocks and pericardial effusion, often presenting in the first few years after the development of Raynauds phenomenon, the disease's hallmark symptom. Increased age and the presence of certain autoantibodies, particularly anti-topoisomerase, significantly increase the risk for these cardiac complications (Boin et al., 2017). Besides, in a study on an African American patient cohort, approximately 10% were found to have severe cardiac manifestations, further highlighting the heterogeneity of the diseases as well as their calamitous impact in multicultural populations (Boin et al., 2017). Thus, early identification and monitoring of the cardiac involvement are critical in systemic sclerosis management, which underscores the need for individualized therapeutic strategies to control these emerging cardiovascular risks.

5.2.5. Renal Implications

In systemic sclerosis (scleroderma), renal implications are particularly concerning as renal crisis is an occasionally lethal manifestation of the illness. Studies indicate the prevalence of scleroderma renal crisis among populations affected is relatively varied; for instance, it has been reported to be as much as 7% in African American individuals, significantly higher than the reported 2% that was discovered in European populations, indicating the need to observe patients closely across groups (Boin et al., 2017). The structural alterations of the kidneys in scleroderma typically lead to hypertension and worsening renal failure, calling for identification of the involved underlying biomarkers like Galectin-3 that may be involved in the renal fibrosis and inflammation pathology mechanisms (Bellotti et al., 2018). Thus, the management of renal complications in systemic sclerosis not only serves to control immediate threats to health but emphasizes the need for patient-specific therapeutic interventions to ensure improved patient outcomes within various populations (Figure 5.8).

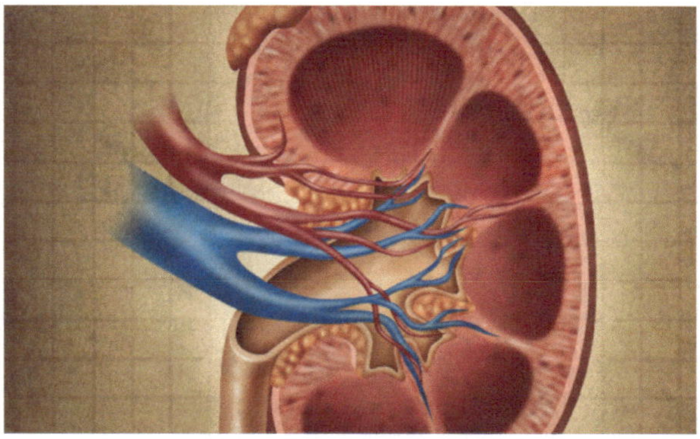

Figure 5.9. In systemic sclerosis (scleroderma), renal implications are particularly concerning, as renal crisis represents a potentially life-threatening manifestation of the disease.

Source: https://d148x66490prkv.cloudfront.net/c360/imported/transfer/kidney_5.png.

5.2.6. Musculoskeletal Symptoms

Musculoskeletal symptoms are the most notable feature of systemic sclerosis (scleroderma), with a severe effect on patient quality of life. Symptomatic joint pain, stiffness, and swelling result from the pathologic fibrosis that defines the disease. Diffuse systemic sclerosis is particularly associated with more widespread musculoskeletal disease, as indicated by a cohort study showing that 57% of African American patients presented with severe disease manifestations, including painful arthralgias that were compounded by abnormalities in the connective tissue (Boin et al., 2017). In addition, the impact of oral manifestations, such as microstomia, may also play a role in making the musculoskeletal symptoms more complex by limiting the capacity of patients to engage proactively in physical activities (Onesti et al., 2016). Such integration of musculoskeletal symptoms highlights the need for comprehensive management plans to address both the physical and psychosocial effects that affect patients with systemic sclerosis. These are required to improve overall patient outcomes and quality of life.

5.2.7. Neurological Effects

Neurological presentations of systemic sclerosis (SSc) can significantly impact patients' quality of life and are expressed through a pattern of symptoms that are physically and emotionally disabling. Cognitive dysfunction, neuropathy, and erectile dysfunction (ED) are frequent complications and, as such, highlight the multi-systemic effect of SSc on neurology. Interestingly, studies indicate that in men with SSc, a shocking 38% have severe ED, typically developing years after the onset of non-Raynauds symptoms, which may suggest a more significant neurological component in the disease process (Mohamed et al., 2012). To that end, environmental exposures , such as the use of organic solvents have also been implicated in autoimmune diseases , such as SSc, further suggesting that reversible risk factors can exacerbate neurological deterioration in patients affected (Anaya et al., 2012). This interlink between environmental and systemic etiologies is a reflection of the multifactorial nature of SSc and its effects on the nervous system, and hence multifaceted management strategies are needed to curtail these interdependent conditions (Figure 5.10).

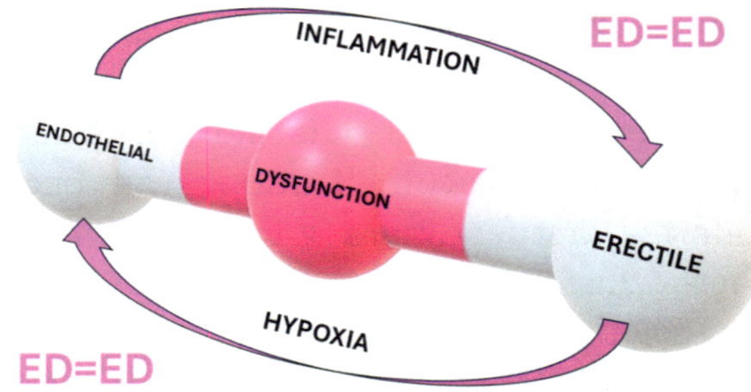

Figure 5.10. Cognitive dysfunction, neuropathy, and erectile dysfunction (ED) frequently emerge as complications, highlighting the multi-systemic impact of SSc on neurological health.

Source: https://www.mdpi.com/ijms/ijms-26-03073/article_deploy/html/images/ijms-26-03073-g002.png.

5.2.8. Raynaud's Phenomenon

Raynaud's Phenomenon, a common clinical presentation in systemic sclerosis, has a significant impact on the quality of life and overall management of patients. It is an intermittent vasospastic response to cold or stress, resulting in digital ischemia and occurring with variable degrees of severity in scleroderma patients. The link between Raynaud's Phenomenon and systemic sclerosis is particularly noteworthy; it often occurs as a presenting feature of the condition, with 60% or greater of patients exhibiting symptoms of limited scleroderma, such as in the CREST syndrome complex (Balamurugan, 2006). Apart from its physical impact, Raynaud's could contribute to psychological distress, exacerbating the emotional burden of an ongoing illness (Reay, 2008). Identification of the complexities of Raynaud's not only aids prognosis in systemic sclerosis but also pinpoints its need for a comprehensive treatment strategy in overcoming its physiological as well as psychosocial consequences.

5.2.9. Quality of Life Considerations

The quality of life of systemic sclerosis (scleroderma) patients is drastically impacted by the multifaceted characteristics of the disease, encompassing physical and psychological features. The patients typically endure disabling symptoms , such as skin tightening, arthralgia, and gastrointestinal tract involvement, which make them have diminished functionality in daily activities. The presence of mouth changes , such as microstomia and restricted mouth opening, exacerbates social and emotional challenges, impacting interpersonal relationships and self-esteem (Onesti et al., 2016). Furthermore, the ambiguity of disease control heightens tension and distress among patients because they are compelled to cope with treatment options and the ambiguity of their condition (Airo et al., 2018). These quality of life issues need to be managed by healthcare professionals, which requires an integrated approach , including both medical care and supportive care interventions addressing the unique needs of systemic sclerosis patients (Figure 5.11).

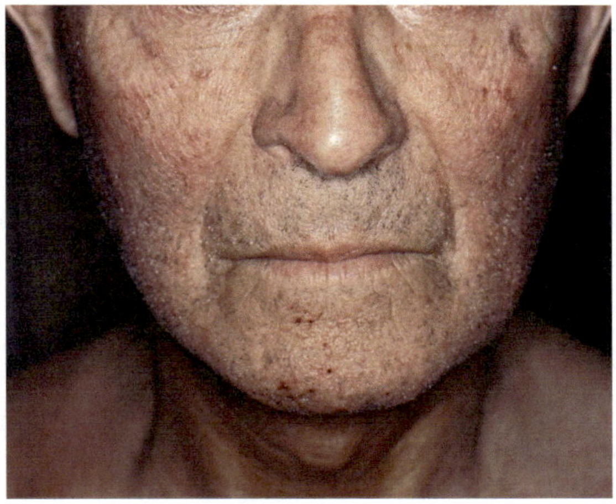

Figure 5.11. The quality of life for individuals diagnosed with systemic sclerosis (scleroderma) is significantly compromised due to the multifaceted nature of the disease, which encompasses both physical and psychological dimensions.

Source: https://www.rarediseaseadvisor.com/wp-content/uploads/sites/25/2023/05/scleroderma_MI_01AEQVWD-scaled.jpg.

Test Your Knowledge

1. What are the typical cutaneous findings in systemic sclerosis?
2. Which gastrointestinal symptoms are most common in systemic sclerosis?

5.3. Diagnosis and Assessment

Learning Outcome

1. Understand clinical evaluation techniques
2. Explain laboratory tests and biomarkers
3. Describe the imaging studies utilized
4. Focus on differential diagnosis considerations
5. Know the role of skin biopsy
6. Perform an assessment of organ function
7. Discuss the use of scoring systems
8. Know the importance of a multidisciplinary approach
9. Identify challenges in early diagnosis

Diagnosis and evaluation of systemic sclerosis (scleroderma) involve a multi-factorial process that takes into account clinical manifestations and advanced imaging techniques. Early identification of microvascular changes, particularly through nailfold videocapillaroscopy, is significant in the evaluation of vascular injury because the procedure effectively quantifies peripheral capillary structure and can predict worsening of disease before more perceptible symptoms (Cutolo et al., 2016). Furthermore, right ventricular function evaluation provides information on potential complications , such as pulmonary arterial hypertension, which is common among systemic sclerosis patients. Utilizing new echocardiographic techniques like 3-dimensional echocardiography and 2-dimensional speckle tracking allows better evaluation of right ventricular function, revealing relevant alterations even in individuals with no evident heart disease (Badano et al., 2015). Thus, an integrated diagnostic strategy involving clinical evaluation and imaging is mandatory for effective management of systemic sclerosis.

5.3.1. Clinical Evaluation Techniques

Clinical evaluation of scleroderma (systemic sclerosis) necessitates a multi-disciplinary evaluation using varying diagnostic modalities to assess organ involvement and microvascular injury. Among these, nailfold video capillaroscopy (NVC) is a precious modality for direct visualization of microvascular remodeling, with clinicians having the capability to detect the disease's pathognomonic findings.

Although NVC remains the gold standard, accessibility issues provide the impetus for a search for other tools , such as dermatoscopy and smartphone attachments, which hold promising potential for facilitating diagnosis from diverse settings (Tervaert et al., 2023).

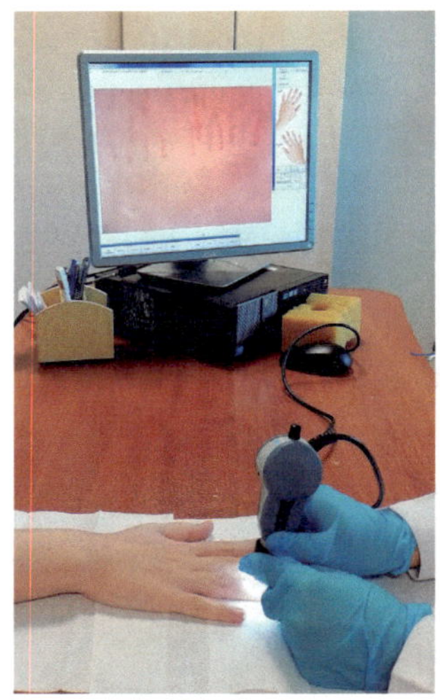

Figure 5.12. Nailfold video capillaroscopy (NVC).

Source: https://minio.scielo.br/documentstore/2359-4292/BZQH57tYYY88XsB7Ttc7LFG/198a33854b749b3e400d49188a92aa3f361857b4.png.

Moreover, recent literature highlights the connection between microvascular injury and pulmonary symptoms in systemic sclerosis, such that morphological as well as functional assessment methods become relevant (Ruaro et al., 2022). These evaluations not only dictate clinical decision-making but also facilitate a greater understanding of the multifaceted interaction between peripheral perfusion deficits and generalized organ dysfunction in such complex patients (Figure 5.12).

5.3.2. Laboratory Tests and Biomarkers

Laboratory testing and biomarker analysis continue to be of critical relevance in the understanding of systemic sclerosis (scleroderma) as well as its diverse manifestations. Modern studies have established that traditional clinical assessments often fall short of providing a true reflection of the disease's complexity; therefore, advanced imaging and molecular testing are now increasingly utilized. For instance, quantitative high-resolution computed tomography (HRCT) has been helpful in evaluating lung fibrosis progression, where improver patients based on gene expression subsets have pulmonary function stability relative to non-improvers, who have reduced lung function and greater fibrosis (Bogatkevich et al., 2017). Furthermore, multiplex cytokine analysis of dermal interstitial fluid also allows the examination of localized inflammatory processes that shed light on the current disease's pathogenesis (Clark et al., 2015). These new laboratory techniques could ultimately lead to more personalized therapeutic interventions and improved patient outcomes for systemic sclerosis.

5.3.3. Imaging Studies Utilized

Evaluation of systemic sclerosis (scleroderma) involves an integrated approach with the application of advanced imaging tests to diagnose microvascular changes and involvement of organs. Nailfold video capillaroscopy (NVC) is the gold standard for the documentation of capillary modifications because it allows direct observation of scleroderma-related microvascular remodeling.

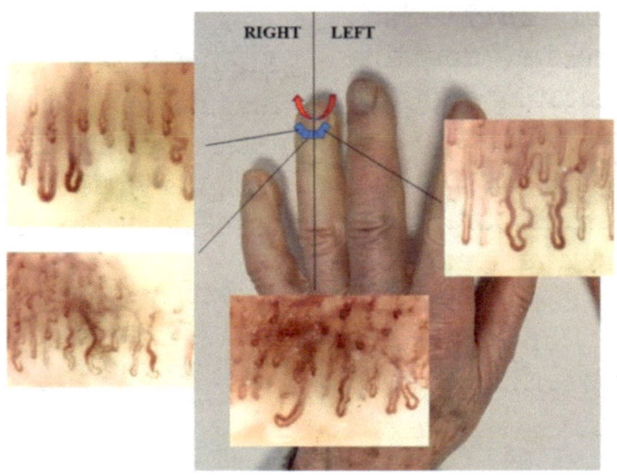

Figure 5.13. Nailfold video capillaroscopy (NVC) stands as the gold standard for visualizing capillary alterations, enabling direct observation of microvascular remodeling specific to scleroderma patients.

Source: https://ars.els-cdn.com/content/image/1-s2.0-S1521694223000359-gr6.jpg.

Even though NVC is very sensitive and specific, its unavailability requires exploring alternative methods, such as digital microscopy and dermatoscopy, which have produced varying degrees of correlation with NVC findings (Tervaert et al., 2023). Furthermore, recent evidence suggests a close relationship between microcirculatory impairment and pulmonary complications, reinforcing the supreme importance of integrating both morphological and functional imaging modalities in clinical practice (Ruaro et al., 2022). With the help of such imaging modalities, clinicians are able to derive valuable information regarding the gravity of disease manifestation, allowing timely interventions as well as personalized patient management protocols (Figure 5.13).

5.3.4. Differential Diagnosis Considerations

When performing differential diagnosis of systemic sclerosis (scleroderma), doctors must distinguish between the present complex state and other imitative diseases. Localized scleroderma, such as morphea, presents with unique clinical features that distinguish it from systemic conditions; morphea lacks the characteristic features of Raynaud's phenomenon and sclerodactyly, which are frequent in systemic sclerosis (Ardeleanu et al., 2020). Also, some systemic sclerosis patients are rare and may occur without the usually associated features of circulating antinuclear antibodies (ANA) or Raynaud's phenomenon, complicating the diagnosis (Carreira et al., 2017). Such absence of such markers presents daunting diagnostic challenges, necessitating rigorous clinical examinations and investigations to rule out other autoimmune or connective tissue diseases. As precise diagnosis is paramount to appropriate management and treatment strategies, familiarity with these differential considerations is significant for healthcare providers taking care of scleroderma.

5.3.5. Role of Skin Biopsy

Skin biopsy has a pivotal role in diagnosing and managing systemic sclerosis (scleroderma) treatment, and it offers critical information on the pathophysiologic changes of the disease. Through analysis of skin samples, and more specifically from the dorsal forearm, researchers have utilized confocal laser scanning microscopy to quantify fibrosis of the skin. There is evidence of elevation of collagen type I and III, and fibronectin, in the skin of patients compared to healthy controls, and this indicates the fibrotic characteristic of systemic sclerosis (Busquets et al., 2010). Moreover, the ability to measure the effectiveness of therapeutic intervention by skin biopsy attests to its clinical potential; a reduction in fibrosis score was observed among patients after treatment, which showed promise for skin biopsy as a worthwhile endpoint for clinical trials (Gambardella et al., 2018). Last but not least, skin biopsy is not merely a diagnostic procedure but also an instrument to track disease course and response to treatment (Figure 5.14).

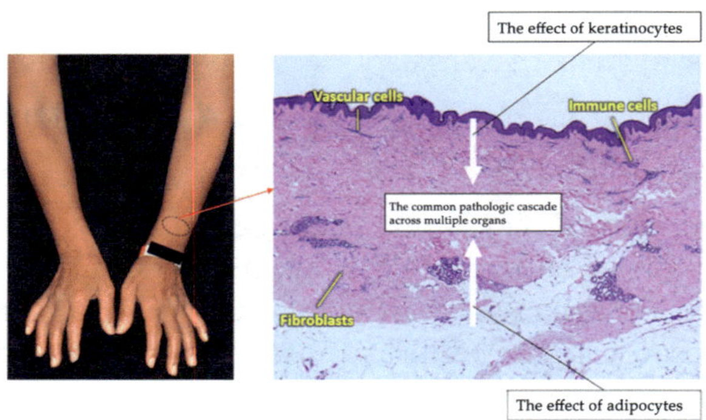

Figure 5.14. The role of skin biopsy in the diagnosis and management of systemic sclerosis (scleroderma) is paramount, offering critical insights into the pathophysiological changes associated with the disease.

Source: https://pub.mdpi-res.com/jcm/jcm-09-02687/article_deploy/html/images/jcm-09-02687-g003.png?1597838223.

5.3.6. Assessment of Organ Function

Organ function evaluation in systemic sclerosis (scleroderma) is relevant since the disease has a multi-systemic impact on all major organ systems. Due to the potential for pulmonary complications, such as pulmonary arterial hypertension (PAH), advanced echocardiographic techniques like 3-dimensional echocardiography (3DE) and 2-dimensional speckle tracking (2DSTE) have become crucial in the evaluation of right ventricular (RV) function in asymptomatic patients without a history of heart disease (Badano et al., 2015). These modalities enable practitioners to detect early alteration in RV anatomy and function, showing that even without PAH, patients prefer increased systolic pulmonary arterial pressure. Furthermore, studies have revealed that treatments , such as mycophenolate mofetil not only promote improvement in skin disease but also stabilize pulmonary status, emphasizing observation on a continuous basis (Jimenez et al., 2012). Thus, thorough organ function evaluations are crucial in the management of systemic sclerosis and improving patient outcomes.

5.3.7. Use of Scoring Systems

The application of score systems in the management and assessment of systemic sclerosis (scleroderma) is key in assessing the severity of disease and response to treatment. The most extensively validated is the modified Rodnan Skin Score (MRSS), which assesses thickening of the skin and is a highly relevant indicator of disease progression. The MRSS not only enables the tracking of outcomes over time but also aids in the stratification of patients according to their disease subsets, which is valuable for individualized therapeutic approaches. Current studies have reported that scoring systems, in combination with imaging biomarkers like high-resolution computed tomography (HRCT), could allow for improved comprehension of interstitial lung disease (ILD) in systemic sclerosis, as suggested by correlations between inflammatory gene expression subsets and clinical outcomes (Afeltra et al., 2017; Bogatkevich et al., 2017). Such a scoring system integration ultimately benefits more efficient management planning in a condition recognized for its heterogeneity of presentation (Figure 5.15).

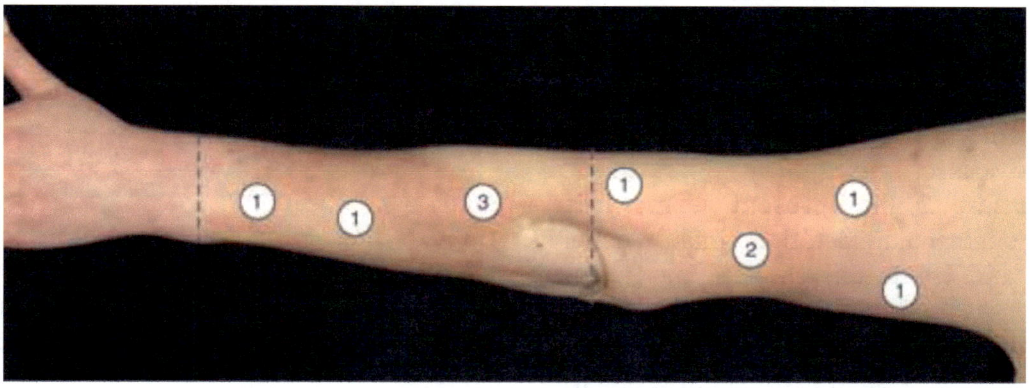

Figure 5.15. Most established method is the modified Rodnan Skin Score (MRSS), which quantitatively measures skin thickening and serves as a critical indicator of disease progression.

Source: https://journals.sagepub.com/cms/10.5301/jsrd.5000231/asset/cb217c40-f7a4-421d-ac18-851a0160e1ce/assets/images/large/10.5301_jsrd.5000231-fig4.jpg.

5.3.8. Importance of Multidisciplinary Approach

The multidisciplinary type of systemic sclerosis (scleroderma) requires a coordinated multidisciplinary approach to the treatment of its multiple aspects. Because this chronic autoimmune disease involves the skin and various internal organs to a significant extent, therapy needs to be diverse and cover a range of branches of medicine, including rheumatology, dermatology, pulmonology, and psychiatric services. Integration among healthcare providers, researchers, and patients is crucial to the design and provision of intervention approaches to improve health-related quality of life (HRQoL) in persons with the disease, according to the Scleroderma Patient-centered Intervention Network (SPIN) (Arthurs et al., 2012). Moreover, the appreciation of the interaction between immune-inflammatory mechanisms and resulting organ-specific complications highlights the significance of integrating data from more than one medical field to realize the best patient outcomes (Denton, 2016). Therefore, the development of a cooperative environment not only maximizes the efficacy of treatment but also ensures an all-around approach towards mitigating the effects of systemic sclerosis.

5.3.9. Challenges in Early Diagnosis

Systemic sclerosis (scleroderma) is difficult to diagnose early due to the superimposed presentation of its symptoms over those of other autoimmune diseases. Nonspecific symptoms , such as fatigue, arthralgia, and skin changes, are common and readily mistaken or delayed in diagnosing the etiologic condition. Most importantly, microangiopathy, a feature of systemic sclerosis, may present years earlier than other clinical manifestations, making timely diagnosis and treatment challenging (Cutolo et al., 2016). Techniques like nailfold video capillaroscopy have helped identify preclinical changes in the vasculature characteristic of the disease; their availability and use, however, remain strikingly inconsistent among healthcare providers (Cutolo et al., 2016). This is compounded by the fact that some of the manifestations of systemic sclerosis are subtle and initially misdiagnosed as benign, hence, even accurate diagnosis becomes more challenging. Consequently, patients remain untreated for a prolonged period, thereby worsening their prognosis and overall quality of life (Figure 5.16).

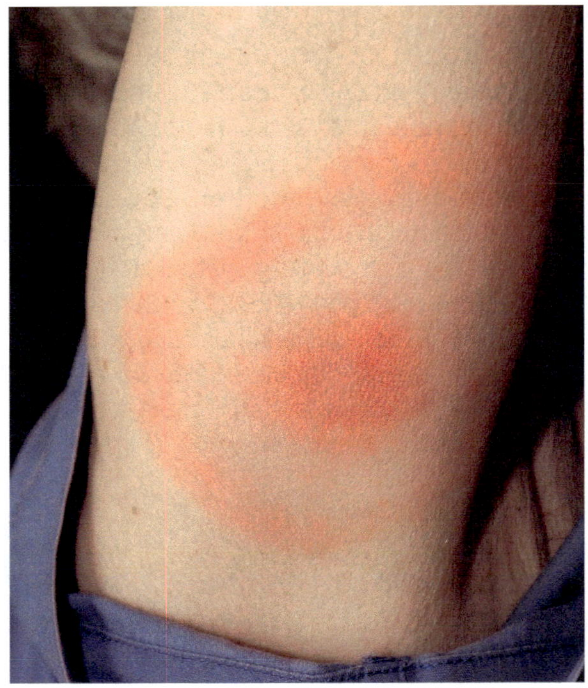

Figure 5.16. Patients often exhibit nonspecific signs , such as fatigue, joint pain, and skin changes, which can easily lead to misdiagnosis or delayed recognition of the underlying condition.

Source: https://aldf.com/wp-content/uploads/2023/11/Symptoms-of-Lyme-Disease-1.jpg.

Test Your Knowledge

1. What imaging techniques are used to assess pulmonary fibrosis in systemic sclerosis?
2. How is pulmonary arterial hypertension diagnosed in patients with systemic sclerosis?

5.4. Treatment and Management

Learning Outcome

1. Explain pharmacological interventions
2. Discuss non-pharmacological therapies
3. Focus on the role of physical therapy
4. Understand the management of specific symptoms
5. Know the importance of patient education
6. Describe psychological support and counseling
7. Identify emerging therapies and clinical trials
8. Focus on lifestyle modifications
9. Learn long-term management strategies

Effective management and treatment of systemic sclerosis (scleroderma) demand intricate interplay tailored to each patient's individual needs because the disease is heterogeneous. Rheumatologists must distinguish systemic sclerosis from other scleroderma syndromes, including localized scleroderma and other autoimmune conditions, that manifest similarly yet require a different therapeutic strategy (Kodet & Oreská, 2019). In the instance of localized scleroderma patients, for instance, the initial inflammatory phase is paramount to successful therapy; utilizing powerful topical corticosteroids and phototherapy is capable of yielding the best outcomes if treatment begins early (Ardeleanu et al., 2020). Furthermore, controlling individual symptoms, such as gastrointestinal abnormalities, pulmonary hypertension, and skin manifestations, by pharmacological and non-pharmacological measures, is a crucial aspect in improving quality of life. This combined management strategy stresses the necessity for early diagnosis and regular monitoring to ensure adaptive therapeutic regimens that align with individual patients' evolving clinical presentation.

5.4.1. Pharmacological Interventions

Pharmacologic treatment is also a central component in the management of systemic sclerosis (scleroderma), particularly in symptom alleviation and in enhancing patients' quality of life. A systematic literature review highlighted the efficacy and safety of several drugs, such as calcium channel blockers, phosphodiesterase-5 inhibitors, and intravenous prostacyclin analogues, that demonstrate remarkable efficacy and effectiveness on the frequency and severity of Raynaud's phenomenon (RP) and healing of digital ulcers (DUs) (Cordeiro et al., 2024). Nifedipine is the preferred drug as a first-line agent for RP, and sildenafil and bosentan are efficient second-line medications in patients with severe and refractory disease (Barbosa et al., 2024). Although promising results are discovered in connection with these pharmacologic modalities, it must be emphasized that non-pharmacologic therapy, though generally less supported by robust evidence, has the capacity to confer added advantage when used concurrently with these medications, lending evidence for the need for a multimodal treatment approach.

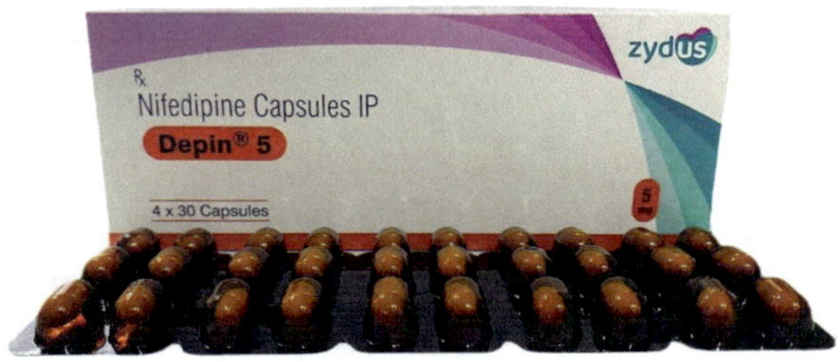

Figure 5.17. Nifedipine is recommended as a first-line therapy for RP, while sildenafil and bosentan serve as effective second-line treatments for patients experiencing severe and refractory cases

Source: https://5.imimg.com/data5/SELLER/Default/2023/8/338104025/GE/NB/VI/91766502/5mg-nifedipine-capsules-ip.jpeg.

5.4.2. Non-Pharmacological Therapies

Treating systemic sclerosis (scleroderma) using non-pharmacologic interventions is a multi-aspect approach that can alleviate symptoms and enhance the quality of life for patients. Psychological interventions, particularly cognitive-behavioral therapy, have proven effective in decreasing pain that is associated with a wide range of conditions, including those most prevalent among patients with systemic sclerosis, making for an integrated system of treatment that addresses both mental and physical health (Agostini et al., 2016). In addition, modalities , such as spa therapy have gained much consensus among professionals as being suitable to reduce musculoskeletal symptoms, which are highly prevalent in patients with scleroderma (Paoloni et al., 2017). They profit not only from pain relief but also from the empowerment of patients with their active participation in their own recovery. By implementing non-pharmacological measures into the regimen, healthcare practitioners can create a more holistic model that addresses physical and emotional requirements, ultimately leading to improved outcomes for individuals who endure this complex autoimmune disease.

5.4.3. Role of Physical Therapy

The role of physical therapy in the management of systemic sclerosis, also referred to as scleroderma, is central to maximizing quality of life and minimizing the disabling effects of the disease. Physical therapy interventions are designed to enhance mobility, relieve pain, and maximize physical function as a whole, which can be severely compromised as a result of the symptoms of the disease. In particular, as fatigue can be a chronic and persistent symptom in scleroderma patients, resolution of the same by tailored physical therapy modalities can positively impact patients' functioning on a day-to-day basis as well as their overall quality of life (Assassi et al., 2011). Moreover, incorporation of psychological therapies within the physical therapy management has been shown to effectively mitigate pain, thereby ensuring a comprehensive treatment regime (Agostini et al., 2016). Consequently, multidisciplinary treatment incorporating physical therapy not only controls the physical impairment resulting from systemic sclerosis but also controls psychological health, enhancing resilience and encouraging patient compliance with ongoing rehabilitation (Figure 5.18).

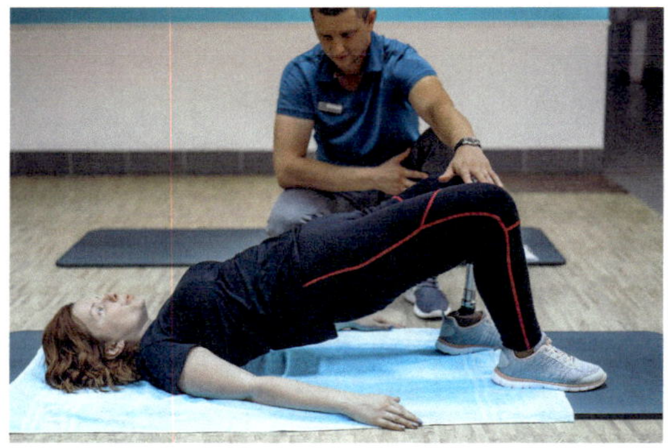

Figure 5.18. Physical therapy interventions focus on improving mobility, reducing pain, and enhancing overall physical function, which can be significantly compromised due to the diseases symptoms.

Source: https://vitalitytulsa.com/wp-content/uploads/2024/11/Physical-Therapy-for-Hip-Pain-12-Best-Exercises-Stretches.jpg.

5.4.4. Management of Specific Symptoms

Adequate control of some systemic sclerosis (scleroderma) symptoms is necessary in order to improve the quality of life in patients. The altered mobility of the mouth is one of the significant presentations, with conditions , such as microstomia, affecting everyday functions , such as eating and communication. Recent studies have explored new treatments, such as autologous fat transplant and adipose-derived stromal cells (ADSCs) injection, that have been reported to enhance mouth opening function in affected patients. Notably, even though both treatments achieved significant improvement, there was no evident first-line method, prompting a call for further investigation into this area of study (Onesti et al., 2016). Furthermore, management of non-lethal complications—i.e., fatigue and calcinosis—is also required, as these are capable of largely impacting daily functioning as well as health overall. Though treatments are symptomatic rather than curative, rigorous management regimens must be in place in order to adequately balance benefit with risk (Denton, 2016).

5.4.5. Importance of Patient Education

Effective patient education is central to the management of systemic sclerosis (scleroderma), particularly given the multifaceted nature of this disease. Systematic education allows for the patient to be aware of their diagnosis, feel symptoms, and become actively engaged in treatment regimens. As systemic sclerosis also demonstrates extensive racial disparities, particularly in African American patients who present with more aggressive disease presentations, individualized educational programs will help close these disparities in care. This education should not only teach the clinical presentation of the disease but should also incorporate psychosocial counseling in order to enhance patients' quality of life and medication compliance. Further, research , such as the Genome Research in African American Scleroderma Patients (GRASP) cohort is important for designing targeted interventions that consider the unique requirements of various groups with scleroderma (Boin et al., 2017). Overall, enhanced patient education is an important element in optimizing outcomes and resilience building in patients living with systemic sclerosis (Bassel et al., 2014) (Figure 5.19).

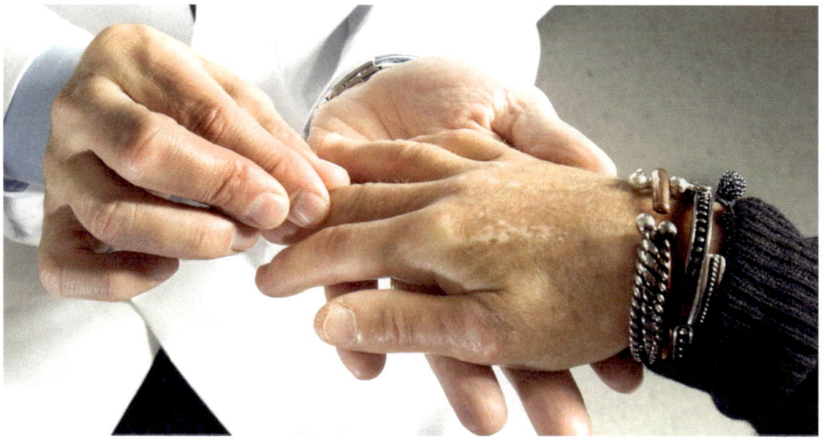

Figure 5.19. Effective patient education plays a pivotal role in managing systemic sclerosis (scleroderma), particularly given the complexity of this chronic condition.

Source: https://www.hss.edu/globalassets/images/conditions/scleroderma-hss-rheumatology-1200x628.jpg.

5.4.6. Psychological Support and Counseling

Proper psychological and counseling support are integral components of treating Systemic Sclerosis (Scleroderma) because the severe emotional and psychological pain associated with this long-term condition should not be underestimated. These individuals typically experience anxiety, depression, and disturbance in their body image, all of which significantly impact life quality. It has been observed that psychological counseling can provide coping mechanisms for the patients to deal with feelings of isolation and uncertainty, thus enhancing the overall resilience. Therapy and support groups for facilitating open discussion about their experiences also lessen the emotional burden of the disease. Furthermore, the addition of psychological care to routine medical treatment offers a better-rounded experience, addressing the physical and emotional side of care. This combined strategy emphasizes the value of making mental well-being a key aspect of therapy, as the understanding that only through collaborative effort in the management of sophisticated conditions , such as systemic sclerosis, is an optimal outcome achieved (Benea et al., 2016; Georgescu et al., 2016).

5.4.7. Emerging Therapies and Clinical Trials

Among the complexities of systemic sclerosis (scleroderma), emerging drugs and clinical trials are a promising frontier in the quest for effective treatments. New developments have helped to detail the multifaceted pathogenesis of the disease with a focus on the two-pronged mechanism involving immune-mediated inflammatory processes and the fibrotic lesions that destroy multiple organ systems (Denton, 2016). Surprisingly, these discoveries have prompted novel therapeutic strategies aimed at specific pathways of fibrosis, such as myofibroblast activation and the regulatory mechanisms involving growth factors and cytokines (Jimenez et al., 2013). These new methods are subject to clinical trials regarding safety and efficacy, such as immunosuppressive therapy and potential antifibrotic medications. While researchers continue to explain and evaluate these new therapies, there is hope for severely improving the late complications of systemic sclerosis, ultimately enhancing patient outcome and quality of life (Figure 5.20).

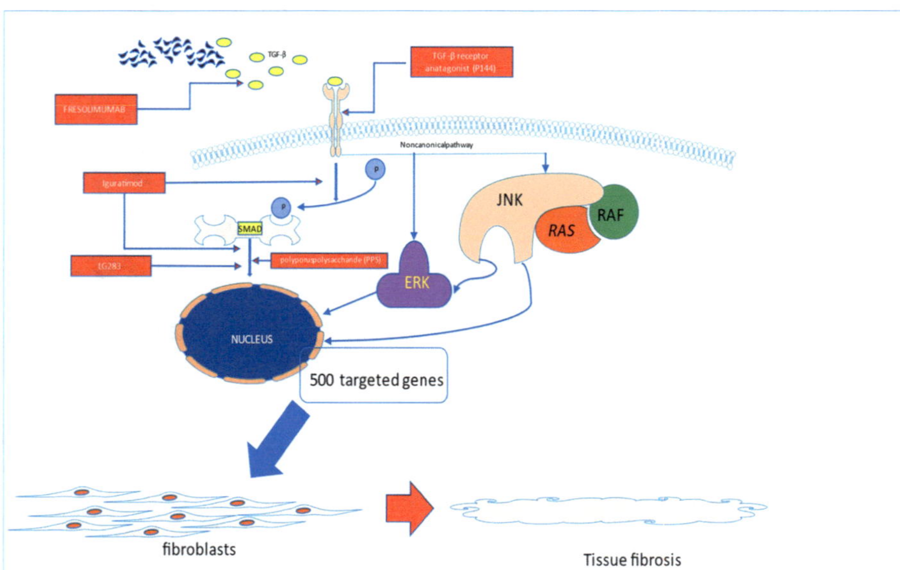

Figure 5.20. Clinical trials are integral to assessing the safety and efficacy of these innovative approaches, including immunosuppressive therapies and potential antifibrotic agents.

Source: https://www.mdpi.com/pharmaceuticals/pharmaceuticals-16-01066/article_deploy/html/images/pharmaceuticals-16-01066-g001.png.

5.4.8. Lifestyle Modifications

Lifestyle adjustments are a key component of systemic scleroderma (scleroderma) management aimed at improving patient outcomes and quality of life. It has been proven that diet modification, for example, adhering to an anti-inflammatory diet rich in omega-3 fatty acids and antioxidants, can successfully reverse disease activity and improve immune regulation, as mandated by recent research (Sobek et al., 2024). Equally significant is exercise regularly; not only does it help in managing symptoms, but it also enhances mental health, presenting a holistic approach to care. Further, good quality sleep and stress reduction through mindfulness interventions can also reduce systemic inflammation, a key concern in scleroderma management (Balanescu et al., 2022). By considering these changes, patients become more actively involved in their own health, and ultimately increase disease control and overall well-being. Thus, the inclusion of lifestyle changes is not just an adjunct but is crucial in the integrated treatment of systemic sclerosis.

5.4.9. Long-term Management Strategies

Effective long-term management of Systemic Sclerosis (Scleroderma) involves a multidisciplinary treatment approach involving pharmacologic therapies, physical therapy, and psychological support. Due to the complex nature of the autoimmune condition, the treatment plan must be tailor-made to tackle isolated symptoms , such as thickening of the skin, pulmonary hypertension, and gastrointestinal involvement. For instance, disease-modifying therapies that suppress immune system activity are essential, particularly for those with severe complications, as documented in recent research of similar illnesses , such as multiple sclerosis, where drug treatment approaches vary significantly in nature and efficacy (Kay et al., 2015). Furthermore, incorporation of psychological therapy, including Cognitive-Behavioral Therapy and mindfulness training, can sufficiently alleviate pain and improve patients' quality of life (Agostini et al., 2016). Such an integrative approach guarantees that both the physical and emotional aspects of care are included, finally contributing to enhanced results in individuals living with Systemic Sclerosis (Figure 5.21).

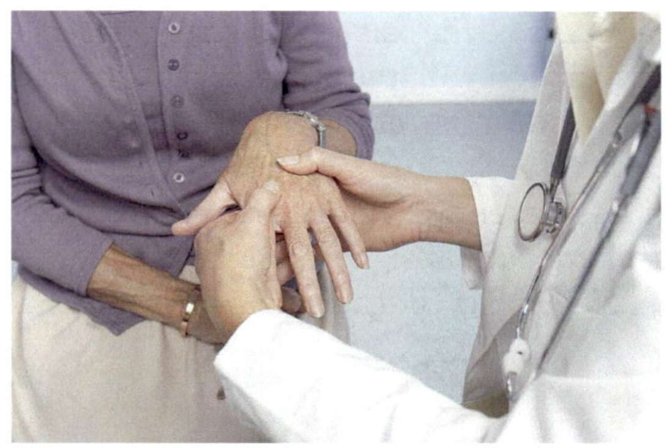

Figure 5.21. Effective long-term management strategies for Systemic Sclerosis (Scleroderma) necessitate a multidisciplinary approach that encompasses pharmacological interventions, physical therapies, and psychological support.

Source: https://drmaggieyu.com/wp-content/uploads/2024/05/Functional-Medicine-Scleroderma-1184x789.jpg.

Test Your Knowledge

1. How is pulmonary fibrosis in systemic sclerosis managed?
2. What are the treatment options for gastrointestinal dysmotility in systemic sclerosis?

Summary

Understanding the complexities of systemic sclerosis, or scleroderma, involves an integrated approach that considers both the physiological and psychosocial factors of the illness. The interplay between early stressors, coping mechanisms , such as self-compassion, and the evolution of hyper-arousal can significantly influence disease trajectory and symptom perception, highlighting the importance of early intervention strategies (Kearney & Hicks, 2016). Also, novel diagnostic instruments like nailfold capillaroscopy (NFC) have been discovered to differentiate between different interstitial lung diseases (ILDs) related to connective tissue diseases, paving the way for more precise and prompt interventions (Altınışık et al., 2015). As we learn more about these relationships and diagnostic tools, it is increasingly clear that psychological care and improved diagnostics are part of comprehensive management of scleroderma, ultimately benefiting patients through outcomes and quality of life.

In highlighting the features in summary points pertinent to systemic sclerosis (scleroderma), one has to stress the complex interplay of genetic and environmental determinants acting on the pathophysiology of the disease. Recent studies have highlighted the caveolin 1 function in modulating transforming growth factor beta (TGFbeta) signaling, a critical pathway implicated in the process of fibrosis in systemic sclerosis. Specifically, CAV1 is highly reduced in fibrotic tissue, an association with the scleroderma fibroblast fibrotic phenotype, suggesting therapeutic relevance to the restoration of caveolin 1 function (de Almeida et al., 2008). Furthermore, initial clinical trial data, such as from trials of the tyrosine kinase inhibitor dasatinib, are promising for lung fibrosis prevention but show relatively limited overall efficacy. This overlap of pathophysiology and therapeutic insight is the beauty of systemic sclerosis and the complexity that still confronts its management (Bogatkevich et al., 2017).

KEY TERMS FROM THIS CHAPTER

- Anti-topoisomerase
- Autoimmunity
- Connective tissue growth factor (CTGF)
- Cytokines
- Echocardiography
- Extracellular matrix proteins
- Fibrosis
- Immune dysfunction
- Molecular mechanisms
- Reactive oxidizing species (ROS)
- Audiovestibular manifestations
- Cellular senescence
- Cosmetic complaints
- Dysmotility
- Erectile dysfunction (ED)
- Fibroproliferative vasculopathy
- Gastro-intestinal manifestations
- Microvascular changes
- Morbidity
- Vascular alterations

CRITICAL THINKING QUESTIONS

1. **Which of the following is a hallmark clinical feature of systemic sclerosis?**
   a. Muscle weakness
   b. Skin thickening and fibrosis
   c. Lymphadenopathy
   d. Blistering rash
2. **Which autoantibody is most commonly associated with diffuse cutaneous systemic sclerosis?**
   a. Anti-centromere antibody
   b. Anti-Ro (SSA) antibody
   c. Anti-topoisomerase I (Scl-70) antibody
   d. Anti-dsDNA antibody
3. **Limited cutaneous systemic sclerosis is often associated with which syndrome?**
   a. CREST syndrome
   b. Felty's syndrome
   c. Goodpasture's syndrome
   d. Cushing's syndrome
4. **Which of the following is typically the earliest clinical manifestation in systemic sclerosis?**
   a. Renal crisis
   b. Digital ulcers
   c. Raynaud's phenomenon
   d. Telangiectasia
5. **What is the most serious potential complication of scleroderma renal crisis?**
   a. Pulmonary embolism
   b. Hemolytic anemia
   c. Malignant hypertension
   d. Hypercalcemia

Answers to Critical Thinking Questions

1. (b) 2. (c) 3. (a) 4. (c) 5. (c)

Short Answer Questions

1. What are the primary pathological processes involved in systemic sclerosis?
2. How does endothelial cell injury contribute to the development of systemic sclerosis?
3. What is the difference between limited and diffuse cutaneous systemic sclerosis?
4. How does Raynaud's phenomenon present in systemic sclerosis?
5. What are the diagnostic criteria for systemic sclerosis?
6. Which autoantibodies are associated with limited vs. diffuse systemic sclerosis?
7. What is the role of immunosuppressive therapy in systemic sclerosis?
8. How are calcium channel blockers used in the treatment of Raynaud's phenomenon?

References

1. Clark, K. E., Lopez, H., Abdi, B. A., Guerra, S. G., Shiwen, X., Khan, K., Etomi, O., Martin, G. R., Abraham, D. J., Denton, C. P., & Stratton, R. J. (2015). Multiplex cytokine analysis of dermal interstitial blister fluid defines local disease mechanisms in systemic sclerosis. *Arthritis research & therapy*, *17*(1), 73. https://doi.org/10.1186/s13075-015-0575-8 (accessed on 17th June 2025).
2. Abraham, D., Assandri, D., Assassi, S., Auluck, A., Bacher, M., Baron, M., Baron, M., et al. (2017). Review article: Pathogenesis and clinical manifestations of gastrointestinal involvement in systemic sclerosis. https://core.ac.uk/download/83049880.pdf (accessed on 17th June 2025).
3. Adler, S., Airò, P., Allanore, Y., Ananieva, L., et al. (2016). Incidences and risk factors of organ manifestations in the early course of systemic sclerosis: A longitudinal EUSTAR study. https://core.ac.uk/download/74235777.pdf (accessed on 17th June 2025).
4. Afeltra, A. M. V., Barbano, B., Cianci, R., Gigante, A., et al. (2017). Intrarenal arterial stiffness is increased in systemic sclerosis patients with anti-ribonucleic acid polymerase III antibodies. https://core.ac.uk/download/98339896.pdf (accessed on 17th June 2025).
5. Agostini, M., Alfonsi, E., Aloisi, A. M., Alvisi, E., et al. (2016). Psychological treatments and psychotherapies in the neurorehabilitation of pain: Evidences and recommendations from the Italian consensus conference on pain in neurorehabilitation. https://core.ac.uk/download/54538696.pdf (accessed on 17th June 2025).
6. Airó, P., Alarcón-Riquelme, M., AlKassab, F., et al. (2014). Immunochip analysis identifies multiple susceptibility loci for systemic sclerosis. https://core.ac.uk/download/42360789.pdf (accessed on 17th June 2025).
7. Airó, P., Alegre-Sancho, J. J., Allanore, Y., Caimmi, C., et al. (2018). Smoking in systemic sclerosis: A longitudinal European Scleroderma Trials and Research Group study. https://core.ac.uk/download/188823578.pdf (accessed on 17th June 2025).
8. Airó, P., Alexander, T., Allanore, Y., Bombardieri, S., et al. (2018). *Systemic Sclerosis: State of the Art on Clinical Practice Guidelines.* https://core.ac.uk/download/188621024.pdf (accessed on 17th June 2025).
9. Akin, C., Alvarez-Twose, I., Bankova, L., Bodemer, C., Brockow, K., Brockow, K., Caughey, G., et al. (2018). Diffuse cutaneous macrocytosis with novel somatic KIT mutation K509I and association with tuberous sclerosis. https://core.ac.uk/download/323063103.pdf (accessed on 17th June 2025).
10. Alabrudziński, K., Biernikiewicz, J., Biernikiewicz, M., Borowiec, A., et al. (2025). A comprehensive review of systemic sclerosis: Diagnosis, clinical features and management strategies. https://core.ac.uk/download/646080063.pdf (accessed on 17th June 2025).
11. Allanore, Y., Chung, L., Denton, C. P., Hughes, M., et al. (2021). Author correction: Raynaud phenomenon and digital ulcers in systemic sclerosis. https://core.ac.uk/download/394996977.pdf (accessed on 17th June 2025).
12. Altınışık, G., Balkarli, A., Çakmakçi Karadoğan, D., Çobankara, V., et al. (2015). The role of nailfold capillaroscopy in interstitial lung diseases: Can it differentiate idiopathic cases from collagen tissue disease associated interstitial lung diseases? https://core.ac.uk/download/227075151.pdf (accessed on 17th June 2025).

13. Anaya, J. M., Barragán Martínez, C., Mantilla, R. D., Montoya-Ortiz, G., et al. (2012). Organic solvents as risk factor for autoimmune diseases: A systematic review and meta-analysis. https://core.ac.uk/download/86444243.pdf (accessed on 17th June 2025).

14. Ardeleanu, V., Constantin, V. D., Radaschin, D. S., Stana, C., et al. (2020). Laser therapy in superficial morphea lesions–indications, limitations and therapeutic alternatives. https://core.ac.uk/download/304672910.pdf (accessed on 17th June 2025).

15. Arthurs, E., Assassi, S., Bartlett, S. J., Bassel, M., et al. (2012). New directions for patient-centered care in scleroderma: The Scleroderma Patient-centered Intervention Network (SPIN). https://core.ac.uk/download/55621462.pdf (accessed on 17th June 2025).

16. Assassi, S., Fischbach, M., GENISOS Study Group, Gonzalez, E. B., et al. (2011). Predictors of fatigue severity in early systemic sclerosis: A prospective longitudinal study of the GENISOS cohort. https://core.ac.uk/download/323073807.pdf (accessed on 17th June 2025).

17. Badano, L., Bourji, K. I., Cozzi, F., Miatton, M., et al. (2015). Evaluation of right ventricular function performed by 3D-echocardiography in scleroderma patients. https://core.ac.uk/download/80154728.pdf (accessed on 17th June 2025).

18. Balamurugan, S. (2006). Study on pulmonary hypertension and diastolic dysfunction in scleroderma. https://core.ac.uk/download/235665438.pdf (accessed on 17th June 2025).

19. Balanescu, A., Gwinnutt, J. M., Rodríguez Carrio, J., Wieczorek, M., et al. (2022). 2021 EULAR recommendations regarding lifestyle behaviors and work participation to prevent progression of rheumatic and musculoskeletal diseases. https://core.ac.uk/download/635115938.pdf (accessed on 17th June 2025).

20. Balla, M. P., De Vincentiis, M., Di Stadio, A., Greco, A., et al. (2018). Otolaryngologic symptoms in multiple sclerosis: A review. https://core.ac.uk/download/188830242.pdf (accessed on 17th June 2025).

21. Barbosa, L., Barreira, S., Boleto, G., Castro, C., et al. (2024). Portuguese recommendations for the management of Raynaud's phenomenon and digital ulcers in systemic sclerosis and other connective tissue diseases. https://core.ac.uk/download/614519814.pdf (accessed on 17th June 2025).

22. Bassel, M., Brown, A., Fries, J. F., Hibbard, R., Joachim, R., Kwakkenbos, L., et al. (2014). Taking charge of systemic sclerosis: A pilot study to assess the effectiveness of an internet self-management program. https://deepblue.lib.umich.edu/bitstream/2027.42/106842/1/acr22192.pdf (accessed on 17th June 2025).

23. Bellotti, C., De Francesco, G. P., Lavra, L., Magi, F., et al. (2018). Galectin-3: One molecule for an alphabet of diseases, from A to Z. https://core.ac.uk/download/153369169.pdf (accessed on 17th June 2025).

24. Benea, V., Georgescu, S. R., Mitran, C. I., Mitran, M., et al. (2016). The current treatment of erectile dysfunction. https://core.ac.uk/download/144552982.pdf (accessed on 17th June 2025).

25. Bernstein, E. J., Denton, C. P., Flaherty, K. R., Kazerooni, E. A., et al. (2021). Systemic sclerosis–associated interstitial lung disease: How to incorporate two Food and Drug Administration–approved therapies in clinical practice. https://core.ac.uk/download/480391357.pdf (accessed on 17th June 2025).

26. Bogatkevich, G. S., Du, S., Ganguly, B. J., Goldin, J., et al. (2017). Novel lung imaging biomarkers and skin gene expression subsetting in dasatinib treatment of systemic sclerosis-associated interstitial lung disease. https://core.ac.uk/download/323078738.pdf (accessed on 17th June 2025).

27. Boin, F., Carns, M., Chung, L., Criswell, L. A., et al. (2017). Clinical and serological features of systemic sclerosis in a multicenter African American cohort: Analysis of the genome research in African American scleroderma patient's clinical database. https://core.ac.uk/download/323074312.pdf (accessed on 17th June 2025).

28. Busquets, J., Del Galdo, F., Jimenez, S. A., Kissin, E., et al. (2010). Assessment of tissue fibrosis in skin biopsies from patients with systemic sclerosis employing confocal laser scanning microscopy: An objective outcome measure for clinical trials? https://core.ac.uk/download/129190940.pdf (accessed on 17th June 2025).

29. Onesti, M. G., Fioramonti, P., Carella, S., Fino, P., Marchese, C., & Scuderi, N. (2016). Improvement of Mouth Functional Disability in Systemic Sclerosis Patients over One Year in a Trial of Fat Transplantation versus Adipose-Derived Stromal Cells. *Stem cells international*, *2016*, 2416192. https://doi.org/10.1155/2016/2416192(accessed on 17th June 2025).

30. Carreira, P. E., Derk, C. T., Deuschle, K., Kay, J., et al. (2017). Systemic sclerosis without antinuclear antibodies or Raynaud's phenomenon: A multicenter study in the prospective EULAR Scleroderma Trials and Research (EUSTAR) database. https://core.ac.uk/download/85209415.pdf (accessed on 17th June 2025).

31. Castro, S. V., Jimenez, S. A., & Piera-Velazquez, S. (2010). Role of growth factors in the pathogenesis of tissue fibrosis in systemic sclerosis. https://core.ac.uk/download/83050041.pdf (accessed on 17th June 2025).

32. Sobek, K. Łucja, Mazur, M., Waz, D., Szarłowicz, J., Goliszek, Z., Tabin-Barczak, W., ... Samuła, S. (2024). The Impact of Diet and Lifestyle on the Course of Autoimmune Diseases. *Quality in Sport*, *36*, 56879. https://doi.org/10.12775/QS.2024.36.56879(accessed on 17th June 2025).

33. Cohen Tervaert, J. W., Gniadecki, R., Ma, Z., Mulder, L., et al. (2023). Methods of assessing nailfold capillaroscopy compared to video capillaroscopy in patients with systemic sclerosis: A critical review of the literature. https://core.ac.uk/download/597521356.pdf (accessed on 17th June 2025).

34. Cordeiro, A., Costa, E., Cunha-Santos, F., Dourado, M., et al. (2024). Systematic literature review to inform the Portuguese recommendations for the management of Raynaud's phenomenon and digital ulcers in systemic sclerosis and other connective tissue diseases. https://core.ac.uk/download/614518814.pdf (accessed on 17th June 2025).

35. Cortese, A., Francisci, S., Gauzzi, M. C., Gessani, A., et al. (2015). Increased circulating levels of vitamin D binding protein in MS patients. https://core.ac.uk/download/54522329.pdf (accessed on 17th June 2025).

36. Richard-Miceli, C., & Criswell, L. A. (2012). Emerging patterns of genetic overlap across autoimmune disorders. *Genome medicine*, *4*(1), 6. https://doi.org/10.1186/gm305(accessed on 17th June 2025).

37. Croce, A., D'Aguanno, V., De Vincentiis, M., De Virgilio, A., et al. (2018). Audio-vestibular symptoms in systemic autoimmune diseases. https://core.ac.uk/download/188823057.pdf (accessed on 17th June 2025).

38. Cutolo, M., Llado, A., Paolino, S., Pizzorni, C., et al. (2016). Capillaroscopy in 2016: New perspectives in systemic sclerosis. https://core.ac.uk/download/74613576.pdf (accessed on 17th June 2025).

39. de Almeida, C. J., Del Galdo, F., Jasmin, J. F., Jimenez, S. A., et al. (2008). Decreased expression of caveolin 1 in patients with systemic sclerosis: Crucial role in the pathogenesis of tissue fibrosis. https://core.ac.uk/download/83050044.pdf (accessed on 17th June 2025).

40. Denton C. P. (2016). Advances in pathogenesis and treatment of systemic sclerosis. *Clinical medicine (London, England)*, *16*(1), 55–60. https://doi.org/10.7861/clinmedicine.16-1-55(accessed on 17th June 2025).

41. Piera-Velazquez, S., & Jimenez, S. A. (2015). Role of cellular senescence and NOX4-mediated oxidative stress in systemic sclerosis pathogenesis. *Current rheumatology reports*, *17*(1), 473. https://doi.org/10.1007/s11926-014-0473-0(accessed on 17th June 2025).

42. Gabrielli, A., Milano, A., Skol, A. D., Kreuter, A., Voskuyl, A. E., Schuerwegh, A. J., Herrick, A., et al. (2013). The systemic lupus erythematosus IRF5 risk haplotype is associated with systemic sclerosis. https://core.ac.uk/download/9653223.pdf (accessed on 17th June 2025).

43. Gambardella, L., Giovannetti, A., Malorni, W., Pietraforte, D., et al. (2018). Oxidative stress in the pathogenesis of systemic scleroderma: An overview. https://core.ac.uk/download/188830467.pdf (accessed on 17th June 2025).

44. Georgescu, S. R., Mitran, C. I., Mitran, M. I., Sârbu, M., et al. (2016). Vulvodynia: An under-recognized disease. https://core.ac.uk/download/144552984.pdf (accessed on 17th June 2025).

45. Kearney, K. & Hicks, R. E. (2016). Early nurturing experiences, self-compassion, hyperarousal and scleroderma: The way we relate to ourselves may determine disease progression. https://www.ccsenet.org/journal/index.php/ijps/article/view/63646(accessed on 17th June 2025).

46. Jimenez, S. A., Lee, J. B., Mendoza, F. A., et al. (2012). A prospective observational study of mycophenolate mofetil treatment in progressive diffuse cutaneous systemic sclerosis of recent onset. https://core.ac.uk/download/129190941.pdf (accessed on 17th June 2025).

47. Jimenez, S. A., Mendoza, F. A., & Rosenbloom, J. (2013). Strategies for anti-fibrotic therapies. https://core.ac.uk/download/83049954.pdf (accessed on 17th June 2025).

48. Kay, K. A. (2015). *Relapsing-Remitting Multiple Sclerosis: Advances in Disease-Modifying Therapies*. https://open.bu.edu/bitstream/2144/13960/10/Kay_bu_0017N_11509_WEB.pdf (accessed on 17th June 2025).

49. Kodet O, Oreská S. Systemic Sclerosis Mimics [Internet]. New Insights into Systemic Sclerosis [Working Title]. IntechOpen; 2019. Available from: http://dx.doi.org/10.5772/intechopen.88546(accessed on 17th June 2025).

50. Macia, A., Muotri, A. R., & Saleh, A. (2019). Transposable elements, inflammation, and neurological disease. https://core.ac.uk/download/323065096.pdf (accessed on 17th June 2025).

51. Mohamed, A. A. W., Airó, P., Allanore, Y., Caramaschi, P., et al. (2012). Erectile dysfunction is frequent in systemic sclerosis and associated with severe disease: A study of the EULAR Scleroderma Trial and Research group. https://core.ac.uk/download/14524326.pdf (accessed on 17th June 2025).

52. Oreska S, Tomcik M. Gastrointestinal Involvement in Systemic Sclerosis: Overview, Neglected Aspects, Malnutrition, Body Composition and Management [Internet]. New Insights into Systemic Sclerosis [Working Title]. IntechOpen; 2019. Available from: http://dx.doi.org/10.5772/intechopen.88286(accessed on 17th June 2025).

53. Paoloni, M., Bernetti, A., Brignoli, O., Coclite, G. M., et al. (2017). Appropriateness and efficacy of spa therapy for musculoskeletal disorders: A Delphi method consensus initiative among experts in Italy. https://core.ac.uk/download/84928671.pdf (accessed on 17th June 2025).

54. Reay, N. (2008). *The Quality of Life in Patients with Diffuse and Limited Systemic Sclerosis*. https://core.ac.uk/download/288395350.pdf (accessed on 17th June 2025).

55. Ruaro, B., Salton, F., Gandin, I., Confalonieri, M., D'Oria, M., Hughes, M., Confalonieri, P., et al. (2022). Correlation between microvascular damage and internal organ involvement in scleroderma: Focus on lung damage and endothelial dysfunction. https://core.ac.uk/download/566469592.pdf (accessed on 17th June 2025).

IDIOPATHIC INFLAMMATORY MYOPATHIES

6

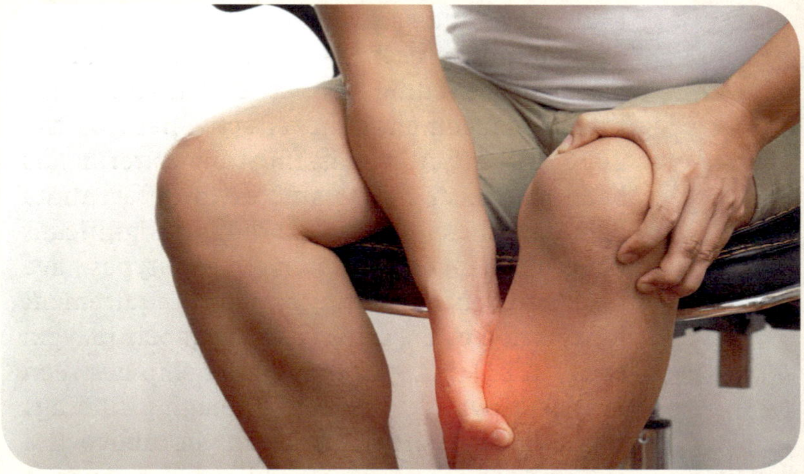

LEARNING OBJECTIVES

After studying this chapter, you will be able to:

1. Identify types of idiopathic inflammatory myopathies
2. Explain pathophysiology and mechanisms
3. Discuss diagnosis and assessment
4. Focus on treatment and management strategies

Introduction

Idiopathic Inflammatory Myopathies (IIM) is a heterogeneous collection of autoimmune diseases characterized by muscle inflammation, weakness, and variable levels of muscle damage. Such illnesses, e.g., polymyositis, dermatomyositis, and inclusion body myositis, are difficult to diagnose and treat owing to their complex clinical presentation and overlap with other disorders. The introduction of newer imaging techniques, such as ultrasound modalities, has much to contribute towards the improved comprehension and management of IIM. Shear wave elastography and power Doppler imaging have shown promise in muscle pathology estimation in IIM, although their accuracy and efficiency have to be substantiated by large-scale studies (Dankó et al., 2018; Paramalingam et al., 2023). This chapter will address the clinical features, diagnostic approach, and emerging treatment strategies for IIM, emphasizing a requirement for continued research and global collaboration in order to maximize outcomes for patients (Figure 6.1).

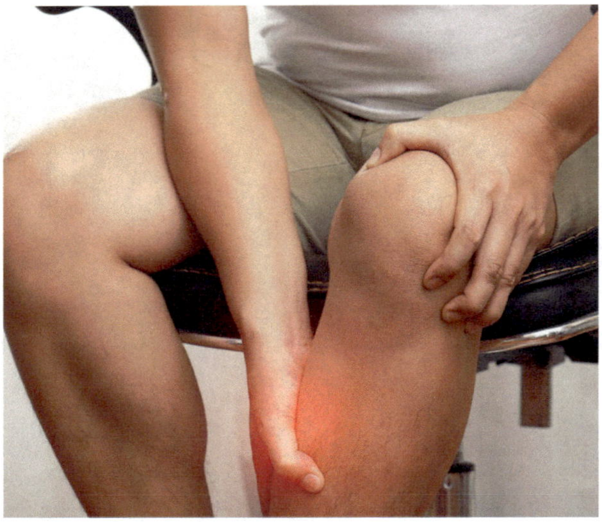

Figure 6.1. Idiopathic Inflammatory Myopathies (IIM) represent a diverse group of autoimmune diseases characterized by muscle inflammation, weakness, and varying degrees of muscle damage.

Source: https://ameripharmaspecialty.com/wp-content/uploads/2021/10/myositis.jpg.

6.1. Types of Idiopathic Inflammatory Myopathies

Learning Outcome

1. Understand polymyositis, and dermatomyositis
2. Focus on inclusion body myositis
3. Discuss necrotizing autoimmune myopathy
4. Learn overlap myositis
5. Describe juvenile idiopathic inflammatory myopathy
6. Explain the classification criteria
7. Know the differences in clinical features
8. Discuss the prognosis for each type

The clinicopathological range of idiopathic inflammatory myopathies (IIMs) consists of several different subtypes, each possessing its own clinical and pathological characteristics. The two most renowned varieties, for the most part, are polymyositis and dermatomyositis; these both present with symmetrical proximal weakness of muscles, but dermatomyositis is distinguished by skin manifestations as well. More recently, the onset of immune-mediated necrotizing myopathy has also been reported because of its distinctive histological changes and often severe muscle weakness. Notably, there are subtypes , such as intermittent antisynthetase syndrome and overlap myositis that also add complexity to the clinical presentation, presenting themselves in multiple ways and needing proper classification for their management. The effectiveness of the 2017 EULAR/ACR classification criteria has been shown in recent studies to differentiate between these subtypes, though significant flaws when it comes to some IIM subtypes have been noted, necessitating a radical requirement for revision of the criteria for diagnosis (Saygin et al., 2024). Further, the relationship between muscle magnetic resonance imaging findings and clinical characteristics in the above IIM subtypes is promising for enhanced diagnostic sensitivity (Shimoyama et al., 2024).

6.1.1. Polymyositis

Polymyositis (PM) is a familiar idiopathic inflammatory myopathy subtype characterized by symmetrical proximal weakness of the muscles and inflammation. While its pathogenesis remains unclear, it has previously been believed to be caused by an interplay between genetic susceptibility and environmental factors that stimulate the immune system against the muscle fibers. Similar to the other forms of myositis, PM is most often accompanied by specific autoantibodies, which may facilitate diagnosis and prognosis establishment (Bhardwaj et al., 2024). According to a retrospective analysis, patients with PM, particularly those with cardiac involvement or other autoimmune disease, were at higher risk of death, with infections being the main cause of death in this group of patients

(Opinc-Rosiak et al., 2025). Thus, prompt diagnosis and tailored treatment strategies are the key to achieving optimal results in patients suffering from polymyositis, reflecting the complexity and severity of this autoimmune illness in the broader landscape of idiopathic inflammatory myopathies (Figure 6.2).

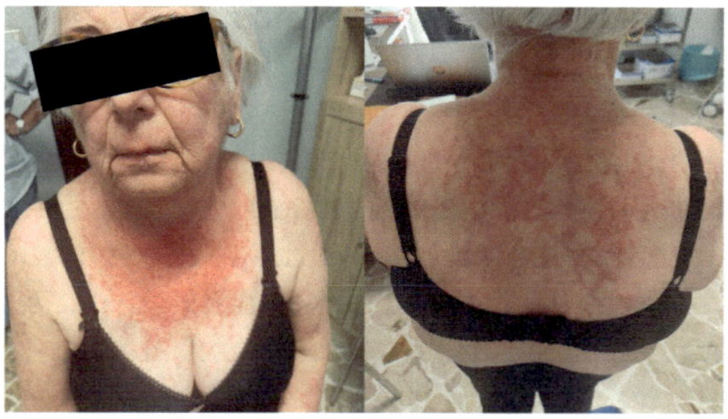

Figure 6.2. Polymyositis (PM) is a prominent subtype of idiopathic inflammatory myopathies characterized by symmetrical proximal muscle weakness and inflammation.

Source: https://www.mdpi.com/diagnostics/diagnostics-15-00275/article_deploy/html/images/diagnostics-15-00275-g001.png.

6.1.2. Dermatomyositis

Among patients with idiopathic inflammatory myopathies, dermatomyositis is not only differentiated by its typical cutaneous manifestations but also by its severe impact on muscle function and quality. The autoimmune condition predominantly affects the skin and skeletal muscle, most often with characteristic rashes coupled with progressive muscle weakness. Of interest, the epidemiological information indicates that dermatomyositis is the most prevalent subtype of idiopathic inflammatory myopathies, with 71% of the cases included in a Chilean referral center study had an annual incidence of 0.58 per 100,000 adults (Ramirez et al., 2025). Furthermore, dermatomyositis also has a direct relationship with interstitial lung disease (ILD), where up to 60% of patients may present with ILD as the first symptom. Identification of the risk for ILD in such patients is crucial, as early detection might enable successful treatment, which may help stabilize lung function and prevent worsening of dermatomyositis manifestations (Morina et al., 2025).

6.1.3. Inclusion Body Myositis

Inclusion body myositis (IBM) is a distinctive form of idiopathic inflammatory myopathy, one which occurs most frequently in older adults, typically individuals over the age of 50.

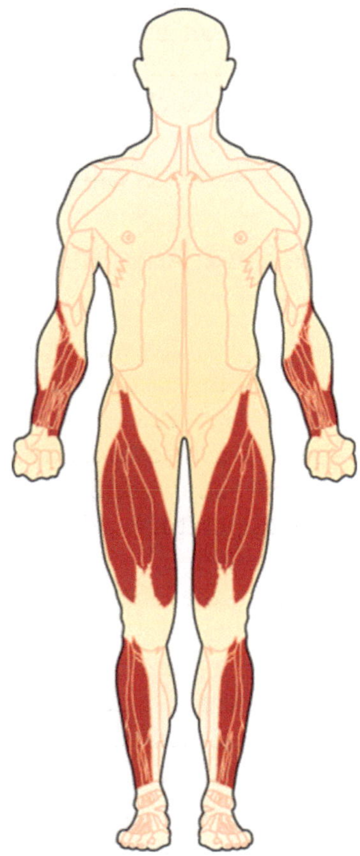

Figure 6.3. Inclusion body myositis (IBM) stands out as a distinct form of idiopathic inflammatory myopathy, predominantly affecting older adults, typically those over the age of 50.

It is characterized by progressively increasing muscle weakness and atrophy and affects proximal and distal muscle groups asymmetrically, in contrast to the distribution of other inflammatory myopathies , such as dermatomyositis and polymyositis. Unfortunately, your treatments for IBM are limited in number and unsuccessful; while corticosteroids are used for most inflammatory diseases, they have no proven benefit in IBM. More recently, the use of intravenous immunoglobulin has been reported to slow disease progression and some improvement may occur, though efficacy has not yet been established over the long term (Aggarwal et al., 2012). The issues in treating it are compounded by IBM's lengthy progression, which renders therapeutic efficacy an evaluation nightmare (Bohan et al., 2011). As a result, ongoing research into more effective interventions is still necessary to improve outcomes in those afflicted with this illness (Figure 6.3).

6.1.4. Necrotizing Autoimmune Myopathy

As a large subgroup of idiopathic inflammatory myopathies, necrotizing autoimmune myopathy (NAM) is characterized by rapid muscle weakness and typical pathological features, including widespread muscle fiber necrosis with sparse inflammatory infiltration. NAM is often accompanied by significant clinical heterogeneity, and therefore, diagnosis and treatment can be difficult. NAM patients may be resistant to standard immunosuppressive therapy, and thus, there is value in exploring new treatment modalities. Actually, the association of NAM with comorbidities is a trend to worry about; patients with IIMs like NAM also have a high prevalence of comorbidities that negatively impact their health and overall quality of life. For instance, studies establish that patients with IIMs have far higher rates of intricate multimorbidity than healthy controls, and as such, have more severe physical and mental health outcomes (Fornaro et al., 2023). Effective NAM management involves a multidisciplinary approach to addressing these diverse health conditions to tailor treatment to the individual patient (Jasper F Nies et al., 2024).

6.1.5. Overlap Myositis

Overlap myositis constitutes a significant subgroup among the idiopathic inflammatory myopathies, characterized by the concomitant presence of myositis and systemic autoimmune diseases, such as systemic lupus erythematosus and scleroderma. Overlap myositis challenges traditional paradigms in diagnosis due to its nonspecific clinical presentation and variable symptomatology. It shares the features of both myositis and other autoimmunity in patients, making therapeutic regimens complicated. The immunologic and genetic underpinnings of overlap myositis remain to be explored, with evidence for shared autoantibodies across related syndromes (Bianchi et al., 2024). Overlap myositis cannot be distinguished from the pure clinical forms of dermatomyositis or pure polymyositis on a clinical basis without diligent autoantibody panel evaluation and clinical history, as corticosteroid response may vary significantly across different subtypes (Okikiade et al., 2023). Understanding overlap myositis thus highlights the interconnectedness and complexity of autoimmune disorders, influencing both treatment and diagnosis (Figure 6.4).

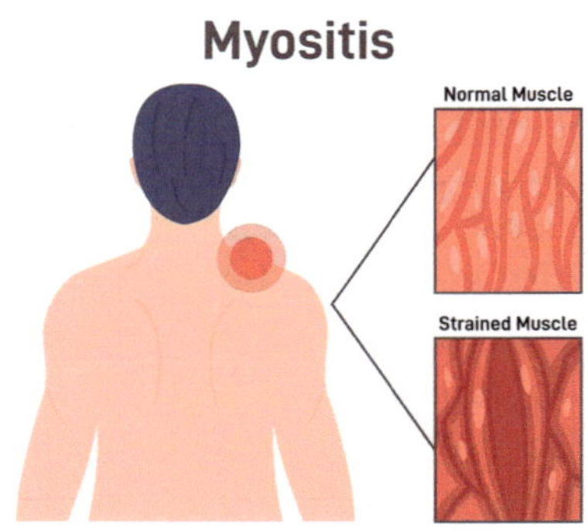

Figure 6.4. Overlap myositis.

Source: https://aarc.sg/wp-content/uploads/2023/10/shutterstock_2179418729.jpg.

6.1.6. Juvenile Idiopathic Inflammatory Myopathy

Juvenile idiopathic inflammatory myopathy (JIIM) is a group of autoimmune diseases characterized by muscle weakness and inflammation, most frequently found in children and early adolescents. The JIIM pathophysiology involves intricate processes involving transcription factors , such as nuclear factor κB (NF-κB) and nuclear factor of activated T-cells (NFAT), having a dualism of their function in both muscle damage and regeneration. Activation of NF-κB in blood vessel endothelium is important for the influx of inflammatory cells into muscle tissue, more relevant in dermatomyositis than in other forms of myositis, and NFAT activation is an indicator of the localized tissue injury seen in inflamed muscle fibers. Although strides towards elucidating these pathways have been made, identification and utilization of valid biomarkers for JIIM remain in their early stages, with proof to support their routine clinical use still absent, thus emphasizing the importance of ongoing research in this new field (De Paepe & Zschüntzsch, 2015; Benveniste et al., 2019).

6.1.7. Classification Criteria

The classification of idiopathic inflammatory myopathies (IIM) has been significantly advanced with the utilization of the EULAR/ACR criteria, formulated under the supervision of an expert panel to maximize diagnostic precision. Even though they are extensive, recent evidence has shown limitations in these criteria in terms of excluding specific IIM subtypes, such as immune-mediated necrotizing myopathy and antisynthetase syndrome, that make classification and disease treatment more difficult (Saygin et al., 2024).

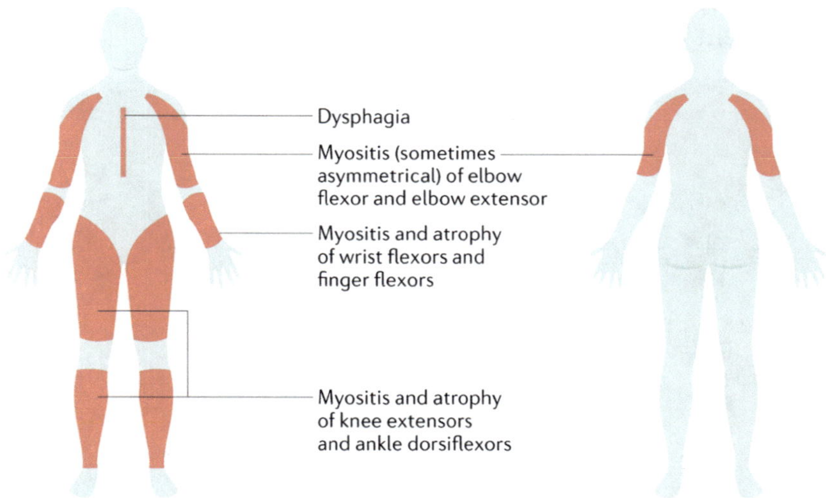

Figure 6.5. The classification of idiopathic inflammatory myopathies (IIM) has been significantly advanced through the implementation of the EULAR/ACR criteria, which were established by a consortium of experts aimed at improving diagnostic accuracy.

Source: https://media.springernature.com/lw1200/springer-static/image/art%3A10.1038%2Fs41572-021-00321-x/MediaObjects/41572_2021_321_Fig6_HTML.png.

Furthermore, the role of electromyography (EMG) in IIM diagnosis has been virtually obviated in the context of these classification criteria despite evidence that fibrillation potentials and positive sharp waves are ubiquitous even in partially meeting cases (Hokkoku et al., 2024). These developments underscore the necessity for revising the classification criteria to make them encompass the heterogeneity of IIM and be sensitive to developments in diagnostic methods (Figure 6.5).

6.1.8. Differences in Clinical Features

The clinical presentation of idiopathic inflammatory myopathies (IIMs) is extremely heterogeneous, particularly among the various subtypes , such as dermatomyositis (DM), polymyositis (PM), and inclusion body myositis (IBM). DM is characterized by typical skin features along with muscle weakness, while PM is normally characterized by symmetrical proximal muscle weakness without any dermatological findings. In contrast, IBM uniquely presents in older persons with its proximal and distal muscle involvement, asymmetrically in the majority, and is notoriously resistant to standard immunotherapies, unlike the responsiveness to DM and PM therapy (Aggarwal et al., 2012). Secondly, the rarity of these diseases complicates clinical understanding, and multicenter registries become a necessity for extensive studies and improved patient care (Bohan et al., 2011). These differences in clinical manifestations not only affect diagnosis and treatment strategies but also necessitate individualized therapeutic interventions to treat the diverse presentations of IIMs properly.

6.1.9. Prognosis for Each Type

An understandable knowledge of the prognosis for the two forms of idiopathic inflammatory myopathy (IIM), the most common of which are polymyositis and dermatomyositis, is crucial to optimal patient management and care.

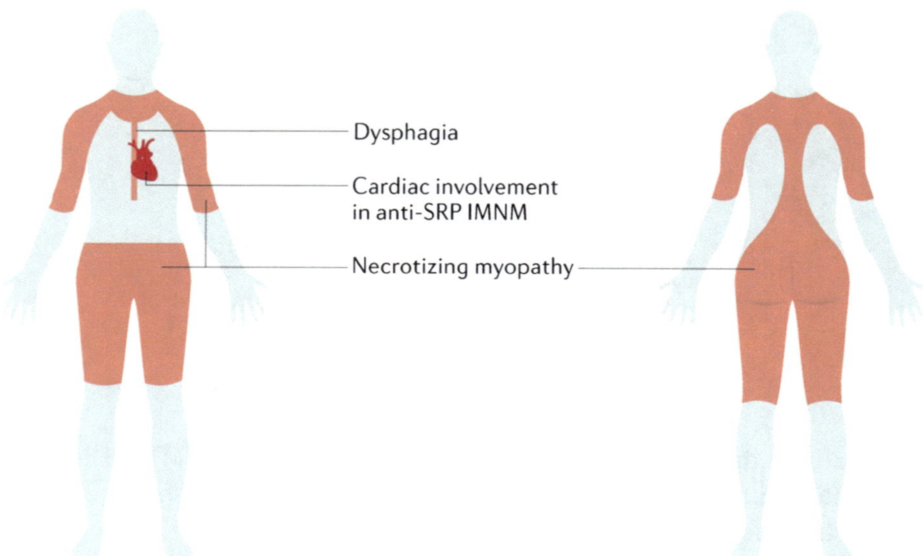

Figure 6.6. Understanding the prognosis for each type of idiopathic inflammatory myopathy (IIM), primarily polymyositis and dermatomyositis, is critical for patient management and care optimization.

Source: https://media.springernature.com/lw1200/springer-static/image/art%3A10.1038%2Fs41572-021-00321-x/MediaObjects/41572_2021_321_Fig5_HTML.png.

There is evidence that the two conditions have similar survival curves, with estimated five- and ten-year survival rates of 77% and 62% respectively, indicating an intermediate long-term prognosis for patients. Nonetheless, issues of age at diagnosis, sex, and race have significant impacts on outcomes, with increased survival risk in older patients and non-Caucasian races. In addition, the treatment approaches, specifically the corticosteroids used, also affect mortality, indicating that disease severity at treatment initiation has an impactful role (Benveniste et al., 2019). With ongoing progress in research, the incorporation of biomarkers in the prognostic algorithm is important, though their usage presently is limited because of a need for further validation (Benveniste et al., 2019). In the end, there needs to be a multifaceted approach to the improvement of prognostic estimates in IIM (Figure 6.6).

Test Your Knowledge

1. What are the characteristic skin findings in dermatomyositis?
2. What are overlap myositis syndromes, and which autoimmune diseases are commonly associated?

6.2. Pathophysiology and Mechanisms

Learning Outcome

1. Focus on the immune system involvement
2. Discuss the role of autoantibodies
3. Understand muscle fiber damage
4. Explain inflammatory processes
5. Describe genetic predispositions
6. Identify environmental triggers
7. Discuss the role of cytokines and chemokines
8. Understand muscle regeneration and repair mechanisms
9. Focus on current research on pathophysiological mechanisms

Idiopathic inflammatory myopathies (IIMs) pathophysiology involves complex interactions of autoimmune mechanisms leading to inflammation and damage of the muscles. Central to the process are autoantibodies, such as those directed against aminoacyl-tRNA synthetases, which are implicated in antisynthetase syndrome and correlate with interstitial lung disease and other distinct clinical phenotypes (Wu et al., 2024). Aside from that, the occurrence of specific antibodies, like anti-Mi-2 in dermatomyositis, not only indicates classic skin manifestations but also impacts disease prognosis (Wu et al., 2024). On a cellular level, dysregulation of major histocompatibility complex (MHC) molecules, as highlighted in newer studies, amplifies autoimmune responses, with methods applied to quantify the proteins quantitatively, excluding observational bias while improving diagnostic sensitivity. Lastly, knowledge of these mechanisms is paramount to understanding targeted therapies and improved patient outcomes in IIMs (Figure 6.7).

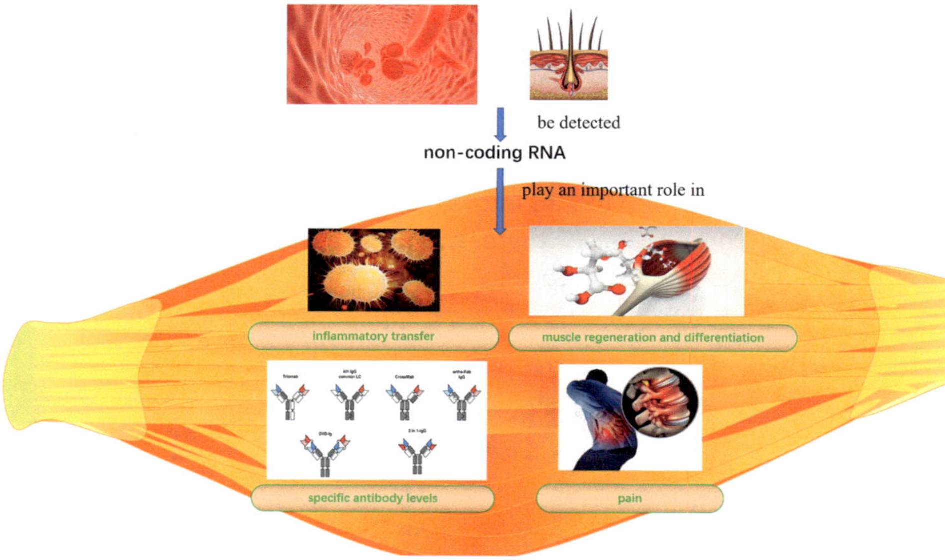

Figure 6.7. The pathophysiology of idiopathic inflammatory myopathies (IIMs) is marked by a complex interplay of autoimmune mechanisms that lead to muscle inflammation and damage.

Source: https://www.frontiersin.org/files/Articles/1227945/fimmu-14-1227945-HTML/image_m/fimmu-14-1227945-g001.jpg.

6.2.1. Immune System Involvement

The immune system plays a central role in the pathogenesis of idiopathic inflammatory myopathies (IIM), wherein an unbalanced immune response contributes significantly to inflammation and damage in muscle tissues. Foremost among these is the activation of specific transcription factors, i.e., nuclear factor κB (NF-κB) and nuclear factor of activated T-cells (NFAT), which are responsible for mediating expression of most pro-inflammatory cytokines and chemokines. Such shared activation not only propagates inflammatory cell recruitment but also reflects tissue damage patterns in specific IIM subtypes. In dermatomyositis, for instance, inflammation tends to amass mostly perimysially, while in polymyositis, infiltrating immune cells penetrate nonnecrotic muscle fibers, which exhibits an intricate relationship between immune activation and muscle pathology. A wide-ranging cytokine network, involving tumor necrosis factors (TNFs) and interleukins, further underscores the immune mediator function in IIM, with potential therapeutic targets for modulating these inflammatory pathways (De Paepe & Zschüntzsch, 2015; De Paepe, 2017).

6.2.2. Role of Autoantibodies

In idiopathic inflammatory myopathies (IIM), the role of autoantibodies is better appreciated to be central in diagnosis and understanding of underlying immunopathogenesis. Autoantibodies may not only be key biomarkers that contribute to the diagnosis of some subtypes, such as polymyositis and dermatomyositis, but also in disease course prediction and response to treatment. Their presence is typically associated with specific muscle pathologies and with the degree of inflammation, and therefore, they provide information about the clinical heterogeneity of these diseases. Moreover, their detection makes possible the creation of targeted therapeutic approaches towards the intricate cytokine networks involved in IIM, comprising a wide variety of immune mediators like TNF and interleukins (De Paepe & Zschüntzsch, 2015). The establishment of large registries, for example, the studies in pediatric populations, also mirrors the role that autoantibodies will have to play in guiding clinical trials and improving patient outcomes (Bohan et al., 2011) (Figure 6.8).

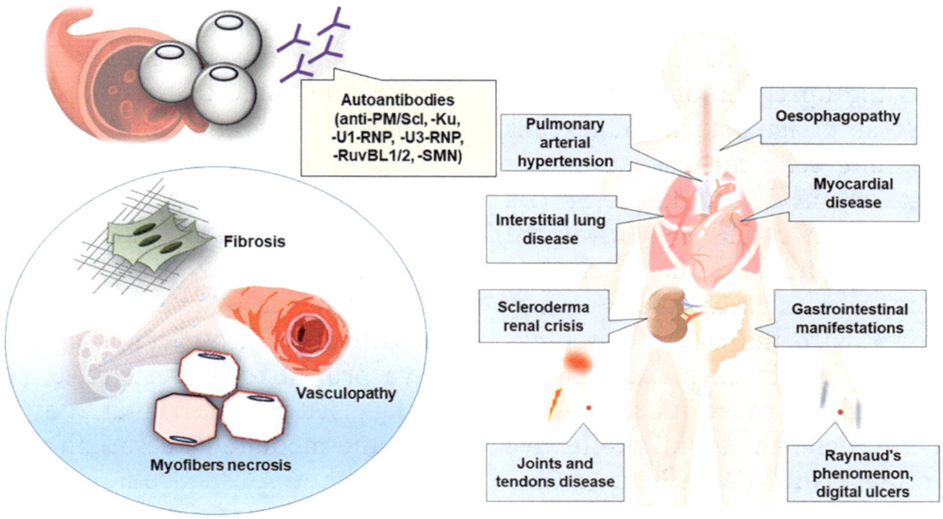

Figure 6.8. Autoantibodies can serve as important biomarkers that not only assist in confirming the diagnosis of various subtypes, such as polymyositis and dermatomyositis, but also help in predicting disease progression and treatment response.

Source: https://www.frontiersin.org/files/Articles/974078/fimmu-13-974078-HTML-r1/image_m/fimmu-13-974078-g002.jpg.

6.2.3. Muscle Fiber Damage

Muscle fiber damage is an integral part of the IIMs' pathology, immune-mediated muscle diseases. The inflammation induced by these conditions triggers a cascade of cellular and molecular events leading to profound muscle damage. In this environment, inflammatory cell invasion, e.g., macrophages and lymphocytes, amplifies tissue damage and disrupts normal regenerative processes in muscles. Evidence indicates that cytokines and chemokines play a central role in mediating this inflammatory response, both as proactivators and recruiters of immune cells. Remarkably, studies have documented that in chronic inflammation, such as that observed in Duchenne muscular dystrophy, these signaling molecules can regulate the management of muscle fiber damage and regeneration, highlighting their dual role in disease and therapeutic potential (Bleecker et al., 2013). It is crucial to understand these mechanisms to create specific treatments to reduce muscle fiber damage in IIMs (Cappelletti et al., 2011).

6.2.4. Inflammatory Processes

The inflammatory pathways in idiopathic inflammatory myopathies (IIMs) are complex and multifunctional, with a cacophony of cellular and molecular interactions. At the heart of them is the activation of transcription factors , such as nuclear factor κB (NF-κB) and nuclear factor of activated T-cells (NFAT) and are central to the regulation of cytokine and chemokine expression. These signal molecules are most important in the recruitment and activation of inflammatory cells, which cause the damage to muscle fibers and weakness seen in IIMs. One such example is the upregulation of NF-κB in endothelial cells as a signal to immune cells so that the immune cells can accumulate in muscles, particularly in dermatomyositis (De Paepe, 2017). Further, cytokine involvement in inflammation and healing during chronic inflammation, as seen in Duchenne muscular dystrophy, directs us to the role of cytokines as therapeutic targets (Bleecker et al., 2013). Hence, understanding these pathways of inflammation is crucial in defining effective management protocols for IIMs (Figure 6.9).

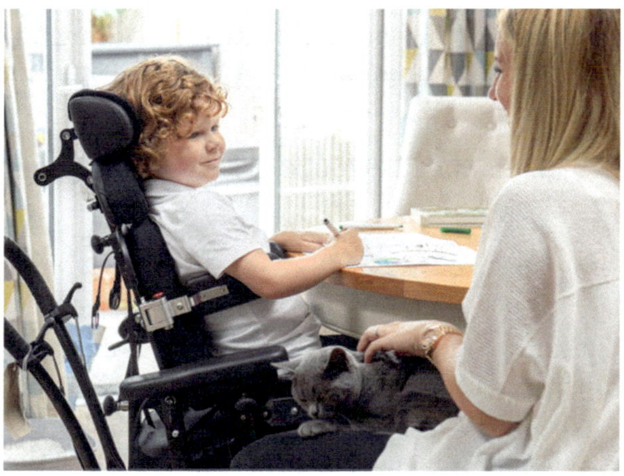

Figure 6.9. The inflammatory processes underlying idiopathic inflammatory myopathies (IIMs) are complex and multifaceted, involving a myriad of cellular and molecular interactions.

Source: https://www.utsouthwestern.edu/newsroom/articles/year-2020/assets/duchenne-muscular-header.jpg.

6.2.5. Genetic Predispositions

Explaining genetic predispositions is essential while studying idiopathic inflammatory myopathies (IIM), which are complex autoimmune diseases characterized by inflammation and muscle weakness. It has been suggested that certain genetic determinants contribute to the pathology of IIM to a great extent. For instance, gene variations that regulate immune responses would make one more vulnerable to these diseases, indicating a heritable component that needs further investigation. This genetic basis not only allows for an understanding of disease pathogeneses but also affects classification efforts, such as with the creation of the 2017 EULAR/ACR criteria, which tried to offer a format for IIM subtype classification. However, the current criteria have proven to be restrictive, particularly in being used for individual subtypes , such as immune-mediated necrotizing myopathy and antisynthetase syndrome, thus emphasizing the need for ongoing improvement with the development of new genetic data (Conticini et al., 2024; Saygin et al., 2024). This is required for the purposes of improving diagnostic accuracy and therapeutic approaches.

6.2.6. Environmental Triggers

The role of environmental stimuli in developing and causing idiopathic inflammatory myopathies (IIM) is a complex interaction of variables warranting careful examination. Current evidence suggests that these triggers, from infections to inhalants to even geoclimatic forces, have the potential to dysregulate immune tolerance, thereby inducing disease onset in genetically predisposed individuals. However, study populations have been small and diverse, yielding fragmented and nonconclusive evidence on individual contributions of the environment (Cardelli et al., 2024). Notably, autoimmune responses are believed to be initiated due to the exposures, with muscle and lung injury characteristic of IIM (Martins et al., 2025). Identifying these environmental triggers is of major significance to better manage patients and tailor preventive interventions, and this is where more research is to be conducted to establish more certain correlations between such triggers and the various expressions of idiopathic inflammatory myopathies (Figure 6.10).

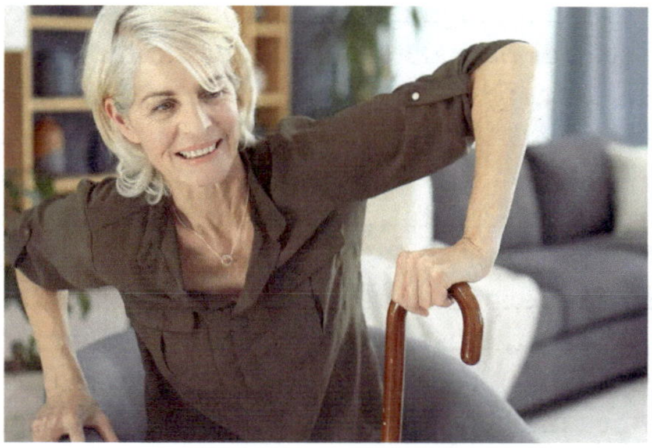

Figure 6.10. The role of environmental triggers in the onset and progression of idiopathic inflammatory myopathies (IIM) presents a complex interplay of factors that warrant careful examination.

Source: https://medicinetoday.com.au/sites/default/files/styles/wide/public/2024-10/1024Idiopathic_inflammatory_myopathies_CH.jpg.webp?itok=_C2JxJxb.

6.2.7. Role of Cytokines and Chemokines

Cytokines and chemokines play a pivotal role in the pathogenesis of idiopathic inflammatory myopathies (IIM), orchestrating the immune response and controlling muscle inflammation. Immune signaling molecules, these cytokines and chemokines are responsible for recruiting and activating key immune cells to mediate the inflammatory milieu of IIM. For example, in conditions , such as dermatomyositis and polymyositis, cytokines like interleukin-6 (IL-6) and TNF-alpha (TNF-α) are elevated, enhancing an inflammatory state that causes muscle fiber damage. Furthermore, chemokines act as chemoattractants, drawing inflammatory cells to sites of tissue damage and thereby exacerbating disease. Worthy of note are the nuclear factor κB (NF-κB) and nuclear factor of activated T-cells (NFAT) signaling pathways, which play a central role in this process as they regulate the expression of most immune mediators after damage to muscles and inflammation, and indicate their complex interaction in disease pathogenesis (Bleecker et al., 2013; De Paepe, 2017).

6.2.8. Muscle Regeneration and Repair Mechanisms

Muscle repair and regeneration processes are a vital part of idiopathic inflammatory myopathies (IIMs) pathogenesis, since the involved autoimmune pathology markedly influences these processes. Immune-mediated damage to the muscle fibers in IIMs needs a successful response in order to maintain muscle homeostasis. Macrophages, a central player in muscle inflammation, have a dual role; they can promote damage by secreting proinflammatory cytokines and reactive oxygen species, but also tissue repair and regeneration. Some macrophage subsets, specifically, promote muscle fiber regeneration by secreting growth factors that induce satellite cell activation and proliferation, which are crucial in muscle healing. Dysregulation of these processes, as typically seen with IIMs, leads to impaired muscle recovery and prolonged weakness. Understanding of these intricate interactions, and more importantly, the macrophage polarization phases, is imperative to the development of focused therapeutic approaches that aim to repair muscle function and prevent disease progression (Li et al., 2024; Izuka et al., 2025) (Figure 6.11).

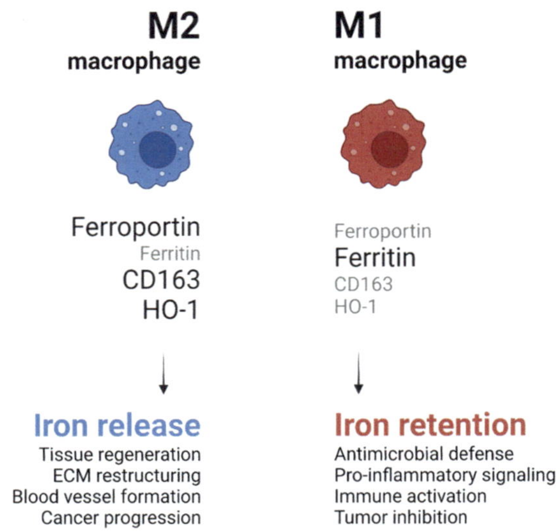

Figure 6.11. Macrophages, as central players in muscle inflammation, have dual roles; they can exacerbate damage through the release of proinflammatory cytokines and reactive oxygen species while also facilitating tissue repair and regeneration.

Source: https://pub.mdpi-res.com/ijms/ijms-26-02107/article_deploy/html/images/ijms-26-02107-g004.png?1740734396.

6.2.9. Current Research on Pathophysiological Mechanisms

Recent studies of the pathophysiologic mechanisms of idiopathic inflammatory myopathies (IIM) have uncovered significant complexities to present diagnostic paradigms. Studies have highlighted the role of biomarkers as central parameters in understanding these conditions; however, clinical application of biomarkers is presently limited by a paucity of validation in large patient populations, and careful interpretation of findings is needed (Benveniste et al., 2019). IIM classification has also been expanded to include phenotypes, such as antisynthetase syndrome and autoimmune necrotizing myopathy, which characterize the refined interplay between clinical, immunologic, and histologic features of the diseases (A'Callaghan et al., 2011). This ongoing research is crucial not only for the establishment of better diagnostic criteria but also for individualized therapy, since myositis pathophysiology is only partially known. Hence, studies currently seek to deepen our knowledge of such mechanisms, eventually facilitating progress in both diagnostics and treatments for those so affected.

Test Your Knowledge

1. How does the pathophysiology of inclusion body myositis involve degenerative mechanisms?
2. How do cytokines and chemokines contribute to muscle inflammation and damage?

6.3. Diagnosis and Assessment

Learning Outcome

1. Explain clinical evaluation and history
2. Discuss laboratory tests and biomarkers
3. Define electromyography (EMG)
4. Understand muscle biopsy techniques
5. Focus on imaging studies
6. Describe differential diagnosis considerations
7. Know the role of multidisciplinary teams
8. Identify challenges in early diagnosis
9. Learn advances in diagnostic technologies

Correct diagnosis and thorough examination are crucial in the treatment of idiopathic inflammatory myopathies (IIMs). The disease typically presents with muscle weakness and overlaps with other autoimmune diseases, hence complicating diagnosis. Clinicians utilize a combined approach, including careful patient history, clinical presentation, and laboratory testing , such as muscle enzyme levels and autoantibody titers. Electromyography (EMG) and magnetic resonance imaging (MRI) are also valuable tools for the detection of characteristic muscle inflammation. In recent times, the formation of guidelines by bodies like the American College of Rheumatology has raised diagnostic precision, keeping in mind the importance of interdisciplinary treatment by specialists to develop strategies based on patient-specific scenarios. Furthermore, evolving evidence emphasizes the importance of individually crafted diagnostic pathways to differentiate IIMs from other syndromes, particularly those that accompany viral infections like COVID-19, where frequent testing and novel evidence continually inform management strategies (Henderson et al., 2020; Glikson et al., 2021) (Figure 6.12).

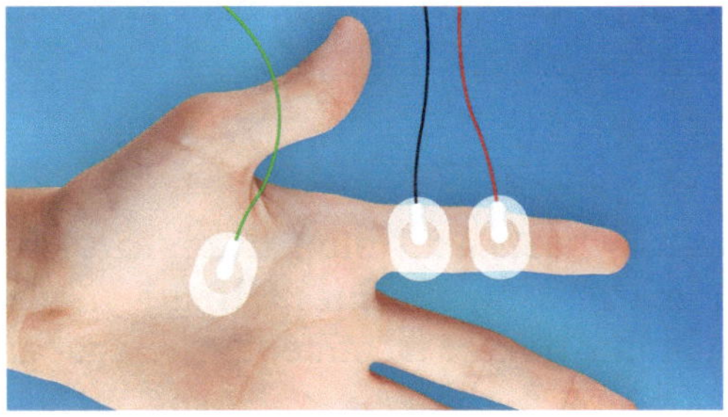

Figure 6.12. Electromyography (EMG) and magnetic resonance imaging (MRI) also play crucial roles in identifying characteristic muscle inflammation.

Source: https://d2yjegym0lbr1w.cloudfront.net/thumbs/electromyography_1280.jpg?v=201701103.

6.3.1. Clinical Evaluation and History

The clinical evaluation and history taking in suspected idiopathic inflammatory myopathies (IIM) patients is a critical process, which serves for decision-making and guiding diagnosis. The assessment typically involves a comprehensive evaluation that includes the quantification of muscle strength, skin manifestations, and joint symptoms since the disease is associated with heterogeneous manifestations overlapping other diseases. In addition, careful patient history is critical in establishing possible environmental triggers or concomitant autoimmune disease that can affect the course of the disease. Recent advances have identified the importance of multicenter associations to broaden our understanding of these rare disorders; for example, a national registry that was initiated in the UK has been able to collect detailed clinical and biological data from children significantly expanding the body of information available for juvenile myositis (Bohan et al., 2011).

The complexities of cytokine involvement also underscore the importance of vigilant clinical evaluations, as they can reveal distinctive pathogenic pathways and inform targeted therapeutic interventions in the treatment of IIM (De Paepe & Zschüntzsch, 2015).

6.3.2. Laboratory Tests and Biomarkers

Laboratory tests and biomarkers are important in the diagnosis and treatment of idiopathic inflammatory myopathies (IIMs) in that they contribute to a better understanding and individualization of treatment. They act as markers of pathophysiological conditions that exist at the core, and hence, clinicians can make effective diagnostic and prognostic assessments. While their clinical usage is on the rise, evidence supporting routine use is still sparse, as emphasized by Benveniste et al. (2019). Further, development of multicenter registries and biobanks, for example, of pediatric IIMs, is a tool for efficient data collection and further studies, which is in acute need due to the rarity of the diseases (Bohan et al., 2011). As investigation proceeds, confirmation of some of these biomarkers across different groups of patients will be increasingly significant, ultimately translating into improved patient outcomes for those suffering from these complex illnesses (Figure 6.13).

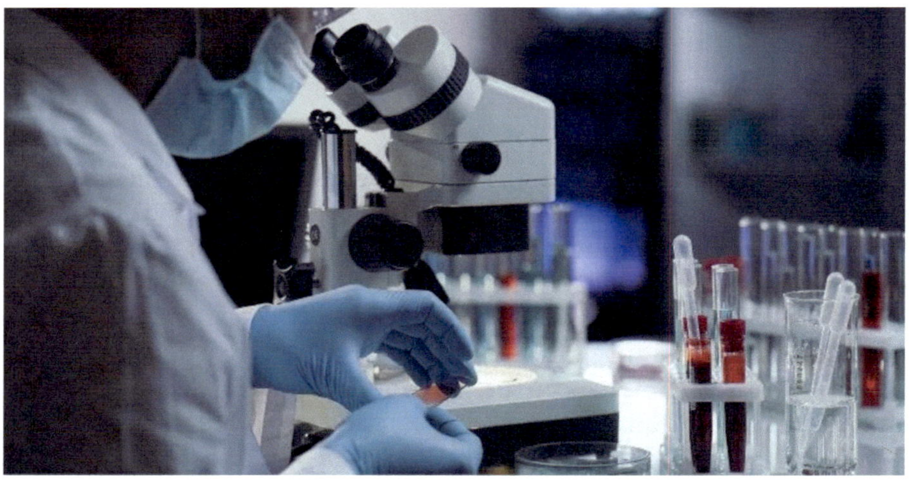

Figure 6.13. In the diagnosis and management of idiopathic inflammatory myopathies (IIMs), laboratory tests and biomarkers play a crucial role in enhancing understanding and tailoring treatment strategies.

Source: https://eu-images.contentstack.com/v3/assets/blt485767b4a9c4cef5/blte2c4fe1ec2f83c11/673f01166f38b329b375b254/diagnostics_2.webp?width=1280&auto=webp&quality=95&format=jpg&disable=upscale.

6.3.3. Electromyography (EMG)

Electromyography (EMG) is an important diagnostic tool in the diagnosis of idiopathic inflammatory myopathies (IIM), providing critical information regarding muscle function and pathology. By assessing electrical muscle activity, EMG identifies abnormalities that indicate inflammation and muscle tissue damage. For instance, a pilot study conducted more recently developed an EMG-scoring protocol to optimize the assessment of disease activity in juvenile idiopathic inflammatory myopathies, focusing on the relationship between EMG and muscle strength measures (Cappellari et al., 2021). Apart from that, EMG has also played an important role in differentiating myopathies from other neuromuscular diseases, like statin-associated autoimmune myopathy, with EMG showing spontaneous activity due to muscle damage (Dokukin et al., 2017). This inclusion of EMG within the diagnostic procedure gives an integrative picture of muscle involvement, thereby enhancing the management and treatment of patients with IIM.

6.3.4. Muscle Biopsy Techniques

Muscle biopsy techniques are pivotal to the diagnosis and management of idiopathic inflammatory myopathies (IIM). With the procurement of a specimen of muscle tissue, clinicians can assess histological features of inflammatory reactions, such as the presence of necrotic fibers and infiltrating immune cells. The tests not only help distinguish between the different types of IIM but also help rule out other muscular diseases. The newer advances in imaging modalities, such as ultrasound, enhance the biopsy process through facilitating real-time visualization and enhancing the accuracy of the procedure. Studies have proven that the efficacy of ultrasound techniques like shear wave elastography has the potential to detect significant differences in muscle properties between controls and IIM patients and thereby inform future treatment (Aggarwal et al., 2012; Paramalingam et al., 2023). Overall, muscle biopsy remains a foundational tool in the diagnostic arsenal against IIM, contributing significantly to patient outcomes (Figure 6.14).

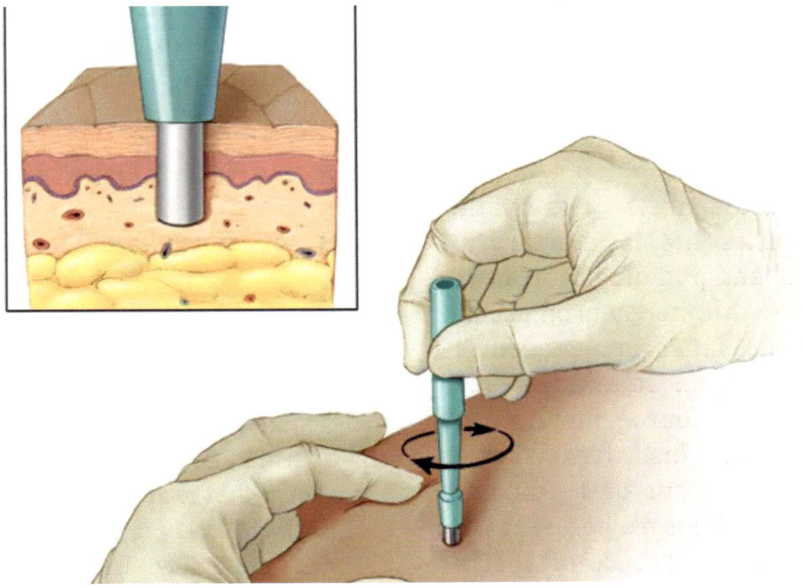

Figure 6.14. Muscle biopsy techniques play a crucial role in the diagnosis and management of idiopathic inflammatory myopathies (IIM).

Source: https://thelifesciencesmagazine.com/wp-content/uploads/2024/09/2.-Understanding-Soft-Tissue-Biopsy_-Procedure-Types-and-What-to-Expect-source-.mayoclinic.org_.jpg.

6.3.5. Imaging Studies (MRI, CT)

Technological improvements in imaging studies, particularly magnetic resonance imaging (MRI) and computed tomography (CT), have significantly advanced the evaluation and management of idiopathic inflammatory myopathies (IIMs). MRI is a valuable imaging tool for the imaging of muscle inflammation and damage and for assessment of large muscle groups and identification of abnormalities related to clinical manifestations. It not only aids in diagnosis but also in tracking response to treatment and disease progression. Additionally, CT scans prove beneficial in providing valuable information, especially when exploring associated pulmonary findings. However, despite these imaging modalities' efficacy, their application is generally plagued by factors of cost and accessibility. As suggested, imaging biomarkers are increasingly at the forefront of IIM management, complementing traditional assessment and the way ahead for more integrated care for patients (Aggarwal et al., 2012; Dimachkie et al., 2023). In the end, these novel imaging modalities are particularly promising as a direction for the future of diagnosing and treating IIMs.

6.3.6. Differential Diagnosis Considerations

Accurate differential diagnosis of idiopathic inflammatory myopathies (IIM) is necessary due to the shared clinical and pathological features of these conditions with other neuromuscular conditions. Clinicians must make accurate differentiation of IIM from conditions, such as muscular dystrophies, neurogenic diseases, and systemic autoimmune disorders , such as systemic lupus erythematosus or rheumatoid arthritis, where the conditions may present with myopathic features. The presence of specific autoantibodies can also play a huge role in this process because studies indicate that specific autoantibody profiles correlate with specific clinical subsets of IIM and thus further improve diagnostic specificity (Leclair, 2023). Further, varying responses to therapy, such as with rituximab in anti-aminoacyl tRNA synthetase-positive individuals, further underscore the importance of accurate classification in therapy (De Paepe & Zschüntzsch, 2015). Hence, systematic clinical evaluation, laboratory examinations, and advanced imaging tests are crucial in establishing a proper diagnosis and effective treatment for IIM patients (Figure 6.15).

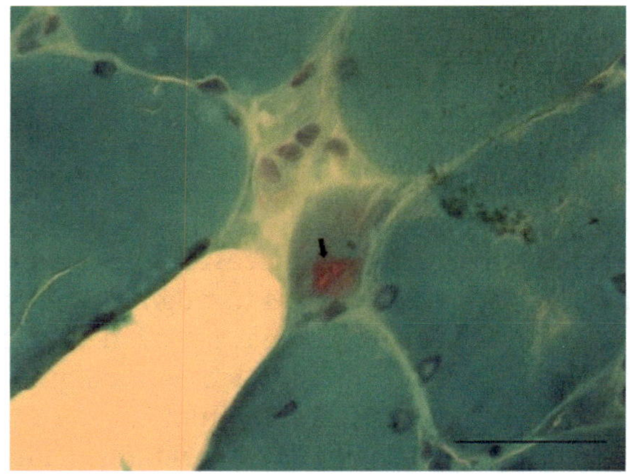

Figure 6.15. Accurate differential diagnosis in idiopathic inflammatory myopathies (IIM) is critical due to the clinical and pathological similarities these conditions share with other neuromuscular disorders.

Source: https://www.tandfonline.com/cms/asset/a4450502-1fbe-4c32-86d5-8ef8784d2034/ilab_a_2000584_f0009_c.jpg.

6.3.7. Role of Multidisciplinary Teams

The management of idiopathic inflammatory myopathies (IIMs) involves a multi-disciplinary approach that is able to leverage the expertise of multidisciplinary teams. Such multidisciplinary teams typically include rheumatologists, neurologists, physical therapists, and occupational therapists, all of whom play definitive roles in managing the intricate and varied presentations of the condition. Together, they can devise individualized treatment plans that take not just the patients' medical needs into consideration but also the psychosocial factors affecting their health. Also, the development of standardized treatment protocols is crucial because it upholds the importance of consensus among healthcare workers to deliver uniform and efficient treatment of IIMs (Paik et al., 2025). Here, the adoption of digital health solutions can augment self-management practices for patients through the use of personalized treatment plans as well as enhanced communication between team members and patients, bridging existing research and practice gaps (Battista et al., 2024).

6.3.8. Challenges in Early Diagnosis

Early diagnosis of IIM is particularly difficult because idiopathic inflammatory myopathies have a heterogeneous and complex etiology. Clinical features , such as weakness, fatigue, and dysphagia are non-specific and overlap with other disorders and therefore delay diagnosis. Additionally, the pathogenic processes of these conditions are poorly understood, which makes diagnostic criteria development complicated.

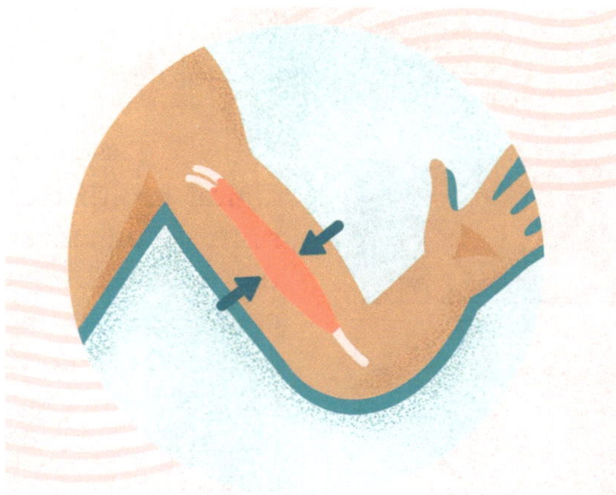

Figure 6.16. Symptoms , such as muscle weakness, fatigue, and dysphagia are often non-specific and can overlap with other conditions, delaying accurate identification.

Source: https://images.everydayhealth.com/images/2025-gateway-illustrations/eh-muscular-dystrophy-gg-1440x810.png?sfvrsn=dae618d9_4.

As highlighted in recent publications, identification of autoantibody profiles can be used to define individual IIM subgroups and possibly enhance diagnostic specificity, but these advances are not currently being translated to widespread clinical practice (Leclair et al., 2023). Access to specialty testing and diagnostic marker interpretation is also significant impediment for clinicians. Given these issues, increased awareness and education regarding the intricacies of IIM are called for with a focus on intervention and the best possible outcome for the patient (De Paepe & Zschüntzsch, 2015) (Figure 6.16).

6.3.9. Advances in Diagnostic Technologies

The recent developments in diagnostic technology have deeply influenced our understanding and management of idiopathic inflammatory myopathies (IIM). The integration of high-resolution imaging modalities, such as MRI, with advanced biomarker analysis has facilitated more precise identification of the diseases presentation and discrimination between a number of myopathic subtypes. For instance, new genomic sequencing technologies are increasingly being employed to uncover genetic susceptibility related to IIM, thus facilitating early diagnosis and customized treatment modalities. In addition, improvements in immunological profiling allow clinicians to have an increased understanding of autoimmune mechanisms leading to disease.

These technologies not only aid in diagnosing IIM but also increase our knowledge about concomitant autoimmune disorders and their complexity, for example, those caused by complement deficiencies, as enumerated in recent reviews of autoimmune disorders, for instance, the significance of genetic factors in systemic lupus erythematosus (Coss et al., 2022). Moreover, expanded diagnostic capacity can lead to earlier intervention, which may improve patient outcomes and quality of life (Rapezzi et al., 2022).

Test Your Knowledge

1. How is muscle biopsy used in the diagnosis and classification of IIMs?
2. What findings on MRI support a diagnosis of inflammatory myopathy?

6.4. Treatment and Management Strategies

Learning Outcome

1. Discuss corticosteroids and immunosuppressants
2. Understand physical therapy and rehabilitation
3. Explain the role of biologic therapies
4. Focus on nutritional considerations
5. Describe the management of comorbidities
6. Focus on patient education and support
7. Know long-term monitoring and follow-up
8. Identify emerging therapies and clinical trials
9. Discuss the impact of treatment on quality of life

Effective therapy and management strategies for idiopathic inflammatory myopathies (IIMs) are based on an interdisciplinary strategy that intersects conventional therapy with emerging self-management technologies. Conventional therapies, including corticosteroids and other immunomodulatory medications, have been the pillars of therapy for a long time; however, advances in disease pathogenesis have necessitated targeted interventions. Notably, digital health technologies provide a possible route to enhancing patient outcomes through the potential for engaging individuals in self-management by means of personalized treatment plans, symptom tracking, and education content that is aimed at facilitating long-term care plans (Battista et al., 2024). Existing research emphasizes the importance of establishing effective self-management interventions, with the study suggesting that there is a wide gap in research that must be filled in order to optimize patient participation and outcomes (Battista et al., 2024). Furthermore, continued research into novel therapies, such as targeted biologic agents, continues to change the paradigm of treatment, holding out promise for individualized treatment of these multifactorial disease entities.

6.4.1. Corticosteroids and Immunosuppressants

In the management of idiopathic inflammatory myopathies (IIMs), both corticosteroids and immunosuppressants play a key role in the suppression of the autoimmune process that characterizes these conditions. Corticosteroids, typically the first-line therapy, are invaluable due to their anti-inflammatory properties, with rapid reduction of symptoms and improvement in muscle strength. However, long-term corticosteroid administration has severe adverse effects for which the advent of immunosuppressive medications like mycophenolate mofetil and cyclosporine A is required to minimize steroid treatment and optimize the effectiveness of treatment (Gabrielli et al., 2011). While beneficial, their administration is quite heterogeneous across global regions, depending on gross national product as well as certain disease phenotypes (Agarwal et al., 2024). This disparity underscores the necessity to develop standardized treatment protocols emphasizing patient-focused care and considering differential access to therapeutic modalities across the world (Figure 6.17).

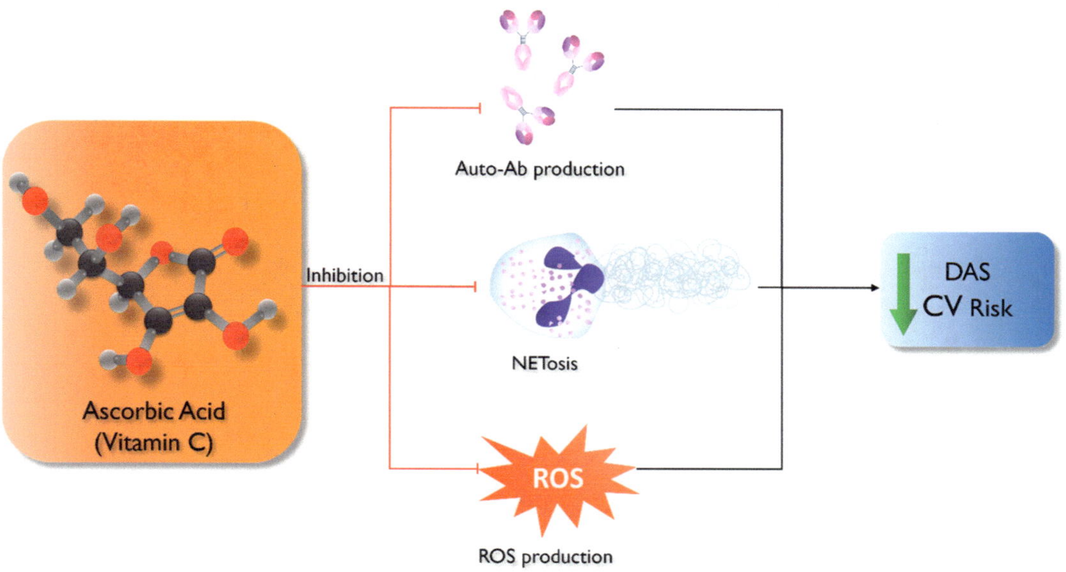

Figure 6.17. Corticosteroids and immunosuppressants play a pivotal role in mitigating the autoimmune response that characterizes these conditions.

Source: https://www.mdpi.com/ijms/ijms-25-07284/article_deploy/html/images/ijms-25-07284-g001.png

6.4.2. Physical Therapy and Rehabilitation

Physical rehabilitation and therapy are extremely crucial in the management of idiopathic inflammatory myopathies (IIM) as they play a great part in alleviating muscular weakness and also functional impairments typically seen with IIM. Rehabilitation therapy for IIM patients typically comprises a regimen consisting of a combination of exercise therapies to improve strength, endurance, and overall physical function. These treatments are extremely beneficial post-treatments like Rituximab (RTX), which has been shown to be beneficial in refractory IIM, evidenced by diminished glucocorticoid reliance and improved muscle function in patients (Gamba et al., 2024). Furthermore, novel modalities , such as transcranial direct current stimulation have also been investigated, with potential to further enhance pain reduction and fatigue decrease when combined with aerobic exercise (Missé et al., 2024). A multimodal approach using physical therapy, thus, not only aids rehabilitation but also allows patients to gain greater control over their disease and improve their quality of life.

6.4.3. Role of Biologic Therapies

Biologic agents have also proven to be a viable option for the treatment of idiopathic inflammatory myopathies (IIM) since they can target specific immunopathogenic mechanisms responsible for such diseases. The intricate cytokine network in IIM, wherein the activities of such factors as TNF and Interleukins are imbalanced, signals that a particular solution would prove more effective for patients. While conventional therapy, like corticosteroids, has been of limited benefit, biologic agents that repress these cytokines have been either partially or entirely successful. For instance, research has found that anti-IFN drugs have been able to diminish the type 1 interferon gene expression by far in dermatomyositis and polymyositis, thereby leading to improved muscle strength (Aggarwal et al., 2012). However, challenges are experienced, as in inclusion body myositis, with poor outcomes to the treatment, as a reflection of a need for more studies and clinical trials in order to determine the efficacy and safety of these biologic medications (Aggarwal et al., 2012) (Figure 6.18).

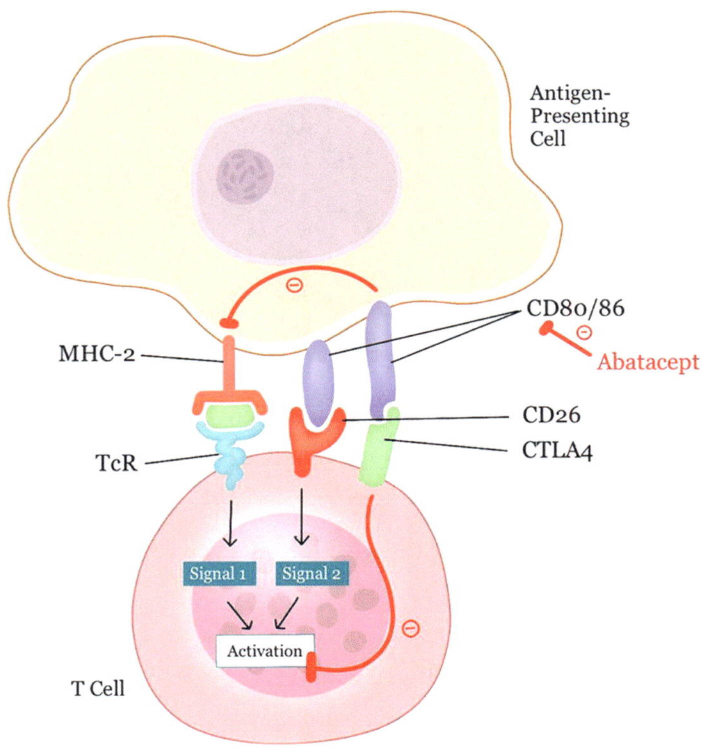

Figure 6.18. Mechanism of action of abatacept. MHC-2 – major histocompatibility complex – 2, TcR – T cell receptor.

Source: https://cdnintech.com/media/chapter/83765/1678862543/media/F3.png.

6.4.4. Nutritional Considerations

Nutritional implications form a critical part of Idiopathic Inflammatory Myopathies (IIM) treatment, with muscle inflammation potentially having a great influence on nutritional needs as well as overall well-being. A proper diet can alleviate symptoms, raise muscular strength, and lower the side effects of medication. For instance, an anti-inflammatory diet that includes fruits, vegetables, and omega-3 fatty acids can help support immune system function and combat inflammation. In addition, meeting protein requirements is critical for muscle mass maintenance, particularly in patients with muscle wasting.

Employing specific dietary strategies, as suggested by clinical guidelines, can also be employed to enhance gastrointestinal motility, typically deranged in IIM patients, and consequently their nutritional status and quality of life, as emphasized by recent studies on gastrointestinal motor disorders (Keller et al., 2018). Hence, a tailored nutritional plan is essential for improved results in patients with IIM and addressing the multi-factorial challenges that they pose (Klionsky et al., 2021).

6.4.5. Management of Comorbidities

Comorbidities in idiopathic inflammatory myopathies (IIMs) patients are significant to manage for the best outcomes of health and for enhancing the quality of life. Comorbidities are prevalent in IIM patients and contribute to morbidity, as well as complicate the treatment process. Studies have illustrated that physical and mental health among this population is significantly impaired, particularly in individuals with other comorbidities, which could further deteriorate their condition (Agarwal et al., 2024).

Effective management methods will have to be multi-disciplinary in scope, integrating rheumatology, neurology, and rehabilitation skills. Furthermore, consideration of specific needs regarding age, race, and sex can facilitate improved outcomes, as the survival distinction between polymyositis and dermatomyositis groups has demonstrated (Crofford et al., 2012). Thus, management of comorbidities not only controls the primary IIM but also becomes absolutely crucial in enhancing the overall health and survival of the patients (Figure 6.19).

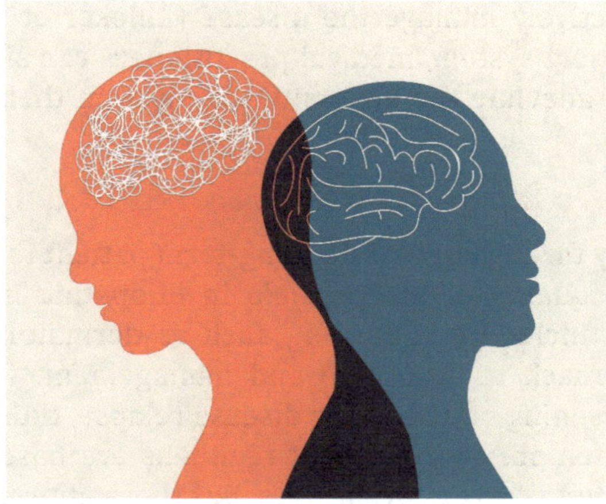

Figure 6.19. Physical and mental health in this population are significantly impaired, particularly in individuals with additional comorbidities, which can exacerbate their overall health status

Source: https://www.news-medical.net/images/Article_Images/ImageForArticle_22028_16430272124432966.jpg.

6.4.6. Patient Education and Support

Effective patient education and support are both essential components of the treatment of idiopathic inflammatory myopathies (IIMs), as they empower patients to become active participants in their treatment. Individualized education programs have the potential to enhance patients' understanding of their disease, their treatment plan, and compliance with recommended therapies. Recent controversies highlight the potential of digital health interventions, which offer symptom monitoring and messaging tools to engage with healthcare providers, eventually empowering patients with IIMs to self-manage and plan in the long term (Battista et al., 2024). Further, collective data within the EuroMyositis Registry also capture IIM heterogeneity, determining associations between clinical subtypes and extramuscular features that patients must be aware of to effectively manage the disease (Lilleker et al., 2017). With such resources and a comprehensive support system, medical practitioners can significantly improve the quality of life for IIM sufferers and alleviate the adversity they face in their daily living.

6.4.7. Long-term Monitoring and Follow-up

Only through successful long-term patient follow-up and monitoring is an optimal therapy outcome and quality of life possible in idiopathic inflammatory myopathies (IIM). The heterogeneity of IIM, including subtypes , such as dermatomyositis and polymyositis, requires a patient-tailored approach to follow-up and management. Regular assessment facilitates prompt recognition of worsening of disease or disease relapse, thus allowing proper adjustment in therapeutic strategies. Contemporary treatment regimens are based primarily on high-dose corticosteroids and add-on immunosuppressive agents, but these approaches need to be modified repeatedly according to the patient's reaction and secondary effects (Alves et al., 2016). Furthermore, the emerging discipline of cytokine profiling opens the door to targeted treatments and places a challenge on continuous research into the efficacy of treatment and patient stratification (De Paepe & Zschüntzsch, 2015). Thus, systematic follow-up visits not only improve clinical results but also drive insight into IIM pathogenesis and management (Figure 6.20).

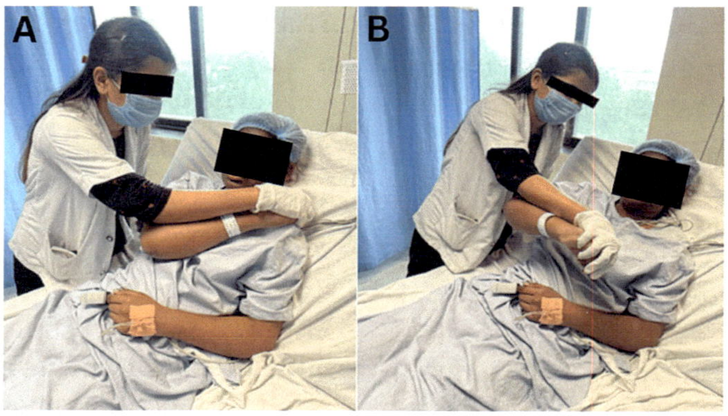

Figure 6.20. Effective long-term monitoring and follow-up of patients with idiopathic inflammatory myopathies (IIM) are crucial for optimizing treatment outcomes and enhancing quality of life.

Source: Waghe V R, Sasun A R, Raghumahanti R (January 24, 2024) Targeting Weakness With a Combination of Isotonic Exercises in Dermatomyositis With Polyneuropathy: A Case Report. Cureus 16(1): e52873. doi:10.7759/cureus.52873

6.4.8. Emerging Therapies and Clinical Trials

Exploring novel therapies for idiopathic inflammatory myopathies (IIM) is critical because of the limitations of current therapies, particularly the excessive use of glucocorticoids and immunosuppressants with high incidences of long-term toxicity risks. There is an urgent need for new therapeutic approaches, particularly one that not only improves patient outcomes but also reduces the side effects of conventional therapies. The Drug Rediscovery in IMIDs (DRIMID) consortium has already initiated trials into the efficacy of filgotinib, a Janus kinase (JAK) inhibitor, which is promising in other inflammatory conditions. The phase 2 trial will assess the impact of filgotinib on disease activity and quality of life in patients with refractory IIM, as well as corticosteroid toxicity and other biomarkers (Geertsema-Hoeve et al., 2025). Additionally, although few clinical trials over the years have resulted in unmet endpoints, current biologics abatacept and aldesleukin are under evaluation for their capacity to manage IIM, with progress in the field (Neves et al., 2024).

6.4.9. Impact of Treatment on Quality of Life

The treatment of idiopathic inflammatory myopathies significantly affects patients' quality of life, a result of the disease's multifaceted nature and the treatment employed. Traditional immunosuppressive therapy, mostly with glucocorticoids and other immune-modulating agents, more often results in mixed outcomes among patients, leading to continued muscle weakness and inflammation despite treatment (Loell et al., 2012). This limitation highlights the necessity to address not only the physical symptoms but also the overall effect on everyday functioning, emotional well-being, and social relationships. Moreover, prevention of the interaction between chronic inflammatory processes and muscle integrity must be achieved in order to promote muscle well-being and avoid complications (Chiba et al., 2019). Thus, an integrated treatment strategy with both drug therapy and supportive care can enhance overall patient outcomes worldwide by enhancing both physical function and psychosocial status, thus identifying the critical interrelationship between effective treatment and quality of life in patients with these myopathies (Figure 6.21).

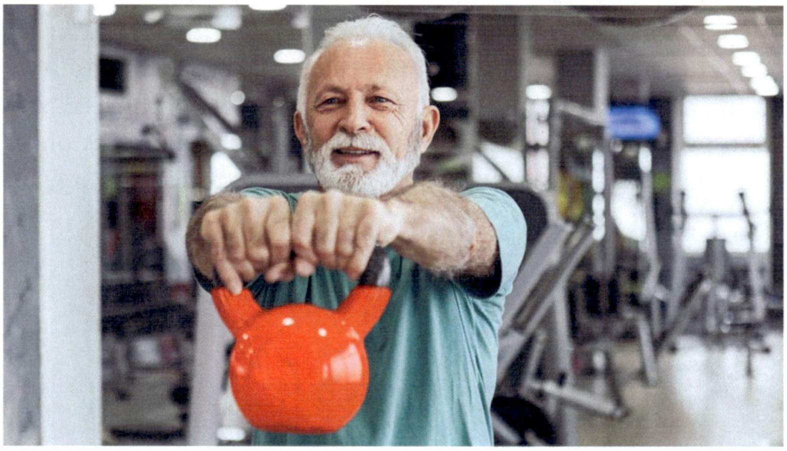

Figure 6.21. The interplay between chronic inflammatory processes and muscle integrity necessitates preventive strategies to maintain muscle health and ward off complications

Source: https://i0.wp.com/post.healthline.com/wp-content/uploads/2019/11/Older_Male_Working_Out_1296x728-header-1-1296x728.jpg?w=1155&h=1528.

Test Your Knowledge

1. What are the treatment strategies for interstitial lung disease in antisynthetase syndrome?
2. What are the supportive therapies (e.g., physical therapy, nutrition) important in IIM?

Summary

Idiopathic inflammatory myopathies present a bewildering clinical scenario of disease presentation and response to treatment, which needs ongoing research to optimize the benefit to patients. The findings emphasize that the diseases of juvenile and adult dermatomyositis are heterogeneous in their courses, with numerous patients potentially developing monophasic or polycyclic disease courses that eventually determine the treatment approach and prognosis (Balogh et al., 2005). Furthermore, the identification of specific myositis-associated antibodies, such as NXP-2, offers predictive evidence about disease course and diagnosis, indicating the need for tailored management plans (Cartron et al., 2020). As the survival rates appear to be favorable, notably in pediatric patients, the importance of long-term follow-up emerges to monitor potential relapses and implement required therapeutic adjustments. Greater awareness and holistic care models can remarkably enhance the quality of life for those suffering from such debilitating conditions, hence emphasizing the need for advancements in clinical practice and research efforts.

The diagnosis of idiopathic inflammatory myopathies (IIM) represents a multifaceted interaction between clinical presentation and diagnostic challenge, especially for juvenile patients. One key challenge still remains the identification of reliable, non-invasive diagnostic procedures capable of correctly following disease progression (Hilário et al., 2000). Recent studies have shown the utility of magnetic resonance imaging (MRI) in diagnosing active disease in muscle, most notably in juvenile dermatomyositis and its variants (Hilário et al., 2000). Surprisingly, MRI features are typically marked by heterogeneous muscle involvement with variation in acute and chronic symptoms based on the etiology such as dermatomyositis and systemic lupus erythematosus. With ongoing improvement in MRI protocols and analysis, the prospect of these developments enhancing diagnostic accuracy and patient management becomes clear. The application of advanced imaging modalities is, therefore, a critical area for future study of the pathophysiology and treatment of IIM.

KEY TERMS FROM THIS CHAPTER

- Autoantibody
- Clinical presentation
- complexity
- Corticosteroids
- Elastography
- Electromyography (EMG)
- Fibrillation potentials
- Lengthy progression
- Muscle fibers
- Polymyositis
- chemokines
- Clinicopathological
- Computed tomography (CT)
- Distal muscle involvement
- Electromyography
- Erythematosus
- Heterogeneity
- Muscle damage
- Muscle inflammation
- Prognostic algorithm

Critical Thinking Questions

1. Which of the following is a hallmark clinical feature of polymyositis and dermatomyositis?

a. Muscle hypertrophy

b. Distal muscle weakness

c. Symmetric proximal muscle weakness

d. Muscle spasms

2. Which dermatologic finding is pathognomonic for dermatomyositis?

a. Malar rash

b. Heliotrope rash

c. Psoriatic plaques

d. Oral ulcers

3. Which of the following autoantibodies is most specific for dermatomyositis?

a. Anti-dsDNA

b. Anti-Jo-1

c. Anti-Mi-2

d. Anti-Ro

4. Inclusion body myositis differs from other inflammatory myopathies because:

a. It is more common in women

b. It primarily affects children

c. It often shows asymmetric, distal muscle weakness

d. It has a rapid onset and responds well to steroids

5. Which test is most useful in confirming a diagnosis of idiopathic inflammatory myopathy?

a. Chest X-ray

b. Muscle biopsy

c. ANA testing

d. Skin biopsy

Answers to Critical Thinking Questions

1. (c) 2. (b) 3. (c) 4. (c) 5. (b)

Short Answer Questions

1. What are the major subtypes of idiopathic inflammatory myopathies?
2. How does polymyositis differ clinically and pathologically from dermatomyositis?
3. What immune cells are primarily involved in the pathogenesis of polymyositis?
4. How do humoral (antibody-mediated) mechanisms contribute to dermatomyositis?
5. What are the diagnostic criteria for polymyositis and dermatomyositis?
6. What is the clinical significance of elevated creatine kinase (CK) in suspected IIM?
7. What is the first-line therapy for polymyositis and dermatomyositis?
8. When should corticosteroids be tapered, and what steroid-sparing agents are used?

References

1. Adedeji Okikiade, O., Afolayan-Oloye, O., Browne-Caesar, T., Agboola, R., Olojede, O., & Oyewole, A. (2023). Dermatomyositis: A case report and review of a rare autoimmune inflammatory disease. *Advances in Research*. https://www.semanticscholar.org/paper/12347d50b18617c60fb98d8ea3943ecaaf0be750 (accessed on 17th June 2025).
2. Agarwal, V., Agarwal, V., Aggarwal, R., Aharonov, O., Ajmani, S., Aoude, M., Asranna, A., et al. (2024). Global disparities in the treatment of idiopathic inflammatory myopathies: Results from an international online survey study. https://core.ac.uk/download/614148021.docx (accessed on 17th June 2025).
3. Aggarwal, R., & Oddis, C. V. (2012). Inclusion body myositis: Therapeutic approaches. https://core.ac.uk/download/12213811.pdf (accessed on 17th June 2025).
4. Battista, S., Giardulli, B., Sieiro Santos, C., Aharonov, O., Puttaswamy, D., Russell, A.-, & Gupta, L. (2024). Digital Health and Self-Management in Idiopathic Inflammatory Myopathies: A Missed Opportunity?. *Current rheumatology reports*, *26*(11), 383–391. https://doi.org/10.1007/s11926-024-01157-6 (accessed on 17th June 2025).
5. Alves, S. C., Fasano, S., & Isenberg, D. A. (2016). Current pharmacological treatment of idiopathic inflammatory myopathies. https://core.ac.uk/download/79552795.pdf (accessed on 17th June 2025).
6. Lilleker, J. B., Vencovsky, J., Wang, G., Wedderburn, L. R., Diederichsen, L. P., Schmidt, J., Oakley, P., Benveniste, O., Danieli, M. G., Danko, K., Thuy, N. T. P., Vazquez-Del Mercado, M., Andersson, H., De Paepe, B., deBleecker, J. L., Maurer, B., McCann, L. J., Pipitone, N., McHugh, N., Betteridge, Z. E., ... all EuroMyositis contributors (2018). The EuroMyositis registry: an international collaborative tool to facilitate myositis research. *Annals of the rheumatic diseases*, *77*(1), 30–39. https://doi.org/10.1136/annrheumdis-2017-211868 (accessed on 17th June 2025).
7. Balogh, Z., Borgulya, G., Constantin, T., Dankó, K., et al. (2005). Disease course, frequency of relapses and survival of 73 patients with juvenile or adult dermatomyositis. https://core.ac.uk/download/11855978.pdf (accessed on 17th June 2025).
8. Battista, S., Giardulli, B., Sieiro Santos, C., Aharonov, O., Puttaswamy, D., Russell, A. M. & Gupta, L. (2024). Digital health and self-management in idiopathic inflammatory myopathies: A missed opportunity? *Current Rheumatology Reports, 26*, 383–391. https://www.semanticscholar.org/paper/b6db3f2cf6ff2977bac7a8343394ecc83273be59 (accessed on 17th June 2025).
9. Benveniste, O., Goebel, H. H., & Stenzel, W. (2019). Biomarkers in Inflammatory Myopathies-An Expanded Definition. *Frontiers in neurology*, *10*, 554. https://doi.org/10.3389/fneur.2019.00554(accessed on 17th June 2025).
10. Bhardwaj, M., Khamankar, S. G., Sinwal, A., Ishu, Poonia, R., Sharma, V. S., & Sinwal, V. (2024). A review of recent advances in the classification, pathogenesis, diagnosis, and treatment of idiopathic inflammatory myopathies. *Journal of Pharma Insights and Research*. https://www.semanticscholar.org/paper/7f0a702325cf2c279d4e78ded51fb191a368fe1c (accessed on 17th June 2025).
11. Bianchi, M., Kozyrev, S. V., Notarnicola, A., Sandling, J., Pettersson, M., Leonard, D., Sjöwall, C., et al. (2024). Unraveling the genetics of shared clinical and serological manifestations

in patients with systemic inflammatory autoimmune diseases. *Arthritis & Rheumatology (Hoboken, N.J.), 77*, 212–225. https://www.semanticscholar.org/paper/9d1ee9c0f96614455e33c60dee788090e294d88b (accessed on 17th June 2025).

12. Bohan, B., Brown, G., Chinoy, H., Christen-Zaech, S., Pilkington, C. A., et al. (2011). A national registry for juvenile dermatomyositis and other pediatric idiopathic inflammatory myopathies: 10 years' experience; the Juvenile Dermatomyositis National (UK and Ireland) Cohort Biomarker Study and Repository for Idiopathic Inflammatory Myopathies. https://core.ac.uk/download/10413.pdf (accessed on 17th June 2025).
13. Cappellari, A., Petaccia, A., Consonni, D., Minoia, F., Filocamo, G., & Picca, I. (2021). Development and preliminary validation of an electromyography-scoring protocol for the assessment and grading of muscle involvement in patients with juvenile idiopathic inflammatory myopathies. https://core.ac.uk/download/589948516.pdf (accessed on 17th June 2025).
14. Cappelletti, C., Salerno, F., Morandi, L., Mora, M., Confalonieri, P., Bernasconi, P., & Mantegazza, R. (2011). Idiopathic inflammatory myopathies: A review of immunopathological features and current models of pathogenesis. https://core.ac.uk/download/322399059.pdf (accessed on 17th June 2025).
15. Cardelli, C., Trentin, F., Fattorini, F., Diomedi, M., Laurino, E., Barsotti, S., Mosca, M., et al. (2024). Environmental triggers for idiopathic inflammatory myopathies: Unravelling the known and unknown. *Clinical and Experimental Rheumatology*. https://www.semanticscholar.org/paper/5d8b4a23c0242e07376595f92129f56b7aef82b8 (accessed on 17th June 2025).
16. Cartron, A. M., Chung, C., Osler, M., Trinidad, E., et al. (2020). Nuclear matrix protein 2 antibody-positive adult dermatomyositis: A case report and review of the literature. https://core.ac.uk/download/322493868.pdf (accessed on 17th June 2025).
17. Chiba, F. Y., de Lima Coutinho Mattera, M. S., & Sumida, D. H. (2019). Inflammatory muscle diseases. https://core.ac.uk/download/322442805.pdf (accessed on 17th June 2025).
18. Conticini, E., Dourado, E., Bottazzi, F., Cardelli, C., Bruno, L., Schmidt, J., Carli, L., et al. (2024). Idiopathic inflammatory myopathies: One year in review 2023. *Clinical and Experimental Rheumatology, 42*(2), 213–224. https://www.semanticscholar.org/paper/2dfe327935a7ab2896f7c45587ff4578c94e5ec4 (accessed on 17th June 2025).
19. Coss, S., Zhou, D., Chua, G. T., Abdul-Aziz, R., Hoffman, R. P., Wu, Y. L., Ardoin, S. P., et al. (2022). The complement system and human autoimmune diseases. *Journal of Autoimmunity, 137*, 102979–102979. https://doi.org/10.1016/j.jaut.2022.102979 (accessed on 17th June 2025).
20. Crofford, L. J., MacDonald, P. M., Phillips, K., Schiopu, E., et al. (2012). Predictors of survival in a cohort of patients with polymyositis and dermatomyositis: Effect of corticosteroids, methotrexate and azathioprine. https://core.ac.uk/download/232562235.pdf (accessed on 17th June 2025).
21. Dankó, K., Griger, Z., & Nagy-Vincze, M. (2018). Pharmacological management of dermatomyositis. https://core.ac.uk/download/161059537.pdf (accessed on 17th June 2025).
22. De Paepe, B., & De Bleecker, J. L. (2013). Cytokines and chemokines as regulators of skeletal muscle inflammation: presenting the case of Duchenne muscular dystrophy. *Mediators of inflammation, 2013*, 540370. https://doi.org/10.1155/2013/540370 (accessed on 17th June 2025).

23. Boel De Paepe. A recipe for myositis: nuclear factor κB and nuclear factor of activated T-cells transcription factor pathways spiced up by cytokines[J]. AIMS Allergy and Immunology, 2017, 1(1): 31-42. doi: 10.3934/Allergy.2017.1.31(accessed on 17th June 2025).

24. De Paepe, B., & Zschüntzsch, J. (2015). Scanning for Therapeutic Targets within the Cytokine Network of Idiopathic Inflammatory Myopathies. *International journal of molecular sciences, 16*(8), 18683–18713. https://doi.org/10.3390/ijms160818683(accessed on 17th June 2025).

25. Dimachkie, M. M., Machado, P. M., Roy, B., Salam, K., et al. (2023). Imaging biomarkers in the idiopathic inflammatory myopathies. https://core.ac.uk/download/566653678.pdf (accessed on 17th June 2025).

26. Dokukin, A. N., Farjami, S., Kaiser, C. J., Leung, R., et al. (2017). A case of statin-associated autoimmune myopathy. https://core.ac.uk/download/323075656.pdf (accessed on 17th June 2025).

27. Fornaro, M., Venerito, V., Iannone, F., Ravichandran, N., Nikiphorou, E., Joshi, M., Tan, A., et al. (2023). POS1216 Multimorbidity and PROMIS health outcomes in patients with idiopathic inflammatory myopathies: Data from a large, global e-survey (COVAD Study). *Annals of the Rheumatic Diseases*. https://www.semanticscholar.org/paper/077b15e487bd1666f8b1cecf61f43a608a183222 (accessed on 17th June 2025).

28. Gabrielli, A., Logullo, F., Pettinari, L., Danieli, M. G., & Moretti, R. (2011). Immunoglobulin treatment in polymyositis and dermatomyositis. https://core.ac.uk/download/322399068.pdf (accessed on 17th June 2025).

29. Gamba, A., Depascale, R., Zanatta, E., Ienna, L., Cruciani, C., Gatto, M., Zen, M., et al. (2024). Effectiveness and safety of low dose Rituximab as remission-maintenance treatment for patients with refractory idiopathic inflammatory myopathies: Results of a retrospective study from a monocentric cohort. *Clinical Rheumatology, 43*, 3167–3174. https://www.semanticscholar.org/paper/f880a009861d13b4e3421c16cc271b9043120922 (accessed on 17th June 2025).

30. Geertsema-Hoeve, B. C., van Laar, J. A. M., Raaphorst, J., Tas, S., Welsing, P., Goekoop, R. J., Magro Checa, C., et al. (2025). Multicenter, 26-week, open-label phase 2 trial of the JAK inhibitor filgotinib in Behçet's disease, idiopathic inflammatory myopathies and IgG4-related disease: DRIMID study protocol. *BMJ Open, 15*. https://www.semanticscholar.org/paper/97b9000987424b979a22abad958a1feb0d41a256 (accessed on 17th June 2025).

31. Glikson, M., Nielsen, J. C., Kronborg, M. B., Michowitz, Y., Auricchio, A., Barbash, I. M., Barrabés, J. A., et al. (2021). 2021 ESC Guidelines on cardiac pacing and cardiac resynchronization therapy. *European Heart Journal, 42*, 3427–3520. https://doi.org/10.1093/eurheartj/ehab364 (accessed on 17th June 2025).

32. Henderson, L. A., Canna, S., Friedman, K. G., Gorelik, M., Lapidus, S., Bassiri, H., Behrens, E. M., et al. (2020). American College of Rheumatology clinical guidance for multisystem inflammatory syndrome in children associated with SARS–CoV-2 and hyperinflammation in pediatric COVID-19: Version 1. *Arthritis & Rheumatology, 72*, 1791–1805. https://doi.org/10.1002/art.41454 (accessed on 17th June 2025).

33. Hilário, M. O. E., Lederman, H. M., Len, C. A., Lutti, M., et al. (2000). Juvenile idiopathic inflammatory myopathies: The value of magnetic resonance imaging in the detection of muscle involvement. https://core.ac.uk/download/37704297.pdf (accessed on 17th June 2025).

34. Hokkoku, K., Yamamoto, J., Uchida, Y., Kondo, A., Mukai, T., Hatanaka, Y., Kono, H., et al. (2024). Frequency of EMG abnormalities in idiopathic inflammatory myopathies under the EULAR/ACR classification criteria. *Medicine, 103*. https://www.semanticscholar.org/paper/b556f86976095e238bb0b553aa1903fc3eb14c7a (accessed on 17th June 2025).

35. Izuka, S., Komai, T., Tsuchida, Y., Tsuchiya, H., Okamura, T. & Fujio, K. (2025). The role of monocytes and macrophages in idiopathic inflammatory myopathies: Insights into pathogenesis and potential targets. *Frontiers in Immunology, 16*. https://www.semanticscholar.org/paper/d9dc35d5d64ba2d991e01bf871eda852f8a73596 (accessed on 17th June 2025).

36. Keller, J., Bassotti, G., Clarke, J. O., Dinning, P. G., Fox, M., Grover, M., Hellström, P. M., et al. (2018). Advances in the diagnosis and classification of gastric and intestinal motility disorders. *Nature Reviews Gastroenterology & Hepatology, 15*, 291–308. https://doi.org/10.1038/nrgastro.2018.7 (accessed on 17th June 2025).

37. Klionsky, D. J., Petroni, G., Amaravadi, R. K., Baehrecke, E. H., Ballabio, A., Boya, P., Bravo-San Pedro, J. M., et al. (2021). Autophagy in major human diseases. *The EMBO Journal, 40*. https://doi.org/10.15252/embj.2021108863 (accessed on 17th June 2025).

38. Leclair, V. (2023). Risk factors and outcomes in inflammatory myopathies. https://core.ac.uk/download/570950851.pdf (accessed on 17th June 2025).

39. Li, Z., Liu, H., Xie, Q. & Yin, G. (2024). Macrophage involvement in idiopathic inflammatory myopathy: Pathogenic mechanisms and therapeutic prospects. *Journal of Inflammation (London, England), 21*. https://www.semanticscholar.org/paper/09d9a05d832fbef4accb5ff2431cab5a37b76460 (accessed on 17th June 2025).

40. Loell, I. (2012). Polymyositis and dermatomyositis–Inflammation, muscle structure & immunosuppressive treatment. https://core.ac.uk/download/70340221.pdf (accessed on 17th June 2025).

41. Martins, E. F., Cappello, C., Shinjo, S., Appenzeller, S., & de Souza, J. M. (2025). Idiopathic inflammatory myopathies: Recent evidence linking pathogenesis and clinical features. *International Journal of Molecular Sciences, 26*. https://www.semanticscholar.org/paper/0f4a01eecc74c8e32a66eeaa7053b4b26b8f09f7 (accessed on 17th June 2025).

42. Missé, R. G., dos Santos, A. M., Borges, I., Grecco, M. V., Faria, M. S. M. S., da Silva, L. R. S., Correia, B. L., et al. (2024). Impact of transcranial direct current stimulation in pain, fatigue, and health quality of life of patients with idiopathic inflammatory myopathies: A randomized, double-blind, sham-controlled crossover clinical trial. *International Journal of Rheumatology, 2024*. https://www.semanticscholar.org/paper/7c40ddee3414ad3d9e6ed32007e0fe9cd03ef6da (accessed on 17th June 2025).

43. Morina, G., Sambataro, D., Libra, A., Palmucci, S., Colaci, M., La Rocca, G., Ferro, F., et al. (2025). Recognition of idiopathic inflammatory myopathies underlying interstitial lung diseases. *Diagnostics, 15*. https://www.semanticscholar.org/paper/c9937a96c108c1b9b52451d84344f2e3e013955c (accessed on 17th June 2025).

44. Neves, A., Viveiros, L., Venturelli, V., & Isenberg, D. (2024). Where are we now in biological drugs for myositis? *Rheumatology*. https://www.semanticscholar.org/paper/37d989f44614234e4a187b9f0aca1e5d519752a7 (accessed on 17th June 2025).

45. Nies, J. F., Hendrix, C., Bartram, M. P., Spear, R., Hagmann, H., Benzing, T., & Kubacki, T. (2024). Effectiveness and safety of immunoadsorption as a rescue treatment of inflammatory

myopathies: Report of three cases and literature review. *Therapeutic Advances in Musculoskeletal Disease, 16*. https://www.semanticscholar.org/paper/6069bfa004191877213a878b5e092e0266f234d8 (accessed on 17th June 2025).

46. Nishimura, A., Nelke, C., Huber, M., Mensch, A., Roth, A., Oberwittler, C., Zimmerlein, B., et al. (2024). Differentiating idiopathic inflammatory myopathies by automated morphometric analysis of MHC-1, MHC-2 and ICAM-1 in muscle tissue. *Neuropathology and Applied Neurobiology, 50*. https://www.semanticscholar.org/paper/c87d560b4ba76b2a99c661783422a8594a6e4214 (accessed on 17th June 2025).

47. Opinc-Rosiak, A., Kulesza, E. M., Mikosińska, A. J., Brzezińska, O., & Makowska, J. (2025). Infections as a predominant cause of death in adult patients with idiopathic inflammatory myopathies. *Clinical and Experimental Rheumatology, 43*(2), 290–299. https://www.semanticscholar.org/paper/14bfd1ce9cc59c48ea87ac20172d472c88b27883 (accessed on 17th June 2025).

48. Paik, J. J., Werth, V. P., Chinoy, H., Masri, K. R., Jambekar, A., Hasan, F., Borlenghi, C., et al. (2025). Treatment guidelines for idiopathic inflammatory myopathies in adults: A comparative review. *Rheumatology*. https://www.semanticscholar.org/paper/75a67bce9bff0946c9273d3282d949b946f8f170 (accessed on 17th June 2025).

49. Paramalingam, S. (2023). Exploring shear wave elastography and B-mode ultrasound measurements as potential biomarkers in the diagnosis and monitoring of patients with idiopathic inflammatory myopathies: A novel approach. https://core.ac.uk/download/621574812.pdf (accessed on 17th June 2025).

50. Ramirez, P., Giglio, A., Dominguez, I., Garrido, F. & Gutierrez, F. (2025). Snapshot of a decade: Idiopathic inflammatory myopathies in Chile—a 10-year short report. *Journal of Clinical Rheumatology: Practical Reports on Rheumatic & Musculoskeletal Diseases*. https://www.semanticscholar.org/paper/a73b433cc407ae08ffa82afe7c11c85df393ac94 (accessed on 17th June 2025).

51. Rapezzi, C., Aimo, A., Barison, A., Emdin, M., Porcari, A., Linhart, A., Keren, A., et al. (2022). Restrictive cardiomyopathy: Definition and diagnosis. *European Heart Journal, 43*, 4679–4693. https://doi.org/10.1093/eurheartj/ehac543 (accessed on 17th June 2025).

52. Saygin, D., Glaubitz, S., Zeng, R., Bottai, M., de Visser, M., Dimachkie, M., Fiorentino, D. F., et al. (2024). Performance of the 2017 EULAR/ACR classification criteria for adult and juvenile idiopathic inflammatory myopathies and their major subgroups: A scoping review. *Clinical and Experimental Rheumatology*. https://www.semanticscholar.org/paper/89d6a022fec26a126f397438ab6ab221886c4d8f (accessed on 17th June 2025).

53. Selva-O'Callaghan, A., Trallero-Araguás, E., Grau, J. M., Prieto-González, S., & Lazo, V. (2011). Myositis and cancer. https://core.ac.uk/download/322399065.pdf (accessed on 17th June 2025).

54. Shimoyama, T., Yoshida, K., Muro, Y., Ito, H., Matsushita, T., Oto, Y., Ukichi, T., et al. (2024). Magnetic resonance imaging patterns revealing muscle pathology and clinical features in idiopathic inflammatory myopathies. *Rheumatology*. https://www.semanticscholar.org/paper/94a8db235fbe246630c7be18757fe920d1f9dd0d (accessed on 17th June 2025).

55. Wu, Y., Luo, J. & Duan, L. (2024). Pathogenic mechanisms of disease in idiopathic inflammatory myopathies: Autoantibodies as clues. *Frontiers in Immunology, 15*. https://www.semanticscholar.org/paper/1fb7d05a56fba7a7d41f292a7febb13b7ead0fbe (accessed on 17th June 2025).

VASCULITIDES

7

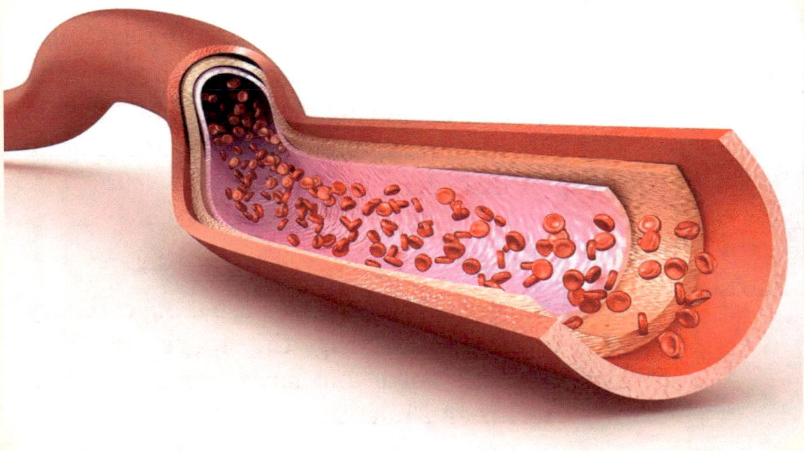

LEARNING OBJECTIVES

After studying this chapter, you will be able to:

1. Understand the classification of vasculitides
2. Explain the pathophysiology of vasculitides
3. Discuss clinical manifestations and diagnosis
4. Explain treatment and management strategies

Introduction

Vasculitides are a category of heterogeneous and multifactorial disorders involving inflammation of the blood vessels, potentially culminating in severe organ damage and systemic disease. Their etiology is still poorly understood, involving environmental and genetic factors that determine their pathogenesis. Recent evidence has explained genetic predisposition to different forms of vasculitis, with shared susceptibility loci among them, such as the ones close to the HLA genes and the KDM4C locus, which plays a role in epigenetic regulation (Carmona et al., 2018). Additionally, external factors, such as exposure to levamisole-contaminated cocaine, have been associated with particular clinical syndromes, including autoimmune events that could lead to severe renal implications (Butcher et al., 2014). Understanding these intricate interactions will be necessary to improve diagnosis, treatment, and outcomes of the patient with these rare but significant diseases (Figure 7.1).

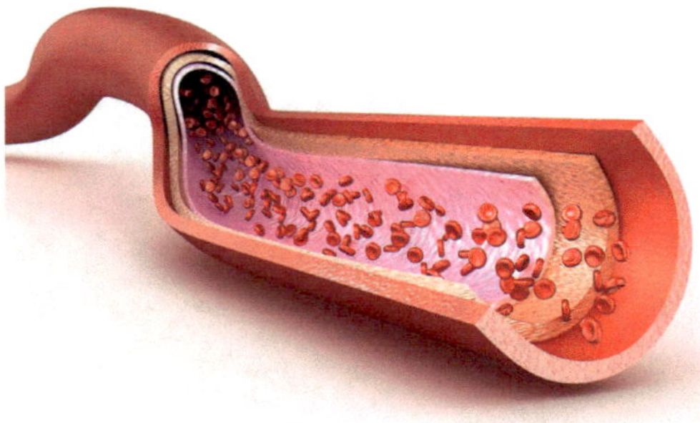

Figure 7.1. Systemic vasculitides.

Source: https://medicinetoday.com.au/sites/default/files/styles/wide/public/2023-11/0520VasculitidesCH.jpg.webp?itok=ZgfZC-MA

7.1. Classification of Vasculitides

Learning Outcome

1. Understand large vessel vasculitides;
2. Explain medium vessel vasculitides;
3. Discuss small vessel vasculitides;
4. Focus on primary vs. secondary vasculitides;
5. Learn systemic vs. localized vasculitides;
6. Identify granulomatous vs. non-granulomatous vasculitides;
7. Learn classification criteria and guidelines;
8. Describe the role of the American College of Rheumatology;
9. Know the importance of accurate classification.

The classification of vasculitides is essential in order to make the appropriate diagnostic and therapeutic approach because they can present with different manifestations and can potentially be systemic. Vasculitides are basically classified predominantly based on the caliber of the affected vessel, into small, medium, and large vessels. This classification helps clinicians deduce the etiology and pathology underlying them, because the clinical presentation and potential complications bear significant differences between these categories. For instance, the small vessel vasculitides, such as ANCA-associated vasculitis, may have typical cutaneous lesions that are prognostic of the underlying vasculitis and accompanying histopathological alterations (Ho et al., 2023).

On the other hand, medium and large vessel vasculitides may have more extensive complications, and consequently, alternative treatments have to be applied (Ralli et al., 2020). With an understanding of these categories, not only is accurate diagnosis facilitated, but also the development of specific management protocols that will optimize outcomes in this challenging group of disorders.

7.1.1. Large Vessel Vasculitides

The great vessel vasculitides are a big category of vasculitis affecting the large arteries, especially the aorta and large branches. Giant cell arteritis and Takayasu arteritis are two such diseases, which have characteristic systemic manifestations of fever, malaise, and weight loss that overshadow the actual underlying vascular disease. Initiation of active therapy is necessary because involvement of major vessels can lead to severe complications like ischemia, aneurysm, and even organ failure, and therefore, early detection is necessary to improve patient outcomes.

Large vessel vasculitides are diagnosed by virtue of their nonspecific presentation, highlighting the imperative necessity for primary care doctors to recognize a wide range of signs and symptoms that can indicate these conditions (Conte et al., 2020). Early interventions with immunosuppressive therapy can significantly reduce morbidity and mortality, highlighting the importance of a multi-disciplinary approach in their management (Conte et al., 2020) (Figure 7.3).

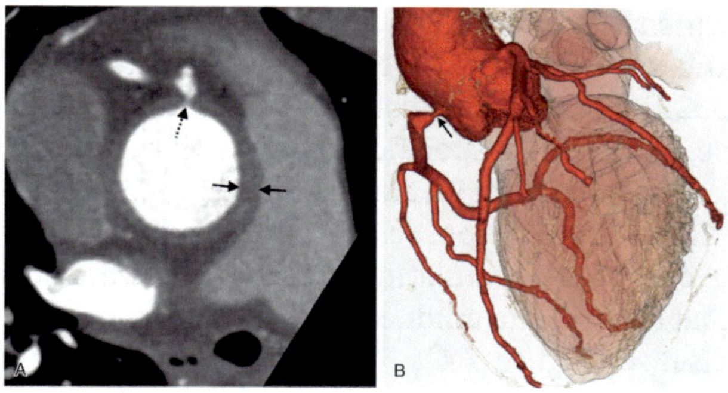

Figure 7.2. Large vessel vasculitides represent a significant subset of vasculitis disorders that primarily affect the major arteries, notably the aorta and its major branches.

Source: https://radiologykey.com/wp-content/uploads/2021/11/f30-06-9780323763035.jpg.

7.1.2. Medium Vessel Vasculitides

Medium vessel vasculitides represent a large subgroup of the more overarching category of vasculitides that involve medium-sized vessels and both systemic inflammation as well as target organ damage. Polyarteritis nodosa and Kawasaki disease are both prototypical of this subgroup, where an immune system abnormality leads to inflammation of the wall of the artery with the potential to cause resultant severe ischemic complications. The clinical picture may be erratic, ranging from generalized symptoms of fever and malaise to more local issues based on the organs involved and diagnosis is particularly challenging. Even though immune events are well known, the role of neutrophils has also gained attention, showing that they can sustain inflammatory responses in the vascular bed and contribute further to tissue damage. It is important to understand these dynamics because medium vessel vasculitides patients can have an increased neutrophil-to-lymphocyte ratio, and so there should be increased vigilance by healthcare providers to be able to manage these multifactorial conditions adequately (Conte et al., 2020; Amsler et al., 2022).

7.1.3. Small Vessel Vasculitides

Small vessel vasculitides represent a distinctive group of diseases with small vessel inflammation and an enormous range of clinical manifestations. These diseases, including eosinophilic granulomatosis with polyangiitis (EGPA) and cryoglobulinemic vasculitis, may lead to life-threatening complications if the conditions are not recognized and treated early and adequately. For instance, EGPA is also associated with unexplained but relevant central nervous system involvement, like PRES cases complicating its prognosis and management (Barilaro et al., 2015). Similarly, cryoglobulinemia, typically secondary to hepatitis C virus infection, may lead to severe vascular and renal complications, like glomerulonephritis resulting in renal failure (Braun et al., 2007). The multifaceted nature of small vessel vasculitides underscores the necessity for tailored therapeutic approaches addressing not only the inflammatory processes themselves but also their systemic impact, advising clinicians on how to maximize patient benefits (Figure 7.3).

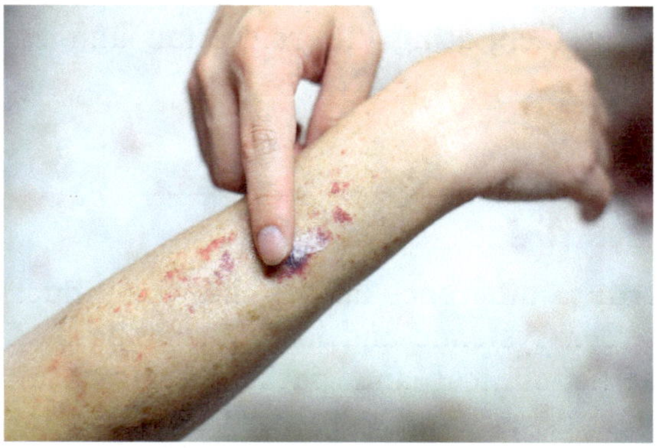

Figure 7.3. Small vessel vasculitides represent a distinct group of disorders characterized by inflammation of the small blood vessels, leading to a diverse array of clinical manifestations.

Source: https://www.verywellhealth.com/thmb/QnuQ8TSNWM6FghCuikWkid8pB7I=/1500x0/filters:no_upscale():max_bytes(150000):strip_icc()/GettyImages-1368041284-d2ae1e72d91c40b1a854bff87c686f89.jpg.

7.1.4. Primary vs. Secondary Vasculitides

It is crucial to differentiate between primary and secondary vasculitides to diagnose and treat properly. Primary vasculitides are autoimmune conditions with inflammation of blood vessels without a known etiology, commonly with a heterogeneous collection of symptoms impacting more than one organ system. Examples are Granulomatosis with polyangiitis and Microscopic polyangiitis, which must be treated specifically with immunosuppression. In contrast, secondary vasculitides are associated with known conditions like infections, malignancies, or reactions to drugs, and these causes are implicated in the inflammatory process. For instance, patients of ANCA-associated vasculitis have increased risks of infection, as defined by a national survey reporting extraordinarily high infection rates among such patients versus controls (Amft et al., 2020). Besides this, the overlap of symptoms between primary and secondary causes complicates clinical diagnosis, which is all the more reason why advanced imaging techniques like PET/CT play an indispensable role in facilitating differentiation and early diagnosis (Taimen, 2021).

7.1.5. Systemic vs. Localized Vasculitides

A critical difference among the vasculitides is between systemic and local forms, both with specific clinical and pathological features. Systemic vasculitides, such as Granulomatosis with Polyangiitis (GPA) or Eosinophilic Granulomatosis with Polyangiitis (EGPA), are defined by diffuse inflammatory reactions involving potentially more than one organ system and, if left untreated, result in significant morbidity and mortality. For instance, recent data indicate that systemic types, i.e., Antineutrophil Cytoplasmic Antibodies (ANCA)-associated vasculitides (AAV), have exhibited steady rates of incidence as well as mounting prevalence, which partly is due to improved treatment and survival rates among patients (Rathmann, 2023). Conversely, localized vasculitides tend to be limited to a specific area or organ and are less systemic but just as hazardous if untreated (Clarke, 2009). Appreciation of such differences is crucial in formulating therapeutic strategies that address the unique pathophysiology of each disease (Figure 7.4).

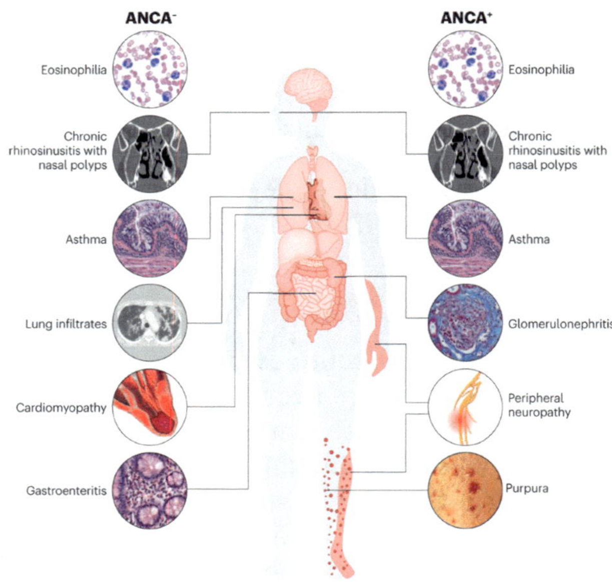

Figure 7.4. Systemic vasculitides, such as Granulomatosis with Polyangiitis (GPA) or Eosinophilic Granulomatosis with Polyangiitis (EGPA), involve widespread inflammatory responses that can affect multiple organ systems, leading to significant morbidity and mortality if left untreated.

Source: https://media.springernature.com/lw1200/springer-static/image/art%3A10.1038%2Fs41584-023-00958-w/MediaObjects/41584_2023_958_Fig1_HTML.png.

7.1.6. Granulomatous vs. Non-granulomatous Vasculitides

The distinction between granulomatous and non-granulomatous vasculitides is significant with regards to their clinical presentation and pathophysiology. Granulomatous vasculitides , such as granulomatosis with polyangiitis (GPA), are characterized by the formation of granulomas, organized aggregates of macrophages, in response to chronic inflammation, also exhibited by ANCA positivity. Alternatively, non-granulomatous vasculitides, such as microscopic polyangiitis, do not characteristically have granuloma formation and are mostly distinguished by their impact on smaller vessels, causing extensive tissue injury with or without such organized inflammation. The distinctions are more than morphologic; for example, AAVs, including GPA and eosinophilic granulomatosis with polyangiitis, have a common autoimmune element and are mediated by anti-neutrophil cytoplasmic antibodies that cause vessel damage (Berti et al., 2020). Furthermore, more recent research indicates that microvascular alterations can be identified in patients with AAV through contemporary imaging, eliciting information about disease progression and potential therapeutic goals (Bergamini et al., 2023).

7.1.7. Classification Criteria and Guidelines

Categorization of vasculitides lies in the foundation of accurate diagnosis and treatment, given the heterogeneity of the diseases. Definite guidelines developed by the American College of Rheumatology constitute integral tools for clinicians to interpret the complexities of vasculitis syndromes, particularly in disorders like eosinophilic granulomatosis with polyangiitis (EGPA).

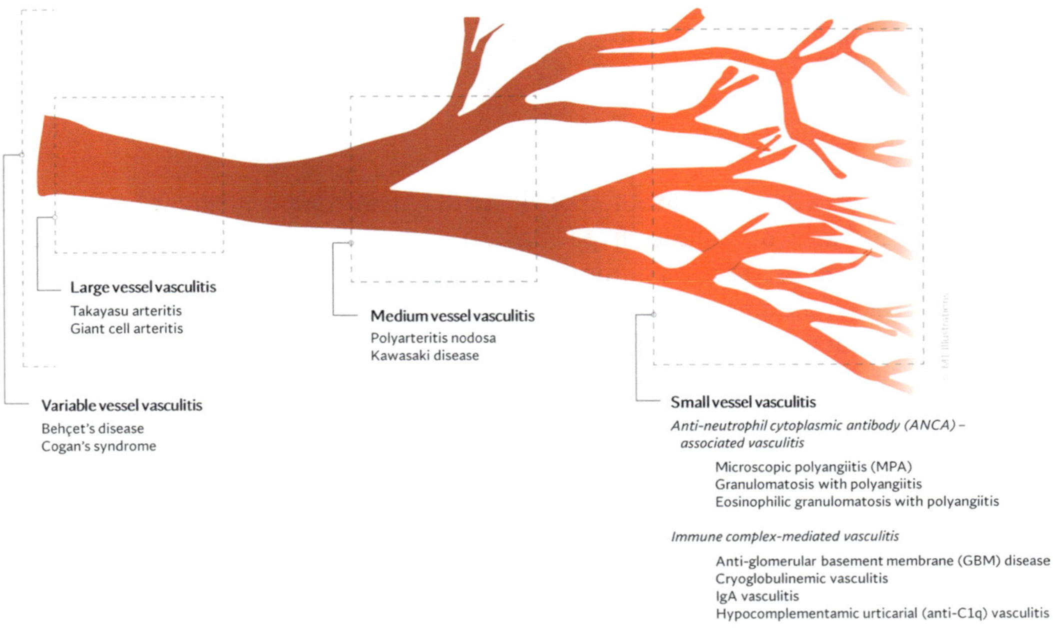

Figure 7.5. The classification of vasculitides is foundational for accurate diagnosis and treatment, given the heterogeneous nature of these conditions.

Source: https://www.hopkinsvasculitis.org/wp-content/uploads/2023/12/Website-blood-vessel-1.png.

For example, a systematic review revealed that head and neck presentations of EGPA patients typically fulfill an average of 4.6 of the criteria of this classification system, highlighting the utility of standardized classification in day-to-day practice (Basnyat et al., 2016). In addition, the awareness of the heterogeneity among various forms of vasculitis, such as ANCA-associated vasculitides, adds further utility for both therapeutic and prognostic considerations. Without reference to prevailing classification criteria, the potential for misdiagnosis is heightened, something that can have a profound influence on patient outcomes and complicate treatment plans (Yates & Watts, 2017). With this in mind, strict classification criteria are necessary in delivering effective clinical decision-making (Figure 7.5).

7.1.8. Role of the American College of Rheumatology

The American College of Rheumatology (ACR) plays an important role in enhancing the treatment and awareness of vasculitides, a group of diseases that affect the inflammation of the blood vessels. By establishing comprehensive diagnostic criteria and treatment guidelines, ACR assists clinicians in diagnosing and treat conditions , such as eosinophilic granulomatosis with polyangiitis (EGPA) that have a severe impact on the patients' quality of life. Research highlighted in recent meta-analyses reveals that ACR criteria play a crucial role in informing diagnosis and therapeutic management, particularly among patients with certain symptoms for manifestations of EGPA in the head and neck, where adherence to such guidelines has mirrored improved patient outcomes and sensitivity to steroid treatments (Basnyat et al., 2016). Further, the ACR continually reports on ANCA-associated vasculitides' pathogenesis and treatment options, which reflects its commitment to the alleviation of the associated morbidity and mortality characteristic of these multifactorial diseases (Yates & Watts, 2017).

7.1.9. Importance of Accurate Classification

Correct vasculitides classification is critical for accurate diagnosis and treatment because it directly affects therapy practices and outcomes in patients. The heterogeneity with blood vessel wall inflammation complicates differentiation among types, making differentiation critical. Classification typically depends on vessel diameter and related clinical features, such that individual syndromes and particular therapy practices can be identified.

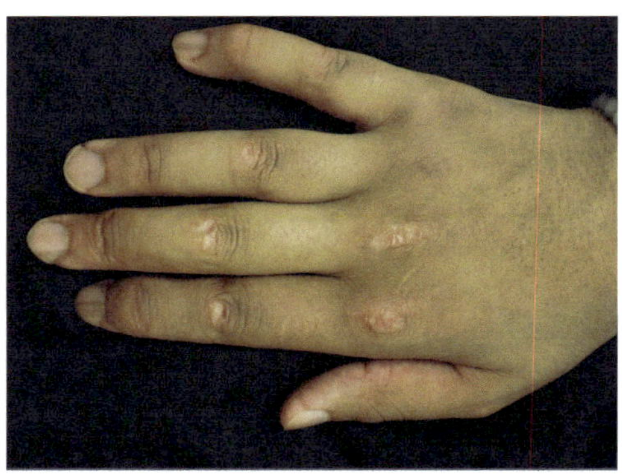

Figure 7.6. Accurate classification of vasculitides is crucial for effective diagnosis and management, as it directly influences therapeutic strategies and patient outcomes.

Source: https://www.medical.theclinics.com/cms/10.1016/j.mcna.2021.04.011/asset/5c9e4a7e-260a-4049-bca5-c2fa80e0499c/main.assets/gr3_lrg.jpg.

Furthermore, early and correct classification can diminish diagnostic delay, which is commonly associated with elevated healthcare costs and potential complications, including multiorgan failure. New advances, such as the use of imaging techniques , such as positron emission tomography with computed tomography (PET/CT), have achieved maximum diagnostic accuracy and demonstrated clinically important results in the majority of cases (Ralli et al., 2020). Therefore, emphasis on accurate classification not only helps in the provision of timely intervention but also helps improve long-term patient outcomes, making it important in vasculitides (Ralli et al., 2020) (Figure 7.6).

Test Your Knowledge

1. Which diseases fall under the medium vessel vasculitis category?
2. What are the most common types of small vessel vasculitis?

7.2. Pathophysiology of Vasculitides

Learning Outcome

1. Understand immune system involvement
2. Focus on genetic predispositions
3. Define environmental triggers
4. Explain inflammatory processes
5. Focus on vascular damage mechanisms
6. Discuss the role of cytokines and chemokines
7. Describe endothelial dysfunction
8. Understand organ involvement and complications

The pathophysiology of vasculitides is the complex interplay of genetic, immunologic, and environmental processes causing inflammation of the blood vessels. Recent studies have underlined the fundamental role of genetic predisposition, with findings indicating that intergenic polymorphisms close to HLA-DQB1 and HLA-DQA2 are associated with disease patterns of vasculitis, emphasizing the importance of human leukocyte antigen (HLA) class II genes in disease manifestation (Carmona et al., 2018). In addition, the recognition of KDM4C as a shared risk locus underscores the significance of epigenetic mechanisms in disease etiology. The categorization of the vasculitides by vessel size, utilized in the Chapel Hill classification, allows for an appreciation of the varying immunopathogenic processes that underlie the illnesses (Brouwer et al., 2021). Furthermore, production of biologic therapies targeted against specific cytokines proves heterogeneity of immune responses in different forms of vasculitis and fosters knowledge of their pathophysiologic rationale.

7.2.1. Immune System Involvement

The immune system plays a central role in the pathogenesis of vasculitides, where abnormal immune activity initiates inflammation and injury of blood vessels. In granulomatosis with polyangiitis (GPA) kind of diseases, the immune system becomes abnormally activated and generates granulomatous inflammation and vasculitis that are mainly localized to the respiratory tract and kidneys. The availability of anti-neutrophil cytoplasmic antibodies (ANCA) can facilitate this immune dysregulation, and it acts as a biomarker for diagnosis and disease activity monitoring (Greco et al., 2016). The distinctive pathology of levamisole-adulterated cocaine abuse also implicates an interesting role of immune involvement, where patients report perinuclear anti-neutrophil cytoplasmic antibodies that target atypical antigens with dramatic cutaneous and renal manifestations (Jen et al., 2015). These figures emphasize the complex interplay between immune regulation and vascular inflammation in determining the requirement for efficient immune modulation of vasculitides (Figure 7.7).

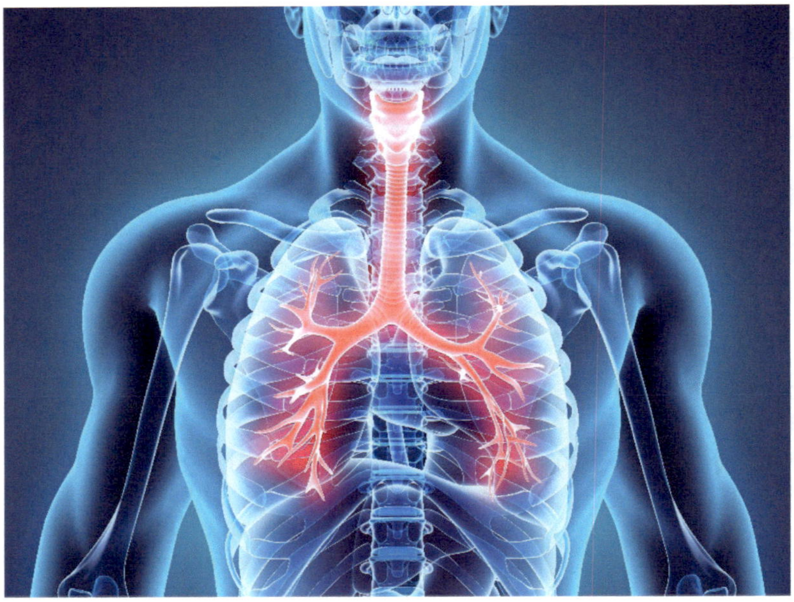

Figure 7.7. Granulomatosis with polyangiitis (GPA).

Source: https://medlineplus.gov/images/GranulomatosiswithPolyangiitisandTracheal%20Disorders_share.jpg.

7.2.2. Genetic Predispositions

The role of genetic predispositions to vasculitides is a key area of research, as certain genetic factors have been known to play a decisive role in deciding susceptibility to such autoimmune diseases. Research has demonstrated that individuals with a history of autoimmune diseases in the family may present a higher risk for developing ANCA-associated vasculitis (AAV), which reflects the genetic etiology of these conditions. Specifically, overlapping conditions , such as rheumatoid arthritis (RA) have been observed to occur alongside AAV and raise diagnostic concerns that can delay treatment and worsen patient outcomes (Draibe et al., 2015). Moreover, vasculitides in children , such as IgA vasculitis and Kawasaki disease, will generally have distinct presentation patterns that can be traced back to the genetic profile. Early detection of these predispositions is imperative, as it allows for timely intervention, which will have a significant impact of limiting renal or cardiac-related complications (Bailey et al., 2024). Lastly, understanding the genetic basis of vasculitides will be key to furthering diagnostic accuracy and therapeutic strategies.

7.2.3. Environmental Triggers

Environmental stimuli play a fundamental role in the pathogenesis of vasculitides, serving as triggers for an abnormal immune reaction against the blood vessels. In large part, exposure to specific pollutants, infections, or other environmental stimuli can lead to the immune dysregulation of such diseases. For instance, neutrophil activation with environmental stressors has been observed to increase vascular inflammation and perpetuate vascular damage and disease progression. Research has proven that elevated circulating neutrophil-to-lymphocyte ratios are prevalent among patients with vasculitis, with the suggestion that environmental triggers could augment neutrophil activity to play a role in the inflammatory milieu in the vascular compartment (Amsler et al., 2022). Also, studies supported by initiatives , such as the Italian Ministry of Health and AIRC highlight the necessity of exploring such environmental interactions, in which understanding them may provide entry to targeted therapeutic approaches when dealing with various forms of vasculitis (Allen et al., 2018) (Figure 7.8).

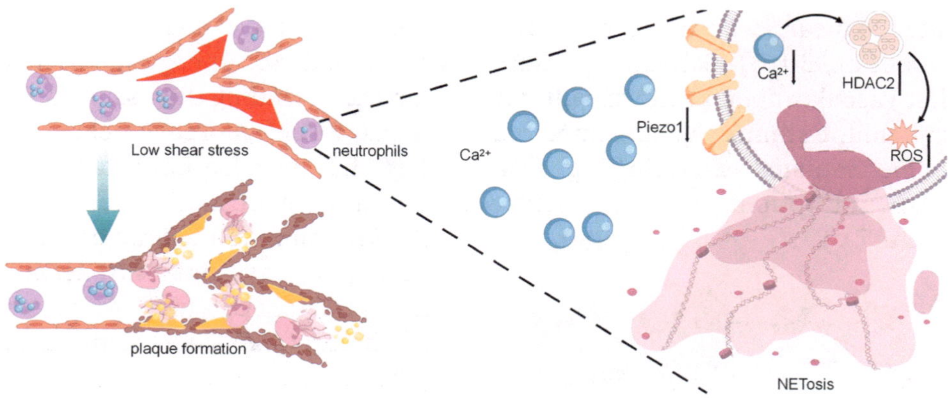

Figure 7.8. The interaction between neutrophils and environmental stressors has been shown to amplify vascular inflammation, contributing to vascular damage and disease progression.

Source: https://www.atherosclerosis-journal.com/cms/10.1016/j.atherosclerosis.2024.117473/asset/712f02b8-c4c0-43f4-9d75-338cc7d4cbd0/main.assets/ga1_lrg.jpg.

7.2.4. Inflammatory Processes

It is essential to grasp inflammatory mechanisms in the comprehension of the pathophysiology of vasculitides since these diseases are fundamentally vascular inflammation on the basis of immunologically mediated processes. In most other systemic autoimmune diseases, CD4(+) T lymphocytes, particularly effector memory T (T-EM) cells, have been found to be implicated in tissue damage and disease progression. These T-EM cells release pro-inflammatory cytokines that enhance the recruitment and activation of other immune cells, such as macrophages and neutrophils, that enhance the inflammatory response in blood vessels (Abdulahad et al., 2014). Moreover, the deregulation of cytokine homeostasis, particularly on interleukin-17 (IL-17), has been included in a number of rheumatic disorders, demonstrating its involvement in the inflammatory environment essential for vasculitis development (Altab et al., 2020). Thus, blocking these inflammatory pathways might provide new therapeutic potential to reduce vascular inflammation in vasculitides.

7.2.5. Vascular Damage Mechanisms

It is essential to understand the pathophysiology of vascular damage in the context of understanding vasculitides, which have a tendency to engage complex interactions between immune cells and the vascular endothelium. The population of CD4(+) T cells, known as effector memory T (T-EM) cells, is critical to this process. The T-EM cells secrete various pro-inflammatory cytokines that enhance endothelial damage, which in turn initiates a cascade of immune responses that are part of vasculitic expressions (Abdulahad et al., 2014). Furthermore, endothelial progenitor cells (EPCs) are increased in children with systemic vasculitis; however, their functional capacity is severely impaired during periods of active disease. This impairment could potentially disrupt the process of repair of the endothelium and exacerbate the disarray between injury and repair (Brogan et al., 2015). Collectively, these data show that vascular damage in vasculitides is due to both immune stimulation and impaired regenerative mechanisms, shedding light on potential therapeutic options to regain vascular integrity (Figure 7.9).

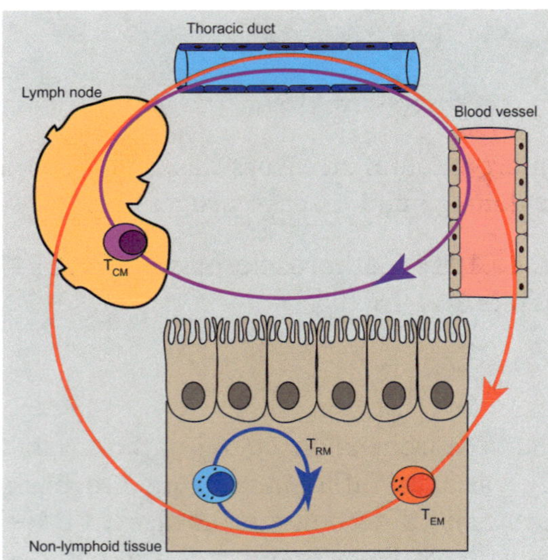

Figure 7.9. A key player in this process is the subset of CD4(+) T cells known as effector memory T (T-EM) cells.

Source: https://www.amjtransplant.org/cms/10.1111/ajt.14101/asset/ac6d725e-b341-4d14-81cf-66550c67d2b4/main.assets/gr1_lrg.jpg.

7.2.6. Role of Cytokines and Chemokines

The role of chemokines and cytokines in vasculitides pathogenesis is most important, since these signaling molecules are capable of recruiting and activating immune cells, thereby perpetuating inflammatory processes in the blood vessels. In particular, cytokines , such as interleukin-6 (IL-6) and tumor necrosis factor-alpha (TNF-α) contribute to the inflammatory setting leading to vascular damage, with data illustrating that perivascular adipose tissue (PVAT), which is in healthy conditions, secretes excess of these cytokines, which are attracted by T cells and macrophages to the inflammatory site, further extending the tissue damage (Nosalski & Guzik, 2017). Moreover, chemokines like MCP-1 (CCL2) are also important for mediating the recruitment of monocytes, thereby spreading the inflammation characteristic of vasculitides. Such pathways not only account for disease mechanisms but also point towards targets for better management of vasculitic diseases (Abraham et al., 2017).

7.2.7. Endothelial Dysfunction

Endothelial dysfunction constitutes a key element of vasculitides' pathogenesis, being the result of a lack of balance between endothelial injury and repair. An imbalance has been proven to exist in active systemic vasculitis of children, even though the circulating levels of endothelial progenitor cells (EPCs) are still high, their functionality is greatly impaired and contribute to more severe vascular pathology and inflammation-related damage (Brogan et al., 2015). Such dysfunction may be further reinforced by inflammatory responses at a systemic level, as pro-inflammatory cytokines , including TNF-α, have been shown to inhibit the reparative potential of EPCs, thus leading to a compromised ability to repair endothelial damage (Brogan et al., 2015). Furthermore, the interaction between thrombosis and inflammation means that endothelial dysfunction is not merely a disease severity marker that can be used diagnostically, but also a pathogenetic event in thrombotic disease in conditions , such as ANCA-associated vasculitis. Reversal of this dysfunction could be the solution to preventing the more remote consequences of vasculitic disease (Figure 7.10).

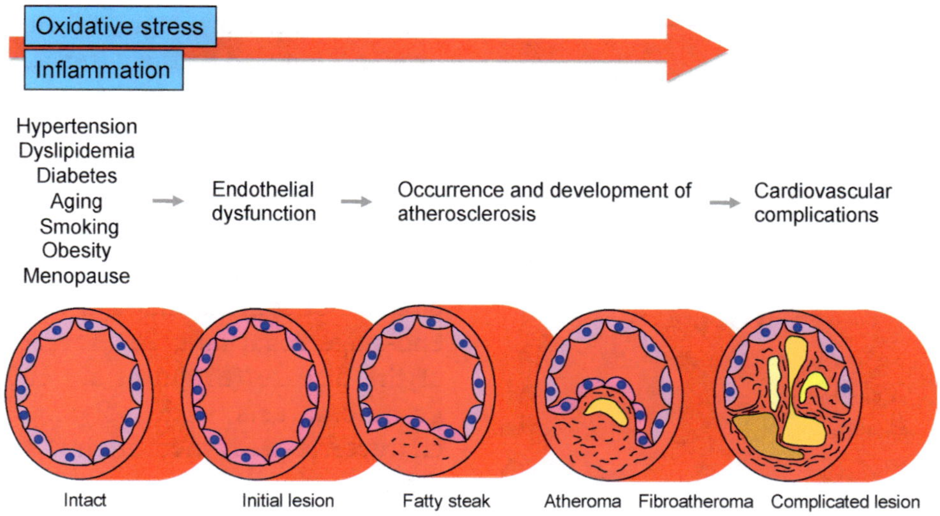

Figure 7.10. Endothelial dysfunction is a crucial factor in the pathogenesis of vasculitides, characterized by an imbalance between endothelial injury and repair.

Source: https://www.mdpi.com/antioxidants/antioxidants-11-01958/article_deploy/html/images/antioxidants-11-01958-g001.png.

7.2.8. Organ Involvement and Complications

The implication of organs in various forms of vasculitides typically leads to significant and even life-threatening complications, particularly of the skin and kidneys. Cryoglobulinaemia, for instance, can induce cutaneous vasculitis and severe glomerulonephritis, with further end-stage renal failure, particularly in those related to hepatitis C virus infection, in which new treatment modalities presented by emerging antiviral therapies provide promising avenues for successful intervention (Braun et al., 2007). Moreover, levamisole-contaminated cocaine abuse complications exhibit a characteristic pathophysiology in the form of skin and renal impairments involving leukocytoclastic vasculitis. It encompasses crescentic and necrotizing pauci-immune glomerulonephritis, further outlining the diverse presentations of vasculitides as well as the requirement for specific therapeutic measures (Jen et al., 2015). Thus, knowledge of these organ involvements and complications is crucial for optimal management of patients afflicted with vasculitides.

Test Your Knowledge

1. What is the role of immune complex deposition in small vessel vasculitis?
2. How does granulomatous inflammation develop in diseases like giant cell arteritis and GPA?

7.3. Clinical Manifestations and Diagnosis

Learning Outcome

1. Identify common symptoms across types
2. Explain organ-specific manifestations
3. Focus on laboratory tests and biomarkers
4. Learn imaging techniques for diagnosis
5. Describe biopsy and histopathological findings
6. Know differential diagnosis considerations
7. Discuss the role of rheumatologists in diagnosis
8. Identify challenges in early diagnosis
9. Know the importance of patient history and examination

Clinical presentation of vasculitides may vary significantly depending on the type and severity of the condition, such that diagnosis may be challenging at times. Some of the symptoms are fever, malaise, weight loss, and arthralgias, which might conceal the underlying inciting vascular inflammation. In eosinophilic granulomatosis with polyangiitis, for instance, neurological complications of posterior reversible encephalopathy syndrome (PRES) with vasogenic edema on MRI complicate treatment with immunosuppressive therapy (Barilaro et al., 2015). Further, cryoglobulinaemia can produce diverse presentations in the form of cutaneous vasculitis and glomerulonephritis that can lead to severe renal failure if treated late (Braun et al., 2007). The intricate relationship between systemic signs and organ involvement requires the use of an integrative diagnostic strategy, often needing serological tests and imaging studies to determine the appropriate underlying vascular disease and guide proper treatment modalities.

7.3.1. Common Symptoms Across Types

Vasculitides exhibit a variety of common symptoms that have a far-reaching impact on patient outcomes. Patients typically present with systemic symptoms , such as fever, fatigue, and malaise, which are signs of an inflammatory process underlying the disease. Dermatologic symptoms, including rashes and purpura, also frequently appear in every type of vasculitis, and this is indicative of the disease's impact on skin integrity and vascular function. Typically, conditions like cryoglobulinaemia can cause even more severe complications like glomerulonephritis that can ultimately lead to end-stage renal failure, a severe development of the disease (Braun et al., 2007). Similarly, granulomatosis with polyangiitis (GPA) is characterized by necrotizing granulomatous inflammation of the respiratory tract and kidneys and otorhinolaryngologic manifestations that are prone to be initial indicators of the onset of the disease (Greco et al., 2016). Thus, recognition of these general symptoms is crucial to attain early diagnosis and proper therapeutic management in the diverse forms of vasculitides (Figure 7.11).

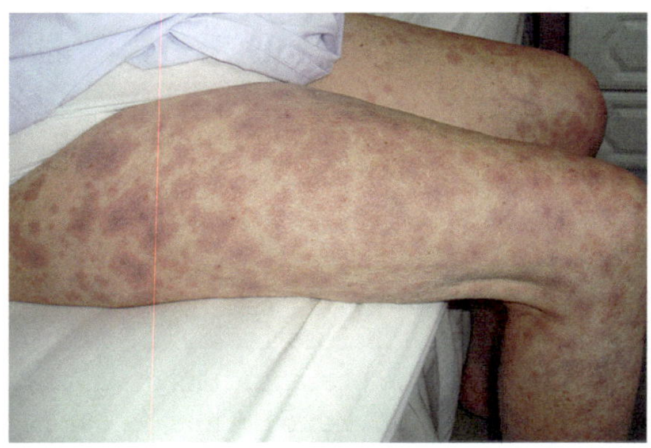

Figure 7.11. Dermatological symptoms, including rashes and purpura, are frequently observed across various forms of vasculitis, highlighting the condition's impact on skin integrity and vascular health.

Source: https://cached.imagescaler.hbpl.co.uk/resize/scaleWidth/815/cached.offlinehbpl.hbpl.co.uk/news/PGH/vascfig1-20170517095510691.jpg.

7.3.2. Organ-specific Manifestations

Organ-specific manifestations of vasculitides underscore the interplay between systemic inflammation and organ-specific tissue damage. Various forms of vasculitis can lead to severe impairment of organ function, e.g., in cryoglobulinaemia, which can result in cutaneous vasculitis and glomerulonephritis that can cause end-stage renal disease, frequently complicated by hepatitis C infection (Braun et al., 2007). Similarly, Granulomatosis with polyangiitis (GPA) shows how the destruction of nasal cartilage can lead to symptoms , such as nasal septum perforation resulting in respiratory problems and necessitating early intervention to avoid damaging organs further (Ralli, 2018). These organ-specific presentations should be recognized to provide accurate diagnosis and treatment, underlining clinicians' need for an increased index of suspicion in evaluating patients with potential vasculitic syndromes. Lastly, understanding such manifestations enhances the therapeutic interventions and results in improved patient outcomes in affected individuals.

7.3.3. Laboratory Tests and Biomarkers

The vasculitide diagnosis and management, including follow-up, have become fundamental elements, particularly through laboratory examinations and biomarkers. Laboratory examination is indispensable to distinguish among various forms of vasculitides, as only one cannot be confirmed by a single test; ultimate assessment may necessitate being addressed from several directions to rule out other mimicking diseases (Ralli et al., 2020). Here, biomarkers , such as antineutrophil cytoplasmic antibodies (ANCA) are notably of diagnostic and prognostic value. For example, in antineutrophil cytoplasmic antibody-associated vasculitis (AAV), elevated levels of extracellular vesicles carrying proteins , such as pentraxin-3 and tissue factor correlate with disease severity and renal involvement and are thus potential non-invasive markers of disease status (Jónasdóttir et al., 2022). These laboratory investigations not only enhance the accuracy of diagnosis but also influence therapeutic decisions and contribute to enhanced patient outcomes in vasculitides care (Figure 7.12).

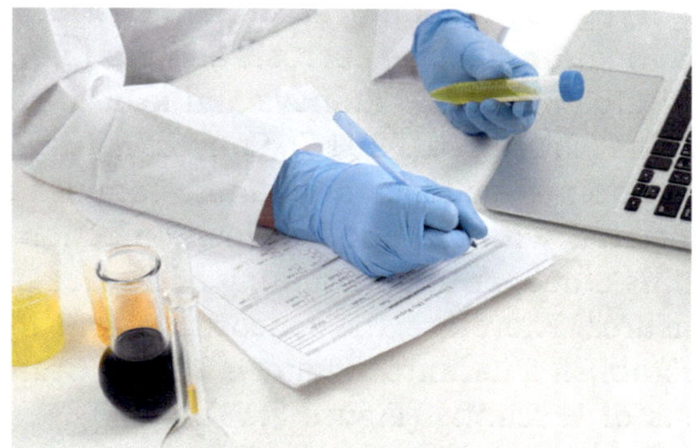

Figure 7.12. Laboratory diagnostics are essential for distinguishing between various types of vasculitides.

Source: https://primemedlabs.in/wp-content/uploads/2024/07/Vasculitis-Sub-2-Lab.png.

7.3.4. Imaging Techniques for Diagnosis

Accurate diagnosis of vasculitides is crucial due to the complex nature and varied presentation of the conditions, from focal to widespread systemic disease. Imaging modalities are at the core of this diagnostic process, and advances , such as positron emission tomography-computed tomography (PET/CT) are now being utilized more frequently in the evaluation of cases suspected of vasculitides. Efficacy of PET/CT in the diagnosis of vasculitis has been proven by studies, where the method provides clinically useful information in a large proportion of patients, thus halting delays in diagnosis that are responsible for higher healthcare costs and complications (Taimen, 2021). Furthermore, in diseases like Takayasu arteritis, imaging allows accurate assessment of large-vessel disease and aids early treatment (Al-Obaidi et al., 2015). Combined, these imaging modalities enhance diagnostic accuracy and treatment of vasculitis, ultimately improving patient care in an environment in which early detection is paramount.

7.3.5. Biopsy and Histopathological Findings

In the context of vasculitides, histopathological analysis and biopsy represent significant features in the accurate diagnosis of diseases , such as granulomatosis, also known as polyangiitis (GPA), and cryoglobulinaemic vasculitis. Histopathological features typically indicate typical patterns of inflammation, such as necrosis and granulomatous inflammation in GPA, which primarily affect the respiratory tract and kidneys and lead to striking clinical manifestations involving multiple organ systems (Greco et al., 2016). Conversely, cryoglobulinaemic vasculitides biopsies often demonstrate deposition of evidence of immune complex and secondary changes in the vessels, most classically associated with hepatitis C virus infection (Braun et al., 2007). Not only do these assist us in gaining a deeper understanding of disease processes, but they also help guide targeted therapeutic measures. Therefore, the concordance of clinical, serological, and histopathological data is required to establish a definite diagnosis and institute proper and effective therapy in patients with various forms of vasculitis (Figure 7.13).

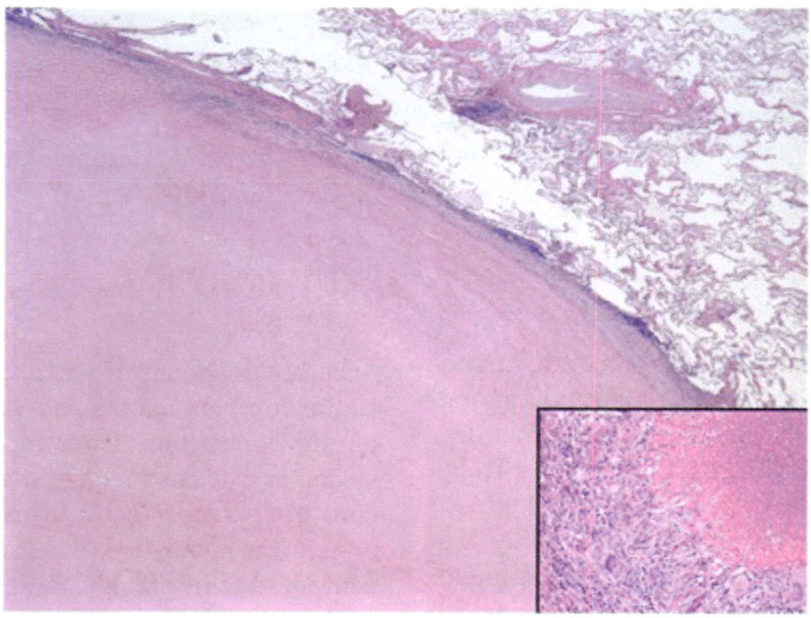

Figure 7.13. In the context of vasculitides, biopsy and histopathological findings serve as crucial elements in accurately diagnosing conditions , such as granulomatosis with polyangiitis (GPA) and cryoglobulinaemic vasculitis.

Source: https://media.springernature.com/full/springer-static/image/art%3A10.1038%2Fmodpathol.2011.155/MediaObjects/41379_2012_Article_BFmodpathol2011155_Fig1_HTML.jpg.

7.3.6. Differential Diagnosis Considerations

The differential diagnosis in presumed vasculitides is essential, particularly because there are shared clinical characteristics with other conditions. For instance, Granulomatosis with polyangiitis (GPA) can cause symptoms , such as nasal obstruction and epistaxis, which mimic more common upper respiratory tract infections, hence making diagnosis tricky if not considered from the outset (Ralli, 2018). In addition to this, conditions like cardiac myxomas can even present with systemic symptoms and skin involvement in the form of purpuric rashes, with the risk of misdiagnosis (Anwar et al., 2018). The challenge is in identifying these presentations early enough to prevent such consequences as organ damage or systemic failure. This indicates the importance of thorough clinical assessment and addition of a broad differential, as immediate intervention can be critical in the avoidance of life-threatening consequences of various vasculitides as well as their mimics.

7.3.7. Role of Rheumatologists in Diagnosis

Rheumatologists play a very important role in the diagnosis and management of vasculitides, particularly in distinguishing diseases , such as granulomatosis with polyangiitis (GPA) from other autoimmune conditions. Their proficiency is part of conducting a complete clinical assessment integrating patient history, physical examination, and ancillary laboratory tests, including serology for anti-neutrophil cytoplasmic antibodies (ANCA) for GPA, an autoimmune illness resulting from systemic inflammation of many organs, most frequently the respiratory system and kidneys (Greco et al., 2016). Besides, rheumatologists collaborate with other specialists , such as nephrologists and otorhinolaryngologists, to ensure patients receive a multidisciplinary diagnosis and management (Belino et al., 2024). The collaboration maximizes the accurate diagnosis process, leading to effective and timely management regimens. Given that vasculitides are a heterogeneous group of diseases, the role of rheumatologists is invaluable in ensuring maximum patient outcomes through diagnostic competence and collaborative management (Figure 7.14).

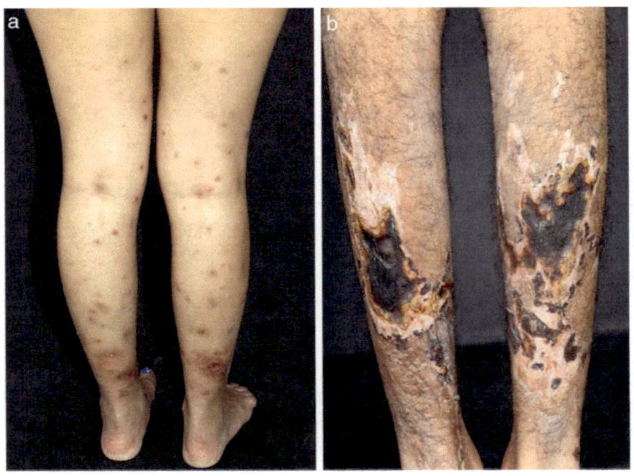

Figure 7.14. Rheumatologists play a critical role in the diagnosis and management of vasculitides, particularly in distinguishing conditions , such as granulomatosis with polyangiitis (GPA) from other autoimmune disorders.

Source: https://static.elsevier.es/multimedia/03650596/0000009500000003/v4_202007210853/S0365059620300969/v4_202007210853/en/main.assets/gr3.jpeg.

7.3.8. Challenges in Early Diagnosis

The diagnostic challenge in vasculitides during their early stages presents significant challenges, most commonly resulting from their heterogeneous clinical presentation. The patients typically present with unremarkable and nonspecific symptoms , such as fever and weight loss that are common in numerous diseases. This makes them similar to each other and thus exposes them to misdiagnosis or delayed intervention, which exacerbates disease progression and morbidity and mortality rates (Yates & Watts, 2017). Furthermore, the employment of specific autoantibodies, such as IgG antineutrophil cytoplasmic autoantibodies, is also problematic. While these antibodies have been associated with granulomatosis with polyangiitis and microscopic polyangiitis, the renal histopathologic changes of the two entities are often indistinguishable, making diagnosis difficult (Bettinelli et al., 2018). Thus, the lack of absolute early diagnostic markers emphasizes the need for enhanced awareness among clinicians and advances in diagnostic methods to maximize patient outcomes in vasculitides.

7.3.9. Importance of Patient History and Examination

A thorough physical examination and patient history are critical components in the diagnosis of vasculitides, where the presentation can be nonspecific and variable. Familiarity with the patient's previous conditions, including infections or autoimmune disorders, can give clues to potential precipitating factors for the challenging diseases. For instance, in cases like Henoch-Schönlein purpura (HSP), identification of gastrointestinal symptoms and recent infection can assist in making an early diagnosis, such as that illustrated through the case management of an elderly patient whose symptoms were blamed on rotavirus infection (Adderley et al., 2017). Also, the presence of eosinophilic granulomatosis with polyangiitis underlines the significance of meticulous medical history, as its atypical presentations can be obscured by prior self-medication with corticosteroids, thereby complicating the diagnosis (Andolina et al., 2014). Such cases highlight the fact that a systematic approach to patient history and physical examination not only assists proper diagnosis but also leads to proper treatment planning (Figure 7.15).

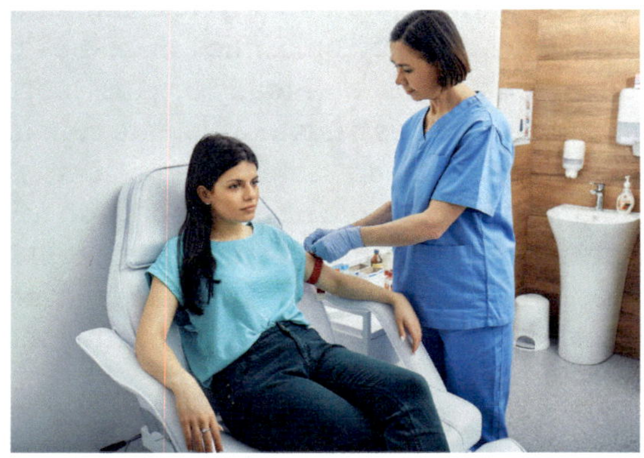

Figure 7.15. Understanding the patients' prior health conditions, including infections or autoimmune disorders, can offer insights into potential triggers for these complex diseases.

Source: https://drmaggieyu.com/wp-content/uploads/2023/08/a-closer-look-at-rare-autoimmune-diseases-and-their-management-1184x834.jpg.

Test Your Knowledge

1. What imaging techniques are used to diagnose large vessel vasculitis?
2. What role does tissue biopsy play in confirming vasculitis?

7.4. Treatment and Management Strategies

Learning Outcome

1. Focus on corticosteroids in treatment
2. Learn immunosuppressive therapies
3. Understand biologic agents and targeted therapies
4. Discuss supportive care and symptom management
5. Explain the role of multidisciplinary teams
6. Monitor for treatment efficacy
7. Explain long-term management strategies
8. Focus on patient education and self-management
9. Learn future directions in treatment research

The therapy and management of vasculitides need to be tailored based on the subtype and etiology of the disease, which is critically important for determining patient outcomes. For instance, cryoglobulinaemia-associated vasculitis, which could be secondary to hepatitis C virus infection, needs to be treated with an integrated strategy combining both immunosuppression and antiviral agents. Current advances in the antiviral treatments offer an opportunity for causal therapy, particularly for such patients where their cryoglobulinaemia relates to viral infections, hence curing both the expression of vasculitis and etiology of underlying pathosis (Braun et al., 2007). Successful treatment further involves ongoing monitoring of renal function and potential complications , such as renal failure, highlighting the complex presentation of such diseases (Aminde et al., 2016). Last but not least, a tailored approach integrating pharmacological treatment and diligent monitoring is required to maximize the results in patients with various forms of vasculitides.

7.4.1. Corticosteroids in Treatment

Corticosteroids form the hub of management in most vasculitides due to their potent anti-inflammatory action. They are particularly useful for managing acute flare by rapidly suppressing the immune response that characterizes them. In the context of eosinophilic granulomatosis with polyangiitis (EGPA), corticosteroids are effective in reducing complications like posterior reversible encephalopathy syndrome (PRES), an uncommon but severe manifestation of central nervous system involvement of ANCA-associated vasculitides. Judicious use of corticosteroids, coupled with careful surveillance of blood pressure, can soothe symptoms while addressing causative inflammatory processes (Barilaro et al., 2015). In addition, recent advances highlight the necessity to optimize corticosteroid therapy among children with vasculitides since new clinical trials focus on limiting glucocorticoid toxicity and improving patient outcome (Brogan et al., 2016). Hence, corticosteroids remain a mainstay of therapy in the treatment of vasculitides (Figure 7.16).

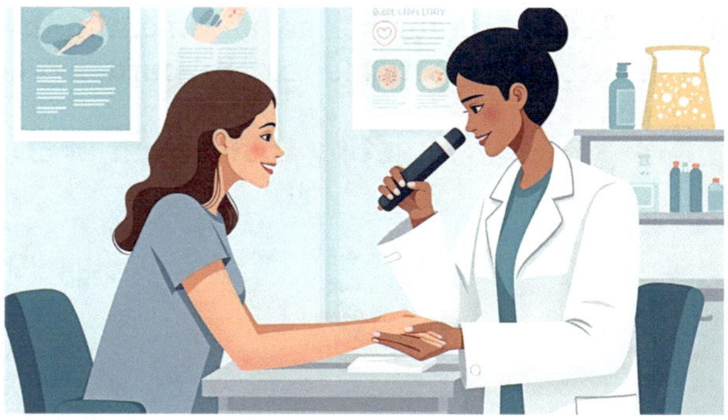

Figure 7.16. Judicious use of corticosteroids, coupled with careful monitoring of blood pressure, may alleviate symptoms while addressing underlying inflammatory processes

Source: https://www.kaya.in/media/mageplaza/blog/post/b/e/betamethasone-uses-benefits-side-effects-guide.jpg.

7.4.2. Immunosuppressive Therapies

The treatment of vasculitides typically involves the prescription of immunosuppressive drugs, which are critical in managing inflammation and preventing tissue destruction. For eosinophilic granulomatosis with polyangiitis (EGPA), this is further complicated when complicating conditions like posterior reversible encephalopathy syndrome (PRES) arise; this makes it challenging to use immunosuppressant medications safely, given their capacity to aggravate endothelial injury and hypertension (Barilaro et al., 2015). As new evidence illustrates, the development of individually tailored treatment regimens has revolutionized the treatment landscape for pediatric vasculitis patients, particularly through recognition that specific conditions, including Kawasaki Disease, can be assisted by adjunctive corticosteroid use alongside traditional therapies , such as intravenous immunoglobulin (IVIG) (Brogan et al., 2016). A thoughtful understanding of these treatments and their implications is essential in order to optimize patient outcomes for differing presentations of vasculitis.

7.4.3. Biologic Agents and Targeted Therapies

Introduction of biologic agents and targeted therapy revolutionized the treatment of vasculitides, particularly in children and those diseases involving eosinophilic dysregulation. Some newer trends include clinical trials for employing biologics to selectively target offending inflammatory pathways and reduce dependency on glucocorticoids and their resistant side effects. For instance, interleukin-5 therapy has been promising in the management of eosinophilic granulomatosis with polyangiitis and hyper eosinophilic syndrome so that their complex conditions can be managed customarily (Mateo et al., 2023). Further, the addition of targeted therapy has shed some light on the pathogenesis of disease, with a pressing requirement for well-designed randomized controlled trials to assess the efficacy of these novel treatments in the majority of vasculitis syndromes (Brogan et al., 2016). With further advancement in therapy, it can greatly benefit the outcomes of patients and reduce glucocorticoid toxicity burden, particularly among vulnerable patients (Figure 7.17).

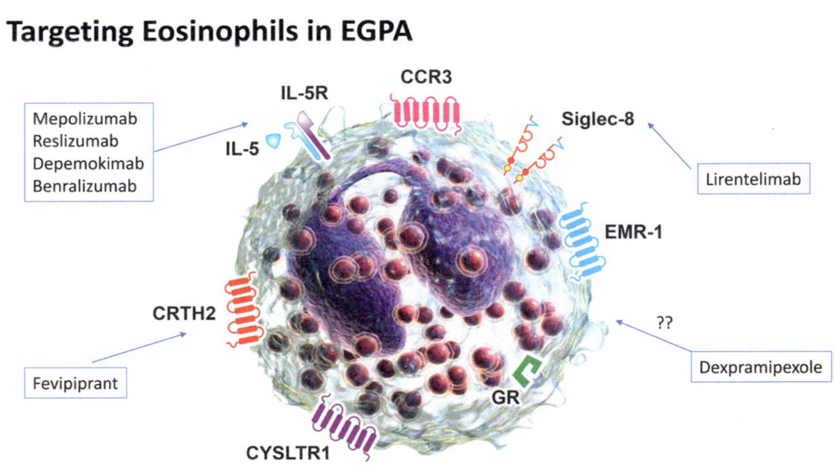

Figure 7.17. Therapies aimed at interleukin-5 have shown promise in treating eosinophilic granulomatosis with polyangiitis and hyper eosinophilic syndrome

Source: https://www.rheumatic.theclinics.com/cms/10.1016/j.rdc.2023.03.006/asset/6b936064-7ec6-40d9-ba12-5abbf41e4510/main.assets/gr2_lrg.jpg.

7.4.4. Supportive Care and Symptom Management

Symptom control and supportive care are also critical aspects of the treatment of vasculitides, given the complex and often disabling nature of these illnesses. Many of these patients have a variety of symptoms that significantly impair their quality of life, necessitating a multidisciplinary management of both physical and psychological demands. Efficient management strategies involve pain mitigation, dietary supplementation, and counseling to alleviate psychological distress, all of which serve to alleviate the symptom burden of symptoms , such as fatigue, pain, and depression. Moreover, improvements in imaging technologies, e.g., PET/CT, have improved vasculitis diagnosis through reducing diagnostic delay and improving response to therapy, thereby optimizing supportive care strategies (Taimen, 2021). In particularly challenging cases, such as primary CNS vasculitis in patients with other compromising illnesses, such as HIV, early and effective drug therapy in combination with supportive care is important to obtain the best quality of results (Pellinen et al., 2016). Hence, a multimodal approach to care remains important in the treatment of such complex cases.

7.4.5. Role of Multidisciplinary Teams

Treatment of vasculitides often involves teamwork, making multidisciplinary teams very important. Because of the complexity of these diseases, in which various organ systems may be involved and manifest through various clinical features, integrating the knowledge of various medical specialties is called for. For instance, ophthalmologists, pulmonologists, and rheumatologists may all examine a patient with vasculitis and treat complicating conditions , such as pulmonary disease or eye manifestations, such as in the case of Cogan's syndrome, wherein audio-vestibular symptoms are usually accompanied by systemic inflammation (D'Aguanno et al., 2017).

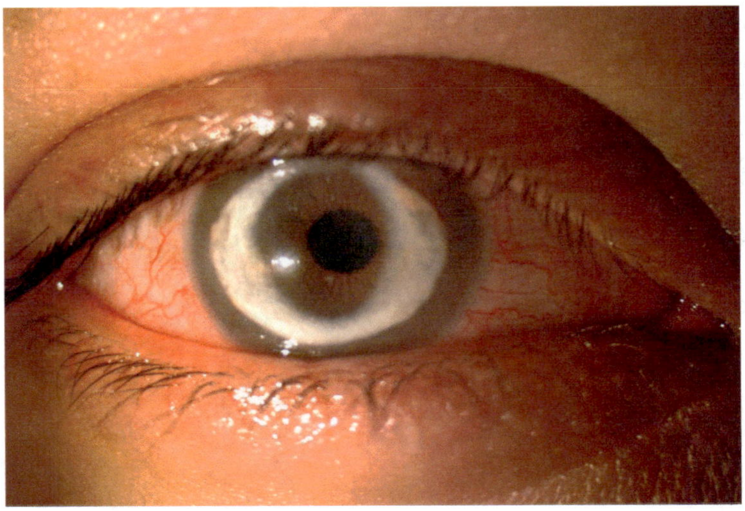

Figure 7.18. Cogan's syndrome.

Source: https://djo.harvard.edu/public/journals/1/submission_465_467_coverImage_en_US.jpg.

Furthermore, the identification and care of interstitial lung diseases, as typically associated with autoimmune manifestations, are facilitated by an integrated effort between pulmonology and rheumatology that can enhance diagnosis and tailor therapy to individual patients (Cerri et al., 2016). Lastly, utilization of multidisciplinary teams not only enhances the quality of care but also makes investigation into the pathophysiology of these complex diseases more feasible (Figure 7.18).

7.4.6. Monitoring for Treatment Efficacy

Effective monitoring of treatment outcomes is important in the management of vasculitides, particularly conditions like granulomatosis with polyangiitis (GPA). Diagnosis and monitoring should be encompassing in their scope , including clinical assessment, serological tests for anti-neutrophil cytoplasmic antibodies (ANCA), and histology, as addressed in the most recent EULAR guidelines. These recommendations emphasize the place of biopsy in making diagnoses and the need for tailored glucocorticoid treatment in an effort to reduce side effects while managing disease (Mukhtyar et al., 2016). An individual should also remember that although rising ANCA levels can indicate relapse, it should not constitute the sole foundation for selecting treatment. Integrated monitoring through structured assessment tools ensures that patients are fully managed, not just for the vasculitis but also for the side effects of drugs. Monitoring in this strict way not only enhances treatment outcomes but also promotes patient involvement in disease management (Greco et al., 2016).

7.4.7. Long-term Management Strategies

The long-term vasculitides management plan is crucial in preventing the acceleration of disease and enhancing the quality of life in patients. Successful strategies typically involve an amalgamation of immunosuppressive drugs tailored to the type and severity of vasculitis, alongside routine monitoring for potential complications. Research indicates that protocolized management enhances outcome significantly, particularly in systemic vasculitides involving multiple organs and risk of organ damage (Ralli et al., 2020). Moreover, if cryoglobulinaemia develops, understanding its association with hepatitis C is important; novel antiviral treatments can provide causal therapy options that can avoid major syndromes like glomerulonephritis and end-stage renal failure (Braun et al., 2007). Thus, a comprehensive management plan not only addresses the initial inflammatory response but also addresses prevention, follow-up on a regular basis, and therapeutic adjustments to achieve maximal long-term well-being in patients with such complex diseases (Figure 7.19).

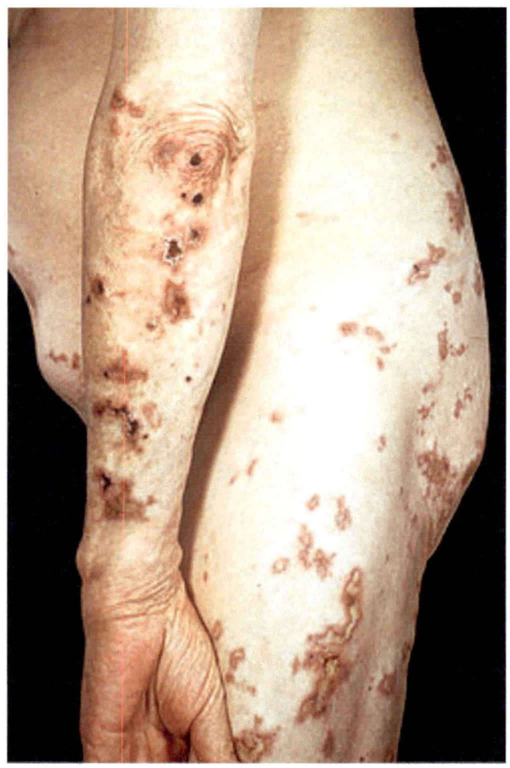

Figure 7.19. Cryoglobulinaemia.

Source: https://upload.wikimedia.org/wikipedia/commons/thumb/f/fc/Cryoglobulinemia2.jpg/250px-Cryoglobulinemia2.jpg.

7.4.8. Patient Education and Self-management

Effective patient education and self-management are key components of management in patients diagnosed with vasculitides, particularly in light of the heterogeneity and unpredictability of such illness. Due to the fact that small vessel vasculitides will often present with nonspecific features, there is a need for medical professionals, most notably general practitioners, to equip patients with information regarding how to recognize initial symptoms and trace the path of the disease (Conte et al., 2020). This empowerment not only enhances patients' compliance with treatment protocols but also inspires a proactive mindset towards taking care of their own health. According to evidence, ANCA-associated vasculitides patients express a significant need for substantial information regarding their diagnosis, treatment, and potential side effects, typically wishing to be informed directly by physicians (Mooney et al., 2014). With enhanced patient education and facilitating self-management practices, clinicians can significantly contribute to the improvement of the quality of life in individuals with vasculitides and improve health outcomes.

7.4.9. Future Directions in Treatment Research

As scientists venture into the complexities of vasculitides, future research into treatments is also becoming more optimistic. One of these concerns the interaction between genetic predispositions and environmental factors, particularly as studies reference a correlation between low vitamin D levels and increased incidences of granulomatous polyangiitis and eosinophilic granulomatosis, and as such, more study of these correlations is called for (Gatenby, 2014). Moreover, emerging imaging techniques , such as PET/CT, are showing potential in increasing diagnostic accuracy and reducing delays in the diagnosis of systemic vasculitides and hence facilitating appropriate therapeutic interventions (Taimen, 2021). These advances are revealing the applicability of personalized medicine, where therapy could be tailored based on individuals' genetic and environmental parameters. Ultimately, multidisciplinary therapy that includes genetic research, environmental assessments, and hi-tech imaging equipment is the future of vasculitis treatment, its promise being to enhance patient outcomes and establish therapeutic protocols.

Test Your Knowledge

1. What are the emerging therapies or biologics being explored in vasculitis treatment?
2. What are the risks and monitoring strategies for immunosuppressive therapy?

Summary

The multifactorial etiology of vasculitides necessitates a comprehensive understanding of their various subtypes and complications. As highlighted by the article, the connection between levamisole-contaminated cocaine abuse and vasculitis identifies an emerging public health problem, which places in the spotlight unique clinical syndromes characterized by renal disease and cutaneous lesions (Butcher et al., 2014). Secondly, the development of medium-sized-artery vasculitides in pediatric groups, including Kawasaki disease and polyarteritis nodosa, emphasizes the need for early diagnosis and personalized therapeutic approaches (Bakkaloglu et al., 2010). The conditions not only have varied clinical manifestations but also intricate pathophysiological mechanisms that are worthy of continued study and improved clinical management protocols. The pending data necessitate greater awareness among medical personnel to facilitate timely intervention and improved patient outcomes in the case of vasculitides. As our knowledge grows, so does our ability to counteract the effects of these severe inflammatory conditions.

Vasculitides are understood through the comprehension of their diverse clinical manifestations and recent advances in research towards improved diagnosis and treatment. Small vessel vasculitides commonly present with a wide range of neurological, renal, pulmonary, and dermatological presentations, necessitating the identification of these nonspecific presentations by healthcare practitioners for effective differential diagnosis and management (Conte et al., 2020). Recent evidence from the European Vasculitis Society indicates the pandemic's adaptability by the medical community, exemplifying worldwide cooperation and virtual communication essential to this era. Progress in clinical trials is revolutionizing steroid minimization and maintenance treatment, whereas large studies on renal pathology and gene-based understanding of illness , such as eosinophilic granulomatosis with polyangiitis (EGPA), provide key evidence for classification and treatment optimization (Greco et al., 2016). Lastly, the incorporation of new research and clinical practice characterizes the evolving world of vasculitis treatment, with the need for constant awareness and adaptation in the field.

KEY TERMS FROM THIS CHAPTER

- Antineutrophil Cytoplasmic Antibodies (ANCA)
- Cryoglobulinaemia
- Disease progression
- Endothelial dysfunction
- Endothelial progenitor cells (EPCs)
- Eosinophilic granulomatosis
- Glomerulonephritis
- hazardous
- Henoch-Schönlein purpura (HSP)
- Histopathological data
- Immunosuppressive therapy
- Leukocytoclastic vasculitis
- Meta-analyses
- Otorhinolaryngologic
- Particular therapy
- Pathophysiology
- Perivascular adipose tissue (PVAT)
- Polyangiitis
- Vasculitic syndromes
- Vasculitides

Critical Thinking Questions

1. **Which of the following vasculitides primarily affects large arteries , such as the aorta and its major branches?**
   a. Microscopic polyangiitis
   b. Takayasu arteritis
   c. Granulomatosis with polyangiitis
   d. Behçet's disease
2. **Which clinical feature is most characteristic of giant cell arteritis?**
   a. Oral ulcers
   b. Hematuria
   c. Temporal headache with jaw claudication
   d. Palpable purpura
3. **Which vasculitis is most strongly associated with anti-neutrophil cytoplasmic antibodies (ANCAs)?**
   a. Polyarteritis nodosa
   b. Henoch-Schönlein purpura
   c. Granulomatosis with polyangiitis (GPA)
   d. Kawasaki disease
4. **Which of the following is a classic feature of Kawasaki disease in children?**
   a. Digital gangrene
   b. Coronary artery aneurysms
   c. Pitting edema
   d. Telangiectasia
5. **Palpable purpura is most commonly associated with which type of vasculitis?**
   a. Large vessel vasculitis
   b. Medium vessel vasculitis
   c. Small vessel vasculitis
   d. Venous thrombosis

Answers to Critical Thinking Questions

1. (b) 2. (c) 3. (c) 4. (b) 5. (c)

Short Answer Questions

1. How are vasculitides classified based on the size of the affected blood vessels?
2. What are the primary examples of large vessel vasculitides?
3. What are the key immune mechanisms that cause inflammation in vasculitides?
4. How do anti-neutrophil cytoplasmic antibodies (ANCAs) contribute to vascular damage?
5. What are the hallmark clinical signs of giant cell arteritis?
6. How does Takayasu arteritis typically present in young adults?
7. What is the first-line treatment for ANCA-associated vasculitis?
8. When should high-dose corticosteroids be initiated in vasculitis?

References

1. Abdulahad, A., Abdulahad, A., Abdulahad, A., Abdulahad, A., Abdulahad, A., Abdulahad, A., Ait-Oufella, H., et al. (2014). T cells in vascular inflammatory diseases. https://core.ac.uk/download/pdf/82869901.pdf (accessed on 17th June 2025).
2. Abraham, D., Assandri, R., Assassi, S., Auluck, A., Bacher, P., Baron, M., Baron, M., et al. (2017). Review article: Pathogenesis and clinical manifestations of gastrointestinal involvement in systemic sclerosis. https://core.ac.uk/download/83049880.pdf (accessed on 17th June 2025).
3. Adderley, C., Adderley, C., Bender, M., Epstein, D., Homberg, M., Kim, J., Mongillo, M., et al. (2017). A case of Henoch-Schönlein purpura associated with rotavirus infection in an elderly Asian male and review of the literature. https://core.ac.uk/download/323078862.pdf (accessed on 17th June 2025).
4. Al-Obaidi, M., Brogan, P. A., Dolezalova, P., Eleftheriou, D., et al. (2015). Takayasu arteritis in childhood: Retrospective experience from a tertiary referral center in the United Kingdom. https://core.ac.uk/download/29415232.pdf (accessed on 17th June 2025).
5. Alamo, B. S., Bajema, I. M., Bettiol, A., Carlson, N., Cid, M. C., Egan, A. C., Emmi, G., et al. (2023). The sound of interconnectivity; The European Vasculitis Society 2022 Report. https://diposit.ub.edu/dspace/bitstream/2445/209228/1/The%20Sound%20of%20Interconnectivity%20the%20European_Kireports.pdf (accessed on 17th June 2025).
6. Allen, M., Almansa, R., Altmeyer, R., Baggiolini, M., Baldini, C., Balhara, K., Balkwill, F., et al. (2018). The long pentraxin PTX3: A prototypical sensor of tissue injury and a regulator of homeostasis. https://core.ac.uk/download/195278097.doc (accessed on 17th June 2025).
7. Altabás, I., Garcia, S., Pérez Gómez, I., Nair, A., Pego Reigosa, J. M., et al. (2020). Blocking IL-17: A promising strategy in the treatment of systemic rheumatic diseases. https://core.ac.uk/download/588395709.pdf (accessed on 17th June 2025).
8. Amedei, E., Amedeo, M., Becatti, M., D,' L., Della Bella, C., et al. (2015). Thrombosis in vasculitis: From pathogenesis to treatment. https://core.ac.uk/download/301569356.pdf (accessed on 17th June 2025).
9. Amft, N., Basu, N., Black, C., Dhaun, N., et al. (2020). Characterizing infection in anti-neutrophil cytoplasmic antibody-associated vasculitis: Results from a longitudinal, matched-cohort data linkage study. https://core.ac.uk/download/293754474.pdf (accessed on 17th June 2025).
10. Aminde, L. N., Dzudie, A., Njim, T., Tsi, E., Noubiap, J. J., et al. (2016). Takayasu's arteritis in an adult female from Cameroon: Diagnosis via Doppler echocardiography. https://core.ac.uk/download/46558990.pdf (accessed on 17th June 2025).
11. Amsler, J., Aymonnier, K., Lamprecht, P., Salama, A., et al. (2022). The neutrophil: A key resourceful agent in immune-mediated vasculitis. https://core.ac.uk/download/548255532.pdf (accessed on 17th June 2025).
12. Andolina, G., Banco, M. A., Bonura, A., Buscemi, S., et al. (2014). An uncommon presentation of eosinophilic granulomatosis with polyangiitis: A case report. https://core.ac.uk/download/53289745.pdf (accessed on 17th June 2025).
13. Ralli, M., Campo, F., Angeletti, D., Minni, A., Artico, M., Greco, A., Polimeni, A., & de Vincentiis, M. (2020). Pathophysiology and therapy of systemic vasculitides. *EXCLI journal*, *19*, 817–854. https://doi.org/10.17179/excli2020-1512 (accessed on 17th June 2025).

14. Anwar, S., Baszis, K., Javidan, C., Macias, C., et al. (2018). Rare presentation of an atrial myxoma in an adolescent patient: A case report and literature review. https://core.ac.uk/download/287888058.pdf (accessed on 17th June 2025).

15. Atienza Mateo, B., Bañas-Conejero, D., Bobolea, I., Crespo-Lessmann, A., et al. (2023). Expert consensus on the use of systemic glucocorticoids for managing eosinophil-related diseases. https://core.ac.uk/download/603961286.pdf (accessed on 17th June 2025).

16. Bailey, K., Breda, L., Chiarelli, F., Ciarelli, S., et al. (2024). The diagnostic role of skin manifestations in rheumatic diseases in children: A critical review of pediatric vasculitis. https://core.ac.uk/download/614994127.pdf (accessed on 17th June 2025).

17. Bakkaloglu, A., Churg, A., Gianviti, A., Harnden, A., Harnden, A., Kawamoto, A., Kussmaul, A., et al. (2010). Medium-size-vessel vasculitis. https://core.ac.uk/download/pdf/8433772.pdf (accessed on 17th June 2025).

18. Barilaro, G., Granata, M., Marra, A. M., Villella, A., et al. (2015). Eosinophilic granulomatosis with polyangiitis (EGPA) and PRES: A case-based review of literature in ANCA-associated vasculitis's. https://core.ac.uk/download/54520276.pdf (accessed on 17th June 2025).

19. Basnyat, S., Goldfarb, J. M., Nyquist, G. G., Rabinowitz, M. R., et al. (2016). Head and neck manifestations of eosinophilic granulomatosis with polyangiitis: A systematic review. https://core.ac.uk/download/83049399.pdf (accessed on 17th June 2025).

20. Belino, C., Ferreira, C., Ferreira, I., Rovisco, J., et al. (2024). Insights from Portuguese nephrologists and rheumatologists concerning the treatment of ANCA vasculitis. https://core.ac.uk/download/639217957.pdf (accessed on 17th June 2025).

21. Bergamini, A., Cesareo, M., Chimenti, M. S., Conigliaro, P., et al. (2023). Subclinical microvascular changes in ANCA-vasculitis's: The role of optical coherence tomography angiography and nailfold capillaroscopy in the detection of disease-related damage. https://core.ac.uk/download/590752199.pdf (accessed on 17th June 2025).

22. Berti, A., Berti, A., Karras, A., Knight, A., Knight, A., Mahr, A., Mahr, A., et al. (2020). ANCA-associated vasculitis. https://core.ac.uk/download/334410844.pdf (accessed on 17th June 2025).

23. Bettinelli, A., Bianchetti, M., Keller, F., Simonetti, G. D., et al. (2018). Vasculitis's associated with IgG antineutrophil cytoplasmic autoantibodies in childhood. https://core.ac.uk/download/159145986.pdf (accessed on 17th June 2025).

24. Braun, G. S., Horster, S., Ihrler, S., Schmid, H., et al. (2007). Cryoglobulinemic vasculitis: Classification and clinical and therapeutic aspects. https://core.ac.uk/download/12175185.pdf (accessed on 17th June 2025).

25. Brogan, P. A., & Eleftheriou, D. (2016). Therapeutic advances in the treatment of vasculitis. https://core.ac.uk/download/79512787.pdf (accessed on 17th June 2025).

26. Brouwer, E., Brüner, M., Hauge, E. M., Keller, K. E., et al. (2021). Vasculitis therapy refines vasculitis mechanistic classification. https://core.ac.uk/download/518775849.pdf (accessed on 17th June 2025).

27. Butcher, B., Carlson, A. Q., Graf, J., Imboden, J. B., et al. (2014). Pauci-immune glomerulonephritis in individuals with disease associated with levamisole-adulterated cocaine: A series of 4 cases. https://core.ac.uk/download/323066873.pdf (accessed on 17th June 2025).

28. Carmona, F. D., González-Escribano, M. F., González-Gay, M. A., Lyons, P. A., et al. (2018). Cross-phenotype analysis of Immunochip data identifies *KDM4C* as a relevant locus for the development of systemic vasculitis. https://core.ac.uk/download/155787568.pdf (accessed on 17th June 2025).
29. Cerri, S., Colaci, M., Della Casa, G., Ferri, C., et al. (2016). Interstitial pneumonia with autoimmune features and undifferentiated connective tissue disease: Our interdisciplinary rheumatology-pneumology experience, and review of the literature. https://core.ac.uk/download/132771526.pdf (accessed on 17th June 2025).
30. Clarke, L. (2009). Endothelial injury and repair in vasculitis of the young. https://core.ac.uk/download/1686273.pdf (accessed on 17th June 2025).
31. Conte, S. M., & Vale, P. R. (2020). Systemic vasculitis's. Part 1: Large, medium and variable vessel diseases. https://core.ac.uk/download/344751841.pdf (accessed on 17th June 2025).
32. Conte, S. M., & Vale, P. R. (2020). Systemic vasculitis's. Part 2: Small vessel diseases. https://core.ac.uk/download/344751842.pdf (accessed on 17th June 2025).
33. Massimo Ralli(2018). Nasal manifestations in granulomatosis with polyangiitis: A case report and review of the literature. OTLOJ 2018; 4 (2) : 22-25; 10.17140/OTLOJ-4-149; (accessed on 17th June 2025).
34. D'Aguanno, V., De Vincentiis, M., Greco, A., Ralli, M., et al. (2017). Optimal management of Cogan's syndrome: A multidisciplinary approach. https://core.ac.uk/download/144473159.pdf (accessed on 17th June 2025).
35. Greco, A., Marinelli, C., Fusconi, M., Macri, G. F., Gallo, A., De Virgilio, A., Zambetti, G., & de Vincentiis, M. (2016). Clinic manifestations in granulomatosis with polyangiitis. *International journal of immunopathology and pharmacology*, *29*(2), 151–159. https://doi.org/10.1177/0394632015617063(accessed on 17th June 2025).
36. Draibe, J., & Salama, A. D. (2015). Association of ANCA-associated vasculitis and rheumatoid arthritis: A lesser recognized overlap syndrome. https://core.ac.uk/download/79496230.pdf (accessed on 17th June 2025).
37. Gatenby, P. A. (2014). The role of environmental factors in the pathogenesis of anti-neutrophil antibody associated vasculitis.
38. Nosalski, R., & Guzik, T. J. (2017). Perivascular adipose tissue inflammation in vascular disease. *British journal of pharmacology*, *174*(20), 3496–3513. https://doi.org/10.1111/bph.13705 (accessed on 17th June 2025).
39. Ho, T., Kang, J. S., Masood, M., Nunley, J. R., et al. (2023). Dermatologic manifestations of rheumatic disease: Cutaneous manifestations of vasculitis's. https://core.ac.uk/download/561013875.pdf (accessed on 17th June 2025).
40. Jen, K. Y., & Nolan, A. L. (2015). Pathologic manifestations of levamisole-adulterated cocaine exposure. https://core.ac.uk/download/323072399.pdf (accessed on 17th June 2025).
41. Jónasdóttir, Á. D. (2022). Inflammatory biomarkers in ANCA-associated vasculitis. https://core.ac.uk/download/543388774.pdf (accessed on 17th June 2025).
42. Mooney, J. (2014). What are the informational needs of patients with ANCA associated vasculitis? A mixed methods study. https://core.ac.uk/download/29109493.pdf (accessed on 17th June 2025).

43. Mukhtyar, C., & Sznajd, J. (2016). How to treat ANCAassociated vasculitis: Practical messages from 2016 EULAR/ERAEDTA recommendations. https://core.ac.uk/download/237699596.pdf (accessed on 17th June 2025).

44. Pellinen, J., Rumore, M. M., & Su, S. (2016). Cyclophosphamide for suspected primary angiitis of the central nervous system in a patient with human immunodeficiency virus: A case report. https://core.ac.uk/download/217327129.pdf (accessed on 17th June 2025).

45. Rathmann, J. (2023). Clinical and epidemiological studies in ANCA-associated vasculitis. https://core.ac.uk/download/553782492.pdf (accessed on 17th June 2025).

46. Taimen, K. (2021). The many faces of vasculitis: Diagnostic challenges and economic burden. ISBN 978-951-29-8558-6 (Print) ISBN 978-951-29-8559-3 (PDF) ISSN 0355-9483 (Print) ISSN 2343-3213 (Online) Painosalama, Turku, Finland 2021. https://core.ac.uk/download/481513323.pdf (accessed on 17th June 2025).

GOUT AND PSEUDOGOUT

8

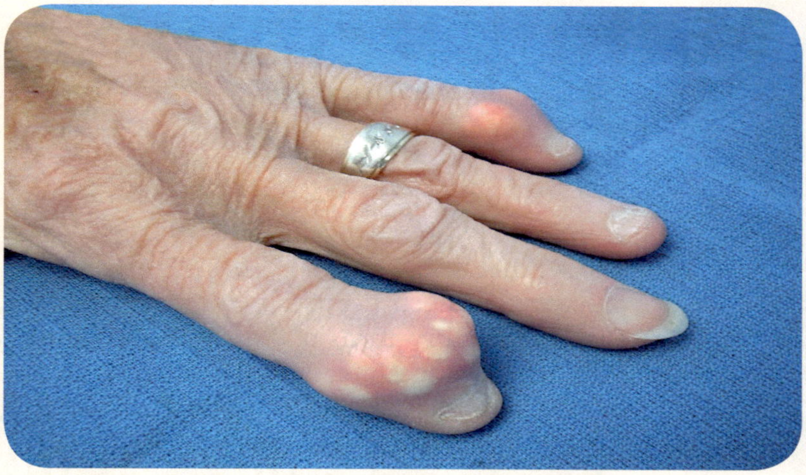

LEARNING OBJECTIVES

After studying this chapter, you will be able to:

1. Understand the pathophysiology of gout
2. Explain the pathophysiology of pseudogout
3. Discuss the diagnosis and treatment of gout
4. Focus on the diagnosis and treatment of pseudogout

Introduction

The background to the two conditions in this discussion involves an in-depth understanding of the two conditions, which are members of the broader category of conditions known as arthritis. Gout has been characterized by the presence of crystals of monosodium urate in joints, leading to intense inflammation, as explained by the induction of production of interleukin-1b (IL-1b) following phagocytosis of such crystals by macrophages (El-Sayed et al., 2023). Conversely, pseudogout is primarily a result of calcium pyrophosphate dihydrate (CPPD) crystal deposition, whose presentation clinically is identical but results from different biochemical processes. Understanding these various processes is important to allow for correct diagnosis and management, especially since arthritis may be observed in diverse forms with similar clinical manifestations, including pain and swelling of affected joints, hence the diagnostic process is challenging (Bhatt, 2014). This identification not only enhances clinical knowledge but also informs treatment strategies for each type of crystal-induced arthritis (Figure 8.1).

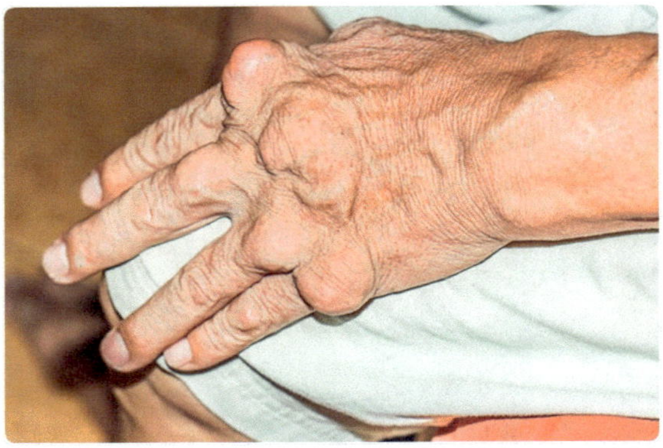

Figure 8.1. Gout and pseudogout.

Source: https://www.news-medical.net/image-handler/picture/2019/7/shutterstock_1205771854.jpg

8.1. Pathophysiology of Gout

Learning Outcome

1. Understand the mechanism of uric acid production
2. Explain the role of purines in gout
3. Focus on crystal formation in joints
4. Learn the inflammatory response to crystals
5. Identify genetic factors influencing gout
6. Explain risk factors associated with gout
7. Discuss the stages of gout development
8. Identify common sites of gout attacks
9. Know the long-term effects of untreated gout

Gout pathophysiology is actually the deposition of monosodium urate (MSU) crystals due to hyperuricemia, i.e., a surplus of uric acid over the solubility level. If the crystals deposit in joint tissues, they are recognized by the innate immune system as signals of danger, and this leads to a severe inflammatory response. This inflammatory cascade is determined mostly by interleukin-1 beta (IL-1β), a pro-inflammatory cytokine whose role has become ever more pivotal in recent years. MSU crystal activation of the NLRP3 inflammasome enhances the expression of IL-1β, enhancing inflammation and resulting in acute gout attacks manifesting with pain and swelling (Kingsbury et al., 2011). Specifically, studies have found that therapies , such as IL-1 inhibitors can effectively alleviate these symptoms, underlining the central role of IL-1β in gout pathophysiology (Busso & So, 2017). Clarification of this intricate crosstalk is significant for the development of novel therapeutic strategies.

8.1.1. Mechanism of Uric Acid Production

The synthesis of uric acid is a basic biochemical process that affects the pathophysiology of gout, an inflammatory form of arthritis associated with an elevated amount of this metabolite in blood. Uric acid is synthesized predominantly from the breakdown of purines, which are intrinsic components found in most foods and cell nucleic acids. Enzymatic reactions, with xanthine oxidase as a key enzyme, catalyze these reactions to yield hypoxanthine and eventually uric acid. When uric acid levels exceed the level of solubility, monosodium urate crystals could precipitate and induce inflammatory responses when deposited in joints. Curiously, the NLRP3 inflammasome was indicated as a key molecule of this inflammatory process, where its activation triggers IL-1β secretion, a potent proinflammatory cytokine involved in gout pathogenesis. Knowledge of such mechanisms not only elucidates the biological processes of gout but also provides an avenue for therapeutic interventions directly addressed to its impact (McCormack et al., 2009; Kingsbury et al., 2011) (Figure 8.2).

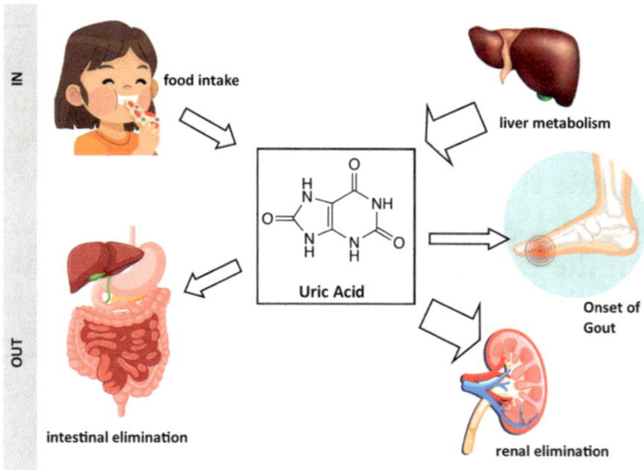

Figure 8.2. Uric acid production is a crucial biochemical process that influences the pathophysiology of gout, a form of inflammatory arthritis marked by elevated levels of this metabolite in the bloodstream.

Source: https://www.mdpi.com/applmicrobiol/applmicrobiol-04-00057/article_deploy/html/images/applmicrobiol-04-00057-g001-550.jpg.

8.1.2. Role of Purines in Gout

The role of purines in the pathophysiology of gout is central since their metabolism determines the body content of uric acid directly. Purines are a group of naturally occurring compounds present in a variety of foods and are metabolized through enzymatic breakdown by xanthine oxidase to the end product, uric acid. Excess uric acid, or hyperuricemia, can also result in the formation of monosodium urate crystals in the joints, which cause inflammation and intense pain characteristic of acute gout attacks. The effect of such acute attacks is profound, with untreated conditions being the cause of chronic arthritis and potential cardiovascular complications, making proper management inevitable. Current therapies are aimed at the inhibition of xanthine oxidase activity to decrease uric acid production and crystal formation and inflammatory modulation by agents that enhance phosphatase activity, which affects inflammation signaling pathways in macrophages (ElSayed, 2023). Because of the interdependence between purines, uric acid, and gout, both diet and drug treatments remain required for effective clinical outcomes (Tikly & Makan, 2013).

8.1.3. Crystal Formation in Joints

Crystal formation in the joints is a common aspect of gout and pseudogout, where the presence of monosodium urate (MSU) and calcium pyrophosphate dihydrate (CPPD) crystals, respectively, leads to significant inflammatory responses. In gout, deposition of MSU crystals triggers acute inflammation through the activation of resident macrophages in the synovium, resulting in the release of interleukin-1b (IL-1b) and other inflammatory mediators, which induce extreme pain and inflammation in the affected joints (El-Sayed et al., 2023).

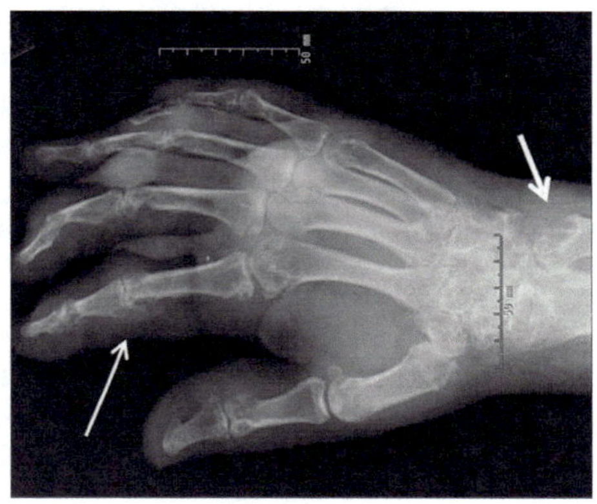

Figure 8.3. The formation of crystals in joints is a central aspect of both gout and pseudogout, where the presence of monosodium urate (MSU) and calcium pyrophosphate dihydrate (CPPD) crystals, respectively, leads to significant inflammatory responses.

Source: https://www.clevelandclinicmeded.com/medicalpubs/diseasemanagement/rheumatology/gout-and-pseudogout/images/figure-5.jpg.

Pseudogout is also linked with CPPD crystal deposition, which also elicits an inflammatory response; the pathways, however, differ in that they do not predominantly involve the same pathway as for MSU crystals (Cronstein et al., 2006). Determination of the specific pathogenic pathways for the formation of crystals and the subsequent inflammation is critical to the construction of effective therapeutic strategies for the relief of these debilitating conditions (Figure 8.3).

8.1.4. Inflammatory Response to Crystals

The inflammatory response to crystals, the hallmark of gout and pseudogout, represents a complex interaction between microcrystals and the endogenous innate immune system. The crystals, such as monosodium urate in gout and calcium pyrophosphate in pseudogout, serve as danger signals to activate inflammatory cascades through inflammasome-dependent and -independent pathways. It is distinguished by the direct interaction between microcrystals and rheumatological cells, leading to the activation of pro-inflammatory mediators, prominently interleukin-1 beta (IL-1β), which has a pivotal function in sustaining pain and inflammation (Busso & So, 2017). IL-1 inhibitor treatment, for instance, anakinra, has been noted to reduce symptoms dramatically in patients with crystal-induced arthritis, with a superior response in gouty patients compared to that in crowned dens syndrome with pseudogout (Aouba et al., 2015). Thus, the elucidation of these mechanisms not only accounts for the pathogenesis of these conditions but also directs therapy in a specific way.

8.1.5. Genetic Factors Influencing Gout

Gout, a multifactorial inflammatory arthritis, is genetically predisposed to be highly influenced by determinants that lead to susceptibility for hyperuricemia—the primary cause for gouty attacks. Genetic factors play a key role in regulating the levels of uric acid, whereby some gene variants affect urate excretion by the kidneys and urate absorption from the intestine. For instance, gene polymorphisms that encode for urate transporters can contribute to the risk of acquiring gout by modifying urate clearance from the circulation. The genetic component is particularly crucial when taking into account the way gout affects various environmental factors, such as diet and lifestyle. Moreover, the intricate interaction of gout with other arthropathies emphasizes the significance of genetic research, through which abnormal immune responses in conditions like rheumatoid arthritis are likely to complicate disease processes further. As gout is often characterized by inflammation of joints, all these genetic foundations further elucidate the pathophysiological processes that accompany crystal-induced arthropathies (Bhatt, 2014) (Figure 8.4).

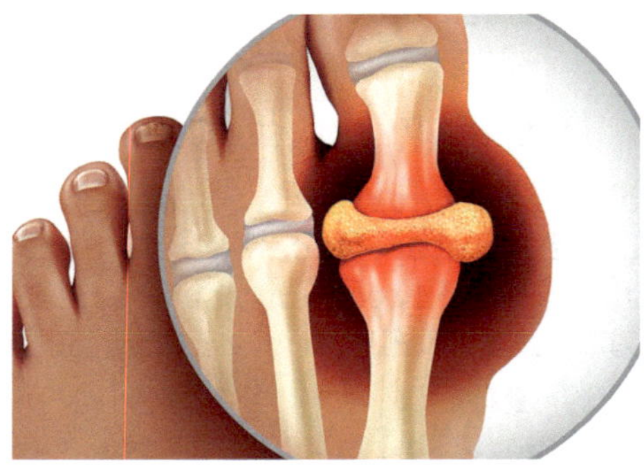

Figure 8.4. Gout, a complex form of inflammatory arthritis, is significantly influenced by genetic factors that predispose individuals to hyperuricemia—the primary cause of gouty attacks.

Source: https://www.hss.edu/globalassets/images/conditions/gout-in-depth-1200x628.jpg.

8.1.6. Risk Factors associated with Gout

Gout, a complex inflammatory arthritis, is driven by several intertwined risk factors that result in the deposition of urate crystals in the joint. One key risk factor is hyperuricemia which may be caused by both enhanced formation and impaired elimination of uric acid. Eating habits, i.e., high consumption of purine-rich foods, such as red meat and seafood, also exacerbate this condition. In addition, lifestyle problems like obesity and alcohol intake have been increasingly associated with high uric acid levels. New evidence also points to the correlation between chronic diseases, like HIV, and gout, which presents differential diagnostic challenges of a distinctive character in arthritic patients with joint pain, as seen in cases of pseudogout with HIV (Id et al., 2010; Wu et al., 2016). Thus, understanding these intricate risk factors is essential for effective prevention and management in gout and other related disorders.

8.1.7. Stages of Gout Development

The path of gout generally occurs in a chain of distinct steps, each characterized by some physiological changes and clinical manifestations. The process starts with an acute episode during which there exists hyperuricemia in the form of high uric acid content in the blood that leads to the formation of monosodium urate crystals. As the condition advances, these crystals can have an inflammatory effect and trigger acute episodes of gout that are commonly associated with intense joint inflammation and pain, usually affecting the great toe. If left untreated, the acute attacks may transfer to intercritical periods, during which patients experience intervals of being free from symptoms, only to have flare-up episodes once again. Fast disease progression may cause the formation of tophi, which are the tissue deposits of urate crystals, and show a chronic stage of the condition. It is crucial to understand these phases for proper management and prevention in patients with gout (Diekhoff et al., 2020; Pineda et al., 2024) (Figure 8.5).

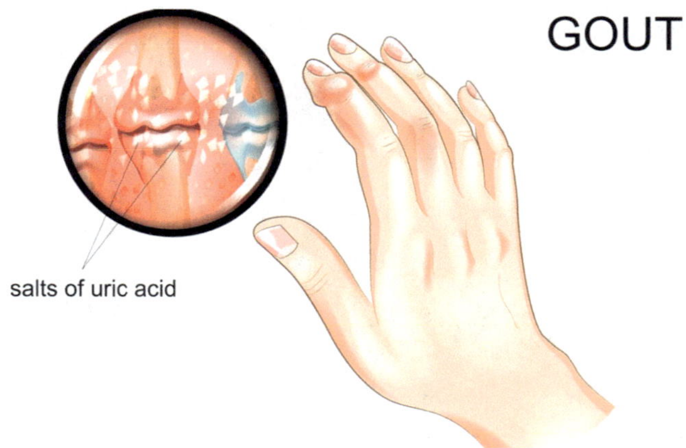

Figure 8.5. The progression of gout typically unfolds in a series of distinct stages, each characterized by specific physiological changes and clinical manifestations.

Source: https://www.pharmacyplanet.com/media/wysiwyg/understanding-the-different-stages-of-gout.JPG.

8.1.8. Common Sites of Gout Attacks

Gout is characterized by the deposition of monosodium urate crystals in the joints and tissues, leading to the acute onset of intense pain and inflammation. The most common site of attacks of gout is the first metatarsophalangeal joint, better known as the big toe, whose symptoms typically manifest as swelling, redness, and immobilizing pain, more commonly at night. Other frequently involved sites are the ankles, knees, and elbows, with swelling sometimes extending to the midfoot and wrists. The anatomical predisposition of these joints may be explained in terms of decreased temperatures and diminished synovial fluid that allow for crystallization and the consequent inflammatory reactions (Bhatt, 2014). Such attacks not only impair mobility but also presage the inherent metabolic derangements of hyperuricemia, requiring sustained management regimens to modulate threats for subsequent flare (Hsieh et al., 2011).

8.1.9. Long-term Effects of Untreated Gout

The ultimate outcome of neglected gout can be extremely disabling and lead to large morbidity and compromised quality of life among patients. Neglected chronic gout often progresses to repeated bouts of acute attacks, which, if continued, will further develop into chronic gouty arthritis with joint destruction and severe disability. As the disease progresses, monosodium urate crystal deposition can result in tophaceous formation, which is painful and causes eventual permanent damage to joints. Curiously, gout has even been characterized as an independent risk factor for cardiovascular disease, contributing to the overall health risk of the disease (Tikly & Makan, 2013). Further, chronic hyperuricemia can predispose the patient to renal insufficiency, a complicating feature in medical management, and possibly lead to kidney damage (Dubchak & Falasca, 2010). Thus, early treatment and diagnosis would be necessary to prevent the chronic consequences of untreated gout, and active management and education of the patient would be indicated (Figure 8.6).

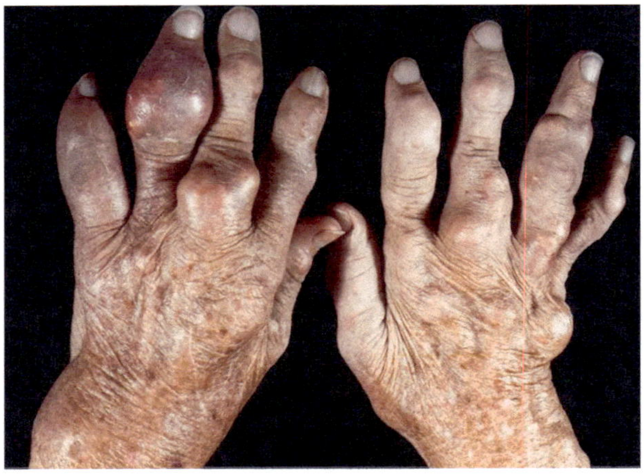

Figure 8.6. Chronic, untreated gout often results in recurrent acute attacks, which, if persistent, may progress to chronic gouty arthritis characterized by joint deformities and severe disability.

Source: https://gouteducation.org/wp-content/uploads/2021/11/very-disfigured-hands-gout-e1635800317852.webp.

Test Your Knowledge

1. What immune cells are activated in an acute gout flare?
2. How does temperature affect urate crystal precipitation in joints?

8.2. Pathophysiology of Pseudogout

Learning Outcome

1. Understand the mechanism of calcium pyrophosphate dihydrate (CPPD) crystal formation
2. Explain the role of calcium metabolism in pseudogout
3. Describe the inflammatory response to CPPD crystals
4. Focus on genetic predisposition to pseudogout
5. Risk factors associated with pseudogout
6. Identify common sites of pseudogout attacks
7. Define stages of pseudogout development
8. Know the differences in symptoms compared to gout
9. Explain the long-term effects of untreated pseudogout

The pathophysiology of pseudogout, characterized primarily by the presence of CPPD crystals in the joints, shares and differs from that of its more fearsome cousin, gout. Whereas the latter is caused by the deposition of monosodium urate crystals secondary to hyperuricemia, pseudogout is a consequence of a change in calcium and phosphate metabolism, typically related to aging and other metabolic disturbances. Research indicates that CPPD crystal deposition triggers inflammatory responses in the synovial fluid, resulting in inflamed and painful joints as well as swelling, as with the activation mechanism in gout, where interleukin-1β is central (El-Sayed et al., 2023). Unlike with gout, the inflammation during pseudogout may have the potential to be of longer duration due to the more complex interaction of inflammatory pathways as well as chondrocyte-derived factors. This divergent mechanism emphasizes the necessity of particular therapeutic approaches in managing the two diseases.

8.2.1. Mechanism of Calcium Pyrophosphate Dihydrate (CPPD) Crystal Formation

Calcium pyrophosphate dihydrate (CPPD) crystal development is a complex biochemical process that focuses on the cross-talk between metabolic state and mineral precipitation. Supersaturation of the pyrophosphate and calcium ions in synovial fluid is essential before nucleation of the crystals.

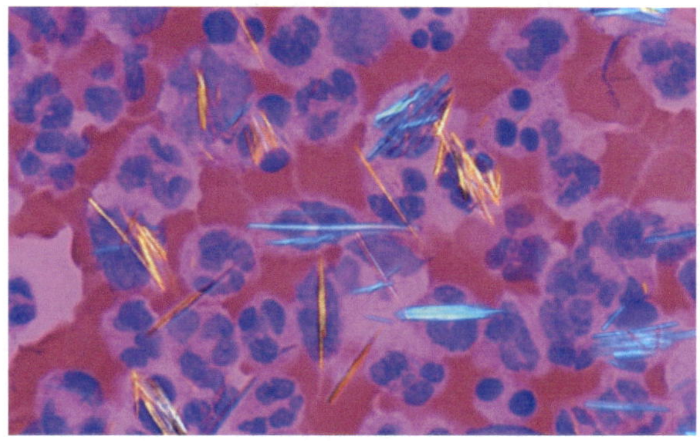

Figure 8.7. The formation of calcium pyrophosphate dihydrate (CPPD) crystals is a complex biochemical process that highlights the interplay between metabolic conditions and mineral deposition.

Source: https://orthopaedia.com/wp-content/uploads/2023/10/ea428521-cedb-4620-956b-1e42af46e4fa-1657247202403.png.

The crystals develop in joints and tendons, typically causing inflammation characteristic of pseudogout. The presence of these crystals triggers a strong immune response, as they cause the resident macrophages to lead to synovial tissue hyperplasia and inflammation. CPPD crystals and basic calcium phosphate crystals, through studies, have been demonstrated to enhance the survival of macrophages and induce DNA synthesis, leading to the tissue hyperplasia that typifies affected joints (Hamilton et al., 2001). Furthermore, bone remodeling cycling and bone marker release attendant on such cycling are critical to the detection of the conditions predisposing to CPPD crystal deposition. This intricate multicfactorial process is a testament to the delicate balance between metabolic derangement and crystal-induced arthropathies (Figure 8.7).

8.2.2. Role of Calcium Metabolism in Pseudogout

Calcium metabolism is a key component in the pathogenesis of pseudogout, a condition that is caused by the deposition of calcium pyrophosphate dihydrate crystals within joints. The disease, also known as calcium pyrophosphate crystal deposition disease (CPPD), occurs when there is disruption of the balance between body calcium and phosphorus homeostasis. Calcium metabolism can be influenced by factors, such as age, hormonal changes, and other metabolic disorders, result in the eventual crystalline deposition in the synovial fluid. The significance of ultrasound and other hi-tech imaging in CPPD diagnosis has been highlighted by recent literature claiming that ultrasound is established to be more sensitive than conventional radiography (Wu et al., 2016). Also, studies on bone markers emphasize the relationship between calcium metabolism and joint health, suggesting that distorted levels may result in the onset and severity of pseudogout. It is vital to comprehend the metabolic processes for optimal management of treated patients.

8.2.3. Inflammatory Response to CPPD Crystals

Inflammatory response to calcium pyrophosphate dihydrate (CPPD) crystals is a key characteristic of pseudogout, recapitulating pathophysiologic mechanisms of gout with monosodium urate crystals. CPPD crystals deposited in the joint provoke a virulent immune response characterized by synovial inflammation that is predominantly mediated by macrophages. These immune cells undergo enhanced survival and proliferation in the presence of CPPD crystals, resulting in synovial hyperplasia, which is a feature of chronic inflammatory arthritis. CPPD crystals have been shown to cause macrophage survival and DNA synthesis, thereby enhancing inflammation and tissue damage (Hamilton et al., 2001). While IL-1β is the hub of the inflammatory cascade of gout, data also indicate its involvement in CPPD-associated inflammation, with a likelihood of shared pathways in the treatment of these crystal-induced arthropathies (Kingsbury et al., 2011). Elucidation of these mechanisms is central to the development of effective therapeutic interventions for patients suffering from pseudogout (Figure 8.8).

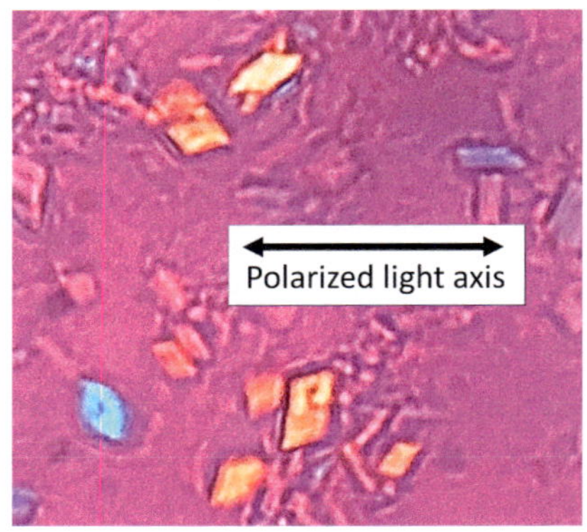

Figure 8.8. The inflammatory response to calcium pyrophosphate dihydrate (CPPD) crystals is a critical aspect of pseudogout, mirroring the pathophysiological mechanisms observed in gout with monosodium urate crystals.

Source: https://upload.wikimedia.org/wikipedia/commons/f/fc/Birefringence_microscopy_of_pseudogout%2C_annotated.jpg.

8.2.4. Genetic Predisposition to Pseudogout

The genetic predisposition to pseudogout, driven primarily by the deposition of calcium pyrophosphate dihydrate crystals in joints, serves to emphasize one of the major areas of study within the big picture of crystal arthropathies. It has been demonstrated that there are certain genetic predispositions that may lead a patient to chondrocalcinosis, an illness closely related to pseudogout. The familial pattern of pseudogout, for instance, suggests a subliminal hereditary component warranting study. After thorough examination, it has been found that age, decreased body mass index, and joint-specific osteoarthritis are also some of the factors associated with such crystal formation (Abhishek et al., 2012). Besides, the association between metabolic syndrome and the systemic predisposition towards such arthropathies proves the multifactorial nature of pseudogout (Dubchak & Falasca, 2010). Elucidation of such genetic bases can offer a guide toward prevention and management strategies, offering a route to more personalized therapeutic interventions for individuals with this painful condition.

8.2.5. Risk Factors Associated with Pseudogout

The onset of pseudogout, which is an inflammatory arthritis, is largely related to several risk factors that can initiate exposure to the condition. The influence of age should be especially considered because the occurrence of pseudogout increases significantly in older individuals, particularly those over the age of 60. Genetically, susceptibility can also be exacerbated, particularly in individuals with a history of chronic arthropathies in their family. The presence of metabolic disorders, such as hyperparathyroidism or those conditions responsible for an excess level of calcium pyrophosphate dihydrate (CPPD) crystals, is also a relevant factor. Joint trauma, hemochromatosis, and hypothyroidism are also known to be other reasons for this condition. Current advances in identifying the concentration of bone markers in synovial fluid and serum samples highlight the etiological ambiguity of pseudogouts and its relationship with systemic processes, calling for early diagnosis and treatment (Cronstein et al., 2006) (Figure 8.9).

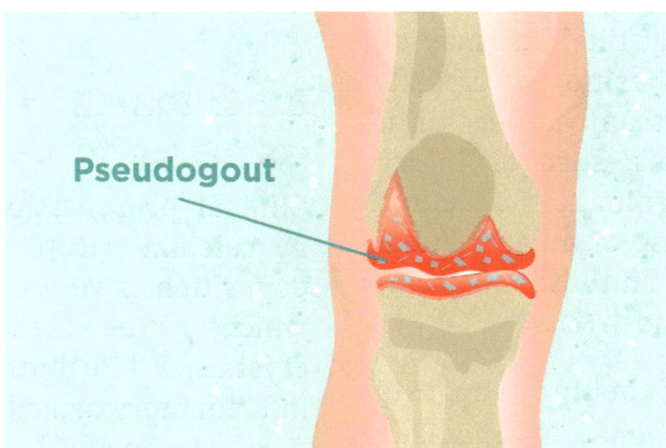

Figure 8.9. The emergence of pseudogout, a form of inflammatory arthritis, is closely linked to various risk factors that can predispose individuals to the condition.

Source: https://creakyjoints.org/wp-content/uploads/2019/02/0219_Pseudogout.jpg.

8.2.6. Common Sites of Pseudogout Attacks

Pseudogout, or calcium pyrophosphate dihydrate (CPPD) crystal deposition disease, typically presents in specific joint sites and produces marked pain and inflammation. The regions most commonly involved are the knees, wrists, and hips, where CPPD crystals deposit and produce sudden attacks of swelling and pain. Unlike gout, which has a dominant impact on the big toe, pseudogout has a tendency to present in acute attacks that may be equivalent to other forms of arthritis. Pseudogout results in joint stiffness and limited mobility, particularly impacting the daily life of individuals. Notably, the anatomical site of pseudogout needs to be identified as the disease in its overlapping presentation is analogous to other arthritic diseases with inflammatory manifestations typically observed in conditions documented in research-based literature on gout and related conditions (Kingsbury et al., 2011; Bhatt, 2014). Thus, proper diagnosis and treatment are instrumental in reducing pain and preserving joint function in patients with the condition.

8.2.7. Stages of Pseudogout Development

The pathogenesis of pseudogout, or calcium pyrophosphate dihydrate (CPPD) crystal deposition disease, follows sequential steps that outline its heterogeneity and problematic nature of diagnosis. Initially, the body may be asymptomatic with the deposition of crystals in joint cartilage, without any notice, until precipitating circumstances, such as injury or surgery, trigger an inflammatory reaction. With the onset of this phase of inflammation, patients develop a sudden and disabling joint pain involving the knees and wrists.

The pathophysiology behind suggests that the inflammatory response is organized by cytokines involved in those of gout, but specifically highlights interleukin-1β as mediating inflammation (Kingsbury et al., 2011). While pseudogout may produce high morbidity, gaps exist in what is known concerning its psychosocial impact on the patient, illustrated in the developing literature concerning CPPD and its broader background concerning the effect on quality of life (Pineda et al., 2024). It is important to recognize these phases for early intervention and management measures (Figure 8.10).

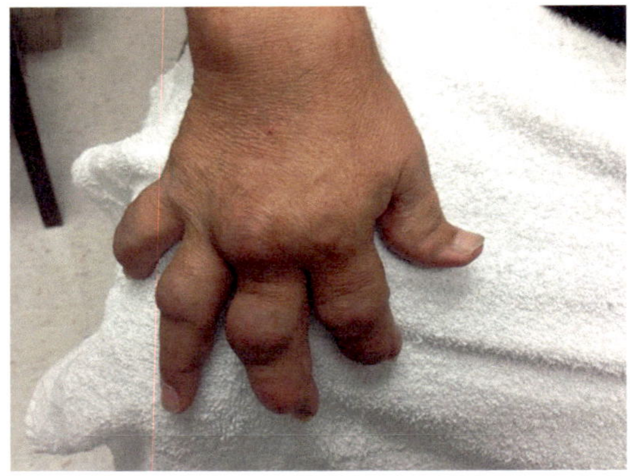

Figure 8.10. The body may exhibit asymptomatic crystal deposition in joint cartilage, often unnoticed until precipitating factors, such as trauma or surgery, trigger an inflammatory response.

Source: https://www.clevelandclinicmeded.com/medicalpubs/diseasemanagement/rheumatology/gout-and-pseudogout/images/figure-1a.jpg.

8.2.8. Differences in Symptoms compared to Gout

Clinical presentation of pseudogout caused by calcium pyrophosphate dihydrate crystal deposition is very different from that of gout, which is preeminent with monosodium urate crystals. While both illnesses have an acute inflammatory arthritis with sudden and severe pain, pseudogout symptomology is more often in larger joints, particularly the knee, as compared to more frequent involvement of metatarsophalangeal joints in gout. In addition, pseudogout attacks will occur infrequently but persist longer than the intermittent gout flares, which are episodically sharp. Importantly, the inflammatory mechanisms behind these conditions also differ; while interleukin-1β plays a central role in gout (explaining why IL-1 inhibitors are effective) (Busso & So, 2017), inflammation in pseudogout may result from other mechanisms, e.g., differences in collagen densities in joint structures (Diekhoff et al., 2020). These symptom and mechanism differences are absolutely vital for accurate diagnosis and treatment of these crystal-induced arthropathies.

8.2.9. Long-term Effects of Untreated Pseudogout

Untreated pseudogout, which is the deposition of calcium pyrophosphate dihydrate crystals within joints, can have many long-term effects that significantly impact the quality of life in a patient. Chronic inflammation within the joints can ultimately lead to persistent pain, stiffness, and reduced mobility, thus leading to functional impairment and an increased risk of falls and fractures in older people. In the course of time, habitual acute attacks may lead to joint damage, worsening osteoarthritis, and making some people unable to carry out everyday activities by themselves. In addition, the systemic effects of untreated pseudogout may correlate with metabolic abnormalities, which may compound the current burden of non-communicable diseases, as noted in the literature on the double burden of health conditions experienced worldwide (Burney et al., 2014). Mitigation of these long-term consequences is crucial because prevention strategies and therapies are available but underused, prompting greater awareness and education on the condition (Dubchak & Falasca, 2010) (Figure 8.11).

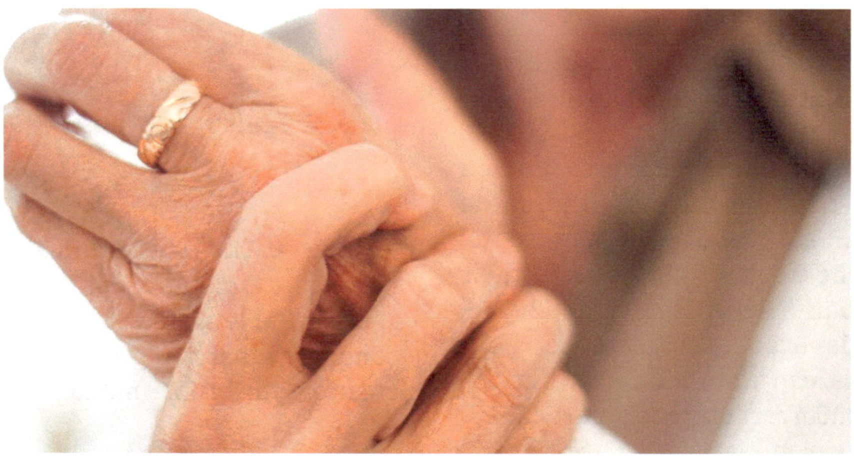

Figure 8.11. Chronic joint inflammation may result in persistent pain, stiffness, and reduced mobility, leading to functional impairments and potentially increasing the risk of falls and fractures in older adults.

Source: https://media.post.rvohealth.io/wp-content/uploads/2020/09/10419-Pseudogout_1200x628-facebook-1200x628.jpg.

Test Your Knowledge

1. What role do aging and cartilage degeneration play in pseudogout?
2. How do CPPD crystals activate the innate immune system?

8.3. Diagnosis and Treatment of Gout

Learning Outcome

1. Identify clinical symptoms and physical examination
2. Explain laboratory tests for uric acid levels
3. Focus on imaging techniques for diagnosis
4. Learn acute treatment options for gout attacks
5. Describe long-term management strategies
6. Focus on dietary modifications and lifestyle changes
7. Discuss medications used in gout treatment
8. Know role of patient education in management
9. Discuss importance of regular follow-up

The clinical diagnosis of gout depends primarily on clinical evaluation, hyperuricemia, and presence of monosodium urate crystals in synovial fluid. Even if the typical presentation is acute monoarticular arthritis, differential diagnoses , such as pseudogout and septic arthritis should be kept in mind due to their imitative symptoms (Aderholdt et al., 2021). Differentiation is exact; for instance, both forms of arthritis can look identical, but the consequences of incorrect diagnosis, particularly where there is a root infection, are severe. Treatment approaches typically include non-steroidal anti-inflammatory drugs (NSAIDs), colchicine, or corticosteroids during acute flares but, for treatment failure, new agents , such as anakinra, proven effective in the management of intricate presentations of crystal-induced arthritis, need to be considered too (Aouba et al., 2015). Accurate knowledge of diagnosis and treatment approaches is hence crucial for effective management of gout, avoiding complications, and patient outcomes.

8.3.1. Clinical Symptoms and Physical Examination

Physical examination and presentation of gout and pseudogout are remarkably similar but are two distinct disorders that must be distinguished with great caution to be treated appropriately. Both have acute inflammation of the joint in the form of swelling, redness, and pain in the majority of cases except in the big toe in gout and larger joints , such as the knee in pseudogout. Physical examination may provide warmth and tenderness over the involved joint and limited range of motion.

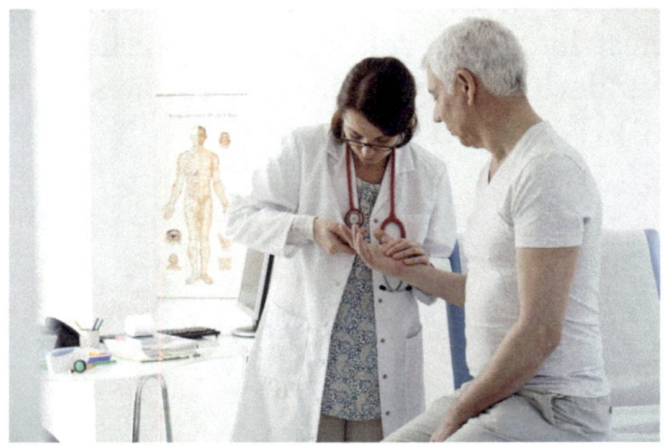

Figure 8.12. The clinical symptoms and physical examination of gout and pseudogout share notable similarities, yet they are distinct conditions requiring careful differentiation to ensure appropriate management.

Source: https://www.verywellhealth.com/thmb/SrxKu1hZU0cmZUTVOMKnF5PPy04=/1500x0/filters:no_upscale():max_bytes(150000):strip_icc()/GettyImages-705006745-57090941387d4095a1b057334f2abfbf.jpg.

Detailed assessment that may include imaging studies or examination of synovial fluid is typically employed by physicians to diagnose these conditions accurately. The advent of musculoskeletal ultrasound (MSUS) has also maximized this diagnostic workup by allowing visualization of joint effusion or crystal deposition, which is indicative of these arthritic conditions (Hsieh et al., 2011). Given that they have overlapping presentations, proper identification of the pathologic process is crucial to avoid mismanagement (Bhatt, 2014) (Figure 8.12).

8.3.2. Laboratory Tests for Uric Acid Levels

The determination of uric acid levels through laboratory tests is the core of diagnosing and treating gout and pseudogout. Hyperuricemia, which is elevated levels of uric acid, is a notable feature of gout and normally leads to monosodium urate crystal deposition in the connective tissue, termed tophi, that can develop years after the initial presentation of the condition (Sendrea et al., 2020). Laboratory examinations not only confirm the phenomenon of hyperuricemia but also allow for an integral assessment of a patient's metabolic status, facilitating correct clinical decisions on treatment and lifestyle adjustment. Moreover, as is indicated by the latest evidence, coordination among laboratory activities is the basis for an improvement in diagnostic accuracy in the case of musculoskeletal conditions like gout and pseudogout (Jokic et al., 2020). Thus, meticulous laboratory testing and uric acid level analysis remain indispensable in optimizing patient care and alleviating the disabling effects of these diseases.

8.3.3. Imaging Techniques for Diagnosis

Both gout and pseudogout diagnosis rely heavily on advanced imaging modalities that enhance the detection capacity compared to older techniques. While older crystal analysis and radiography remain the mainstays, current literature indicates that ultrasonography (U/S) and dual-energy computed tomography (DECT) are rapidly becoming indispensable tools in the field. U/S is more sensitive, over 80%, in identifying calcium pyrophosphate crystals in peripheral joints and therefore superior to radiographic imaging (Wu et al., 2016). Furthermore, DECT has been encouraging, although it has been less studied in the case of pseudogout compared to that in gout, where abundant literature exists (Wu et al., 2016). In addition, bone marker (BM) synovial fluid and serum analysis is another imaging parameter, throwing light into the pathophysiological alterations underlying the arthropathies , such as gout and pseudogout. As an aggregate, these imaging modalities provide more accurate diagnoses, maximally optimizing patient management strategies to these complex diseases (Figure 8.13).

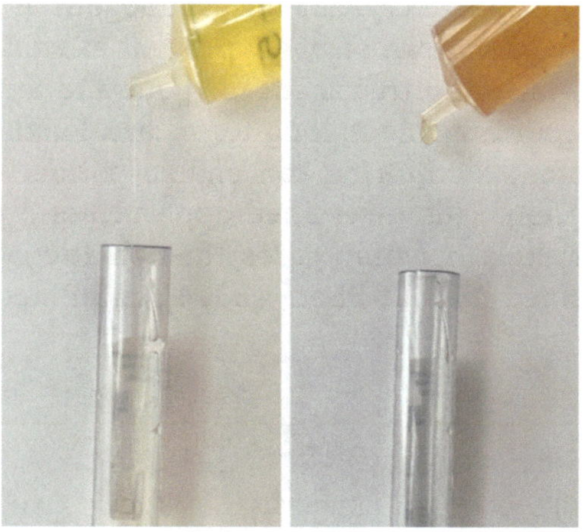

Figure 8.13. The analysis of bone markers (BMs) in synovial fluid and serum represents another dimension in imaging diagnostics, providing insights into the underlying pathophysiology of arthropathies , such as gout and pseudogout .

Source: https://ars.els-cdn.com/content/image/1-s2.0-S1521694223000347-gr4.jpg.

8.3.4. Acute Treatment Options for Gout Attacks

The management of gouty attacks involves a variety of useful treatments for reducing inflammation and pain. Initial management typically includes nonsteroidal anti-inflammatory drugs (NSAIDs), which are well known to treat promptly acute attack and proved as effective as indomethacin, although no randomized, placebo-controlled trials exist for these drugs. For poorly responding or side effect-prone patients treated with NSAIDs, glucocorticosteroids are alternatively administered systemically or intra-articularly with impressive relief of inflammation (Aouba et al., 2015). Colchicine is another second-line effective agent with excellent efficacy if administered early in an attack but is at the cost of gastrointestinal side effects (Aouba et al., 2015). More recent work has revealed anakinra, a novel interleukin-1 inhibitor, which has been reported to relieve rapidly within days in patients with a failure to respond to standard treatment (Aouba et al., 2015). Every treatment offers advantages, emphasizing the need for personalized treatment regimens for optimal management of acute gout.

8.3.5. Long-term Management Strategies

Effective long-term care of gout and pseudogout is essential to alleviate the burden on the patients from these conditions. Central to these care strategies is dietary change, including modification of food to counteract reduced levels of uric acid in the blood for the management of gout and calcium pyrophosphate crystals for pseudogout. A low-purine diet, supplemented by hydration and weight management, can strongly prevent exacerbations. Pharmacologic management, such as the use of urate-lowering treatment for gout and anti-inflammatory medications for pseudogout, also plays an important role in long-term care. Furthermore, ongoing education about disease education and symptom monitoring can enable patients to become active participants in managing their own condition. This diversified approach is crucial, for the management of these arthritides induced by crystals not only cures the somatic symptoms but addresses psychosocial issues as well, as explained in both Bhatt, (2014) and Pineda et al., (2024) (Figure 8.14).

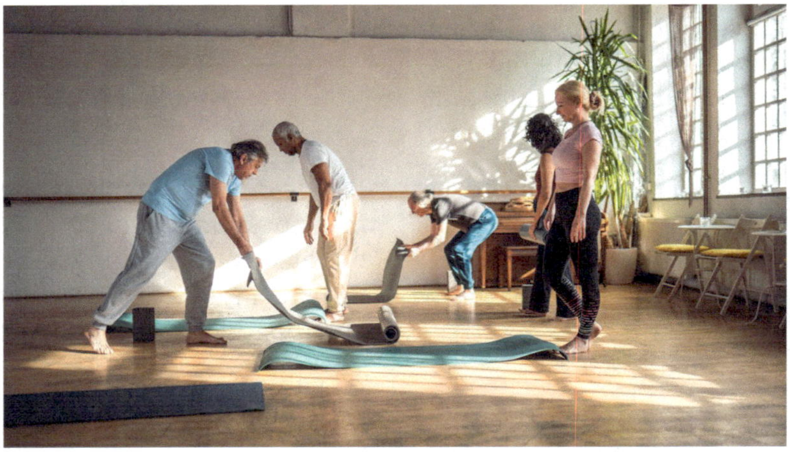

Figure 8.14. Effective long-term management strategies for gout and pseudogout are essential to alleviate the burden these conditions impose on patients' quality of life.

Source: https://media.post.rvohealth.io/wp-content/uploads/2024/02/senior-group-mixed-race-after-yoga-class-1296x728-header.jpg.

8.3.6. Dietary Modifications and Lifestyle Changes

Gout and pseudogout management relies mostly on successful lifestyle and dietary changes, which are critical in preventing symptoms and reducing exacerbations. Because food factors , such as hyperfructose consumption, obesity, and alcohol consumption have been proven to cause the rising prevalence of gout in the modern population, these factors need to be managed by the patients (Dubchak & Falasca, 2010). Adding a diet rich in vegetables, whole grains, and low-fat dairy will reduce uric acid levels, which is important since gout is characterized by hyperuricemia (Abhishek et al., 2017). Maintenance of a healthy weight through regular exercise also reduces the risk of gout attacks and overall health, and, therefore, enhances quality of life in patients. These types of lifestyle changes, when augmented by appropriate medical therapies, form an effective regimen to manage and even cure gout, along with controlling its risk determinants.

8.3.7. Medications used in Gout Treatment

Effective management of gout is largely a matter of employing various drugs that alleviate pain during an attack and prevent future attacks. NSAIDs are most commonly the first line of therapy, inducing relief from severe pain and inflammation immediately by inhibiting the cyclooxygenase enzymes. Colchicine is another key drug that disrupts the inflammatory process by acting on neutrophils, thereby muting symptoms of acute gout attacks. For long-term management, urate-lowering therapy , such as allopurinol or febuxostat is usually prescribed to maintain serum urate in the therapeutic range, preventing repeated attacks and potential joint damage. However, the importance of improved patient education for these medications has been brought into focus in a new study, where knowledge gaps were reportedly hampering adequate self-management of the condition (Russell, 2020). As the incidence of gout increases in different populations, it is important to take medication adherence seriously to enhance patient outcomes and quality of life (Burney et al., 2014) (Figure 8.15).

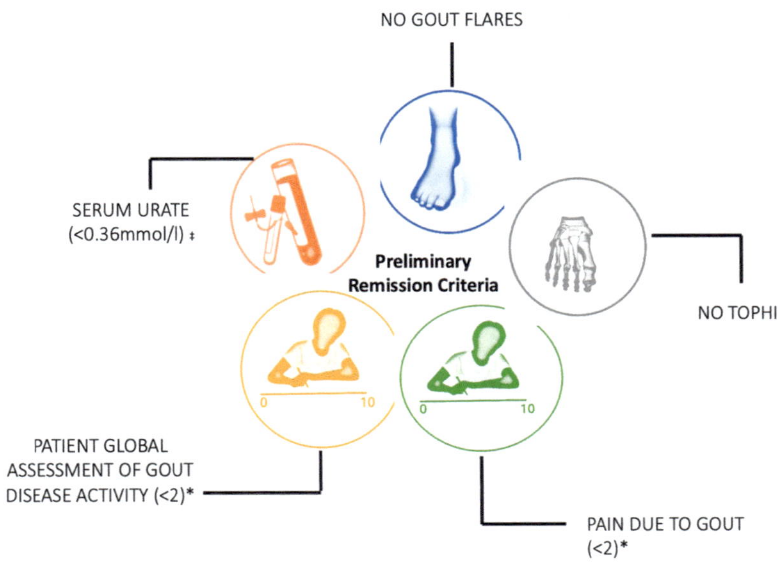

Figure 8.15. For long-term management, urate-lowering therapy , such as allopurinol or febuxostat is often prescribed to maintain serum urate levels within the target range, preventing future episodes and potential joint damage.

Source: https://www.mdpi.com/pharmaceuticals/pharmaceuticals-16-00779/article_deploy/html/images/pharmaceuticals-16-00779-g001.png.

8.3.8. Role of Patient Education in Management

Effective patient education is crucial in the management of gout and pseudogout because it allows patients to understand their conditions and engage in self-management strategies. Comprehensive educational programs can educate patients about the pathological processes involved in these crystal-induced arthropathies, including uric acid deposition in gout and calcium pyrophosphate crystals in pseudogout (Biskupski et al., 2024). By allowing patients to understand the link between lifestyle factors—e.g., nutrition, fluid intake, and medication adherence—and disease flare-up, patients are able to make informed choices that reduce flare-up frequency. In addition, education improves compliance with treatment regimens, including NSAIDs and colchicine therapy, which are components of symptom management and prevention of joint damage (Bhatt, 2014). Finally, informing patients empowers a collaborative mechanism for care that fosters interventionist strategies capable of significantly improving the quality of their lives and reducing the clinical load of these diseases.

8.3.9. Importance of Regular Follow-up

Regular follow-up care is critical in treating gout and pseudogout successfully, as it is a continuous dialogue between patients and healthcare professionals that guarantees treatment protocols are immediately adjusted. Regular monitoring enables healthcare professionals to identify patients at risk of recurrence of symptoms and side effects of drugs, which are equally crucial in preventing acute flare and chronic joint injury. Moreover, as indicated by the findings regarding the need for detailed patient education materials, there may be a systematic follow-up to bridge gaps in information that continually undermine effective self-management among such patients (Russell, 2020). Such interactions also align with broader public health goals, meaning that neglect of certain non-communicable diseases, like gout, can result in significant health burdens (Burney et al., 2014). Therefore, implementing a systematic follow-up protocol not only enhances the quality of patient outcomes but also increases the overall standard of care in treating such inflammatory joint diseases (Figure 8.16).

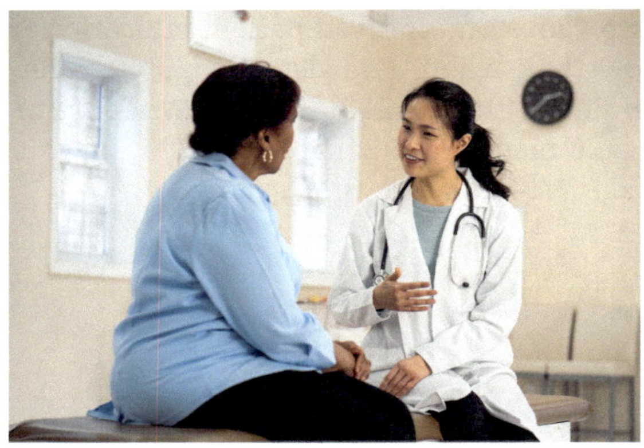

Figure 8.16. Regular follow-up care is paramount in effectively managing gout and pseudogout, as it fosters a continuous dialogue between patients and healthcare providers, ensuring timely adjustments to treatment plans.

Source: https://www.agilonhealth.com/wp-content/uploads/2023/12/iStock-1147429610-1-2-scaled.jpg.

Test Your Knowledge

1. When should imaging (e.g., X-ray, ultrasound, DECT) be used in gout evaluation?
2. What are the first-line medications for acute gout management?

8.4. Diagnosis and Treatment of Pseudogout

Learning Outcome

1. Understand clinical symptoms and physical examination
2. Focus on laboratory tests for CPPD crystals
3. Discuss imaging techniques for diagnosis
4. Explain acute treatment options for pseudogout attacks
5. Describe long-term management strategies
6. Focus on dietary modifications and lifestyle changes
7. Learn medications used in pseudogout treatment
8. Know the role of patient education in management
9. Discuss the importance of regular follow-up

Pseudogout, the deposition of calcium pyrophosphate dihydrate crystals within joints, is a significant diagnostic challenge, particularly in its differentiation from gout. Diagnosis is often based on a combination of clinical evaluation, imaging studies, and aspiration of the joint to examine synovial fluid. The presence of rhomboid-shaped crystals on polarized light microscopy is diagnostic for pseudogout, but more advanced imaging modalities can further define joint changes , such as chondrocalcinosis and subchondral cysts, such as in those with extensive joint destruction and deformities (Ng et al., 2022). The management is based on the control of acute inflammation and promotion of joint function, commonly using NSAIDs and corticosteroids. In more severe cases, when conservative measures fail, surgical intervention like replacement of joints becomes inevitable, but is impossible to achieve due to economic hardships suffered by patients (Ng et al., 2022). Ultimately, early diagnosis and tailoring the treatment are necessary in order to avoid morbidity due to this condition.

8.4.1. Clinical Symptoms and Physical Examination

The clinical presentation of gout and pseudogout is very much alike, presenting with the sudden onset of joint pain, swelling, and redness of the lower extremities. The hyperuricemia in gout leads to the deposition of urate monosodium crystals in the joints and causes sudden inflammatory response of hot red heat and burning pain, commonly occurring in the great toe. In contradistinction, pseudogout due to deposition of calcium pyrophosphate dihydrate crystals may similarly be associated with the same acute symptoms but, at times, with involvement of other joints like the wrists and knees. Physical examination helps differentiate between the two processes. A thorough assessment can identify effusion, erythema, and joint tenderness to warrant further investigation with synovial fluid analysis to identify the crystalline content of the inciting agent. High-tech diagnostic imaging, like MSUS, is helpful to see the changes and enhance clinical examination (Hsieh et al., 2011; Bhatt, 2014) (Figure 8.17).

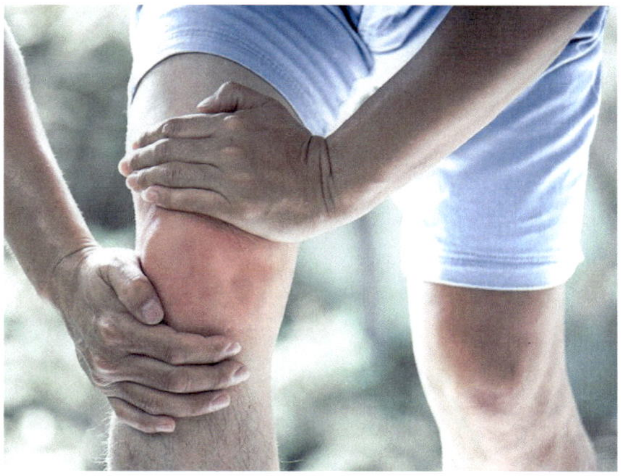

Figure 8.17. The clinical symptoms associated with gout and pseudogout share notable similarities, particularly the sudden onset of joint pain, swelling, and redness, typically affecting the lower extremities.

Source:

8.4.2. Laboratory Tests for CPPD Crystals

The diagnostic evaluation for the detection of calcium pyrophosphate dihydrate (CPPD) crystals, the etiologic agent of pseudogout, relies to a great extent on laboratory tests, primarily synovial fluid examination. It is the most significant procedure since it allows CPPD crystals to be visualized directly under polarized light microscopy to make the diagnosis. In fact, synovial fluid analysis is underutilized, but it has been demonstrated to be a valuable discriminator between forms of joint disease, for example, pseudogout and septic arthritis (Owen, 1974). It is important to realize the clinical nuance of conditions like pseudogout, for instance, in case reports where presentation is subtle and renders diagnosis challenging. For instance, a 76-year-old patient who complained of pain in his feet had a diagnostic pathway which emphasized the importance of proper examination , such as synovial fluid analysis, in distinguishing between different causes of joint inflammation (Karanjia et al., 2013). Hence, such laboratory tests are crucial in managing patients effectively.

8.4.3. Imaging Techniques for Diagnosis

Diagnosis of pseudogout and gout has evolved significantly with improvements in imaging modalities, so clinical evaluation is now important for accuracy. While the conventional crystal analysis and radiography have been the gold standards for decades, newer modalities , such as U/S and DECT are gaining popularity. Research has demonstrated that U/S is greater than 80% sensitive in the detection of calcium pyrophosphate crystals in peripheral joints, a greater rate than traditional radiographic methods (Wu et al., 2016). Further, DECT is beginning to become a possible imaging technique in the differentiation of gout and pseudogout, even as it is still relatively new to this use. The melding of these newer imaging technologies not only increases diagnostic confidence but also addresses unmet clinical needs for the management of crystal arthropathies. With ongoing research, clearly it is a necessity to further solidify these methods and promote randomized, controlled trials to enhance our diagnostic arsenal (Figure 8.18).

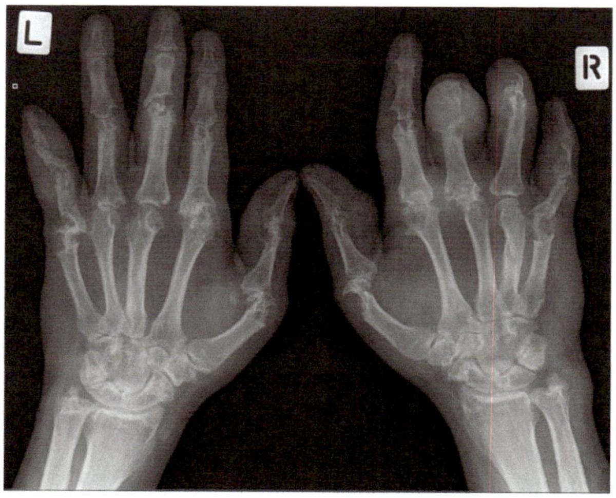

Figure 8.18. The diagnosis of gout and pseudogout has evolved significantly with advancements in imaging techniques, enhancing the accuracy of clinical assessments.

Source: https://media.springernature.com/lw685/springer-static/image/art%3A10.1186%2Far3489/MediaObjects/13075_2011_Article_3234_Fig1_HTML.jpg.

8.4.4. Acute Treatment Options for Pseudogout Attacks

Therapy during an acute attack of pseudogout is primarily with anti-inflammatory medications to suppress pain and inflammation as early as possible. NSAIDs are usually the first line of treatment since they are useful in managing the acute manifestations. If NSAIDs fail or are not indicated, corticosteroids can be administered orally or intra-articularly to suppress the inflammation early. Other studies have also explored the possibility of using interleukin-1 (IL-1) inhibitors, such as anakinra, as promising alternatives in non-responding patients. A study found that anakinra was effective for patients with pseudogout, rendering complete responses in 9 to 11 days, and thereby establishing it as a therapeutic agent when other treatments fail (Aouba et al., 2015). Moreover, IL-1 inhibitors were also promising in the management of resistant crystal-induced arthritis cases, which indicates an emerging dynamic role in pseudogout management (Kingsbury et al., 2011).

8.4.5. Long-term Management Strategies

Effective long-term treatment of gout and pseudogout is crucial to prevent recurrent pain and inflammation secondary to these conditions. A comprehensive treatment plan encompasses pharmacological treatment, lifestyle modifications, and patient education. NSAIDs and corticosteroids are typically employed to treat acute attacks; however, long-term urate-lowering therapy in the case of gout should be initiated to prevent recurrence as well as damage to joints. At the same time, food changes—, such as reducing purine intake and proper hydration, can also impact uric acid levels significantly, hence managing gout more effectively. Treatment of pseudogout is more of a matter of calcium pyrophosphate crystal regulation through similar anti-inflammatory means. Despite advancement, there remain knowledge deficits about the psychosocial impact of such conditions on patients' quality of life, and this indicates that additional research is required to further refine management protocols and improve outcomes for patients, as the literature on arthritis conditions demonstrates (Bhatt, 2014; Pineda et al., 2024) (Figure 8.19).

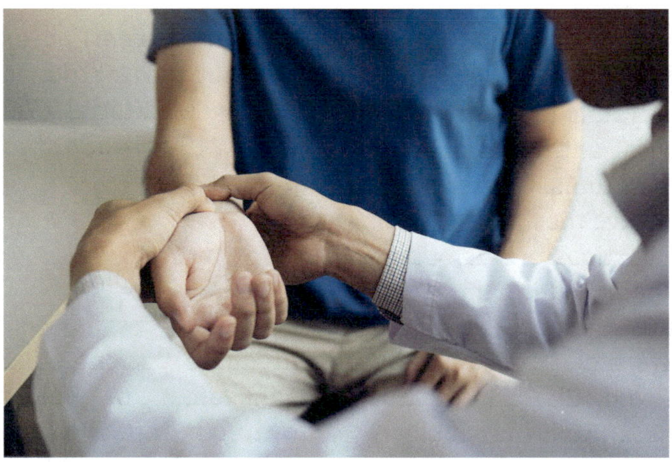

Figure 8.19. Effective long-term management strategies for gout and pseudogout are crucial to mitigate the recurring pain and inflammation associated with these conditions.

Source: https://www.verywellhealth.com/thmb/g2eQEJU4vMopulWm0uWQIaqbc7A=/1500x0/filters:no_upscale():max_bytes(150000):strip_icc()/pseudogout-GettyImages-1152834917-a7bf5a6065c947bd8a587e11e8d85308.jpg.

8.4.6. Dietary Modifications and Lifestyle Changes

Diet and lifestyle modifications are also paramount in the management of gout and pseudogout to relieve symptoms and reduce flare-ups. The increased prevalence of gout in the Western world has been attributed to diet, obesity, and alcohol consumption, highlighting the need for lifestyle interventions. Reduction of intake of purine-rich foods , such as red meat and certain seafood, can reduce serum uric acid levels, a modifiable factor in the control of attacks of gout. Fructose consumption, which is also recognized today as a modifiable risk factor, needs to be limited as it can exacerbate hyperuricemia (Abhishek et al., 2017). Along with food modifications, maintaining a healthy weight through exercise and proper hydration can significantly lower the number of gout attacks and improve joint health overall (Abhishek et al., 2017). Dietary modifications , such as these are not only beneficial in the short term for individuals with gout but also contribute to better health long term.

8.4.7. Medications used in Pseudogout Treatment

The treatment of pseudogout, with deposition of calcium pyrophosphate crystals in joints, relies heavily on the utilization of anti-inflammatory medication to manage symptoms. Conventional pharmacologic options involve the application of NSAIDs, colchicine, and corticosteroids, which are utilized to decrease pain and inflammation during the acute attack. If these standard treatments are not effective, biologic medications like anakinra are employed. Clinical practice has discovered that anakinra is particularly beneficial in those who have been insufficiently responsive to other medications; it has been effective in the treatment of pseudogout and other crystal-induced arthritides, demonstrating a safe profile with rapid resolution of symptoms (Aouba et al., 2015). In addition, recent research indicates the need for an individualized regimen of pseudogout treatment, depending on each patient's unique therapeutic reaction and comorbidities, that might require treatment with other methods (Biskupski et al., 2024) (Figure 8.20).

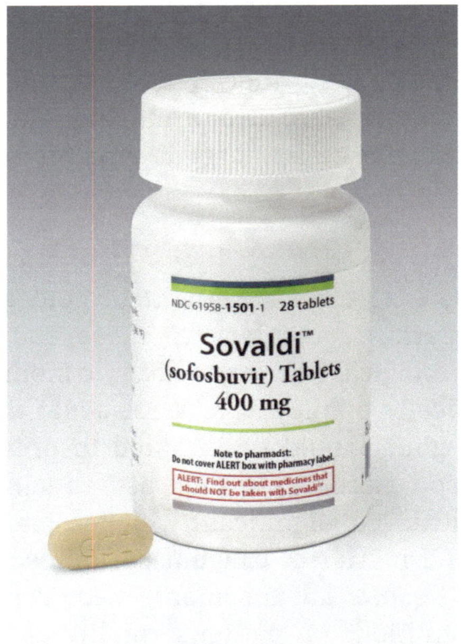

Figure 8.20. Medications used in pseudogout treatment.

Source: https://bloximages.chicago2.vip.townnews.com/tucson.com/content/tncms/assets/v3/editorial/e/c7/ec7e45ae-565b-5999-9b9b-340ec54b54db/565e2aeb6a54e.image.jpg.

8.4.8. Role of Patient Education in Management

Adequate patient education is crucial in the management of gout and pseudogout because it directly influences treatment compliance as well as disease outcomes. Patient education empowers the patient with information about his or her conditions, which encourages the physician and patient to act together and appreciate the imperative for early access to medical care. For instance, patient education on the role of dietary modification in the prevention of acute gout attacks may be able to reduce the frequency and severity of attacks. In addition, education about the distinction between gout and pseudogout, particularly how these two conditions differ in pathogenic pathways and potential comorbidities, will assist in enabling appropriate self-management measures and complication resolution, thus enhancing the quality of life for affected persons. In addition, placing particular stress on the importance of precise adherence to prescribed pharmacotherapies, including NSAIDs and corticosteroids, is of great importance in avoiding the inflammatory responses of these arthropathies and leading to better clinical results (Bhatt, 2014; Biskupski et al., 2024).

8.4.9. Importance of Regular Follow-up

Follow-up visits play a crucial role in the management of gout and pseudogout, which facilitate easy ongoing monitoring and adjustment of treatment. Both conditions, typically characterized by recurrent episodes of joint inflammation and pain, need a keen attitude for avoiding complications as well as enhancing the quality of life in affected patients. Through regular follow-ups, medical practitioners can monitor disease progression, evaluate the efficacy of treatment strategies, and control patients' problems with symptom management. Moreover, the findings of Russell (2020) emphasize that adequate information provision can empower patients to support self-management through active engagement. Because chronic conditions most often translate into sweeping lifestyle modifications, follow-up offers a framework for education and encouragement so that patients are adequately prepared to manage their diseases. Follow-up, thus, is not an empty ritual of booking appointments but a vital component of the integrated method of treating gout and pseudogout (Figure 8.21).

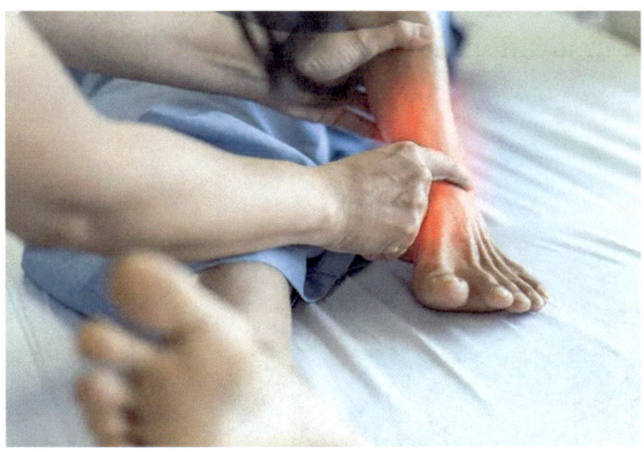

Figure 8.21. Regular follow-up appointments are paramount in the management of gout and pseudogout, as they facilitate ongoing assessment and adjustment of treatment plans.

Source: https://images.medicinenet.com/images/article/main_image/gout-foot-ankle-pain-doctor-physician-treatment.jpg?output-quality=75.

Test Your Knowledge

1. What laboratory tests help exclude secondary causes of pseudogout?
2. What is the role of synovial fluid analysis in diagnosing pseudogout?

Summary

The connection between gout and pseudogout underscores deep diagnostic and management complexities in the field of musculoskeletal disorders. Both conditions, through their characteristic deposition of crystals in joints, are capable of producing disabling manifestations and enormous morbidity, as illustrated in cases that severely impair mobility and quality of life. The intricate dynamic between the disorders, particularly in individuals with complex histories , such as those with HIV infection, highlights the importance of heightened awareness by medical practitioners (Id et al., 2010). Furthermore, the socioeconomic elements of treatment access cannot be overlooked, especially in marginalized communities with issues attaining required surgical interventions as seen in extreme cases of pseudogout (Ng et al., 2022). Lastly, an ultimate comprehension of such conditions, coupled with improved healthcare policies, is essential to enhancing patient outcomes and ensuring the availability and fairness of care among affected populations of gout and pseudogout.

The arthritides associated with crystals, such as gout and pseudogout, have a complexity that demands a coordinated evaluation of their diagnosis and treatment. Effective diagnosis begins with joint fluid analysis, an undertaking commonly complicated by the technical challenge of accurately identifying crystals in a polarized light microscope. Merging new perspectives in technologies, such as Raman spectroscopy, with traditional methods could enhance specificity for the diagnosis of such conditions and further revolutionize patient outcomes and potentially uncover new biomarkers for joint diseases (Niessink, 2024). Another study also emphasized the importance of new information value chain design for gout patients, determining essential data for effective self-management of the disease. Evidence indicated that there are knowledge gaps in patient educational resources that could impede successful disease control (Russell, 2020). Collectively, the findings underscore the imperative for technological innovation and better patient education in the successful management of gout and pseudogout.

KEY TERMS FROM THIS CHAPTER

- Anatomical predisposition
- Bone marker (BM)
- Chronic arthropathies
- Crystal formation
- Crystallization
- Diagnostic process
- Kidney damage
- Monosodium urate (MSU)
- Pathophysiology
- Rheumatological cells
- Biochemical processes
- Calcium pyrophosphate dihydrate (CPPD)
- Crystal deposition
- Crystalline
- Crystals
- Hyperuricemia
- Monosodium urate crystals
- Musculoskeletal ultrasound
- Proinflammatory cytokine
- Subsequent inflammation

Critical Thinking Questions

1. Which substance is responsible for crystal deposition in gout?

a. Calcium phosphate

b. Calcium pyrophosphate

c. Monosodium urate

d. Uric acid dihydrate

2. The most commonly affected joint in an acute gout attack is the:

a. Knee

b. Shoulder

c. First metatarsophalangeal (MTP) joint

d. Wrist

3. Which of the following crystals are seen in pseudogout?

a. Monosodium urate crystals

b. Calcium pyrophosphate dihydrate (CPPD) crystals

c. Calcium oxalate crystals

d. Cholesterol crystals

4. Gout is most often associated with which metabolic abnormality?

a. Hypocalcemia

b. Hyperuricemia

c. Hypouricemia

d. Hyperkalemia

5. Which of the following microscopic features is characteristic of gout crystals?

a. Weakly positive birefringence under polarized light

b. Rhomboid shape

c. Strongly negative birefringence and needle-shaped

d. No birefringence

Answers to Critical Thinking Questions

1. (c) 2. (c) 3. (b) 4. (b) 5. (c)

Short Answer Questions

1. What causes the overproduction or underexcretion of uric acid in gout?
2. How does monosodium urate crystal deposition trigger inflammation?
3. What is the underlying cause of calcium pyrophosphate crystal deposition?
4. How are pyrophosphate crystals formed and deposited in cartilage?
5. What are the typical clinical signs of an acute gout attack?
6. How is serum uric acid level used in the diagnosis of gout?
7. What clinical features help distinguish pseudogout from gout?
8. Which joints are most commonly affected by pseudogout?

References

1. Abhishek, A., Roddy, E., & Doherty, M. (2017). Gout - a guide for the general and acute physicians. Clinical medicine (London, England), 17(1), 54–59. https://doi.org/10.7861/clinmedicine.17-1-54(accessed on 17th June 2025).
2. Aderholdt, D., Patel, R., Schuck, J., Zucconi, M., et al. (2021). Septic arthritis with concomitant pseudogout. https://core.ac.uk/download/482133803.pdf (accessed on 17th June 2025).
3. Aouba, A., Bienvenu, B., Boue, F., Damaj, G., et al. (2015). Efficacy of anakinra for various types of crystal-induced arthritis in complex hospitalized patients: A case series and review of the literature. https://core.ac.uk/download/52192095.pdf (accessed on 17th June 2025).
4. Bhatt, S (2014) *An interactive tool for real time feedback on diagnosis and treatment plan of arthritis based on C++ programing language.* BTech thesis.(accessed on 17th June 2025).
5. Biskupski, M., Cygnarowicz, A., Hosseinnejad, N., Korotko, P., et al. (2024). A review on diagnosis and treatment approaches to calcium pyrophosphate deposition disease. https://core.ac.uk/download/636386088.pdf (accessed on 17th June 2025).
6. Burney, P. G. J., Ferri, C. P., Koob, G., Levin, K., et al. (2014). Remembering the forgotten non-communicable diseases. https://core.ac.uk/download/76995794.pdf (accessed on 17th June 2025).
7. Busso, N., & So, A. (2012). Microcrystals as DAMPs and their role in joint inflammation. Rheumatology (Oxford, England), 51(7), 1154–1160. https://doi.org/10.1093/rheumatology/ker524f (accessed on 17th June 2025).
8. Wu, Y., Chen, K., & Terkeltaub, R. (2016). Systematic review and quality analysis of emerging diagnostic measures for calcium pyrophosphate crystal deposition disease. *RMD open*, *2*(2), e000339. https://doi.org/10.1136/rmdopen-2016-000339(accessed on 17th June 2025).
9. Kingsbury, S. R., Conaghan, P. G., & McDermott, M. F. (2011). The role of the NLRP3 inflammasome in gout. *Journal of inflammation research*, *4*, 39–49. https://doi.org/10.2147/JIR.S11330 (accessed on 17th June 2025).
10. Cronstein, B. N., & Terkeltaub, R. (2006). The inflammatory process of gout and its treatment. https://core.ac.uk/download/323066745.pdf (accessed on 17th June 2025).
11. Dala-Ali, B. M., Atkinson, H. D., Lloyd, M. A., & Welck, M. (2010). Pseudogout associated hip pain in a patient with HIV infection. https://core.ac.uk/download/pdf/8508888.pdf (accessed on 17th June 2025).
12. Di Gesu, M., Iovane, A., Mantia, F., Messina, G., & Thomas, E. (2020). Ultrasound-guided percutaneous treatment of a calcific acromioclavicular joint: A case report. https://core.ac.uk/download/287858674.pdf (accessed on 17th June 2025).
13. Diekhoff, T., Hamm, B., Hermann, K. G. A., Hermann, S., et al. (2020). Dual-energy CT collagen density mapping of wrist ligaments reveals tissue remodeling in CPPD patients: First results from a clinical cohort. https://core.ac.uk/download/533535962.pdf (accessed on 17th June 2025).
14. Dubchak, N., & Falasca, G. F. (2010). New and improved strategies for the treatment of gout. *International journal of nephrology and renovascular disease*, *3*, 145–166. https://doi.org/10.2147/IJNRD.S6048 (accessed on 17th June 2025).

15. ElSayed, S. (2023). PRG4/CD44/PP2A signaling axis: A significant regulator of gout arthritis. https://core.ac.uk/download/552797894.pdf (accessed on 17th June 2025).

16. Hamilton, J. A., McCarthy, G., & Whitty, G. (2001). Inflammatory microcrystals induce murine macrophage survival and DNA synthesis. *Arthritis research*, *3*(4), 242–246. https://doi.org/10.1186/ar308(accessed on 17th June 2025).

17. Hsieh, S. C., & Li, K. J. (2011). Clinical application of musculoskeletal ultrasound in rheumatic diseases. https://core.ac.uk/download/pdf/81179385.pdf (accessed on 17th June 2025).

18. Jokic, A., Kocijan, I., Culej, J., Kopcinovic, L. M., & Bozovic, M. (2020). Laboratory testing of extravascular body fluids: National recommendations on behalf of the Croatian Society of Medical Biochemistry and Laboratory Medicine. Part II–Synovial fluid. https://core.ac.uk/download/335624833.pdf (accessed on 17th June 2025).

19. Karanjia, D. P. M., Lindenmeyer, C. C., Cress, M., Mandel, D., et al. (2013). A case study of pseudo-neuropathic pseudogout. https://core.ac.uk/download/46971956.pdf (accessed on 17th June 2025).

20. Tikly, M., & Makan, K. (2013). Gouty arthritis: an approach for general practice. *South African Family Practice*, *55*(4), 307–312. https://doi.org/10.1080/20786204.2013.10874366 (accessed on 17th June 2025).

21. McCormack, W. J., O'Neill, L. A., & Parker, A. E. (2009). Toll-like receptors and NOD-like receptors in rheumatic diseases. https://core.ac.uk/download/pdf/8355410.pdf (accessed on 17th June 2025).

22. Ng, Y. J., & Velanthren, K. (2022). Windswept deformity from pseudogout: A diagnostic challenge of an extreme presentation–A case report. https://core.ac.uk/download/544154224.pdf (accessed on 17th June 2025).

23. Niessink, T. (2024). A new perspective on crystallizations in rheumatology and orthopedics with Raman spectroscopy. https://core.ac.uk/download/636759734.pdf (accessed on 17th June 2025).

24. Owen, D. S., Jr. (1974). Recent advances in synovial fluid analysis. https://core.ac.uk/download/51294733.pdf (accessed on 17th June 2025).

25. Russell, Maranda, "ANALYSIS OF INFORMATION VALUE CHAINS FOR GOUT SELF-CARE MANAGEMENT" (2020). *Theses and Dissertations--Communication*. 96. https://uknowledge.uky.edu/comm_etds/96(accessed on 17th June 2025).

26. Sendrea, A. M., Salavastru, C., Vrinceanu, D., Copaci, F. I., & Tiplica, G. S. (2020). Tophaceous gout–When the skin comes first. https://core.ac.uk/download/395403574.pdf (accessed on 17th June 2025).

27. Pineda, C., Sandoval, H., Pérez-Neri, I., Soto-Fajardo, C., & Carranza-Enríquez, F. (2024). Calcium pyrophosphate deposition disease: historical overview and potential gaps. *Frontiers in medicine*, *11*, 1380135. https://doi.org/10.3389/fmed.2024.1380135(accessed on 17th June 2025).

OSTEOARTHRITIS

9

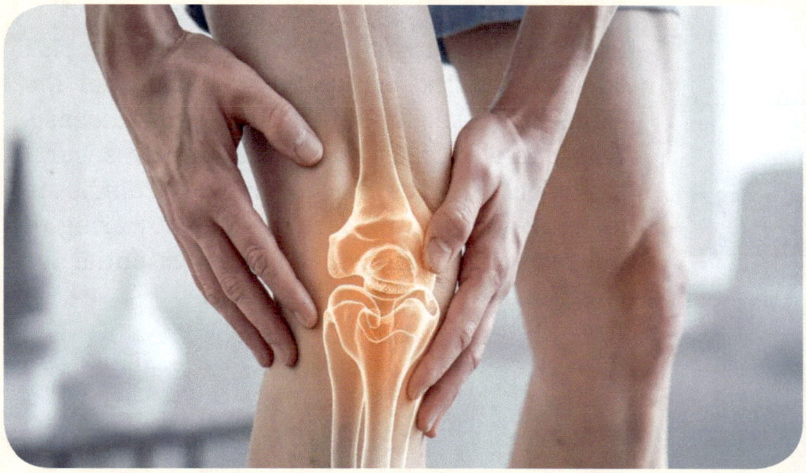

LEARNING OBJECTIVES

After studying this chapter, you will be able to:

1. Identify causes and risk factors
2. Explain symptoms and diagnosis
3. Focus on treatment options
4. Discuss the impact on daily life

Introduction

Osteoarthritis (OA) is a worldwide public health problem and has been ranked as one of the leading causes of chronic pain and disability. The condition encompasses cartilage degeneration and associated inflammatory reactions and often arises as a consequence of accumulated joint wear and tear or following specific forms of injury, referred to as post-traumatic osteoarthritis (Wallace, 2018). This condition, which affects millions and has profound social and economic implications, particularly in aging populations in many nations, highlights the need for effective management strategies. It has been established that arthritis, such as OA, affects an estimated 3 million Australians alone, hence making it not only the most prevalent long-term health condition but also one of the major causes of disability (Bates et al., 2014). With the multifaceted nature of OA and its impact on quality of life, elucidation of the underlying mechanism and exploration of potential treatments are essential for improving patient outcomes (Figure 9.1).

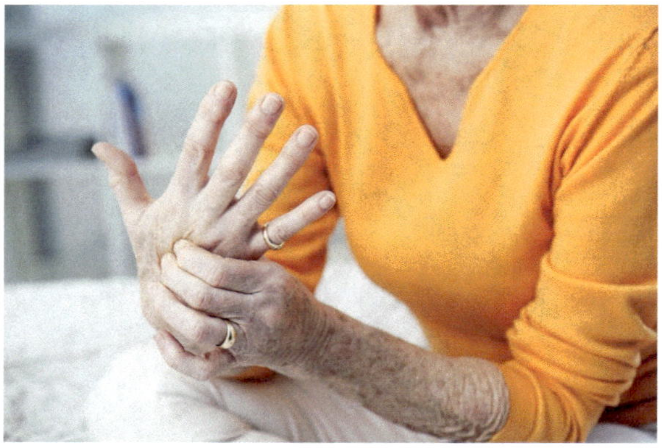

Figure 9.1. Osteoarthritis.

Source: https://www.coastalorthoteam.com/hubfs/Blog_photos/osteoarthritis-hand.jpg.

9.1. Causes and Risk Factors

Learning Outcome

1. Understand age as a primary risk factor
2. Explain genetic predisposition
3. Discuss obesity and its effects
4. Focus on joint injuries and trauma
5. Learn gender differences in prevalence
6. Describe occupational hazards
7. Identify lifestyle factors
8. Explain comorbid conditions
9. Understand environmental factors

Osteoarthritis, a degenerative joint disease, is influenced by a range of causes and risk factors that significantly play a role in its development and progression. Obesity is associated with particular prominence as a major risk factor; with continually rising rates of obesity globally, more than 1.5 billion adults currently being overweight, the disease burden associated with osteoarthritis can likewise be predicted to rise proportionally (Kyrou & Weickert, 2010). Excess weight places additional stress on load-bearing joints, and there is increased wear and tear. Moreover, factors associated with late-life incidence of total joint replacements (TJRs), such as increased body mass index (BMI) and severity of hand osteoarthritis, underscore the complex interaction among these variables and joint health (Aspelund et al., 2016). Even gender is an issue, with females being more susceptible to developing osteoarthritis, particularly after menopause. Concurrently, these factors indicate the complexity of osteoarthritis, emphasizing the need for individualized prevention.

9.1.1. Age as a Primary Risk Factor

Increased age significantly increases the risk of osteoarthritis, hence making it one of the significant risk factors for the joint disease. This correlation is brought about by several biological changes that, over time, contribute to weakening of the cartilage and lowering of the production of synovial fluid, essential for effective functioning of the joint.

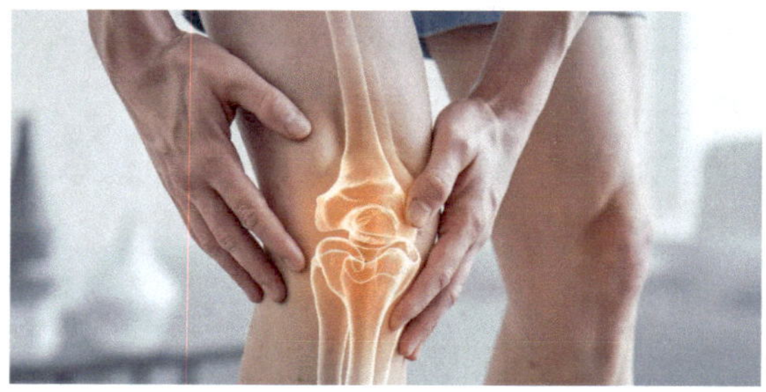

Figure 9.2. As individuals age, the risk of developing osteoarthritis significantly increases, making age a primary risk factor for this degenerative joint disease.

Source: https://geimshospital.com/wp-content/uploads/2025/03/CF59z6Qe-Knee-Arthritis-Symptoms-jpg-1024x512.webp.

Further, the cumulated effect of lifetime mechanical load on joints and hormonal changes with aging can also sustain the degenerative process. Interestingly, investigations have shown that elderly patients with osteoarthritis have higher rates of cardiovascular disease, with one such example of the interconnectedness of healthcare problems in the group. Specifically, osteoarthritis has been linked with heart failure and ischemic heart disease at heightened levels, highlighting the non-negligible impacts of age on patients' health and the need for special intervention (Valdes et al., 2013; Hall et al., 2015) (Figure 9.2).

9.1.2. Genetic Predisposition

Genetic susceptibility is also a clue to osteoarthritis, a degenerative joint condition affecting millions of people around the world. Research has demonstrated that genetics plays a significant role in making a person more susceptible to contracting the disease because there are genes that play a role in maintaining cartilage integrity and joint function. For instance, as indicated in the observation of lumbar disk degeneration, osteoarthritis-susceptibility genetic variants suggest shared pathways that may affect the health of connective tissue (Chan et al., 2011). Furthermore, obesity, which is a strongly established risk factor for osteoarthritis, is progressively linked to genetic factors that contribute to regulating body weight. The epigenetic inheritance of risk for obesity across generations further adds to the complexity by intimating that people can inherit not only genetic susceptibility but also environmental response that predisposes to osteoarthritis (Chen et al., 2016). The interaction between genes and environment thus explains the complex nature of this prevalent joint disorder.

9.1.3. Obesity and its Effects

The prevalence of obesity has risen to epidemic levels around the world, affecting public health and chronic disease dramatically, one of which is osteoarthritis. Based on categories made by the World Health Organization, more than 500 million people are clinically obese, a figure that emphasizes the need for taking immediate action to address this epidemic (Kyrou Weickert, 2010). Obesity is not merely a matter of additional weight; it is also very much related to the development and progression of osteoarthritis because it leads to joints, particularly weight-bearing joints like the hips and knees, to endure additional stress. Studies also indicate that walking gait is adversely affected in individuals with obesity, and impairments are observed that can exacerbate joint pain and movement difficulties (Bashinskaya, 2016). This cycle reveals how the pattern of obesity and osteoarthritis is cyclical, with weight gain on top of decreasing activity levels leading to further joint degeneration and overall health. Obesity treatment is thus the key to osteoarthritis treatment (Figure 9.3).

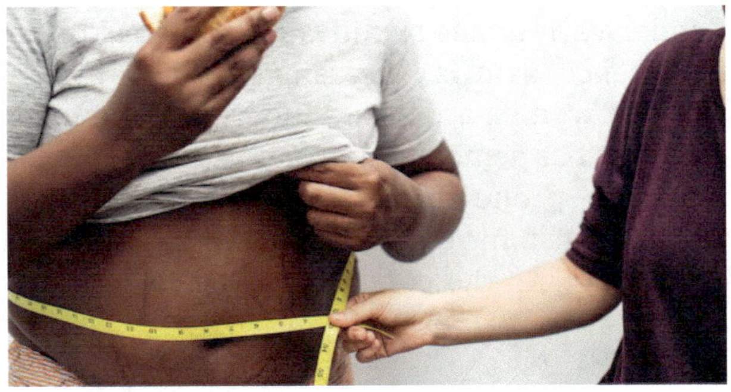

Figure 9.3. The prevalence of obesity has reached alarming levels globally, significantly impacting public health and contributing to various chronic conditions, including osteoarthritis.

Source: https://www.fortishealthcare.com/drupal-data/styles/blog_detail/azblob/2025-04/obesity.png?itok=155oon-f.

9.1.4. Joint Injuries and Trauma

The etiologic link between joint injury and the subsequent development of osteoarthritis (OA) is established. Trauma to the knee, particularly injury of the anterior cruciate ligament (ACL), may initiate a gradual decline in joint function. According to research, ACL injury patients exhibit reduced movement variability, which suggests a stiff loading pattern and potentially contributes to greater cartilage destruction (Breen et al.,

2012). This decline is not immediate; rather, radiologic signs of OA typically emerge approximately ten years following trauma, with patients presenting symptoms earlier depending on age at the time of injury (Ahlbäck et al., 1995). Incidentally, those patients who suffer isolated meniscus tears also exhibit the same trend, with the prior onset of OA in older-aged subjects. It is recognition of these patterns that emphasizes the importance of early intervention and rehabilitation in preserving joint integrity and reducing the long-term implications of injury, particularly among vulnerable groups.

9.1.5. Gender Differences in Prevalence

Gender variation is significant in osteoarthritis occurrence, as it is increasingly proven by the fact that women are more vulnerable than men. Research has demonstrated not only that women are more prone to having osteoarthritis but that they also have greater pain and functional disability with the condition.

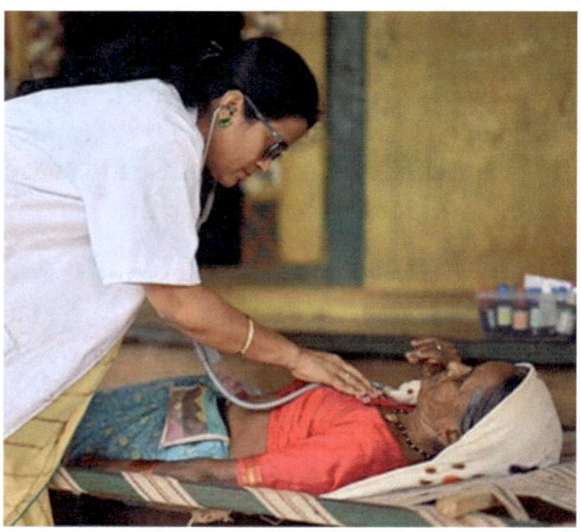

Figure 9.4. Gender differences significantly influence the prevalence of osteoarthritis, with emerging evidence highlighting a higher susceptibility in women compared to men.

Source: https://www.orfonline.org/public/uploads/seo/20240217122627.jpg.

For instance, research has shown that undiagnosed mood disorders, which are more common in women with chronic musculoskeletal pain, increase their perception of pain and comorbidities, emphasizing the need for special interventions among them (Salazar et al., 2013). Moreover, a cross-sectional survey among the disabled population indicates a higher prevalence of musculoskeletal disorders , such as osteoarthritis in women, correlated with anxiety and disturbances in sleep (Salazar et al., 2014). Such findings call for consideration of gender-specific approaches in the treatment and management of osteoarthritis to address its gender-specific impacts on women's health and quality of life (Figure 9.4).

9.1.6. Occupational Hazards

Occupational risk is a significant cause and exacerbation of osteoarthritis, particularly in highly risky professions with repetitive motion, heavy lifting, or prolonged weight-bearing. Workers in such high-risk industries , such as construction and manufacturing expose themselves to various physical stresses that may instigate joint health decline. Workplace safety training cannot be more critical, as it is a necessary preventive intervention to prevent such risks. Such programs not only educate workers in the best ergonomic practices but also enhance awareness of potential psychosocial stressors that may be exacerbating physical injuries by their effects on mental health and quality of life (Mobosi, 2025). Beyond this, higher rates of sick leave attributed to psychosocial causes, reported in the health and education sectors, highlight an alarming trend that interweaves physical with mental occupational hazards (Board, 2025). Therefore, their prevention becomes vital to the promotion of long-term joint health and osteoarthritis prevention in workers.

9.1.7. Lifestyle Factors (e.g., Diet, Exercise)

Osteoarthritis treatment similarly relies to a great extent on aspects of lifestyle, and nutrition and exercise can induce relief of symptoms and improved overall function of the joints. Exercise regularly enhances joint flexibility as well as the strength of the muscles covering the affected joints and consequently reduces stress on the cartilage. Maintenance of a healthy weight through diet and a balanced dietary regimen also prevents undue stress on load-bearing joints, such as the hips and knees. Clinical evidence shows that substantial weight loss, over 15 kg, can lead to remarkable improvement of symptoms and potentially enhance the life expectancy of osteoarthritis patients (Lean, 2011). Furthermore, modification of diet, including anti-inflammatory foods rich in omega-3 fatty acids, can also contribute to joint health. Hence, it is important that a combined strategy of diet control and regular exercise assists in fighting the consequences of osteoarthritis and improves the quality of life for those suffering from it (Figure 9.5).

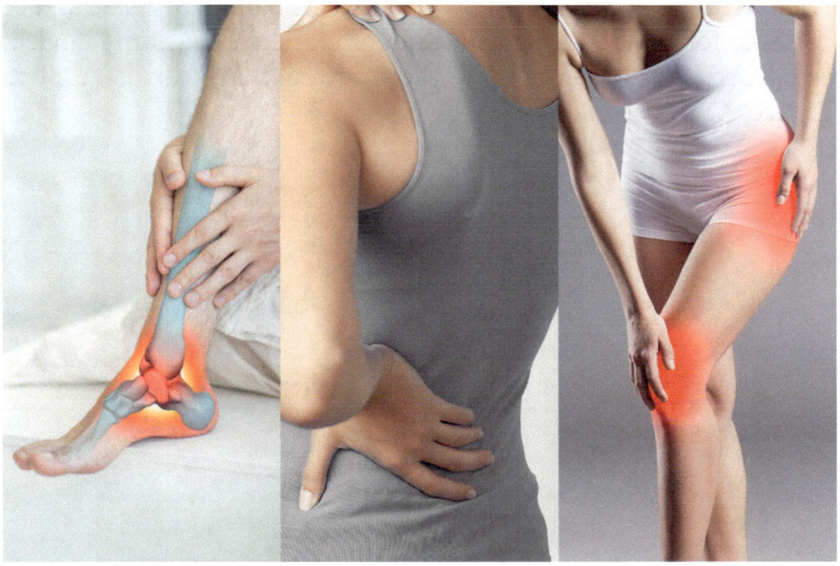

Figure 9.5. Engaging in regular physical activity enhances joint mobility and strengthens the muscles surrounding the affected joints, thereby reducing stress on the cartilage.

Source: https://iulabs.co/cdn/shop/articles/10_Science-Backed_Tips_to_Reduce_Joint_Pain_World_Arthritis_Day.png?v=1713180659&width=1100.

9.1.8. Comorbid Conditions (e.g., Diabetes)

The relationship between osteoarthritis and comorbidities, particularly diabetes, is multifaceted and very deep. Osteoarthritis patients have a greater incidence of chronic diseases , such as diabetes; diabetes can complicate the history of osteoarthritis and increase its symptoms. Evidence is such that there is a greater burden of illness associated with both osteoarthritis and diabetes among more economically disadvantaged individuals, but this doesn't necessarily extend into appropriate diagnosis and treatment outcomes (Steel et al., 2014). Secondly, the comorbidity between the two chronic disorders threatens the quality of diabetes care as comorbid conditions can undermine attainment of primary goals of diabetes control, like blood pressure and glycated hemoglobin control (Bolt et al., 2015). In view of this, an appreciation of comorbidity between osteoarthritis and diabetes not only determines therapy modalities but also calls for consideration of the treatment of the comorbid disease to maximize patient outcomes holistically.

9.1.9. Environmental Factors

Environmental factors are the cause and pathogenesis of osteoarthritis (OA), with nutritional habits playing an important role. It is noted that a diet rich in fruit and vegetables shows an inverse correlation with the development of hip OA, and food groups are protective against joint deterioration (Rowan et al., 2010). Specifically, allium's constituents , such as diallyl disulfide, not only play healthy food functions but also have anti-inflammatory properties via the inhibition of matrix-degrading proteases in chondrocytes, which may lower cartilage destruction (Rowan et al., 2010). Furthermore, the molecular pathways of OA point to the role environmental conditions play; e.g., Proteinase-activated receptor 2 (PAR2) involvement in chondrocytes has been shown to be responsible for osteophyte formation and cartilage degradation, suggesting environmental stimuli may exacerbate these processes. Understanding these interactions in this respect can inform the prevention of OA (Figure 9.6).

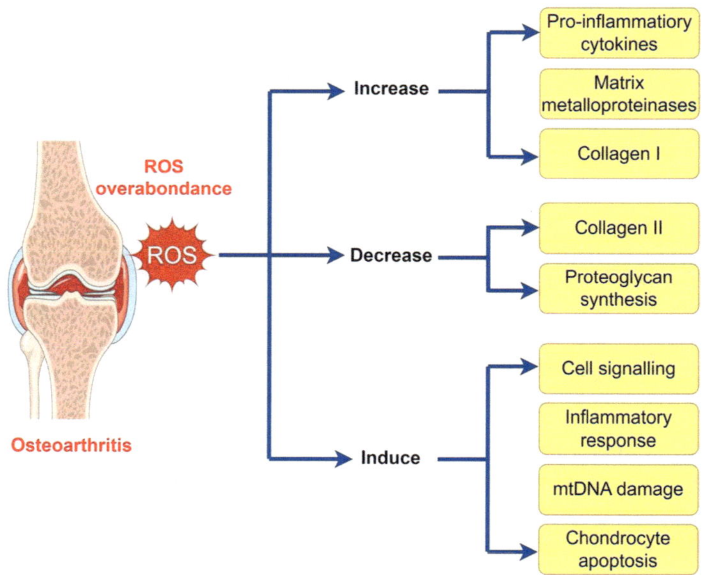

Figure 9.6. Environmental factors play a pivotal role in the development and progression of osteoarthritis (OA), with dietary patterns emerging as a significant influence.

Source: Adam MS, Zhuang H, Ren X, Zhang Y and Zhou P (2024) The metabolic characteristics and changes of chondrocytes in vivo and in vitro in osteoarthritis. Front. Endocrinol. 15:1393550. doi: 10.3389/fendo.2024.1393550

Test Your Knowledge

1. What role does obesity play in OA pathogenesis?
2. How do joint injuries and repetitive stress contribute to OA?

9.2. Symptoms and Diagnosis

Learning Outcome

1. Identify common symptoms of osteoarthritis
2. Focus on pain characteristics
3. Describe stiffness and its implications
4. Explain swelling and inflammation
5. Learn physical examination techniques
6. Describe imaging methods
7. Understand laboratory tests and biomarkers
8. Know the differential diagnosis
9. Discuss the importance of early diagnosis

The symptoms at presentation for osteoarthritis are mostly pain, stiffness, and disability of the joints, which significantly impair quality of life and function. The diagnosis of osteoarthritis is based on clinical assessment supplemented by patient-reported symptoms, although the disease burden is great in comparison with successful management, particularly in susceptible groups. Research indicates that, although the incidence of self-reported knee complaints is very high, only 55.3% of symptomatic osteoarthritis patients are detected by general practitioners, and even fewer are treated appropriately. Further, only a low percentage of diagnosed patients adequately control their symptoms, which are systemic barriers to the healthcare system and do not offer quality services for these patients with this condition (Steel et al., 2014). This discrepancy reflects the key imperative to develop diagnostic methods and methods of treatment that can adequately address complaints experienced by patients, particularly those who are of lower socioeconomic status (Steel et al., 2014).

9.2.1. Common Symptoms of Osteoarthritis

The clinical picture of osteoarthritis (OA) is marked by an overwhelming heterogeneity, indicative of its multifactorial pathology. The most common symptoms are chronic pain, stiffness, and inflammation of the involved joint, particularly after prolonged inactivity or overuse. As highlighted in the literature, their onset is significantly heterogeneous between patients and prefers to be clustered into distinctive phenotypes mirroring distinctive clinical characteristics (Courties et al., 2018). For example, the chronic pain phenotype is usually accompanied by heightened sensitivity and discomfort, mostly in women (Courties et al., 2018). Furthermore, inflammatory markers may be prevalent in some patients, making the usual symptomatology complex. These varied symptoms not only impact daily functioning but also make clinical management of OA complex. Appreciation of such differences is vital for the establishment of individualized treatment regimens that are sensitive to the unique experiences of persons who are afflicted with this disabling disease, leading to enhanced quality of life and function in persons thus affected (Figure 9.7).

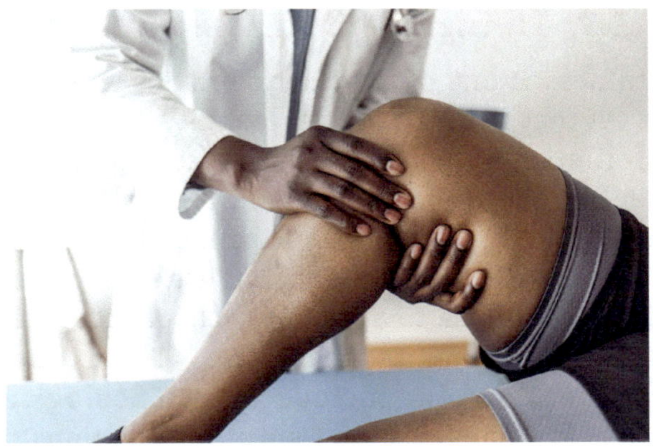

Figure 9.7. Common manifestations include persistent joint pain, stiffness, and swelling, particularly after periods of inactivity or excessive use.

Source: https://www.health.com/thmb/oTfbUk_T7tuT4uQufvhxBUplYr8=/2000x0/filters:no_upscale():max_bytes(150000):strip_icc()/knee-pain-GettyImages-1321088960-839639eb5e9c430e888a77a3a1b8f8f3.jpg.

9.2.2. Pain Characteristics

Knowledge of the pain characteristics of osteoarthritis is important in managing and treating it effectively. Patients present with a multifaceted coexistence of different pain phenotypes that can immensely influence their quality of life. Differences in pain intensity are due to causes , such as disease progression and unique biological responses. For instance, the knee osteoarthritis Chronic Pain (CP) phenotype has been correlated with higher pain scores, defining the crucial role of psychological and social factors in symptom presentation (Courties et al., 2018). Moreover, topical administration of drugs like diclofenac sodium (Pennsaid) emphasizes the value of selective pain intervention, in that it offers similar efficacy to oral medications at lower systemic side effects (Banning, 2009). Through the identification and management of these pain characteristics, health care professionals can more effectively individualize interventions, thereby improving patient outcomes for this disabling disorder.

9.2.3. Stiffness and Its Implications

Stiffness is one of the characteristic symptoms of OA that affects patients' mobility and quality of life significantly. Rigidity is caused by degeneration of cartilage and joint alteration, leading to inflammation and pain on movement. The consequences of stiffness extend beyond pain; it can lead to a vicious cycle of decreased activity and joint progression. Therapeutic regimens often include pharmacological interventions , such as topical formulations of diclofenac sodium, that may be employed to provide localized analgesia without inducing systemic side effects. Research indicates that topically applied diclofenac sodium is equal to the oral form in effectiveness, providing pain relief without gastrointestinal consequences associated with systemic NSAIDs (Banning et al., 2006). Further, the dry skin side effect of normal topically applied use, linked to dimethyl sulfoxide, demonstrates the requirement for careful patient care (Banning, 2009). Awareness and relief of stiffness are important to enhancing patient benefit in OA (Figure 9.8).

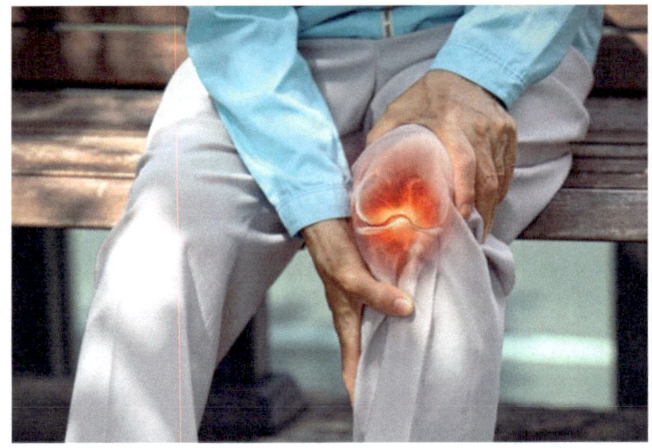

Figure 9.8. Stiffness is a hallmark symptom of osteoarthritis (OA) that significantly affects patients mobility and quality of life.

Source: https://www.sparshhospital.com/wp-content/uploads/2024/10/arthri.jpg.

9.2.4. Swelling and Inflammation

Osteoarthritis (OA) has the inherent involvement of the mechanisms of inflammation and swelling, which are to a significant measure responsible for the disease's development. Cytokines interleukin-1 and tumor necrosis factor-α are released in the inflamed joints, exacerbating cartilage breakdown and promoting synovitis, which is swelling of the joint with pain. The occurrence of these cytokines breaks the balance between cartilage growth and breakdown, and consequently, leads to loss of vital extracellular matrix components like glycosaminoglycans that are crucial to the health of the cartilage (Wallace et al., 2018).

In addition, research highlights that the degree of swelling and inflammation can have a profound effect on the functional capacity and daily activities of patients because the symptoms themselves tend to be associated with the disability level of individuals with osteoarthritis (Bates et al., 2014). Lastly, understanding the etiology of swelling and inflammation in OA is essential for the development of effective treatments for pain relief and joint function improvement.

9.2.5. Physical Examination Techniques

A successful physical examination is most critical in managing and assessing osteoarthritis, as it provides significant information on the course of the condition and the patient's functional limitations. Inspection, palpation, and range of motion are some of the methods employed to determine joint deformity, swelling, or tenderness, which are typical presentations of osteoarthritis. Besides, the use of advanced imaging modalities like quantitative magnetic resonance imaging (qMRI) has also emerged as a valuable diagnostic and monitoring aid for early cartilage degeneration in this condition (Amano et al., 2016). Apart from that, comprehensive assessments with cardiovascular status are also crucial because the prevalence of cardiovascular disease is well-evidenced in patients with osteoarthritis (Hall et al., 2015). With these combined analytical approaches, clinicians can create patient-specific treatment plans that not only address the musculoskeletal effects of osteoarthritis but also consider the overall effects of this chronic disease on every area of health (Figure 9.9).

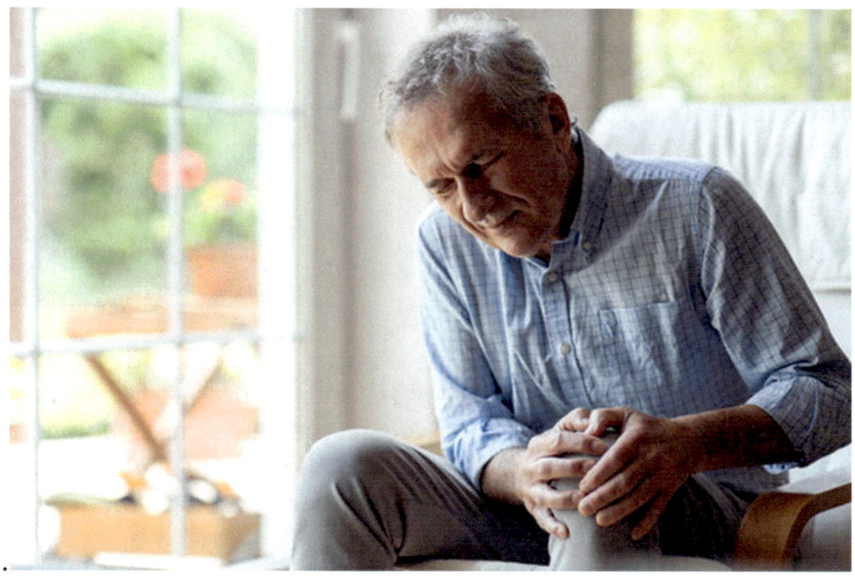

Figure 9.9. An effective physical examination is paramount in the evaluation and management of osteoarthritis, as it provides critical insights into the condition's progression and the patient's functional limitations.

Source: https://static.wixstatic.com/media/4a037c_bd1cd173e9c74ab3a6832add41517bff~mv2.jpg/v1/fill/w_568,h_378,al_c,q_80,usm_0.66_1.00_0.01,enc_avif,quality_auto/4a037c_bd1cd173e9c74ab3a6832add41517bff~mv2.jpg.

9.2.6. Imaging Methods (e.g., X-rays, MRIs)

Imaging procedures like X-rays and magnetic resonance imaging (MRI) play a significant role in managing and diagnosing osteoarthritis (OA). X-rays provide an easy and quick method of viewing changes in bone integrity with observations like joint space narrowing and development of bone spurs, typical of OA progression. Conversely, MRIs give a better image of cartilage and soft tissue, needed for evaluating the condition of the articular cartilage and menisci, the shock-absorbing tissue in the knee (Alexopoulos et al., 2022). Deep learning has also been utilized in high-end MRI for improving diagnostic precision, citing improved predictions in the onset of knee OA when integrating patient data with imaging findings (Alexopoulos et al., 2022). These imaging modalities not only aid in patient diagnosis but also facilitate monitoring for disease progression, thus informing treatment strategies and improving patient outcomes.

9.2.7. Laboratory Tests and Biomarkers

OA diagnosis and treatment are significantly enhanced by advancements in laboratory testing and biomarkers, which provide critical information on disease progression and the efficacy of treatment. Potential urinary proteomic biomarkers have been proven to distinguish between OA and other forms of arthritis and signify a growing trend towards more precise diagnostic methodologies. Research indicates that urinary peptide signatures are able to classify chronic arthropathies with great accuracy, referring to the fact that certain biomarkers are linked with dysregulated collagen synthesis and inflammation as central to OA pathology (Gaya et al., 2017). In addition, nutraceuticals given in OA equine models exerted an anti-inflammatory effect, with clinically significant declines in synovial fluid biomarkers , such as prostaglandin E2 and total protein levels, further pointing to the treatment utility of biochemical markers (van de Water et al., 2017). Such observations point towards a bright future for the inclusion of laboratory tests and biomarkers into standard OA evaluation and treatment protocols.

9.2.8. Differential Diagnosis

Successful differential diagnosis is necessary in the correct diagnosis of osteoarthritis due to the fact that its signs tend to overlap with a number of other musculoskeletal conditions. Symptoms , such as rheumatoid arthritis, gout, and tendonitis can all present identically with joint pain and stiffness, and therefore accurate differentiation must occur in order for correct treatment. Through a detailed clinical examination, including judicious patient history and physical examination, clinicians can distinguish osteoarthritis by noting the insidious onset of symptoms and characteristic patterns of involvement of the joints.

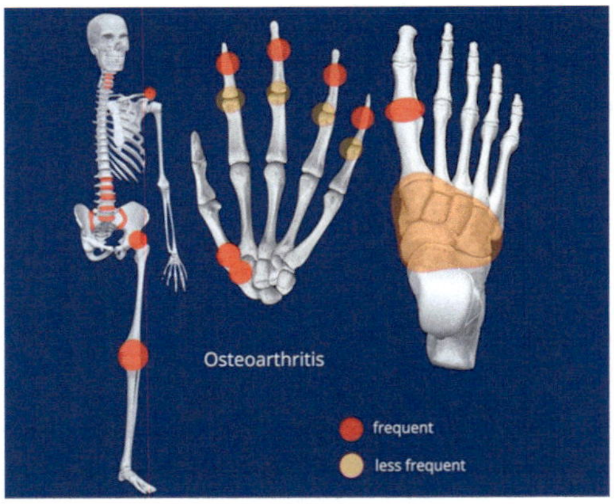

Figure 9.10. Effective differential diagnosis is crucial in the accurate identification of osteoarthritis, as its symptoms frequently overlap with those of various other musculoskeletal disorders.

Source: https://radiologyassistant.nl/img/containers/main/_1tek-osteoarthritis.jpg/1870ea2faa00bc661d4e5d3174adc62e.jpg.

Radiologic studies also aid in recognizing characteristic changes, such as joint space narrowing and osteophyte formation, which are indicative of osteoarthritis as opposed to inflammatory arthritis or degenerative diseases. Identification of these differences also directly influences the choice of treatment, such as topical treatment, such as diclofenac sodium, which can effectively control osteoarthritis pain while minimizing systemic side effects (Banning et al., 2009). Thus, precise differential diagnosis not only chooses the pathology but also optimizes patient outcomes (Altman et al., 2017) (Figure 9.10).

9.2.9. Importance of Early Diagnosis

The significance of early diagnosis of osteoarthritis cannot be overestimated, as it is primarily responsible for determining the overall course of the disease and the quality of life of the subjects. Early diagnosis of osteoarthritis enables healthcare professionals to initiate effective management strategies, including lifestyle modification, physical therapy, and medication, ultimately arresting the disease process and symptom severity. The condition is cited to be among the main contributors to chronic pain and disability and presently affects approximately 3 million Australians, hence the need to address the condition by applying early detection and treatment (Bates et al., 2014). Furthermore, research demonstrates that poor movement in initial development stages can contribute to musculoskeletal disorders, thus amplifying the biomechanical importance of intervening early (Nowlan, 2015). Hence, raising awareness and knowledge about early symptoms can empower patients to access help, supporting improved outcomes and functional independence.

Test Your Knowledge

1. What imaging techniques are commonly used to diagnose OA?
2. What radiographic features are typical of OA?

9.3. Treatment Options

Learning Outcome

1. Understand non-pharmacological interventions
2. Explain pharmacological treatments
3. Focus on physical therapy and rehabilitation
4. Identify surgical options
5. Describe alternative therapies
6. Focus on lifestyle modifications
7. Know the role of nutrition in management
8. Focus on patient education and self-management
9. Learn emerging treatments and research

Osteoarthritis (OA) treatment consists of a variety of interventions whose primary goal is to restore pain relief and mobility. Conventional treatments, such as non-steroidal anti-inflammatory drugs (NSAIDs) and opioids, have long been used symptomatically; however, they do not influence the course of the disease. Recent advances provide encouraging alternatives, like anti-nerve growth factor (anti-NGF) antibodies, which target pain pathways more specifically (Aigner et al., 2014). In addition, new strategies , such as stem cell therapy and growth factor therapy are promising to change the structural components of bone and cartilage, and these are regarded as the potential promise for complete management (Aigner et al., 2014). Unexpectedly, research has identified that the total consumption of dietary fat is not connected with the prevalence of hand osteoarthritis, and it is implied that other factors , such as age and way of life, could play more determining roles in the course of the disease. These results indicate the complexity of OA treatment and demonstrate the significance of customized treatment approaches.

9.3.1. Non-pharmacological Interventions

Non-pharmacologic therapies have been more and more established as a fundamental component of the treatment of osteoarthritis (OA), which addresses both the physical and the psychological aspects of the condition. Such therapies consist of a number of different modalities, like exercise, education, and cognitive-behavioral therapies that may improve function and reduce pain over time. Research indicates that structured exercise regimens work, leading to significant symptom and general quality of life enhancement in the case of OA patients (Fawole et al., 2024). Additionally, weight control and physical therapy are major interventions with vital functions in reducing the effects of skewed joint loading, hence enhancing patient outcomes (Sinha et al., 2024). Most notably, these interventions not only bring immediate relief but also facilitate long-term engagement in health-promoting behaviors, and as such are a major element of an overall treatment regimen. As such, integrating non-pharmacologic approaches is crucial to optimizing treatment for osteoarthritis (Figure 9.11).

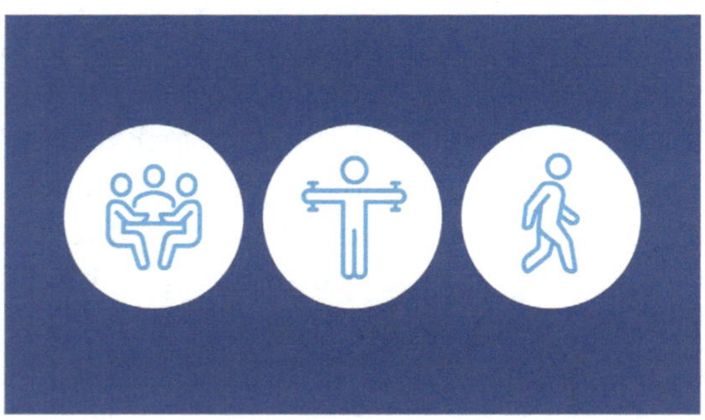

Figure 9.11. Non-pharmacological interventions have gained recognition as vital components in the management of osteoarthritis (OA), addressing both the physical and psychological dimensions of the condition.

Source: https://i.ytimg.com/vi/cGsFcX7Dayg/maxresdefault.jpg.

9.3.2. Pharmacological Treatments

Pharmacologic therapy is centrally relevant in osteoarthritis treatment, with the objectives to restore joint function and alleviate pain. Nonsteroidal anti-inflammatory drugs (NSAIDs) are typically the first drugs of choice, but these provide symptomatic relief by virtue of their analgesic properties. These have come under consideration, however, for prolonged use, namely the risk of gastrointestinal toxicity and cardiovascular side effects, and there has been increasing attention to other modes of therapy. In light of growing opioid addiction and the opioid epidemic of today, medical practitioners are urged to reconsider pain treatment practices. Supporters of national associations call for reduced reliance on opioids with an agenda for focusing on the integration of nonpharmacological therapies along with pharmacotherapy (Swezey, 2018). Moreover, research into adjunct treatments, such as intra-articular corticosteroid or hyaluronic acid injections, may maximize therapeutic effect while addressing the multifaceted osteoarthritis pain (Glennon, 2019). Hence, a balanced knowledge of these drug treatments is required for optimal patient outcomes.

9.3.3. Physical Therapy and Rehabilitation

Rehabilitation and physical therapy play significant roles in the management of osteoarthritis (OA) in enhancing the quality of life for patients. Reduction of pain, improved mobility, and functional independence are possible through successful rehabilitation programs that are tailored to each patient. Various approaches , such as manual therapy, exercise therapies, and educational interventions, have been proven effective for OA management. For instance, inclusion of early mobilization and systematic physical therapy after total knee arthroplasty (TKA) has been identified as essential to maximizing walking potential and recovery, as found in research evidence (Rosenberg, 2025). In addition, advances in digital rehabilitation interventions, such as those based on cognitive behavioral therapy and behavior change theories, have shown promising results in terms of pain reduction and improvement of physical function in OA patients (Zhu et al., 2025). As the modalities continue to evolve, an interdisciplinary approach to rehabilitation remains crucial for maximizing therapeutic results and ensuring long-term patient satisfaction (Figure 9.12).

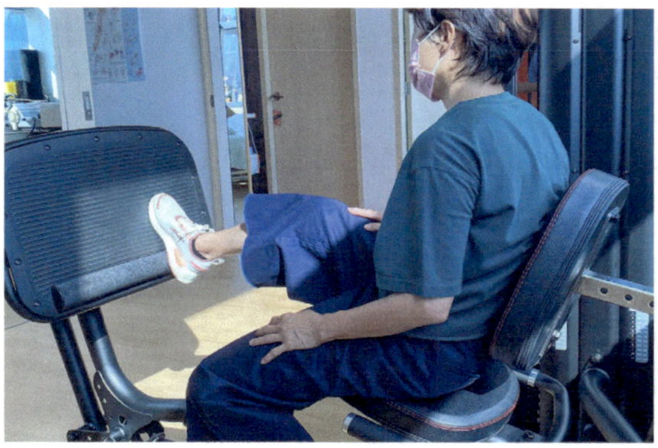

Figure 9.12. Physical therapy and rehabilitation play a critical role in managing osteoarthritis (OA), significantly enhancing patients' quality of life.

Source: https://www.hellophysio.sg/wp-content/uploads/2025/02/knee-osteoarthritis-therapy.jpeg.webp.

9.3.4. Surgical Options (e.g., Joint Replacement)

Progressive osteoarthritis can render the conservative interventions less than adequate, prompting consideration of surgery, such as joint replacement. Joint replacement surgeries, particularly hip and knee arthroplasties, have been highly successful in alleviating pain and restoring function in individuals with severe osteoarthritis. Whether to have surgery is determined by numerous factors , including the severity of symptoms, the overall well-being of patients, and individual preferences. Evidence suggests a worrisome trend in their application; usage rates vary by geographic region and demographic features, including race and ethnicity, and they suggest access inequities to treatment (Esty et al., 2010). Patient and physician education are also important to allow successful shared decision-making, ultimately optimizing outcomes for those considering surgical intervention (Arden et al., 2013). Hence, an understanding of the complexities of joint replacement procedures is essential in osteoarthritis treatment.

9.3.5. Alternative therapies (e.g., Acupuncture)

Other interventions, such as acupuncture, have been viewed as useful adjuncts in the management of osteoarthritis (OA), particularly for pain relief. Conventional drug treatments can have significant side effects, while complementary treatments are more homeostatic in their approach to disease management. Systematic reviews indicate that acupuncture is able to produce clinically relevant relief from pain in a variety of conditions, including musculoskeletal disease, while evidence as to the effectiveness may be contradictory (Lee et al., 2001).

Systematic review of physical agents in osteoarthritis of the knee found that interventions like TENS and EA resulted in clinically significant reductions in pain when used at optimal dosing (Andrianakos et al., 2007). In spite of the heterogeneity of trial quality and outcomes, many clinicians and patients had positive experiences with acupuncture, which suggests its potential as a valuable therapy for OA. With ongoing research, the inclusion of these other therapies may be able to enhance overall treatment plans for patients with this chronic condition (Figure 9.13).

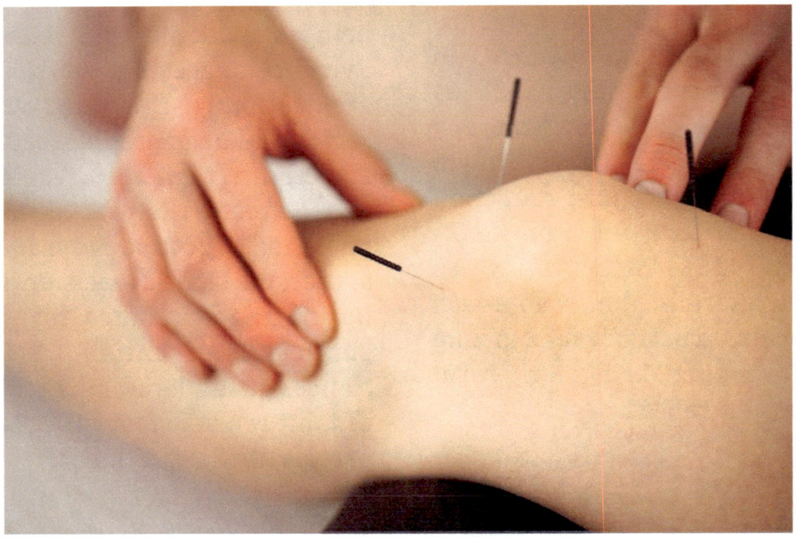

Figure 9.13. Alternative therapies, such as acupuncture, have emerged as potential adjuncts in the management of osteoarthritis (OA), particularly for alleviating pain.

Source: https://images.ctfassets.net/222znibi5gto/ppm_wysiwyg_fid13986_asset/d97978dedb31253e997eee227f9fc428/iStock-154894365.jpg.

9.3.6. Lifestyle Modifications

Osteoarthritis (OA) treatment often extends beyond the utilization of medication to encompass significant lifestyle modifications having potential positive effects on symptoms and overall joint health. Regular exercise is critical in the strengthening of the musculature surrounding a joint, stabilizing it and reducing pain. Additionally, the diet needs to be changed; studies have indicated that diets rich in plant-phenols and omega-3 fatty acids can decrease pain and improve joint function, particularly when they replace saturated fats and refined carbohydrates (Byham-Gray et al., 2024). Further, being a healthy weight is essential because being overweight causes excess stress on weight-bearing joints, aggravating pain and mobility disability. Embracing these lifestyle changes not only promotes active management of OA but also overall health. As more research demonstrates additional benefits of these changes, they are critical components of a holistic treatment regimen for osteoarthritis patients (Wallace et al., 2018).

9.3.7. Role of Nutrition in Management

The management of osteoarthritis (OA) is significantly boosted by certain nutritional treatments, which play a significant role in relieving symptoms and improving patients' quality of life. A balanced diet rich in anti-inflammatory foods has the ability to control weight and subsequently reduce the weight-bearing joints. The growing prevalence of obesity, which the World Health Organization has called a global epidemic, exacerbates the impact of OA by increasing the mechanical loading of the joints and enhancing inflammatory reactions (Weickert et al, 2010). There has also been evidence of a strong link between OA and cardiovascular disease, further reinforcing the complex relationship between these linked disorders (Hall et al., 2015). Dietary foods with high content of omega-3 fatty acids, antioxidants, and vitamins may help to decrease joint pain and enhance mobility, thereby complementing a complete approach to treating both osteoarthritis and its concomitant risks of obesity and cardiovascular diseases. With nutrition, patients can make meaningful steps towards effective management of their OA symptoms (Figure 9.14).

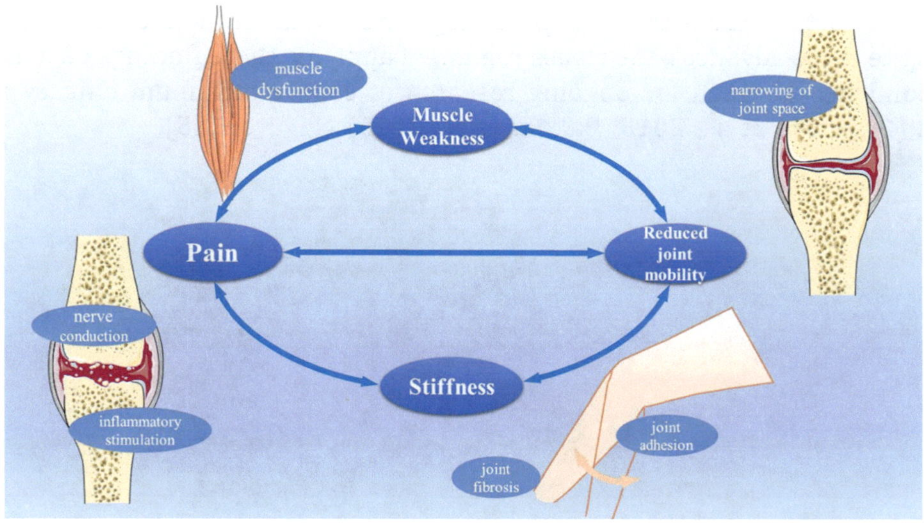

Figure 9.14. The management of osteoarthritis (OA) significantly benefits from targeted nutritional interventions, which play a crucial role in mitigating symptoms and improving patients' quality of life.

Source: https://www.frontiersin.org/files/Articles/794062/fphys-12-794062-HTML/image_m/fphys-12-794062-g002.jpg.

9.3.8. Patient Education and Self-management

Effective patient education and self-management are core aspects of osteoarthritis (OA) management, an influencing factor of quality of life for the majority of individuals, particularly older individuals. Patients who are informed about their condition become key players in symptom management as well as creating feasible health goals. Nonpharmacological treatments, such as lifestyle modification and exercise, were shown to enhance functional outcomes and reduce pain for patients with OA. According to Fayyaz et al (2023), patient education enhances self-management, enabling people to more effectively manage the complexity of their treatment. Furthermore, incorporating novel approaches like peer support and digital health resources, like those included in programs like DM-BOOST, can enhance these self-management strategies and promote treatment plan adherence, illustrating the benefits of tailoring education for healthier outcomes in OA patients (Amante et al., 2024).

9.3.9. Emerging Treatments and Research

With continued research on osteoarthritis (OA), evolving treatments promise to improve patient outcomes. Traditionally, treatment has centered on symptomatic relief through the use of non-steroidal anti-inflammatory drugs and physical therapies that act too frequently by failing to modulate joint disease. New knowledge has brought hope in the form of disease-modifying osteoarthritis drugs (DMOADs) that aim to alter the trajectory through the inhibition of primary pathways to cartilage degeneration. Moreover, regenerative treatments, like platelet-rich plasma and stem cell transplantation, have been promising to augment tissue repair and regeneration and provide longer-term alleviation. Imaging technological advancements, like the high-field magnetic resonance imaging, further clarify the pathophysiology and potentially direct more tailored treatment strategies. Despite these advances, the issues remain of applying these findings on a massive clinical scale, which confirms the need for ongoing research to ensure maximum efficacy and access to new therapies (Crawford et al., 2018; Bakuła et al., 2025) (Figure 9.15).

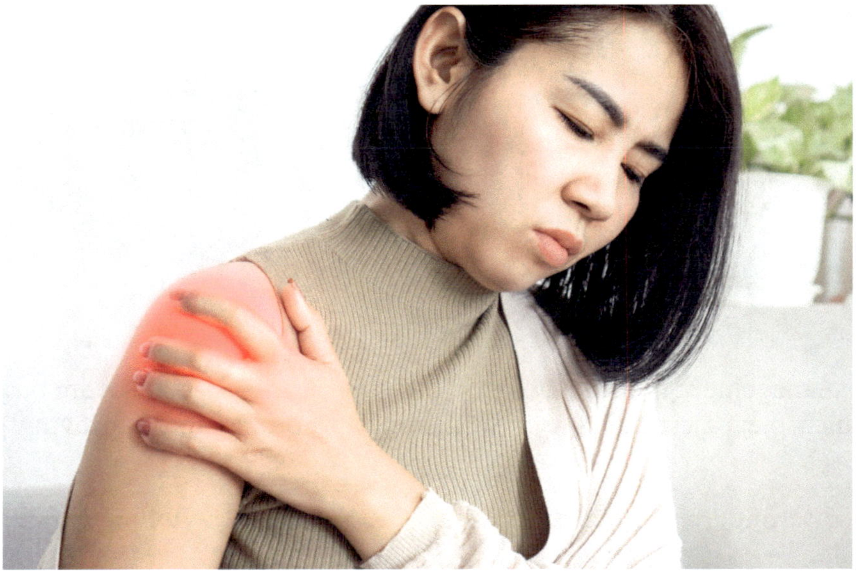

Figure 9.15. Traditionally, therapies have centered around symptom management with non-steroidal anti-inflammatory drugs and physical interventions, which often fail to address the underlying disease progression.

Source: https://www.academyorthopedics.com/wp-content/uploads/2025/05/demystifying-frozen-shoulder-causes-symptoms-and-treatments-scaled.jpeg.

Test Your Knowledge

1. When are corticosteroid or hyaluronic acid injections indicated?
2. What are the surgical options for severe OA?

9.4. Impact on Daily Life

Learning Outcome

1. Know the effects on mobility and physical activity
2. Explain psychological impact
3. Discuss social implications and relationships
4. Know the economic burden on individuals and healthcare
5. Focus on work-related challenges
6. Learn coping strategies for patients
7. Understand support systems and resources
8. Focus on community and family involvement
9. Know the long-term outlook for patients

The impact of knee osteoarthritis on quality of life is tremendous, completely altering the level of ability for individuals to accomplish simple tasks. With a whopping incidence of 240 per 100,000 persons per annum, osteoarthritis severely impairs mobility in up to 80% of patients, rendering one quarter unable to perform simple daily tasks , such as walking, climbing stairs, and even sitting up straight (Pallivalappil, 2022). This restriction not only imposes physical constraints but also imposes psychological burdens, further depreciating health-related quality of life. Consequently, patients end up having higher levels of pain and frustration, which further lead to feelings of helplessness and anxiety towards their condition. Even though patients might choose nonsurgical interventions, these tend to have minimal improvements, prompting some to resort to surgical options that have variable outcomes. Finally, the general impact of knee osteoarthritis underlines the significance of having overall management plans that emphasize physical function and also emotional status (Pallivalappil, 2022).

9.4.1. Effects on Mobility and Physical Activity

The implications of osteoarthritis for physical activity and mobility are far-reaching, with far-reaching effects upon those suffering from the disease. As the joints degenerate, victims typically experience increasing pain and stiffness, grossly impairing their ability for physical activity. This loss of mobility not only adversely affects activities of daily living but also contributes to the development of a sedentary lifestyle, which can lead to a cycle of obesity and ensuing joint complications. Evidence indicates that interventions for optimizing gait patterns, such as obstacle-crossing activities, can optimize mobility before undergoing formal treatments , such as bariatric surgery (Bashinskaya, 2016). Through the enablement of better walking mechanisms, the interventions have the potential to enable patients with osteoarthritis to regain some form of physical activity, which ultimately plays a crucial role in managing the disease and improving overall quality of life (Allan et al., 2017). The addressing of mobility issues in osteoarthritis management strategies is thus crucial to ensuring long-term health and independence (Figure 9.16).

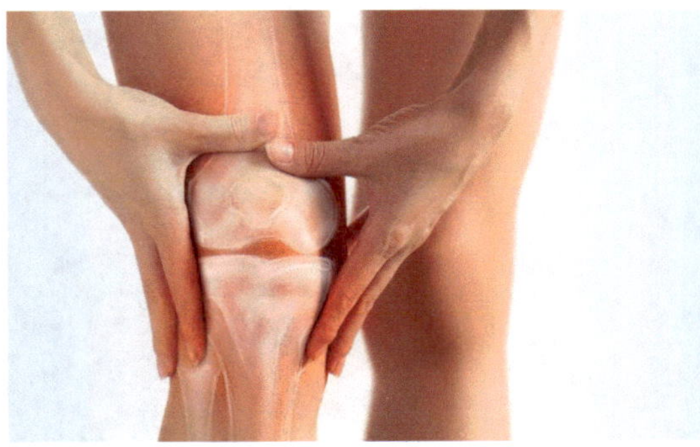

Figure 9.16. As joint degeneration progresses, individuals often experience increased pain and stiffness, which can severely limit their ability to engage in physical activities.

Source: https://www.wellheeledpodiatry.com.au/wp-content/uploads/2023/05/Knocked-Knees-Well-Heeled-Podiatry-scaled.jpg.

9.4.2. Psychological Impact (e.g., Depression, Anxiety)

The psychological effect of osteoarthritis extends beyond the physical disabilities of the condition, affecting the mental health and quality of life of patients dramatically. Osteoarthritis patients often suffer from high rates of depression and anxiety, which can intensify their pain syndromes as well as make them more challenging to treat. It has been shown through research that the rate of psychological distress is considerably higher among chronic pain patients, for example, those with osteoarthritis, and identifies the point at which the physical and mental health intersect (Wride & Bannigan, 2019). The negative influence on treatment outcome of depression and anxiety has been well documented, as they can lead to decreased motivation for self-care and adherence to treatment protocols. Besides that, complementary therapies like Tai Chi and Qi Gong have also been seen to be effective in the alleviation of the mental health issues of osteoarthritis patients, indicating the potential of holistic interventions to improve psychological well-being (Price, 2017). As such, the psychological effects of osteoarthritis need to be addressed in the management and improved outcomes for patients.

9.4.3. Social Implications and Relationships

The social impact of osteoarthritis is far greater than the physical limitations that are normally associated with the condition. Osteoarthritis sufferers often have great emotional and psychological challenges, which can impact interpersonal relationships and decrease overall quality of life. Disability and pain stigmas can result in social isolation, with sufferers avoiding social interaction because they feel judged or cannot keep up with it.

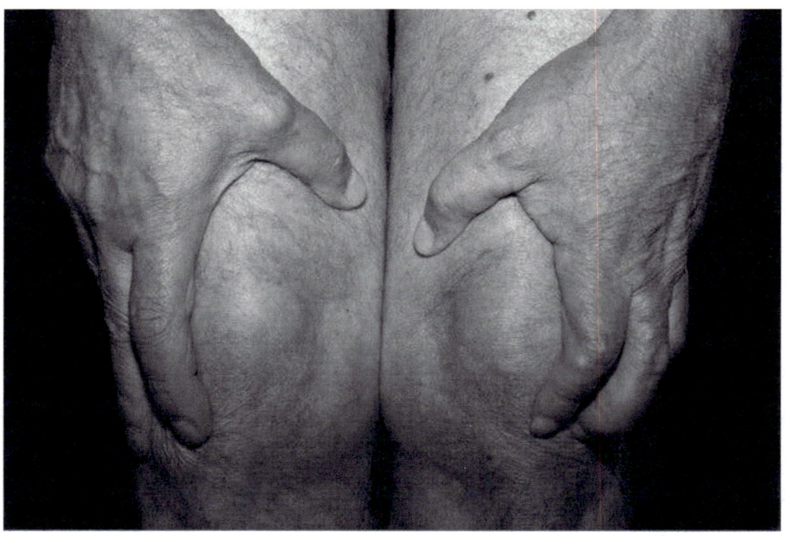

Figure 9.17. The social implications of osteoarthritis extend far beyond the physical limitations commonly associated with the condition.

Source: https://static01.nyt.com/images/2024/05/07/multimedia/WELL-OSTEOARTHRITIS1-jmlk/WELL-OSTEOARTHRITIS1-jmlk-articleLarge.jpg?quality=75&auto=webp&disable=upscale.

Furthermore, disparities in treatment and care services exacerbate these issues because poorer individuals suffer with greater illness burdens that are not proportionally addressed by healthcare interventions, as stated in comparative studies of wealth distribution against self-reported treatment levels and illness burden (Steel et al., 2014). Furthermore, understanding of lived life is utilized in designing better support frameworks, particularly in the case of schemes like the National Disability Insurance Scheme (Bates et al., 2014). Health and social spaces therefore, overlap in addressing the comprehensive needs of people with osteoarthritis (Figure 9.17).

9.4.4. Economic Burden on Individuals and Healthcare

The message of osteoarthritis to the economy of patients and health care systems is considerable, often contributing to the challenges faced by patients in managing their disease. Costs of osteoarthritis include direct medical expenses, such as physician consultations, diagnostic tests, and treatment, and indirect expenses, such as loss of productivity and health-related quality of life. For instance, individuals with osteoarthritis frequently experience chronic pain, which can lead to absence from work and diminished overall labor force participation, placing further burdens on economic resources. According to research, the integration of advanced treatment methods has a deep impact on expenditures for health care, but enhances patient outcomes and satisfaction (Angelini et al., 2004). Moreover, the demand for efficient solutions for pain management highlights the disparity in healthcare access, as unpreferred options could have additional economic costs (Kendall et al., 2001). Hence, it is important to address the economic cost of osteoarthritis to improve the well-being of the people and reduce the overall cost of health care.

9.4.5. Work-Related Challenges

Employees with osteoarthritis (OA) generally experience extreme work-related challenges that hinder their performance and job satisfaction. Physical demands of most workplaces, especially weight-bearing tasks, exacerbate symptoms of lower limb OA and lead to difficulties in maintaining productivity levels.

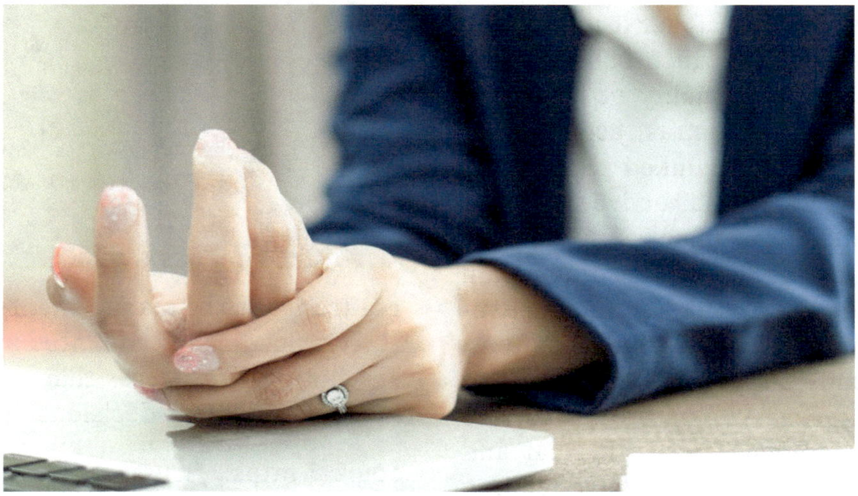

Figure 9.18. Employees afflicted with osteoarthritis (OA) often encounter significant work-related challenges that can hinder their performance and overall job satisfaction.

Source: https://apm.net.au/api/galleryhandler.ashx?moid=2343&dt=3&g=2.

As the study emphasizes, lower limb OA patients experience emotional consequences , such as worries of losing employment and concerns over their futures in the workforce, which may further impact their well-being and efficiency. Additionally, the study reveals that while some employees successfully employ coping mechanisms to manage their condition, their employers play an important role in creating welcoming workplaces (Ginsburg, 2009). Also, addressing systemic healthcare issues is important since embracing changes in the Medicare fee schedule and payment systems can lower some of the cost burdens on workers and employers (Ginsburg, 2009). Thus, it is important to establish consensus among employers and healthcare providers to come up with effective workplace accommodations (Figure 9.18).

9.4.6. Coping Strategies for Patients

Coping strategies also play a critical role in the management of osteoarthritis (OA) as they have a key influence on patients' experience with pain and functional impairment. It has been proven that individuals who employ passive coping strategies manifest higher levels of pain and functional disability, which subsequently compromise their global quality of life (QoL) (Aiyegbusi et al., 2019). In contrast, active coping strategies are noted to be linked with better pain control and lower QoL, as active strategies encourage patients' engagement with adaptive coping activities to build resilience and pain coping (Aiyegbusi et al., 2019). Further, the two-dimensionality in decisions over interventions, such as TKR, lends support to the necessity of integrating effective coping strategies into OA patient management, both physical and emotional needs. Therefore, active coping strategy integration is paramount to improved general well-being and life satisfaction in people with osteoarthritis.

9.4.7. Support Systems and Resources

Osteoarthritis (OA) management is highly facilitated by robust support systems and resources that empower patients to own the treatment decisions. Shared decision-making (SDM) approaches, in this instance via decision aids (DAs), have been shown to facilitate informed decisions regarding surgical versus non-surgical interventions. Evidence indicates that elderly patients and patients with higher levels of pain have individual preferences for treatment strategies, which could be fully addressed through diligent application of DAs across varied care settings (Hurley et al., 2020). Differences in burden of illness according to socioeconomic status also underscore the need for personalized support systems that facilitate equitable access to necessary diagnosis and treatment for osteoarthritis (Steel et al., 2014). Through using these resources, healthcare professionals can develop an interprofessional environment that facilitates patient participation and adherence to care plans, thereby maximizing outcomes for those living with this chronic condition (Figure 9.19).

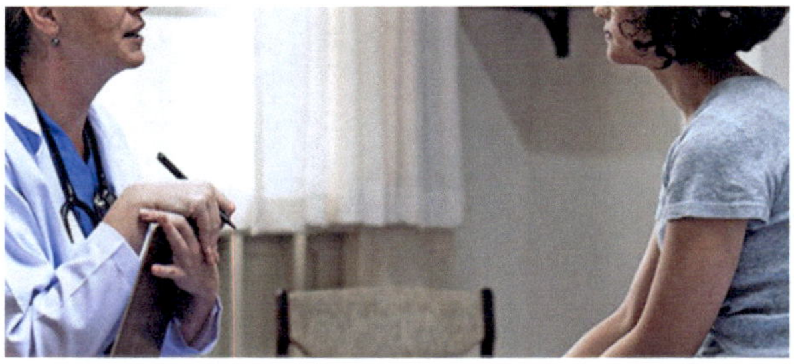

Figure 9.19. The management of osteoarthritis (OA) is significantly enhanced by robust support systems and resources that empower patients in their treatment decisions.

Source: https://trustees.aha.org/sites/default/files/TT_0818_van_dyke_decision_making_900.jpg.

9.4.8. Community and Family Involvement

Family and community involvement is crucial in the management of osteoarthritis, especially in relation to patient recovery and quality of life. The role of family plays a significant contribution in medication compliance and exercise regimens, which are central to pain relief and improvement of mobility. Contact with community resources, such as support groups or health programs in the neighborhood, creates a social environment in which individuals with osteoarthritis are less isolated and in a better position to manage their condition. Also, studies demonstrate that conditions in the physical and social environments are able to affect outcomes of recovery following surgery, such as joint replacements, in support of the value of taking a holistic treatment approach. Both family and social networks establish a framework of support that addresses not only the physical manifestations of osteoarthritis but also the emotional and psychological difficulties faced by patients and thereby enhances overall rehabilitation processes (Ejindu et al., 2012; Sampson, 2016).

9.4.9. Long-term Outlook for Patients

The long-term outcome of osteoarthritis (OA) patients remains an issue, as the natural course of this degenerative joint disorder can significantly affect quality of life. Evidence does exist that shows management programs, including physical therapy and pharmacologic intervention, are critical in alleviating symptoms and enhancing functional ability. For instance, randomized controlled trials , such as those testing the effectiveness of acupuncture reveal that treatment modalities that are tailored to individuals are capable of producing robust pain relief and mobility improvement among OA patients (Becker-Witt et al., 2003). In addition, the shift toward brief hospital stay following joint replacement procedures, despite being cost-reducing, may prove difficult to achieve optimal post-operative rehabilitation, potentially slowing down patients' regaining functional independence (Jones, 2014). Therefore, the integration of holistic long-term care, including ongoing assessment and supportive systems, is needed to improve the prognosis and overall well-being of patients with osteoarthritis.

Test Your Knowledge

1. How does OA affect sleep and overall quality of life?
2. What are the common psychological challenges faced by people living with OA?

Summary

Osteoarthritis treatment, particularly through arthroscopic methods, is one of the most important advances in treatment for such individuals. The systematic review here presents the likely effectiveness of treatments , such as CAM (comprehensive arthroscopic management), which not only provides significant pain alleviation and functional improvement but also can postpone the need for more aggressive procedures like total shoulder arthroplasty. While the findings indicate CAM yields promising outcomes, the variability in conversion rates to shoulder arthroplasty underlines the necessity for further studies in the field to establish standardized treatment protocols that can optimize patient results. The implication of the findings in the study also relates to the necessity of considering patient demographics and some osteoarthritis characteristics when making treatment choices. With the growing literature on osteoarthritis, it is increasingly clear that advanced methods and broad-based evaluations have to be employed to optimize patient care and quality of life for those afflicted with this degenerative condition (Nabergoj et al., 2025; Medviedev et al., 2025).

Knowledge of the management of osteoarthritis (OA) requires a balancing of several therapeutic regimes and current evidence of their effectiveness. A systematic review points to the value of topical medicament products of medicinal plants in that it suggests Arnica gel can be as effective in inducing pain relief as conventional non-steroidal anti-inflammatory medications , such as ibuprofen, but with a slightly less desirable adverse events profile (Cameron et al., 2013). Also, while many interventions based on the application of behavior change techniques in physiotherapy can potentially enhance patient adherence to physical activity in lower limb OA, variation in reporting interventions limits the clarity of conclusions drawn from existing studies (Duda et al., 2019). This convergence of herbal treatment and behavioral therapy illustrates that more high-quality research is required to identify the optimal modalities for the alleviation of symptoms of osteoarthritis and quality of life in patients, proving the complexity of OA treatment.

KEY TERMS FROM THIS CHAPTER

- Antioxidants
- Behavior change
- Body mass index (BMI)
- Chondrocytes
- Chronic disease
- Chronic pain
- Cognitive-behavioral therapies
- Community involvement
- Complexity
- Decision aids (DAs)
- Degenerative joint disease
- Diclofenac sodium
- Disability
- Gender variation
- Genetic susceptibility
- Hand osteoarthritis
- Mechanism
- Mental health
- Movement variability
- Multifactorial pathology

CRITICAL THINKING QUESTIONS

1. **What is the primary pathological feature of osteoarthritis?**
   a. Synovial membrane inflammation
   b. Cartilage degeneration and loss
   c. Bone marrow edema
   d. Autoimmune joint destruction
2. **Which joints are most commonly affected by primary osteoarthritis?**
   a. Distal interphalangeal joints, knees, hips, and lumbar spine
   b. Metacarpophalangeal joints and wrists
   c. Shoulders and elbows
   d. Small joints of the feet only
3. **Which clinical symptom is most characteristic of osteoarthritis?**
   a. Morning stiffness lasting more than 1 hour
   b. Rapid onset of joint swelling
   c. Joint pain that worsens with activity and improves with rest
   d. Symmetrical joint involvement
4. **Which radiographic feature is NOT typical of osteoarthritis?**
   a. Joint space narrowing
   b. Subchondral sclerosis
   c. Marginal osteophyte formation
   d. Juxta-articular erosions
5. **Which of the following is considered a modifiable risk factor for osteoarthritis?**
   a. Age
   b. Female gender
   c. Joint injury and obesity
   d. Genetics

Answers to Critical Thinking Questions

1. (b) 2. (a) 3. (c) 4. (d) 5. (c)

Short Answer Questions

1. What are the primary causes of osteoarthritis?
2. How does age contribute to the development of OA?
3. What are the hallmark clinical symptoms of OA?
4. How does joint pain in OA typically present and progress?
5. What are the first-line pharmacologic treatments for OA?
6. How effective are NSAIDs and topical analgesics in managing OA symptoms?
7. How does OA affect physical mobility and independence?
8. What is the impact of chronic pain from OA on mental health?

References

1. Salazar, A., Dueñas, M., Ojeda, B., & Failde, I. (2014). Association of painful musculoskeletal conditions and migraine headache with mental and sleep disorders among adults with disabilities, Spain, 2007-2008. *Preventing chronic disease*, *11*, E30. https://doi.org/10.5888/pcd11.130144 (accessed on 17th June 2025).
2. Ahlbäck, S., Allen, M., Andersson, G. B. J., Appel, H., Arnold, J. B., Balkfors, B., Buhl-Nielsen, B., et al. (1995). Osteoarthritis of the knee after injury to the anterior cruciate ligament or meniscus: The influence of time and age. https://core.ac.uk/download/pdf/81947525.pdf (accessed on 17th June 2025).
3. Aigner, T., Kuttapitiya, A., Balanescu, A. R., Bannuru, R. R., Chou, R., da Costa, B. R., Danielsson, L., et al. (2014). Future directions for the management of pain in osteoarthritis. https://core.ac.uk/download/29469467.pdf (accessed on 17th June 2025).
4. Aiyegbusi, A. I., Akinbo, S. R. A., & Ishola, T. (2019). Pain coping strategies with functional disability and quality of life in patients with knee osteoarthritis in Lagos, Nigeria. https://core.ac.uk/download/478338871.pdf (accessed on 17th June 2025).
5. Alexopoulos, A., Hirvasniemi, J., & Tümer, N. (2022). Early detection of knee osteoarthritis using deep learning on knee magnetic resonance images. http://arxiv.org/abs/2209.01192 (accessed on 17th June 2025).
6. Allan, J. L., Cooper, C. L., Gray, S., Phillips, A., et al. (2017). Effect of different types of physical activity on activities of daily living in older adults: Systematic review and meta-analysis. https://core.ac.uk/download/77614656.pdf (accessed on 17th June 2025).
7. Allan, R., Dell'Isola, A., Marreiros, S. S. P., Smith, T., et al. (2016). Identification of clinical phenotypes in knee osteoarthritis: A systematic review of the literature. https://core.ac.uk/download/293883849.pdf (accessed on 17th June 2025).
8. Altman, R., Bennell, K., Benson, J., Bjorner, J., Chen, A., Collins, J., et al. (2017). Cross-cultural and construct validity of the Animated Activity Questionnaire. https://core.ac.uk/download/293881766.pdf (accessed on 17th June 2025).
9. Alyousef, Y. S., Johnston, V., Ross, M. H., Smith, T., et al. (2024). Experiences of working with lower limb osteoarthritis: A qualitative study. https://core.ac.uk/download/654321408.pdf (accessed on 17th June 2025).
10. Amano, K., Li, X., Ma, C. B., Pedoia, V., et al. (2016). Persistent biomechanical alterations after ACL reconstruction are associated with early cartilage matrix changes detected by quantitative MR. https://core.ac.uk/download/323079514.pdf (accessed on 17th June 2025).
11. Amante, D. J., Shenette, L. L., Wainaina, S., Balakrishnan, K., Bhatia, S., Lee, J. A., Lemon, S., et al. (2024). Digital health tools and behavioral strategies to increase engagement with diabetes self-management education and support: Design and feasibility of DM-BOOST. *The Science of Diabetes Self-Management and Care, 50*, 497–509. https://www.semanticscholar.org/paper/74debe4d98dab8a73ccacc58c319e35d9e3edce2 (accessed on 17th June 2025).
12. van de Water, E., Oosterlinck, M., Dumoulin, M., Korthagen, N. M., van Weeren, P. R., van den Broek, J., Everts, H., Pille, F., & van Doorn, D. A. (2017). The preventive effects of two nutraceuticals on experimentally induced acute synovitis. *Equine veterinary journal*, *49*(4), 532–538. https://doi.org/10.1111/evj.12629(accessed on 17th June 2025).

13. Andrianakos, A., Fargas-Babjak, A., Gur, A., Khadilkar, A., Molsberger, A., White, A., Shaughnessy, A. F., et al. (2007). Short-term efficacy of physical interventions in osteoarthritic knee pain: A systematic review and meta-analysis of randomized placebo-controlled trials. https://core.ac.uk/download/29019035.pdf (accessed on 17th June 2025).

14. Angelini, G. D., Ascione, R., Caputo, M., Reeves, B., et al. (2004). Monitoring the performance of residents during training in off-pump coronary surgery. https://core.ac.uk/download/pdf/81151153.pdf (accessed on 17th June 2025).

15. Arden, N., Beard, D., Campbell, H., Campbell, T. M., et al. (2013). Total or Partial Knee Arthroplasty Trial – TOPKAT: Study protocol for a randomized controlled trial. https://core.ac.uk/download/19475339.pdf (accessed on 17th June 2025).

16. Aspelund, T., Eiriksdottir, G., Gudnason, V., Harris, T., et al. (2016). Incidence and prevalence of total joint replacements due to osteoarthritis in the elderly: Risk factors and factors associated with late life prevalence in the AGES-Reykjavik Study. https://core.ac.uk/download/38283791.pdf (accessed on 17th June 2025).

17. Avenell, A., Bolland, M., Fraser, C., Hudson, J., et al. (2017). Effects of weight loss interventions for adults who are obese on mortality, cardiovascular disease and cancer: A systematic review and meta-analysis. https://core.ac.uk/download/131025046.pdf (accessed on 17th June 2025).

18. Steel N, Hardcastle AC, Bachmann MO, et al

19. Economic inequalities in burden of illness, diagnosis and treatment of five long-term conditions in England: panel study. BMJ Open 2014;4:e005530. doi: 10.1136/bmjopen-2014-005530

20. (accessed on 17th June 2025).

21. Bakuła, P. R., Jałocha, K., & Zygadło, J. (2025). Exploring Novel Non-Operative Treatments for Osteoarthritis: An Examination of Innovative Therapies. *Quality in Sport*, *38*, 58169. https://doi.org/10.12775/QS.2025.38.58169(accessed on 17th June 2025).

22. Wride, J., & Bannigan, K. (2019). Investigating the prevalence of anxiety and depression in people living with patellofemoral pain in the UK: the Dep-Pf Study. *Scandinavian journal of pain*, *19*(2), 375–382. https://doi.org/10.1515/sjpain-2018-0347 (accessed on 17th June 2025).

23. Banning, M. (2006). The use of topical diclofenac in the pain management of osteoarthritis of the knee. https://core.ac.uk/download/335728.pdf (accessed on 17th June 2025).

24. Banning, M. (2009). Diclofenac solution (Pennsaid) in the management of osteoarthritis of the knee: Patient implications. https://core.ac.uk/download/335974.pdf (accessed on 17th June 2025).

25. Bashinskaya, B. (2016). Effects of obesity on walking patterns and adaptability during obstacle crossing. https://open.bu.edu/bitstream/2144/16125/1/Bashinskaya_bu_0017N_11114.pdf (accessed on 17th June 2025).

26. Becker-Witt, C., Brinkhaus, B., Hummelsberger, J., Irnich, D., et al. (2003). Acupuncture randomized trials (ART) in patients with chronic low back pain and osteoarthritis of the knee: Design and protocols. https://core.ac.uk/download/16432619.pdf (accessed on 17th June 2025).

27. Bennett, L., Crilly, A., Dunning, L., Ferrell, W., et al. (2015). Proteinase-activated

receptor 2 modulates OA-related pain, cartilage and bone pathology. https://core.ac.uk/download/42368902.pdf (accessed on 17th June 2025).

28. Bolt, D. M., Fink, J., Greenlee, R. T., Magnan, S., et al. (2015). The relationship of individual comorbid chronic conditions to diabetes care quality. https://core.ac.uk/download/323070914.pdf (accessed on 17th June 2025).

29. Breen, S., Harrison, A. J., & Kenny, I. C. (2012). The role of previous anterior cruciate ligament injury on the variability of joint kinematics and coordination during a match specific land-cut task. https://core.ac.uk/download/29018778.pdf (accessed on 17th June 2025).

30. Byham-Gray, L., Ghajar, M., Hawes, C., Radler, B., et al. (2024). Diet modification reduces pain and improves function in adults with osteoarthritis: A systematic review. https://core.ac.uk/download/618196760.pdf (accessed on 17th June 2025).

31. Cameron, M., & Chrubasik, S. (2013). Topical herbal therapies for treating osteoarthritis (review). https://core.ac.uk/download/322372947.pdf (accessed on 17th June 2025).

32. Chan, D., Kao, P. Y. P., Samartzis, D., Sham, P. C., et al. (2011). Genetics of lumbar disk degeneration: Technology, study designs, and risk factors. https://core.ac.uk/download/37968810.pdf (accessed on 17th June 2025).

33. Chen, M. Y. R. (2016). Obesity, intergenerational programming, and epigenetics: Emerging concepts and challenges. https://open.bu.edu/bitstream/2144/14400/7/Chen_bu_0017N_10467_web.pdf (accessed on 17th June 2025).

34. Courties, A., Dell'Isola, A., King, C. D., Heinegård, D., et al. (2018). Classification of patients with knee osteoarthritis in clinical phenotypes: Data from the osteoarthritis initiative. https://core.ac.uk/download/293885123.pdf (accessed on 17th June 2025).

35. Crawford, R. J., Elliott, J. M., Hancock, M. J., Smith, A., et al. (2018). Advancing imaging technologies for patients with spinal pain: With a focus on whiplash injury. https://core.ac.uk/download/161704527.pdf (accessed on 17th June 2025).

36. Duda, J., Fenton, S., Gautrey, C., Greig, C., et al. (2019). Effectiveness of behavior change techniques in physiotherapy interventions to promote physical activity adherence in lower limb osteoarthritis patients: A systematic review. https://core.ac.uk/download/287581813.pdf (accessed on 17th June 2025).

37. Ejindu, V., Hermansson, M., Heron, C., Kiely, P., et al. (2012). Quantitative sensory testing in painful hand osteoarthritis demonstrates features of peripheral sensitization. https://core.ac.uk/download/10674768.pdf (accessed on 17th June 2025).

38. Ejohn Editorial Board. (2025). Psychosocial risk prevention strategies in the workplace. *European Journal of Occupational Health Nursing*. https://www.semanticscholar.org/paper/dd902c4e71a2a733f9c145d71385903c9f6c55ac (accessed on 17th June 2025).

39. Esty, A. R., Goodman, D. C., Fisher, E. S., Tomek, I. M., & Bell, J. E. (2010). Trends and regional variation in hip, knee and shoulder replacement. https://core.ac.uk/download/71355430.pdf (accessed on 17th June 2025).

40. Fawole, H., Idowu, O., Osadiaye, O. A., Akinrolie, O., Ibekaku, M., Ojo, M., Kolawole, F. O., et al. (2024). A systematic review on the effects of non-pharmacological interventions for fatigue among people with upper and/or lower limb osteoarthritis. *Rheumatology Advances in Practice,*

8. https://www.semanticscholar.org/paper/f47cc473e9dec5060c4e753fceae5e29e4da67bf (accessed on 17th June 2025).

41. Fayyaz, M., Muneer, B., Iqbal, A., Bilal, M. A., Tabassum, H., & Shahbaz, S. (2023). Mechanical Causes of Osteoarthritis in Adults, its Diagnosis and Treatment : Osteoarthritis in Adults. *THE THERAPIST (Journal of Therapies &Amp; Rehabilitation Sciences)*, *4*(04), 02–07. https://doi.org/10.54393/tt.v4i04.104(accessed on 17th June 2025).

42. Gaya, D., Hampson, R., Latosinska, A., McInnes, I., et al. (2017). Urinary proteomics can define distinct diagnostic inflammatory arthritis subgroups. https://core.ac.uk/download/80696793.pdf (accessed on 17th June 2025).

43. Ginsburg, P. B. (2009). Efficiency and quality: Controlling cost growth in health care reform. https://core.ac.uk/download/71347538.pdf (accessed on 17th June 2025).

44. Glennon, M. K. (2019). Today's fibromyalgia. https://core.ac.uk/download/286697650.pdf (accessed on 17th June 2025).

45. Hall, A. J., Mamas, M. A., Myint, P. K., Smith, T., et al. (2015). Association between osteoarthritis and cardiovascular disease: Systematic review and meta-analysis. https://core.ac.uk/download/41991643.pdf (accessed on 17th June 2025).

46. Hurley, V. B., Kearing, S., Rodriguez, H. P., Savitz, L. A., et al. (2020). Decision aid implementation and patients' preferences for hip and knee osteoarthritis treatment: Insights from the High Value Healthcare Collaborative. https://core.ac.uk/download/323077909.pdf (accessed on 17th June 2025).

47. Jinks, C., O'Neill, T., & Ong, B. N. (2007). Decision-making regarding total knee replacement surgery: A qualitative meta-synthesis. https://core.ac.uk/download/28874669.pdf (accessed on 17th June 2025).

48. Jones, L. J. (2014). The effect of telephone follow-up on pain experienced by patients after knee replacement surgery. https://core.ac.uk/download/144551476.pdf (accessed on 17th June 2025).

49. Kendall, J. M., Latter, V. S., Nasal Diamorphine Trial Group, & Reeves, B. C. (2001). Multicenter randomized controlled trial of nasal diamorphine for analgesia in children and teenagers with clinical fractures. https://core.ac.uk/download/13108486.pdf (accessed on 17th June 2025).

50. Kyrou, Ioannis and Weickert, Martin O. (2010) Clinical problems caused by obesity. Working Paper. Endotext.org : MDText.com, Inc.(accessed on 17th June 2025).

51. Lacy, A. (2017). Dietary fat and the prevalence of hand osteoarthritis: Data from the osteoarthritis initiative. https://core.ac.uk/download/142080935.pdf (accessed on 17th June 2025).

52. Lean, M. (2011). VLED and formula LED in the management of type 2 diabetes: Defining the clinical need and research requirements. https://core.ac.uk/download/9648399.pdf (accessed on 17th June 2025).

53. Lee, A., Vickers, A., MacLennan, A. H., Vickers, A. J., et al. (2001). Systematic reviews of complementary therapies–An annotated bibliography. Part 1: Acupuncture. https://core.ac.uk/download/57903.pdf (accessed on 17th June 2025).

54. Medviedev, Y., Piddubnyi, S., Zaslavska, O., Posvistak, O., & Nalimova, V. (2025). Impact of social media on political campaigns: Management, strategies and results. *Journal of*

Information Systems Engineering and Management. https://www.semanticscholar.org/paper/a2fd668b2a3a899413668468dca6331752af5840 (accessed on 17th June 2025).

55. Mobosi, K. A. (2025). The impact of workplace safety training programs on reducing occupational hazards in high-risk industries. *World Journal of Advanced Research and Reviews*. https://www.semanticscholar.org/paper/063d59ba9ff476dd50a9f7177fef13fc16391ce6 (accessed on 17th June 2025).
56. Nabergoj, M., Denard, P., Collin, P., van Rooij, F., & Lädermann, A. (2025). Arthroscopic management of glenohumeral osteoarthritis: A systematic review of clinical outcomes and treatment durability. *The Hive–Musculoskeletal Journal*. https://www.semanticscholar.org/paper/93bff23107b1f5136a4cf30807164c388ec5221d (accessed on 17th June 2025).
57. Nicholl, B. I., Bedson, J., Broadbent, E., Green, D. J., Dieppe, P., Duncan, R., Dworkin, R., et al. (2014). Osteoarthritis and the rule of halves. https://core.ac.uk/download/9651866.pdf (accessed on 17th June 2025).
58. Nowlan, N. C. (2015). Biomechanics of fetal movement. https://core.ac.uk/download/76995826.pdf (accessed on 17th June 2025).
59. Pallivalappil, F. S. (2022). Quality of life in knee osteoarthritis. https://core.ac.uk/download/544279687.pdf; https://core.ac.uk/download/544279660.pdf (accessed on 17th June 2025).
60. Praba, R., et al. (2023). Prediction of osteoarthritis in the knee by KOA diagnosis using artificial intelligence-based techniques. https://core.ac.uk/download/596247541.pdf (accessed on 17th June 2025).
61. Price, C. A. (2017). Tai Chi/Qi Gong in mental health treatment and prevention: A review of meta-analytic evidence and an analysis of evidence congruence with training practices. https://core.ac.uk/download/84397718.pdf (accessed on 17th June 2025).
62. Rosenberg, N. (2025). Walking ability after total knee arthroplasty: A comprehensive review. *Cureus, 17*. https://www.semanticscholar.org/paper/139f250da83035707752ec18ab909ca7e575c9f3 (accessed on 17th June 2025).
63. Rowan, A. D., Cassidy, A., MacGregor, A. J., Valdes, A. M., Olafsdottir, A. S., Teucher, B., et al. (2010). Dietary garlic and hip osteoarthritis: Evidence of a protective effect and putative mechanism of action. https://core.ac.uk/download/2776285.pdf (accessed on 17th June 2025).
64. Salazar, A., Arnow, B., Baca, R., Badley, E., Ojeda, B., Gleicher, Y., Failde, I., et al. (2013). Undiagnosed mood disorders and sleep disturbances in primary care patients with chronic musculoskeletal pain. https://core.ac.uk/download/161360209.pdf (accessed on 17th June 2025).
65. Sampson, B. A. (2016). Patient outcomes following hip and knee joint replacement surgery: Role of the social and physical environment in recovery. https://core.ac.uk/download/72052957.pdf (accessed on 17th June 2025).
66. Sinha, D., Dash, S. S., & Kachhwaha, R. (2024). Systematic review on treatment of knee osteoarthritis. *Himalayan Journal of Health Sciences*. https://www.semanticscholar.org/paper/d6b1daa1228e21bd964031a0666125dd463d2165 (accessed on 17th June 2025).
67. Bates, S. et al (2014). Arthritis and disability. https://core.ac.uk/download/pdf/30673486.pdf (accessed on 17th June 2025).

68. Swezey, L. (2018). Pain management: A flowsheet for providers. https://core.ac.uk/download/213462537.pdf (accessed on 17th June 2025).

69. Valdes, A. M., Anderson, J. J., arcOGEN Consortium and arcOGEN Collaborators, Brown, M. A., Castaño-Betancourt, M. C., Day-Williams, A. G., Dieppe, P. A., et al. (2013). The genetic contribution to severe post-traumatic osteoarthritis. https://core.ac.uk/download/19210660.pdf (accessed on 17th June 2025).

70. Wallace, C. (2018). Effects of glucocorticoids on chondrocytes and cartilage. https://open.bu.edu/bitstream/2144/31287/5/Wallace_bu_0017N_13687.pdf (accessed on 17th June 2025).

71. Zhu, B., Zhu, D., Xue, X., Yang, H., & Zhang, S. (2025). Behavioral therapy–based digital interventions for treating osteoarthritis: Systematic review and meta-analysis. *Journal of Medical Internet Research, 27*. https://www.semanticscholar.org/paper/df91c672c63eff6e2a6371bd6c6559c03ab5307b (accessed on 17th June 2025).

CALCIUM AND BONE METABOLISM DISORDERS

10

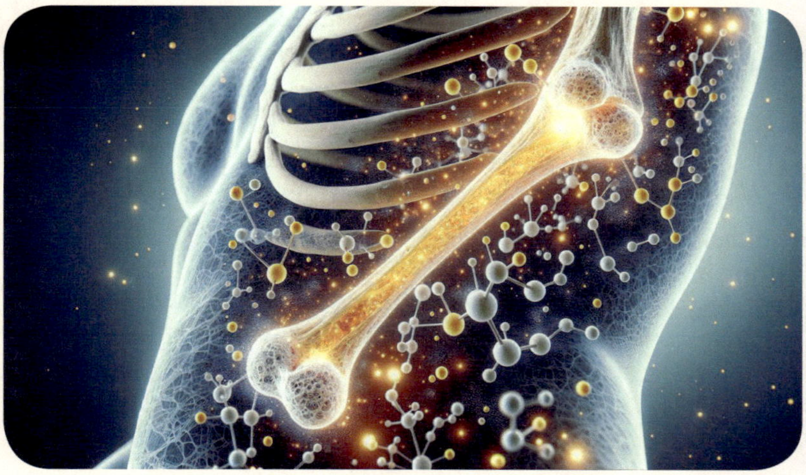

LEARNING OBJECTIVES

After studying this chapter, you will be able to:

1. Understand calcium homeostasis
2. Explain osteoporosis
3. Focus on osteomalacia and rickets
4. Describe hypercalcemia and hypocalcemia

Introduction

Bone metabolism is a complex process that is closely linked to overall health and relies heavily on the preservation of calcium homeostasis, an essential mineral. Dysregulation of calcium homeostasis can potentially lead to serious skeletal disease, expressed as conditions, such as osteoporosis, osteomalacia, and other metabolic bone diseases. The equilibrium between bone resorption and formation is maintained by an interactive dynamics of hormones like parathyroid hormone (PTH) and vitamin D, as well as primary enzymes like alkaline phosphatases. The enzymes play a critical role in ensuring proper mineralization of bone, but simultaneously could be the cause of damaging health effects under circumstances of imbalance (Bover et al., 2018). Moreover, new findings regarding the recognition of the gut microbiota suggest that food components may influence calcium absorption and, thus, bone metabolism (Meheust et al., 2010). Thus, a holistic view of the participation of calcium in bone metabolism is essential to design remedies and understand disorders related to bones (Figure 10.1).

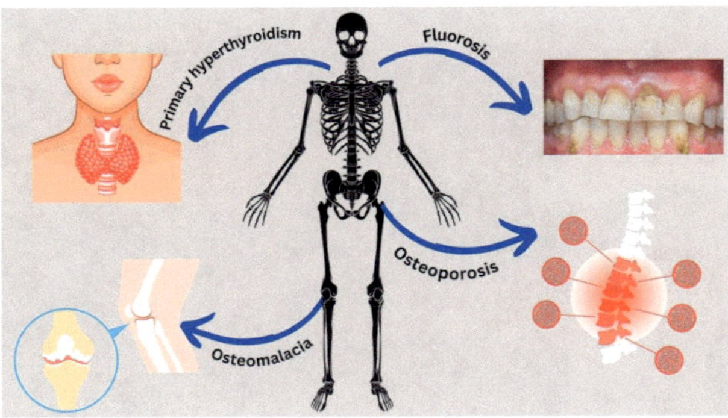

Figure 10.1. Disorders in calcium homeostasis can lead to significant skeletal issues, resulting in conditions , such as osteoporosis, osteomalacia, and various forms of metabolic bone disease.

Source: https://image.oaes.cc/ebedc12b-14af-4b7e-9c28-3d619e5bb933/mtod4038.fig.1.jpg.

10.1. Calcium Homeostasis

Learning Outcome

1. Understand mechanisms of calcium absorption in the intestines
2. Discuss the role of vitamin D in calcium metabolism
3. Explain the hormonal regulation of the calcium level
4. Focus on calcium storage in bones
5. Describe calcium release from bones
6. Identify factors affecting calcium homeostasis
7. Learn the consequences of disrupted calcium homeostasis
8. Understand diagnostic methods for assessing calcium levels
9. Know the importance of maintaining calcium balance

Regulation of calcium homeostasis is not only vital for the integrity of the skeleton but also for physiological function as a whole. The process is complex and involves a cascade of hormonal and cellular events that regulate with precision levels of calcium in the blood and tissues. Hormones , such as PTH and calcitonin play a vital role in stimulating the release of calcium from bone or deposition, respectively. In addition, vitamin D is crucial in maintaining intestinal calcium absorption, and studies have established its broad influence on musculoskeletal integrity (Bover et al., 2017). Dysregulation of these control systems can lead to significant clinical impacts, including hyperparathyroidism or osteoporosis. In farm animals, like dairy cows, the calcium requirement changes during calving are indicative of dynamic regulation of calcium homeostasis. The transition to lactation demands calcium metabolism adaptations that, when suboptimal, can result in such disorders as hypocalcemia, further emphasizing the importance of adequate calcium regulatory mechanisms (Martín-Tereso et al., 2011).

10.1.1. Mechanisms of Calcium Absorption in the Intestines

Calcium uptake mechanisms in the intestines are complex and highly regulated, which is crucial to bone health and general mineral homeostasis. Two transport processes characterize intestinal calcium absorption: passive paracellular and active transcellular transport. The latter process is facilitated by calcium uptake by specific transport proteins, such as TRPV6, which facilitates calcium ion entry into intestinal epithelial cells. This is then mediated by diet, e.g., the presence of prebiotics that can enhance the bioavailability and efficiency of calcium absorption, potentially enhancing gut health markers, including bifidobacteria counts (Meheust et al., 2010). Moreover, diseases that affect calcium homeostasis, e.g., hypocalcemia in milked dairy cows, illustrate that inadequate adaptability in calcium absorption leads to metabolic disturbances. For example, improper reorganization of intestines to address the requirements for calcium can initiate hypocalcemia complications (Martín-Tereso et al., 2011) (Figure 10.2).

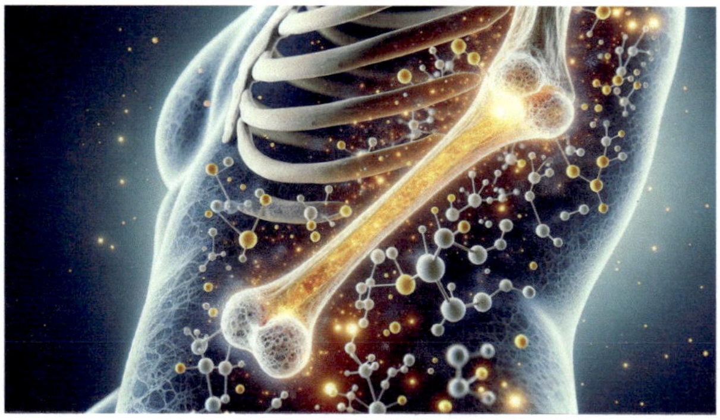

Figure 10.2. The mechanisms of calcium absorption in the intestines are complex and highly regulated, playing a critical role in maintaining bone health and overall mineral balance.

Source: https://drinkharlo.com/cdn/shop/articles/thumbnail_36714808-6c6a-4935-9b4e-59f3e9975e63.jpg?v=1711054405.

10.1.2. Role of Vitamin D in Calcium Metabolism

Vitamin D plays a role in the metabolism of calcium and exerts a profound influence on bone and the skeletal system. Its primary physiological effect is to preserve blood calcium levels by increasing intestinal absorption of calcium and phosphate, two essential minerals for mineralization of the bone. When the body is deprived of vitamins, it is unable to control sufficient calcium in the body, resulting in diseases, such as hypocalcemia and osteoporosis, consequently making the bones weaker and increasing one's risk of breaking them. Moreover, chronic vitamin D deficiency has been associated with a variety of metabolic disorders that affect bone density and rates of turnover, which are essential in preventing disorders of calcium and bone metabolism. Evidence indicates that insufficient vitamin D not only generates systemic disease but also directly impacts the ability of the bones to maintain their architectural integrity, and hence it is essential that optimal calcium metabolism and bone health are afforded sufficient vitamin D synthesis (Dalmaceno et al., 2020).

10.1.3. Hormonal Regulation of Calcium Levels

Hormonal regulation of calcium status is important to maintain bone integrity and overall metabolism, particularly in disorders that interfere with calcium homeostasis. The key hormones involved are PTH, calcitonin, and vitamin D, each playing a unique role in the mobilization and absorption of calcium. PTH secretion occurs in response to low serum calcium, stimulating osteoclasts for bone breakdown and increasing renal reabsorption of calcium. On the other hand, calcitonin lowers calcium by inhibiting osteoclast action and stimulating the deposition of calcium in bones. The effect of dietary factors, including the dietary cation–anion difference (DCAD), can also affect calcium homeostasis. For instance, modifications to dietary ingredients induce systemic acidosis and thus allow for calcium clearance from the circulation and influence metabolic adaptation, and this would be particularly relevant to transition dairy cows with hypocalcemia at calving, as presented in the results in Martín-Tereso et al. (2011). These hormonal relationships are central to the development of therapeutic interventions in calcium and bone metabolism disorders (Figure 10.3).

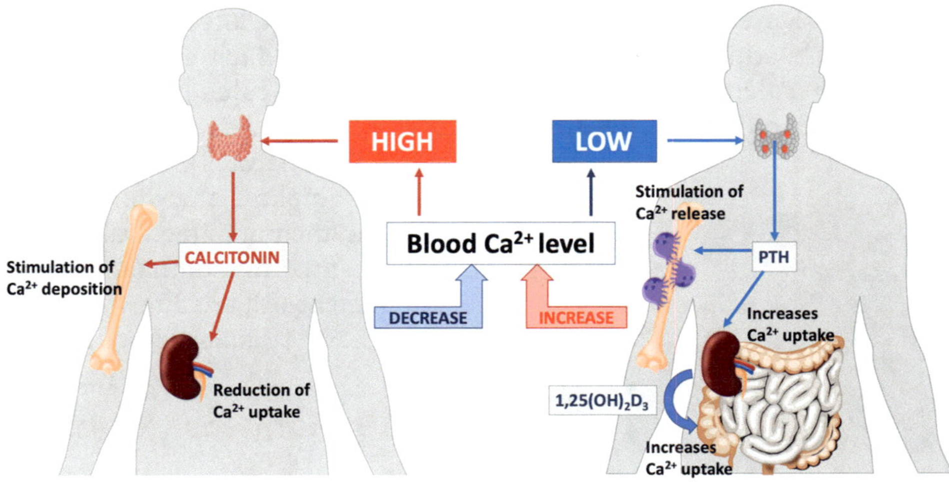

Figure 10.3. The hormonal regulation of calcium levels is crucial for maintaining bone health and overall metabolic functions, particularly in conditions that alter calcium homeostasis.

Source: https://journals.sagepub.com/cms/10.1177/1479973119878713/asset/14487b4c-18d7-4aaa-9675-48fcbbafbeec/assets/images/large/10.1177_1479973119878713-fig1.jpg.

10.1.4. Calcium Storage in Bones

Bone tissue is the primary calcium depot in the human body and maintains calcium homeostasis as well as bone health. Calcium ions are stored in the bone matrix as mineralized structures named hydroxyapatite, which provides the bones with strength and rigidity. The storage of calcium is controlled by various biological processes such as hormonal regulation and nutritional intake. For example, a deficiency in micronutrients like calcium can lead to low bone density, evident in research that compares the levels of calcium in the serum of pregnant versus non-pregnant women (Adriani et al., 2016). Moreover, the insufficiency of calcium intake, combined with over intakes of non-nutritional components, induces a risk to bone health, underlining the necessity of an equilibrium diet in order to maintain adequate calcium levels and prevent bone metabolism disorders (Buckton et al., 2014). Thus, it is important to know how calcium is stored in bones to prevent and treat bone metabolism disorders.

10.1.5. Calcium Release from Bones

Release of bone calcium is a vital physiological process that assists with most of the metabolic activities of the body. Release of PTH is triggered by a decrease in serum concentration of calcium, stimulating osteoclast activity, which promotes bone resorption, thus releasing calcium into the blood. This responsive calcium homeostasis regulation and maintenance of various biological activities, like contraction and nerve function, are contingent on this process. A long-term disruption in this balance can lead to conditions , such as osteoporosis or hypercalcemia. In addition, factors , such as the status of vitamin D and diet overall also exert a significant effect on bone status, illustrating the dependence of skeletal health and nutrition. Understanding these processes is vital in designing interventions to prevent or manage disorders of calcium and bone metabolism, depending on why extensive research has been suggested in this area (Ajbage et al., 2015) (Figure 10.4).

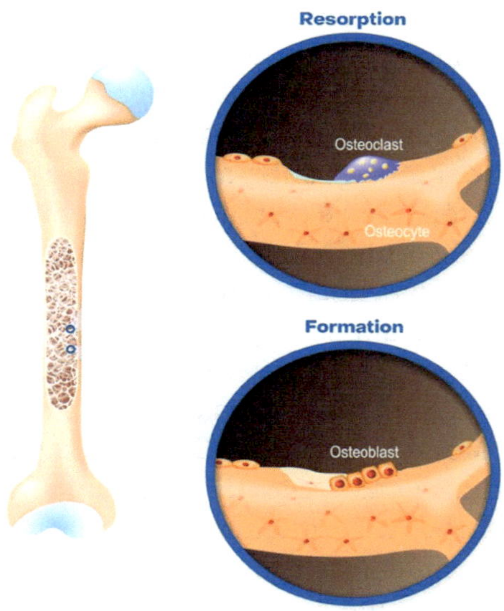

Figure 10.4. The release of calcium from bones is a crucial physiological process that underpins numerous metabolic functions within the body.

Source: https://spinehealth.org/wp-content/uploads/2024/02/SHJ-Special-Edition-Bone-Image-675x1080.jpg.

10.1.6. Factors Affecting Calcium Homeostasis

Calcium homeostasis is a complex physiological process controlled by several factors , including hormonal, dietary, and gut microbiota. The PTH and calcitonin play a central role in controlling serum calcium; they do this by controlling calcium reabsorption in the kidney and osteoclast and osteoblast control in the bones. Moreover, nutrition patterns have an enormous impact on the bioavailability of calcium; shortages can arise due to insufficient consumption, affecting bone density and strength. Current evidence emphasizes the implication of the gut microbiome in the absorption of calcium, where harmonized microbiota are capable of enhancing the bioavailability of calcium from food sources for improving skeletal health. For instance, prebiotic therapy has been found to have favorable impacts on calcium absorption, which is attributed to favorable alterations in gut microbiota , such as increased levels of bifidobacteria, which is critical in a move to attain maximal nutrient absorption and homeostasis (Meheust et al., 2010; Agas et al., 2015). These combined factors illustrate the intricacy of calcium regulation within the body.

10.1.7. Consequences of Disrupted Calcium Homeostasis

Disruption of calcium homeostasis has serious consequences on bone metabolism and overall health, considering the central role that calcium must play in numerous physiological functions. Either hypercalcemia or hypocalcemia normally follows from an imbalance in calcium, resulting in serious structural and density changes in bones. Hypercalcemia may provoke the excessive bone resorption by osteoclasts and lead to weakening of the skeletal system and increased fracture risk, while hypocalcemia may suppress the formation of new bone tissue and provoke the release of parathyroid hormone, stripping the calcium further from bone reserves.

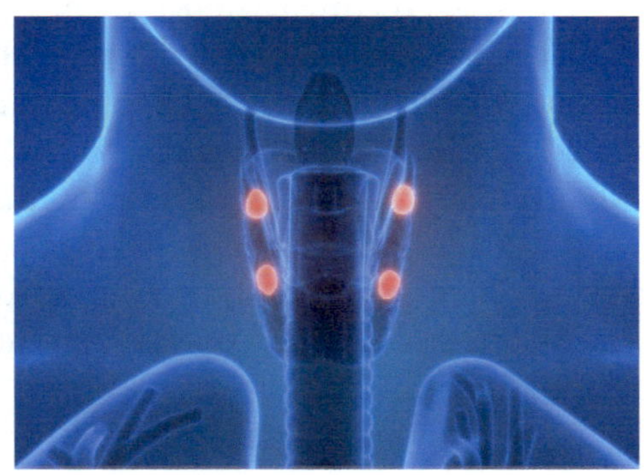

Figure 10.5. Hypercalcemia.

Source: https://cdn-prod.medicalnewstoday.com/content/images/articles/322/322012/diagram-of-parathyroid-glands-which-control-calcium-in-the-blood-and-may-lead-to-hypercalcemia.jpg.

Furthermore, the intricate interaction between bone and hematopoietic systems accentuates the probability that disturbed calcium homeostasis will affect immune function and blood cell production. If these homeostatic mechanisms are broken, the resultant dysfunction can cascade into diseases, highlighting the significance of calcium balance for bone and overall health (Agas et al., 2015) (Figure 10.5).

10.1.8. Diagnostic Methods for Assessing Calcium Levels

Effective diagnostic methods for the determination of calcium levels are significant in the treatment of bone and calcium metabolism disorders. Clinically, the most used method is serum calcium measurement, which measures total calcium and, if necessary, ionized calcium to give a better reflection of the metabolic status. Other examinations, such as the level of alkaline phosphatase, are also valuable since they indicate bone turnover as well as mineralization processes and therefore reflect normal and abnormal states of bone metabolism (Bover et al., 2018). Furthermore, new markers like Gla-rich protein (GRP) are promising in the evaluation of cardiovascular risk due to vascular calcification in patients with chronic kidney disease. It has been established by research that GRP levels correlate with various metabolic markers and are affected negatively as CKD progresses, which suggests their application as an early diagnostic marker of vascular injury (Almeida et al., 2020).

10.1.9. Importance of Maintaining Calcium Balance

Calcium balance maintenance is crucial for both skeletal and systemic health, as calcium is a critical component of bone development and bone remodeling. Changes in calcium status underlie severe disorders, including osteoporosis and rickets, leading to impaired bone quality and fracture hazard. In addition, newer evidence indicates that calcium absorption is food constituent and gut microbiota dependent, and prebiotic activity can enhance calcium absorption and contribute to positive bone density, particularly in adolescent and postmenopausal women (Meheust et al., 2010). Moreover, vitamin D is also significant in calcium metabolism as it not only helps in the absorption of calcium from the intestine but also influences muscle function, which is essential to maintain the bones' and the whole musculoskeletal system's strength (Bover et al., 2017). Thus, proper maintenance and achievement of calcium balance are essential for the prevention of metabolic bone diseases and general well-being (Figure 10.6).

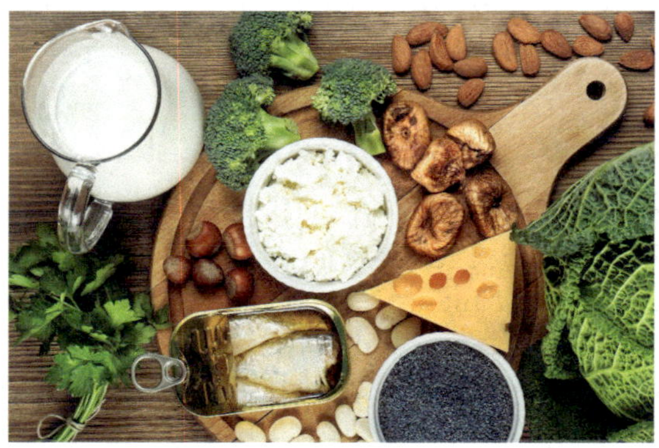

Figure 10.6. The maintenance of calcium balance is crucial for both skeletal and systemic health, as calcium plays a key role in bone formation and remodeling.

Source: https://nutritionsource.hsph.harvard.edu/wp-content/uploads/2020/10/shutterstock_366258461.jpg.

Test Your Knowledge

1. What role does vitamin D play in calcium absorption?
2. How does calcitonin affect calcium levels in the body?

10.2. Osteoporosis

Learning Outcome

1. Know the definition and types of osteoporosis
2. Identify risk factors for developing osteoporosis
3. Discuss symptoms and clinical manifestations
4. Understand the pathophysiology of bone loss
5. Describe diagnostic criteria and imaging techniques
6. Focus on treatment options and management strategies
7. Explain the role of calcium and vitamin D in prevention
8. Discuss lifestyle modifications to reduce risk
9. Know the impact of osteoporosis on quality of life

Osteoporosis, a condition with decreased bone density and increased fracture risk, is significantly influenced by calcium and vitamin D metabolism. Osteoporosis is a significant public health issue, particularly in aging populations, who experience a natural bone mass loss. The modifiable risk factors , such as low levels of serum vitamin D and insufficient calcium intake, have been demonstrated in studies to play central roles in exacerbating osteoporosis. Interventions against such risk factors could lead to a substantial decrease in the burden of osteoporotic fractures, indicating a possible 5% to 17% decline in prevalence where such deficiencies are being targeted (Aghamaleki et al., 2013). Moreover, the interfacing of osteoporosis and renal osteodystrophy highlights the complexity of bone disease in patients with chronic kidney disease, necessitating differential therapeutic approaches favoring bone metabolism effectively (Covic et al., 2017). Consequently, adequate vitamin D and calcium are not only needed for bone development but to forestall the complications of osteoporosis as well.

10.2.1. Definition and Types of Osteoporosis

Osteoporosis is a metabolic bone disorder that leads to low bone density and compromised structure of bone tissue with resultant rise in fracture risk. Osteoporosis is primarily classified into primary and secondary osteoporosis. Primary osteoporosis, which commonly affects postmenopausal women, is caused by endocrine alteration, i.e., menopause-induced loss of estrogen synthesis, the most vital hormone for maintaining bones. For comparison, secondary osteoporosis can occur as a result of other diseases of the medical type or long-term use of drugs that affect bone metabolism, including chronic kidney disease (CKD), which can make diagnosis and treatment challenging (Covic et al., 2017). In addition, the economic cost of hip fractures, a frequent complication of osteoporosis, heightens the need for efficient preventive steps, particularly via controllable risk factor control , such as calcium and vitamin D deficiency and inactivity (Aghamaleki et al., 2013). Such categorization is essential for effective management and treatment among the target individuals (Figure 10.7).

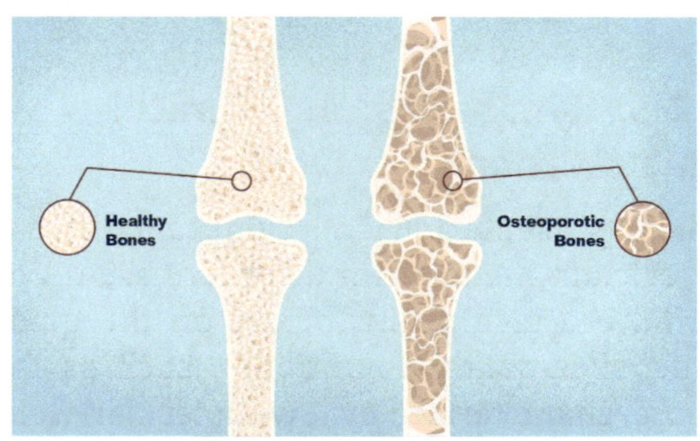

Figure 10.7. Osteoporosis is a metabolic bone disorder characterized by decreased bone density and structural deterioration of bone tissue, leading to increased fracture risk.

Source: https://spinehealth.org/wp-content/uploads/2024/01/Osteoporosis-new.jpg.

10.2.2. Risk Factors for Developing Osteoporosis

Osteoporosis, characterized by decreased bone density and increased fracture risk, is a consequence of an overlap of risk factors that can be categorized broadly as non-modifiable and modifiable risk factors. Age, gender, and family history are non-modifiable; post-menopausal women are particularly vulnerable to osteoporosis because of estrogen deficiencys impact on bone resorption. Modifiable risk factors, conversely, are amenable to intervention. Epidemiological studies are a key body of research that are indicative of the influence of lifestyle, such as inadequate levels of calcium and vitamin D intake, inadequate levels of exercise, and smoking, on the risk of osteoporosis (Aghamaleki et al., 2013). Specifically, inadequate serum vitamin D status and inadequate dietary intake of calcium and vitamin D can lead to a significantly elevated risk of fractures. Successful interventions for these modifiable risk factors can reduce the burden of osteoporotic fractures substantially, and therefore treatment and detection of these risk factors early on are key in the prevention of this disabling disease (Ajbage et al., 2015).

10.2.3. Symptoms and Clinical Manifestations

Clinical presentation and symptoms of bone and calcium metabolism disorders are diverse and have a significant impact on the quality of life of patients. Conditions , such as Dent disease, characterized by low-molecular-weight proteinuria, hypercalciuria, and nephrocalcinosis, possess a specific triad of symptoms that can lead to bone disorders and chronic kidney disease (CKD), particularly in CLCN5 mutation-positive patients. In addition, ectopic mineralization—the harmful precipitation of minerals in soft tissues—is seen in numerous diseases and causes morbidity and mortality by disrupting vascular and organ function. These diseases underscore the importance of understanding the pathogenesis of mineral dysregulation and its implications for the clinician. The various presentations not only require comprehensive diagnostic investigations but also indicate the necessity of individualized therapeutic plans aimed at the relief of symptoms of these metabolic disorders (Figure 10.8).

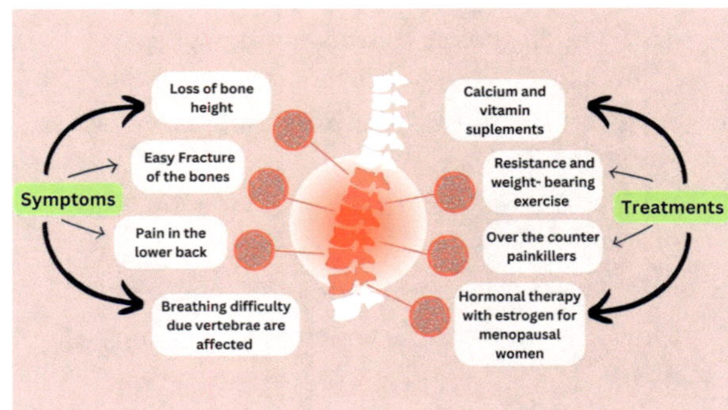

Figure 10.8. The symptoms and clinical manifestations of calcium and bone metabolism disorders are diverse and can significantly impact patient quality of life.

Source: https://image.oaes.cc/ebedc12b-14af-4b7e-9c28-3d619e5bb933/mtod4038.fig.2.jpg.

10.2.4. Pathophysiology of Bone Loss

Bone loss is a multifaceted process that is regulated by a number of physiological and pathologic mechanisms leading to conditions , such as osteoporosis. At the molecular level, the pathophysiology of bone loss is centered on the imbalance between osteoblast activity (bone formation) and osteoclast activity (bone resorption). Modulation of this balance is influenced by factors , such as age, hormonal status, and inflammatory markers. For example, increased galectin-3 levels are involved in osteogenic differentiation and regulation of bone remodeling and thus its potential therapeutic target in bone disorders (Fantauzzi et al., 2017). Further, Cushing's syndrome is just one among the many negative consequences of hypercortisolism that not only disrupts bone turnover but also leads to musculoskeletal disorders , such as osteoporosis and fracture (Biller et al., 2016). Knowledge of these mechanisms is essential to create effective treatments for disorders of calcium and bone metabolism.

10.2.5. Diagnostic Criteria and Imaging Techniques

Proper diagnosis of disorders of calcium and bone metabolism necessitates in-depth awareness of diagnostic criteria as well as cutting-edge imaging techniques. The conventional modalities , such as conventional crystal analysis (CCA) and radiographic imaging have been the gold standard for diagnosing disorders like calcium pyrophosphate crystal deposition disease (CPPD) (Wu et al., 2016). Yet the diagnostic imaging front is revolutionizing at a rapid rate, with newer techniques , such as U/Sand DECT turning out to be valuable assets in its toolkit. It has been discovered that U/S is greater than 80% sensitive for detecting CPPD crystals in peripheral joints compared to conventional radiography (Wu et al., 2016). Also, there is an urgent need for well-controlled studies to test these newer methods, particularly with respect to assessing the majority of patients who have unexplained presentations of bone disorders, frequently challenging the diagnostic process. Eventually, enhancement of diagnostic accuracy by employing these newer technologies can significantly contribute to patient management and outcomes (Figure 10.9).

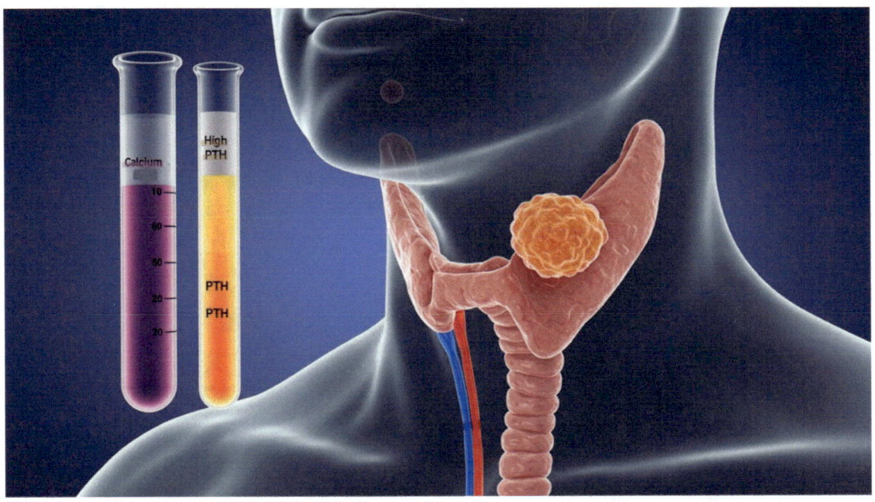

Figure 10.9. The accurate diagnosis of calcium and bone metabolism disorders necessitates a comprehensive understanding of both diagnostic criteria and advanced imaging techniques.

Source: https://media.licdn.com/dms/image/v2/D4E12AQFErYwY99JOUw/article-cover_image-shrink_720_1280/B4EZYMgzyWHUAM-/0/1743966649851?e=2147483647&v=beta&t=1rk0cf0taTcA-Mqf3D6nMA6L8a140Hdy5Dqf5XH-gQw.

10.2.6. Treatment Options and Management Strategies

Effective management modalities and treatment of calcium and bone metabolism disorders require a multidisciplinary approach, particularly in disease conditions , such as osteoporosis and vitamin D deficiency. Among the keystones of management is modification in lifestyle, such as dietary adjustment in increasing calcium intake by fortified food and supplements. Furthermore, weight-bearing exercises are of utmost significance to increase bone density and musculoskeletal integrity as a whole. Pharmacologic treatment, including bisphosphonates and other nonhormonal medications, is essential in the treatment of osteoporosis, especially in individuals with high fracture risk (Davis et al., 2017). Besides, an insight into the underlying biology of such diseases can inform novel therapies, as in more recent research exploring protective measures abstracted from different animal models to highlight promising therapies that may neutralize effects traditionally associated with such chronic diseases as chronic kidney disease (Arnold et al., 2018).

In the end, a personalized therapy program encompassing these steps is essential for optimizing patient benefit.

10.2.7. Role of Calcium and Vitamin D in Prevention

Calcium and vitamin D are key to the prevention of bone metabolism disorders, primarily in bone density increase and overall skeletal health. Vitamin D ensures effective intestinal absorption of calcium to maintain the body in a state of adequate calcium for bone mineralization. Vitamin D deficiency can lead to abnormal calcium levels, contributing to disease in susceptible individuals, such as the elderly and those with limited sun exposure. Evidence stresses that a serum 25(OH)D concentration higher than 30 ng/mL is necessary for overall skeletal well-being and prevention of metabolic diseases from a lack of vitamin D (Caffarelli et al., 2023). Furthermore, adequate vitamin D contributes to immunomodulatory effects that can influence oral health, thereby impacting the prevention and management of dental problems and overall health (Broniec et al., 2024). On that note, it is thus a simultaneous intake of vitamin D and calcium that becomes a crucial method in preventing bone diseases (Figure 10.10).

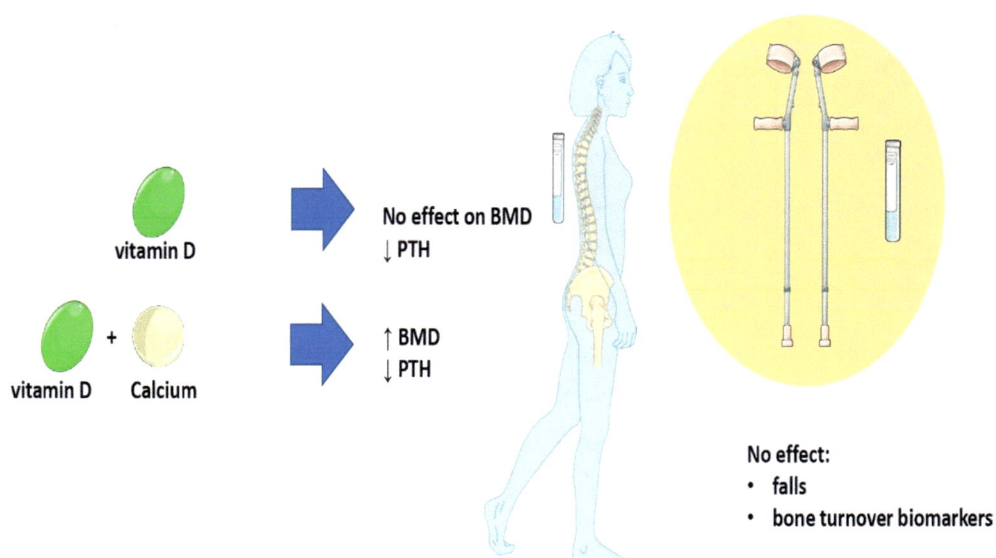

Figure 10.10. Calcium and vitamin D are pivotal in the prevention of bone metabolism disorders, particularly in enhancing bone density and overall skeletal health.

Source: https://www.mdpi.com/diseases/diseases-11-00029/article_deploy/html/images/diseases-11-00029-g001.png.

10.2.8. Lifestyle Modifications to Reduce Risk

Lifestyle modification is also crucial in managing the prevention of calcium and bone metabolism diseases. Nutritional strategies, particularly on the right amount of calcium and vitamin D intake, are the foundation; for instance, enhancing dietary habits to eat foods rich in calcium content should be improved—dairy foods, leafy greens, and fortified foods—can have a good impact in fortifying bones. Aerobic exercise and weight-bearing exercise specifically support bone health by causing osteoblast activity and thus reducing the risk of osteoporosis. Moreover, attention needs to be given to the determinants of the aging gut because changes with advancing age can lead to impaired nutrient absorption, malnutrition, and fracture risk (Bordoni et al., 2015). In addition, awareness of the epigenetic action on bone quality can inform lifestyle adjustments so that both environmental inputs and genetic factors contribute equally to bone metabolism. Facilitating such changes is important in establishing comprehensive preventive strategies in clinical practice (Brandi et al., 2016).

10.2.9. Impact of Osteoporosis on Quality of Life

Osteoporosis has a profound impact on quality of life, not only impairing the integrity of bones but also largely limiting everyday activities and overall well-being. Fractures develop in osteoporotic patients, eventually leading to ongoing pain, reduced mobility, and loss of autonomy. Fear of falling and potential for future harm heighten anxiety and result in social isolation, ultimately impacting mental health. Specifically, exercise is pivotal to maintaining bone density but is undermined in those suffering from osteoporosis due to pain and physical incapacity. Additionally, while high-impact exercise is advantageous in increasing bone turnover among youths, substitutes , such as water exercise present a means of alternative maintenance of bone among older adults predisposed to injury (Climstein et al., 2017). Therefore, every effort must be made to treat the multi-faceted consequences of osteoporosis to enhance the health quality of patients who are suffering from it (Ajbage et al., 2015) (Figure 10.11).

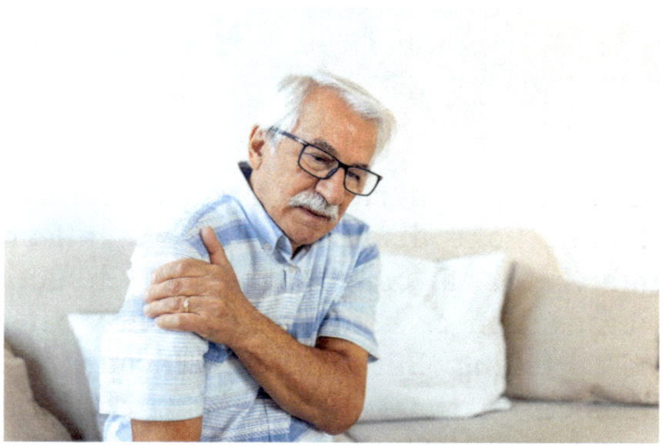

Figure 10.11. Individuals with osteoporosis often experience fractures, which can lead to chronic pain, loss of mobility, and decreased independence.

Source: https://diagnoeasy.s3.ap-south-1.amazonaws.com/1700578224679_old-senior-man-with-shoulder-pain-upset-senior-elder-man-feel-sudden-back-pain-muscles-ache-tension-injury-home-grandfather-touching-shoulder-having-osteoarthritis-arthritis.jpg.

Test Your Knowledge

1. Describe the pathophysiology of osteoporosis.
2. What is the difference between primary and secondary osteoporosis?

10.3. Osteomalacia and Rickets

Learning Outcome

1. Understand the definition and differences between osteomalacia and rickets
2. Know causes and risk factors for osteomalacia and rickets
3. Focus on symptoms and clinical features of both conditions
4. Discuss the pathophysiological mechanisms involved
5. Explain diagnostic approaches and laboratory tests
6. Learn treatment options and nutritional interventions
7. Describe long-term consequences of untreated conditions
8. Focus on public health implications and prevention strategies

Osteomalacia and rickets are two forms of metabolic bone disease that are manifested primarily as a consequence of defective mineralization of bone tissue, which causes bone softening. Both are influenced greatly by defects in the metabolism of phosphate and calcium, and these can be caused by vitamin D deficiency. In adults, osteomalacia is characterized by increased bone pain and susceptibility to fractures, whereas in children, rickets causes deformities of the skeleton and growth abnormalities. Key diagnostic markers include elevated serum alkaline phosphatase, which mirrors increased bone turnover due to defects in mineralization (Chandna et al., 2016). In addition, vitamin D's multifunctional role in calcium absorption and bone metabolism also indicates the systemic nature of the diseases, as recent data indicate the involvement of vitamin D receptors in various cellular processes outside bone health (Bikle et al., 2020). Knowing the etiology and implications of osteomalacia and rickets is crucial for developing effective prevention and treatment strategies in the field of bone metabolism disorders.

10.3.1. Definition and Differences between Osteomalacia and Rickets

Osteomalacia and rickets are two illnesses that are both secondary to abnormal mineralization of bone, but which appear differently depending on the age at onset. Osteomalacia most commonly occurs in adults and is marked by tenderness of bones and weakness of muscles secondary to lack of mineralization in the bone matrix, most often due to vitamin D deficiency or malabsorption syndromes. Contrarily, rickets in children manifests as skeletal deformities, such as bowing of the legs, through comparable mineralization deficits.

While osteomalacia can arise from systemic illnesses that affect calcium and phosphate metabolism, rickets can specifically involve renal phosphate wasting disorders, so that the diagnostic process, as seen in hypophosphatemic rickets, is more complicated. Moreover, the two diseases highlight the central role of vitamin D in bone disease, as indicated in recent articles covering the multifaceted mechanisms of vitamin D metabolism and their clinical implications for skeletal and nonskeletal diseases (Bikle et al., 2020) (Figure 10.12).

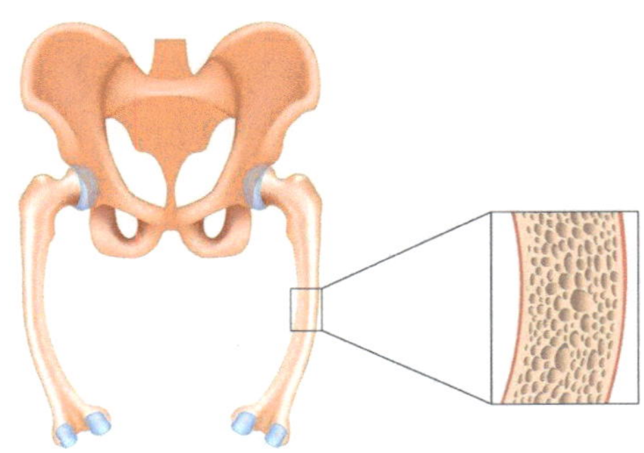

Figure 10.12. Osteomalacia.

Source: https://www.stemcellcareindia.com/wp-content/uploads/2018/06/Stem-Cell-Treatment-Osteomalacia.jpg.

10.3.2. Causes and Risk Factors for Osteomalacia

Osteomalacia, or undermineralization of the bones and resulting softening, has several interrelated causes and risk factors. Prominent among them is a deficiency in vitamins, which has been increasingly prevalent in various demographic groups, particularly elderly persons, individuals with limited sun exposure, and individuals with specific skin diseases or diets (Diamond et al., 2004). The metabolic impairment is also a major contributing factor, as the vitamin D receptor (VDR) and related enzymes play an essential role in bone strength. Mutation of these pathways could enhance the susceptibility to osteomalacia by disrupting calcium and phosphate homeostasis necessary for maximum mineralization (Bikle et al., 2020). Besides, diseases , such as malabsorption syndromes may also increase the weakness in the body's ability to effectively use dietary calcium and vitamins, thereby increasing susceptibility to this disease. Prevention as well as management of these risk factors is imperative for effective prevention and treatment of osteomalacia.

10.3.3. Causes and Risk Factors for Rickets

Rickets, a disease of abnormal mineralization of the bones, is mostly due to a deficiency of vitamins, calcium, and phosphate. The most significant reason for the deficiency is inadequate food intake or improper exposure to sunlight, which is essential for vitamin D production in the skin. Other populations are also at greater risk, particularly the old, those with deeper pigmentation, and those with disease states like coeliac disease that compromise nutrient absorption (Diamond et al., 2004). Furthermore, hereditary mutations that lead to defects in the metabolism of vitamin D can also enhance the susceptibility to rickets, proving that the interaction between genes and environmental factors is complex in the context of bone health (Bikle et al., 2020). The impact of rickets is not just on bone deformity, and it could have an impact on overall health and well-being. Overall, public health intervention thus needs to prevent rickets, particularly through education about sources of vitamin D and sun exposure for vulnerable groups (Figure 10.13).

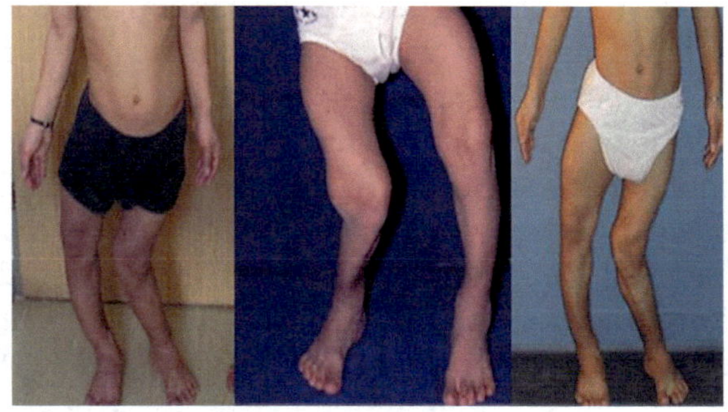

Figure 10.13. Rickets, a condition characterized by impaired bone mineralization, primarily stems from deficiencies in vitamin, calcium, and phosphate.

Source: https://healthjade.com/wp-content/uploads/2018/03/rickets-in-children.jpg.

10.3.4. Symptoms and Clinical Features of Both Conditions

Unraveling the clinical manifestations and symptoms of disorders of calcium and bone metabolism reveals a complex interplay of physiological dysfunction. For instance, Dent disease (DD), characterized by low-molecular-weight proteinuria, hypercalciuria, and nephrocalcinosis, has a characteristic constellation of manifestations, particularly in patients with mutations in the CLCN5 gene. Such patients tend to develop complications , such as nephrolithiasis and chronic kidney disease, showing age-independent associations with these conditions, which are presumably due to proximal tubular dysfunction (Angela D'Angelo et al., 2015). On the other hand, ectopic mineralization disorders tend to manifest as nonspecific soft tissue biomineralization, and this has significant clinical implications, including impairment of mobility and pain (Vilder et al., 2015). They both reference the pressing need for precise genetic and biochemical evaluation to define their unique and shared pathological processes and ultimately to guide appropriate management and treatment interventions in affected patients.

10.3.5. Pathophysiological Mechanisms Involved

Understanding the pathophysiological mechanisms of calcium and bone metabolism disease is crucial in setting effective therapeutic and diagnostic approaches. The homeostasis of calcium is well-controlled through the balance of various hormones, renal function, and the integrity of bone tissues. In particular disorders , such as Dent disease with mutations of the CLCN5 gene, the clinical presentation by the patients includes hypercalciuria and nephrolithiasis due to abnormal tubular reabsorption of phosphate and calcium, highlighting defective proximal tubular function as a prevailing mechanism (Angela D'Angelo et al., 2015). Furthermore, ectopic mineralization observed in aging, as well as in most genetic disorders, demonstrates the complex interaction between cell signaling pathways, apoptosis, and oxidative stress to underscore the multifactorial etiology of such disorders (Vilder et al., 2015). As such, elucidation of these processes not only contributes to understanding disease pathogenesis but also informs targeted intervention strategies (Figure 10.14).

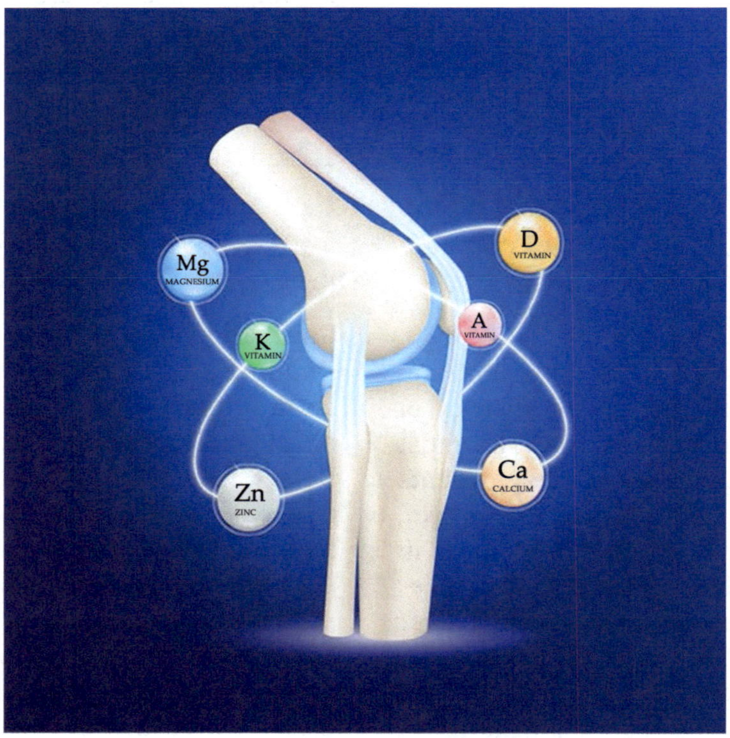

Figure 10.14. Importance of magnesium in bone health.

Source: https://www.apexhospitals.com/_next/image?url=https%3A%2F%2Fbed.apexhospitals.com%2Fuploads%2Fmag_48448bcb34.jpg&w=1920&q=75.

10.3.6. Diagnostic Approaches and Laboratory Tests

Precise diagnostic approaches and laboratory tests are critical to the understanding of disorders within calcium and bone metabolism. Early detection is a product of a combination of biochemical markers, imaging techniques, and patient history evaluation. Blood testing for serum calcium, phosphate, and PTH levels gives useful information about present metabolic activity, while bone mineral density (BMD) tests, such as dual-energy X-ray absorptiometry, quantify bone status and fracture propensity. Besides, advances in automated analysis techniques have boosted the function of healthcare professionals to measure and monitor these parameters more effectively. For example, accuracy monitoring can help parameterize health according to physiological and psychological factors, and eventually inform more individualized treatment protocols in specific populations, like those receiving long-term antipsychotic therapy where high levels of prolactin might be linked with osteoporosis (Cao et al., 2014) (Furukawa et al.). Through the use of such extensive diagnostic methods, clinicians can improve patient outcomes for bone metabolism disorders.

10.3.7. Treatment Options and Nutritional Interventions

Effective management of calcium and metabolic bone disorders involves an inter/trans-disciplinary strategy with both treatment approaches and dietary intervention. Pharmacologic therapies, including bisphosphonates and vitamin D analogs, are essential in neutralizing disorders like osteoporosis through denser bone mass and a reduced fracture risk.

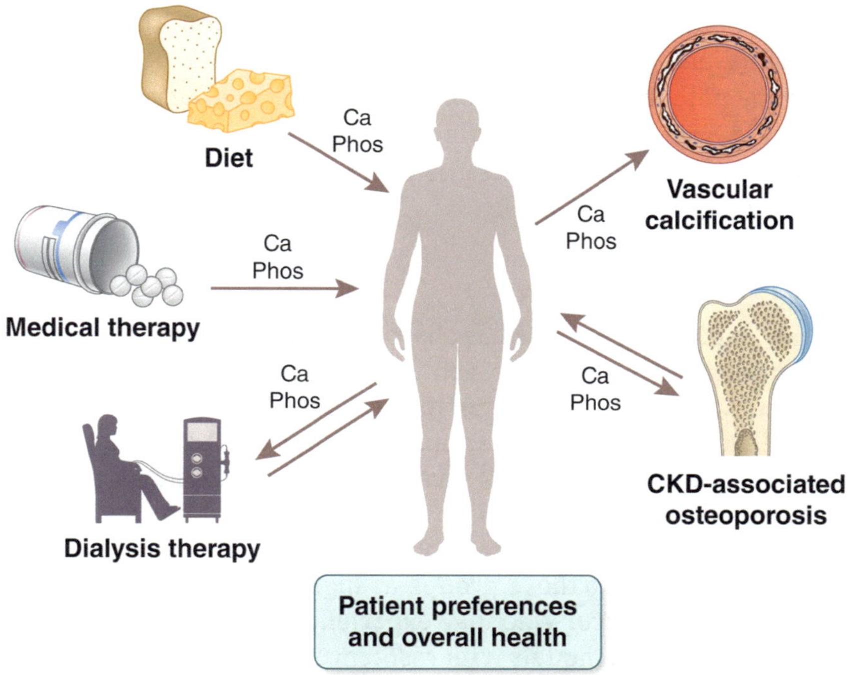

Figure 10.15. Effective management of calcium and bone metabolism disorders necessitates a multifaceted approach encompassing both treatment options and nutritional interventions.

Source: https://www.kidney-international.org/cms/10.1016/j.kint.2024.11.013/asset/56b05264-c092-4726-9a0d-39f7541d70a0/main.assets/gr2_lrg.jpg.

These interventions, however, have to be complemented by nutritional interventions, particularly from adequate dietary consumption of calcium and phosphorus, both of which are responsible for maintaining bone integrity. Current studies highlighted that non-adherence to treatment protocols significantly hinders outcomes, focusing on patient compliance with clinical and dietary advice (Coppo et al., 2014).

Additionally, the incorporation of resistance training was discovered to improve muscle strength, therefore preserving general skeletal integrity, which aligns with the common consensus that lifestyle modification is essential to counteract bone loss as a result of aging (Burton et al., 2010). Thus, an overall method that integrates medication, diet, and exercise can yield the most favorable outcomes in the treatment of these disorders (Figure 10.15).

10.3.8. Long-term Consequences of Untreated Conditions

The eventual sufferer of untreated disorders of calcium and bone metabolism can manifest as severe health problems that drastically affect quality of life. For instance, decreased levels of calcium from untreated hypoparathyroidism have the potential to lead to chronic hypocalcemia, which in turn can result in enhanced risks of osteoporosis and fractures.

These are further compounded by the physical limitations of the affected with a possibility of a cycle of immobility and further deterioration in bone health. Effects involving increased oxidative stress have further been reported in diseases, such as Hailey-Hailey, where cellular metabolic dysfunction impacts overall health and integumental integrity, illustrating the systemic consequences of mineral deficiencies (Cialfi et al., 2018). Furthermore, the lack of effective management for calcium disorders has the potential to create complex clinical situations, necessitating the expertise of specialists, which could have been avoided through timely intervention (Azran et al., 2017). Such long-term implications serve to demonstrate the urgent need for active diagnosis and treatment strategies in managing metabolic disorders.

10.3.9. Public Health Implications and Prevention Strategies

The knowledge of the public health implications of calcium and bone metabolism disorders is critical for the development of the right prevention measures. Calcium is a crucial factor in the maintenance of bone mass, and deficiencies can lead to osteoporosis, elevating the susceptibility to fractures and the consequent health complications in the elderly. As emphasized by recent studies, the incorporation of lifestyle modifications , such as improved nutrition, exercise, and education in public health is essential to neutralize such risks. For instance, a campaign with an emphasis on the requirement of calcium intake can reduce significantly the incidence of osteoporosis and related diseases, particularly among those groups at high risk , such as postmenopausal women and cancer patients with breast cancer who may experience estrogen loss and resulting bone mass loss. In addition, research in animal models with resilience to bone health complexity, as referenced in the review of various species, can help expose new therapeutic interventions and prevention strategies (Arnold et al., 2018). Further, the treatment of osteoporosis needs an overall strategy that includes both lifestyle changes and nonhormonal pharmacologic treatment on the basis of individual needs (Davis et al., 2017) (Figure 10.16).

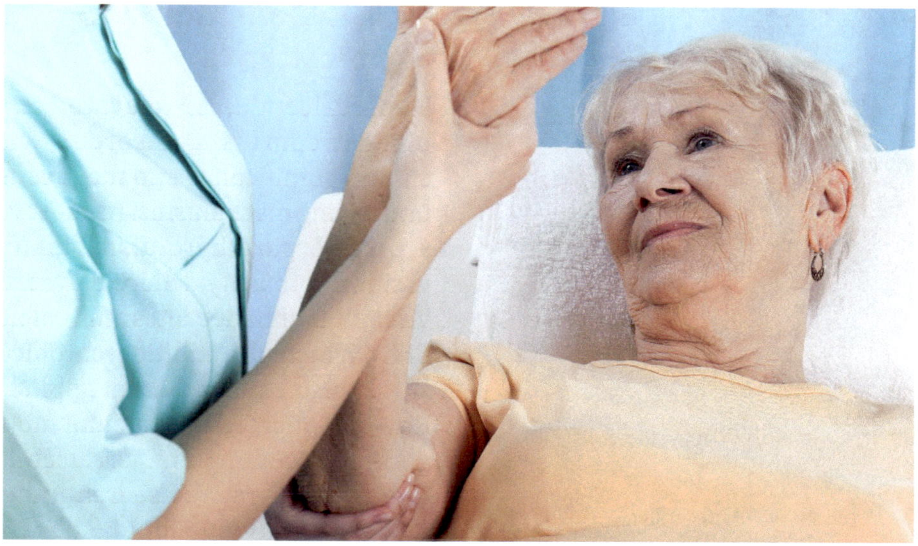

Figure 10.16. Calcium plays a pivotal role in maintaining bone density, and deficiencies can lead to osteoporosis, elevating the risk of fractures and associated health complications in the aging population.

Source: https://womenshealth.gov/sites/default/files/heading-images/Osteoporosis.jpg.

Test Your Knowledge

1. What are the common signs and symptoms of rickets in children?
2. What laboratory findings are typical in osteomalacia?

10.4. Hypercalcemia and Hypocalcemia

Learning Outcome

1. Understand the definition and causes of hypercalcemia and hypocalcemia
2. Discuss symptoms associated with hypercalcemia and hypocalcemia
3. Focus on diagnostic methods for hypercalcemia and hypocalcemia
4. Learn treatment options for hypercalcemia
5. Know treatment options for hypocalcemia
6. Explain the role of calcium supplements in management
7. Describe the importance of monitoring calcium levels in at-risk populations

The control of calcium within the body is essential for numerous physiological processes, and disturbances can lead to severe health issues, as evidenced by hypercalcemia and hypocalcemia. Hypercalcemia, often induced by such disorders as primary hyperparathyroidism or neoplastic diseases, can produce symptoms ranging from altered mentality to cardiac arrhythmias, which demonstrates the key role of calcium in neural and muscular processes. Conversely, hypocalcemia, typical in patients with poor PTH secretion, is accompanied by signs like muscle cramps and seizures that have a heavy burden on quality of life and functional status. Recent studies emphasize the significance of precise diagnosis and tailored treatment strategies for these conditions, particularly in complicated cases like HIV-infected patients. In such a situation, calcium metabolism can be significantly affected by underlying cancers and treatments, and it is difficult to treat conditions like hypercalcemia and hypocalcemia (Grp et al., 2022; Bikle et al., 2019).

10.4.1. Definition and Causes of Hypercalcemia

Hypercalcemia, or elevated calcium in the bloodstream, is a disorder with significant clinical significance and may result from several underlying mechanisms. Its most common causes are hyperparathyroidism, malignancies, and vitamin D toxicity, where elevated hormones or vitamin D enhance intestinal calcium absorption or from bones. In addition, chronic kidney disease (CKD) also emerged as an applicable risk factor that complicated the calcium metabolic balance and produced high hypercalcemia rates among the diseased cats. Research indicates that CKD cats possess a four-fold higher hazard ratio for Total hypercalcemia, indicating the conditions association with renal failure (Abdi et al., 2017). Moreover, other systemic illnesses, such as malignancies or inflammatory conditions, may also impact calcium homeostasis and impair calcium metabolism (Amare et al., 2020). It is therefore important to identify these causative determinants in an effective way to diagnose and treat patients with hypercalcemia (Figure 10.17).

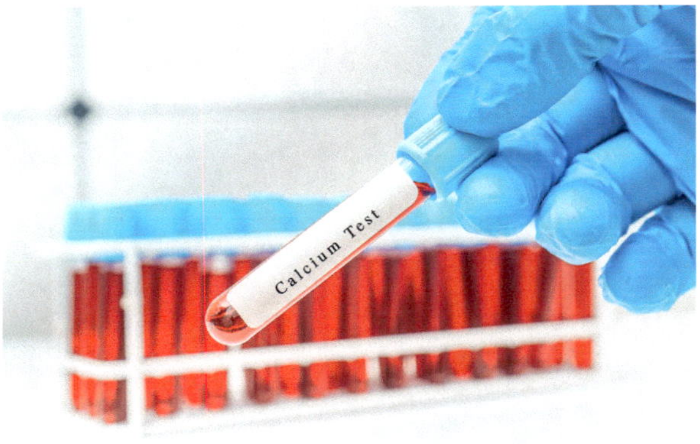

Figure 10.17. Hypercalcemia, characterized by elevated levels of calcium in the bloodstream, poses significant clinical implications and can result from various underlying conditions.

Source: https://img.lb.wbmdstatic.com/vim/live/webmd/consumer_assets/site_images/article_thumbnails/BigBead/what_to_know_ about_hypocalcemia_and_tetany_bigbead/1800x1200_what_to_know_about_hypocalcemia_and_tetany_bigbead.jpg.

10.4.2. Definition and Causes of Hypocalcemia

Hypocalcemia, or serum calcium levels less than normal, is a severe disorder that can have several underlying etiologies with a significant impact on bone metabolism. Hypoparathyroidism is a leading cause of low calcium in which the PTH production is insufficient and leads to reduced reabsorption of calcium by the kidney and reduced bone resorption, and hence low calcium. It is either a post-surgical or a non-surgical disorder; the latter encompasses genetic causes , such as 22q11 deletion syndrome, which is also associated with DiGeorge syndrome, where defective calcium regulation arises due to disrupted hormonal signaling (Astor et al., 2016). Additionally, inadequate intake of nutrients, most notably vitamin D deficiency, can impair calcium absorption in the gastrointestinal tract, hence exacerbating hypocalcemia (Allegrini et al., 2017). Understanding such causes is essential for designing effective treatments and improving patient outcomes in patients suffering from calcium and bone metabolism diseases.

10.4.3. Symptoms Associated with Hypercalcemia

Hypercalcemia, where there is an excess of calcium in the blood, comes with a multitude of symptoms that can have a devastating impact on a person's health and well-being. Neurological symptoms , such as confusion, lethargy, and even psychosis, are not uncommon and may be a direct result of the inhibitory effect of calcium on neuronal excitability.

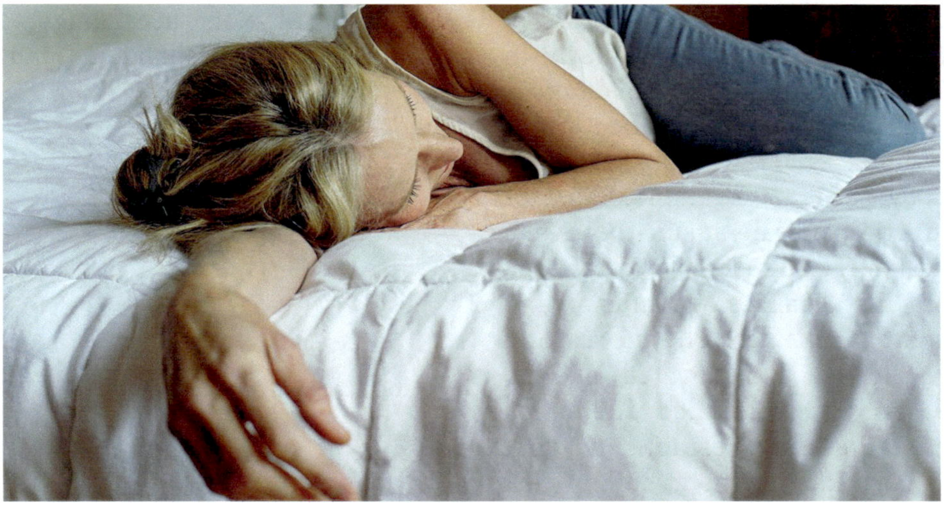

Figure 10.18. Hypercalcemia, characterized by elevated calcium levels in the blood, presents a range of symptoms that can profoundly affect an individual's health and quality of life.

Source: https://media.post.rvohealth.io/wp-content/uploads/2020/08/woman_laying_bed-1200x628-facebook-1200x628.jpg.

Additionally, hypercalcemia tends to lead to gastrointestinal discomfort, including nausea, vomiting, and constipation, since calcium is an integral component of the contraction of muscles and transmission of neuromuscular. Additionally, the patient begins to develop nephrological complications, including polyuria and nephrolithiasis, as a result of excessive elimination of calcium through the urine, which ultimately results in renal impairment if undiagnosed. Chronic conditions like primary hyperparathyroidism (PHPT) are the etiologies of such symptoms and, in general, add to morbidity and mortality if left untreated (Armanini et al., 2015; Grp et al., 2022). Familiarity with these symptoms is necessary to diagnose and treat hypercalcemia in the case of disorders of calcium and bone metabolism on a timely basis (Figure 10.18).

10.4.4. Symptoms associated with Hypocalcemia

Hypocalcemia, with abnormally low serum concentrations of calcium, is expressed through various symptoms, that affect patient physiology and health. Most frequently noted are neuromuscular irritability, with the risk of muscle spasm and cramp, particularly in hands and feet, which is a process called tetany. Additionally, cardiovascular complications , such as arrhythmia or QT prolongation may be developed by patients, a manifestation of the pivotal function of calcium in the heart. Neurotransmission is also sustained by calcium, whereby mental disturbances of confusion and irritability might take place. The correlation between hypocalcemia and elevated alkaline phosphatase (ALP) levels also identifies its intricacy; studies have established that elevated ALP correlates with a higher risk of hypocalcemia, particularly in diseases like secondary hyperparathyroidism due to chronic kidney disease (He et al., 2020). Thus, identification of these signs becomes necessary for early detection and management of calcium metabolism-related diseases (Covic et al., 2017).

10.4.5. Diagnostic Methods for Hypercalcemia and Hypocalcemia

Hypercalcemia and hypocalcemia tests are critical in the diagnosis and successful treatment of calcium and bone metabolism disorders. The initial evaluation typically consists of serum calcium assessment, together with PTH testing, which is used to diagnose primary hyperparathyroidism and other pathologies of hypercalcemia, such as malignancy or granulomatous disease (Bikle et al., 2019). In hypocalcemia, serum analysis of albumin, phosphorus, and magnesium should be evaluated since these electrolytes share an interaction with calcium metabolism (Grp et al., 2022). Ultrasonography and high-resolution CT scans may be employed to identify parathyroid gland abnormalities as well as to evaluate for potential tumors. A patient's clinical history, particularly for parathyroid gland surgeries, is also most critical in making a diagnosis of chronic hypoparathyroidism. These detailed diagnostic techniques enable health professionals to tailor management plans according to the primary cause of calcium imbalance (Figure 10.19).

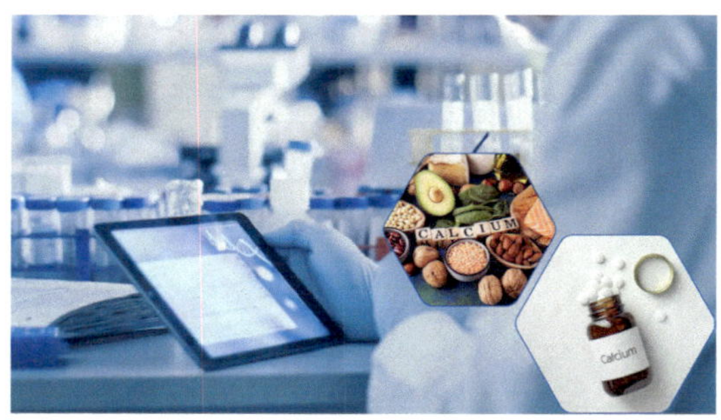

Figure 10.19. Diagnostic methods for hypercalcemia and hypocalcemia.

Source: https://www.wbcil.com/wp-content/uploads/2025/02/The-Role-of-Calcium-Lactate-Gluconate-in-Managing-Low-Blood-Calcium-Levels.jpeg.

10.4.6. Treatment Options for Hypercalcemia

The management of hypercalcemia is multi-modal and tailored to the etiology of the disorder. The initial management can include hydration with intravenous saline to help increase calcium elimination by the kidneys and improve symptoms. In malignancy-related disease, as in breast cancer with bone metastasis, denosumab or bisphosphonates may be employed to block bone resorption and lower serum calcium, thus breaking the cancer's vicious cycle of bone destruction and tumor growth inherent in metastatic disease (Wang et al., 2018). In addition, glucocorticoids can be beneficial, especially in hypercalcemia secondary to granulomatous disease or certain malignancies, by inhibiting vitamin D metabolism and lowering intestinal absorption of calcium. Therapies aimed at the specific malignancy are required in hypercalcemia associated with HIV and concomitant lymphomas, but this has not been our experience (Bikle et al., 2019). Understanding these treatment options is crucial for effective management and optimization of patient outcomes.

10.4.7. Treatment Options for Hypocalcemia

Management of hypocalcemia involves a multi-modal approach that is particular to the etiology of the condition, ranging from post-surgery complications to chronic diseases like hypoparathyroidism. The first line of treatment is usually oral or intravenous supplementation of calcium to correct the serum calcium level quickly. Where hypoparathyroidism is diagnosed, replacement therapy with synthetic PTH is being accepted more and more as a reasonable intervention, most beneficial in patients who have chronic hypoparathyroidism following neck surgery (Grp et al., 2022).

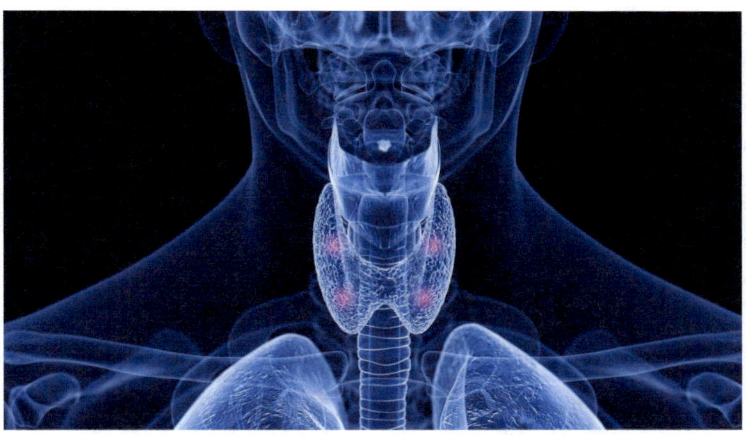

Figure 10.20. In cases where hypoparathyroidism is confirmed, synthetic parathyroid hormone (PTH) replacement therapy is becoming increasingly recognized as a viable option, particularly beneficial for patients with chronic hypoparathyroidism following neck surgery

Source: https://res.cloudinary.com/broadcastmed/image/fetch/ar_16:9,c_fill,g_auto,f_auto,q_auto,w_1300/https%3A%2F%2F55933-bcmed.s3.amazonaws.com%2Fbcp%2Fimages%2FdmImage%2FSourceImage%2Fnew-hypoparathyroidism-guidelines-1920x10802.jpg.

Adjunctive therapy with vitamin D analogs also promotes intestinal calcium absorption, again correcting hypocalcemia. Of special interest, new osteoporosis therapies, such as denosumab, have shown promising outcomes in specific populations and potentially could be of value for patients with select bone turnover disorders (Covic et al., 2017). With increasing understanding of calcium and disorders of bone metabolism, tailored treatment strategies will be critical to optimizing patient health and quality of life (Figure 10.20).

10.4.8. Role of Calcium Supplements in Management

Calcium supplements play a crucial role in the management of diseases of bone metabolism, particularly in individuals at high risk of osteoporosis and fractures. Supplements are required in individuals who may not be able to obtain sufficient calcium from diet, such as postmenopausal women and individuals with certain medical conditions where calcium absorption is compromised. A study indicates that calcium, in combination with vitamin, significantly enhances bone mineral density and, therefore, fractures among osteoporotic patients (Chodkowski et al., 2024). Furthermore, studies have indicated that supplementation is preventive for bone loss in the context of various chronic diseases, and therefore should be recommended accordingly in practice (Azran et al., 2017). However, there has been concern regarding potential harmful effects of over-supplementation with cardiovascular risks, calling for medical professionals to provide calcium supplementation with balanced consideration in mind that respects individual patient needs and circumstances.

10.4.9. Importance of Monitoring Calcium Levels in at-risk Populations

Screening for calcium in risk populations involves the maintenance of calcium within surveillance to avoid and manage disorders of bone metabolism, as alterations in calcium may indicate an imbalance at the systemic level.

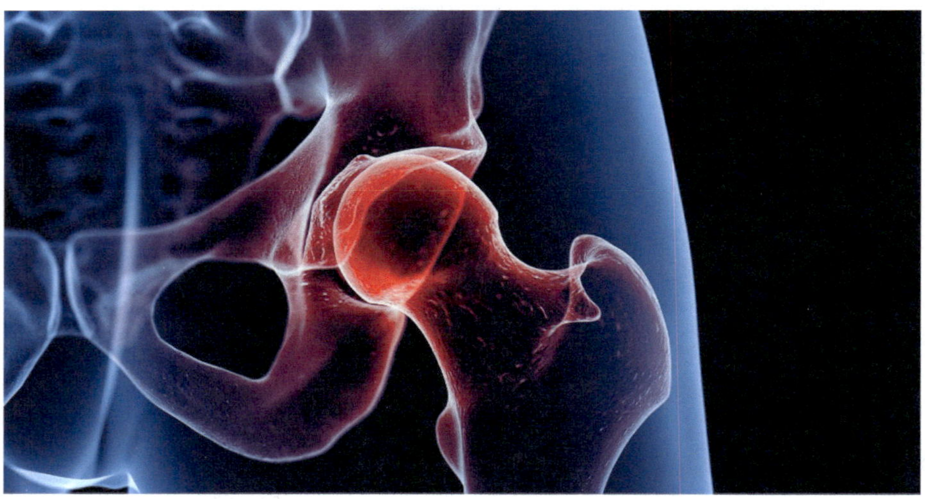

Figure 10.21. Menopause and bone loss.

Source: https://www.endocrine.org/-/media/endocrine/images/patient-engagement-webpage/condition-page-images/female-reproductive-health/menopause_bone_loss_pe_1796x943.jpg.

The risk groups are older persons, postmenopausal females, and patients with CKD because these are susceptible to calcium deficiency or excess, which will exacerbate calcium disorders and lead to increased fracture risk and vascular complications. In CKD, for instance, the abnormal metabolism of calcium is intimately linked with cardiovascular conditions, which highlights the need for continuous monitoring to maintain bone health and prevent vascular calcification (Bover et al., 2018). Furthermore, the cautious assessment of calcium status allows clinicians to tailor treatments, making interventions that may protect against adverse outcomes due to the abnormality of calcium, making it a preventive approach in such vulnerable groups (Ajbage et al., 2015). Lastly, continuous monitoring of calcium levels is a must to achieve maximum health results and reduce the prevalence of debilitating diseases connected to calcium imbalance (Figure 10.21).

Test Your Knowledge

1. How is hypercalcemia managed medically?
2. What are the common causes of hypocalcemia?

Summary

The intricate interplay of calcium and bone metabolism highlights the duality of skeletal illnesses. Full understanding of such interplay is essential to develop prospective treatment strategies. The activity of alkaline phosphatases (APs) is a classic demonstration of the duality of bone metabolism, where they facilitate mineralization but lead to complications like vascular calcification, notably seen in chronic kidney disease (CKD) (Bover et al., 2018). Also, more recent findings on our understanding of the gut microbiota offer an emerging connection to calcium absorption and the consequent bone health, further emphasizing the necessity of enjoying a well-balanced microbiome to prevent dysbiosis and achieve normobiosis, crucial to overall wellness (Meheust et al., 2010). These findings emphasize the need for an interdisciplinary strategies for diagnosing and managing calcium and bone metabolism disorders that includes diet, biochemical, and microbiologic parameters to optimize results in bone health.

In calcium and bone metabolism disorders, several points have been raised that underscore the complexity of such disorders. One of the key points is the interaction between gut microbiota and calcium uptake, with the presence of probiotic microorganisms, particularly bifidobacteria, increasing calcium uptake and bone mass, suggesting nutritional interventions could exploit this interaction in order to have therapeutic benefit (Meheust et al., 2010). In addition, the role played by alkaline phosphatases (APs) in bone metabolism is pivotal as the enzymes facilitate bone mineralization but pose a risk to vascular health during chronic diseases like chronic kidney disease (Bover et al., 2018). The fine balance between the promotive and harmful effects of these biochemical processes underscores the need for multidisciplinary management and treatment with an eye to maximizing the bone's health while minimizing associated risks of systemic disease. Multifaceted strategies like these will play a key role in effectively managing calcium-related disorders.

KEY TERMS FROM THIS CHAPTER

- Apoptosis
- Bone health
- Bone metabolism
- Calcium balance
- Calcium metabolism disorders
- Calcium uptake mechanisms
- Conventional crystal analysis (CCA)
- Diagnostic
- Dietary
- Effective management
- Bone calcium
- Bone matrix
- Bone mineral density (BMD)
- Calcium homeostasis
- Calcium reabsorption
- Chronic kidney disease (CKD)
- Dent disease (DD)
- Diagnostic criteria
- Ectopic mineralization
- Epigenetic action

Critical Thinking Questions

1. **Which hormone is primarily responsible for increasing blood calcium levels?**
   a. Calcitonin
   b. Parathyroid hormone (PTH)
   c. Insulin
   d. Aldosterone
2. **Which of the following is NOT a typical feature of hypercalcemia?**
   a. Polyuria
   b. Constipation
   c. Tetany
   d. Abdominal pain
3. **Vitamin D primarily promotes the absorption of calcium in the:**
   a. Kidneys
   b. Liver
   c. Intestines
   d. Bones
4. **Which condition is commonly associated with decreased bone mineral density?**
   a. Hyperthyroidism
   b. Osteoporosis
   c. Hyperkalemia
   d. Hypoparathyroidism
5. **A patient with chronic kidney disease is at risk of which bone disorder?**
   a. Paget's disease
   b. Osteogenesis imperfecta
   c. Renal osteodystrophy
   d. Osteosarcoma

Answers to Critical Thinking Questions

1. (b) 2. (c) 3. (c) 4. (b) 5. (c)

Short Answer Questions

1. What are the primary hormones involved in calcium homeostasis?
2. How does parathyroid hormone (PTH) regulate blood calcium levels?
3. What are the risk factors for osteoporosis?
4. How is bone mineral density measured?
5. What is the underlying cause of osteomalacia in adults?
6. How is rickets different from osteomalacia?
7. What are the causes of hypercalcemia?
8. What are the clinical signs and symptoms of hypercalcemia?

References

1. Abdi, H., Andress, D., Barber, L., Barber, R., Barber, T., Berend, K., Berry, D., et al. (2017). Chronic kidney disease in cats and the risk of total hypercalcemia. https://core.ac.uk/download/76981028.pdf (accessed on 17th June 2025).
2. Adriani, M. (M.), Setiarsih, D. (D.), & Wirjatmadi, B. (B.). (2016). Bone density status and vitamin D and calcium concentrations in pregnant and non-pregnant women. https://media.neliti.com/media/publications/150299-EN-bone-density-status-and-vitamin-d-and-ca.pdf (accessed on 17th June 2025).
3. Agas, D., Marchetti, L., Douni, E., & Sabbieti, M. G. (2015). The unbearable lightness of bone marrow homeostasis. *Cytokine & growth factor reviews, 26*(3), 347–359. https://doi.org/10.1016/j.cytogfr.2014.12.004(accessed on 17th June 2025).
4. Aghamaleki, A., Dini, M., Keshtkar, A., Khashayar, P., et al. (2013). Estimating the avoidable burden of certain modifiable risk factors in osteoporotic hip fracture using Generalized Impact Fraction (GIF) model in Iran. https://core.ac.uk/download/52204675.pdf (accessed on 17th June 2025).
5. Bover, J., Ureña, P., Aguilar, A., Mazzaferro, S., Benito, S., López-Báez, V., Ramos, A., daSilva, I., & Cozzolino, M. (2018). Alkaline Phosphatases in the Complex Chronic Kidney Disease-Mineral and Bone Disorders. *Calcified tissue international, 103*(2), 111–124. https://doi.org/10.1007/s00223-018-0399-z (accessed on 17th June 2025).
6. Ajbage, J. O., Heijsters, G., Politis, C., Salem, A., et al. (2015). Craniectomy of deeply impacted lower third molar: Incidence of outcomes and complications after one year follow-up. https://core.ac.uk/download/55765860.pdf (accessed on 17th June 2025).
7. Allegrini, D., Autelitano, A., Damante, G., Maver, P., et al. (2017). Cataract and optic disk drusen in a patient with glycogenosis and Di George syndrome: Clinical and molecular report. https://core.ac.uk/download/169434526.pdf (accessed on 17th June 2025).
8. Almeida, E. de, Dias, C., Faísca, M., Guilherme, M., et al. (2020). Gla-rich protein (GRP) as an early and novel marker of vascular calcification and kidney dysfunction in diabetic patients with CKD: A pilot cross-sectional study. https://core.ac.uk/download/322918835.pdf (accessed on 17th June 2025).
9. Amare, B., Kassu, A., Moges, F., Beyene, T., Yabutani, T., et al. (2020). HIV-associated hypocalcemia among diarrheic patients in northwest Ethiopia: A cross-sectional study. https://core.ac.uk/download/326699400.pdf (accessed on 17th June 2025).
10. Anonymous, & White, C. L. (2025). Detection and treatment of mineral nutrition problems in grazing sheep. https://core.ac.uk/download/pdf/6377290.pdf (accessed on 17th June 2025).
11. Armanini, D., Bordin, L., Camozzi, V., Donà, G., et al. (2015). Transient hypercortisolism and symptomatic hyperthyroidism associated to primary hyperparathyroidism in an elderly patient: Case report and literature review. https://core.ac.uk/download/53518371.pdf (accessed on 17th June 2025).
12. Arnold, W., Johnson, R. J., Kuro-o, M., Lanaspa, M., et al. (2018). Novel treatment strategies for chronic kidney disease: Insights from the animal kingdom. https://core.ac.uk/download/150600152.pdf (accessed on 17th June 2025).

13. Astor, M. C., Debowska, A., Eriksen, E. F., Evang, J. A., et al. (2016). Epidemiology and health-related quality of life in hypoparathyroidism in Norway. https://core.ac.uk/download/42625113.pdf (accessed on 17th June 2025).

14. Azran, C., Batterham, R. L., Busetto, L., Dicker, D., et al. (2017). Practical recommendations of the Obesity Management Task Force of the European Association for the Study of Obesity for the post-bariatric surgery medical management. https://core.ac.uk/download/141699962.pdf (accessed on 17th June 2025).

15. Berry, C., Corcoran, D., & Ford, T. J. (2018). Stable coronary syndromes: Pathophysiology, diagnostic advances and therapeutic need. https://core.ac.uk/download/96882082.pdf (accessed on 17th June 2025).

16. Bikle, D. D. (2020). Vitamin D: Newer concepts of its metabolism and function at the basic and clinical level. https://core.ac.uk/download/323063251.pdf (accessed on 17th June 2025).

17. Bikle, D., Kim, S., Kim, S. J., Peluso, M., et al. (2019). Rapid onset of hypercalcemia from high-grade lymphoma in the setting of HIV-related immune reconstitution inflammatory syndrome. https://core.ac.uk/download/323067318.pdf (accessed on 17th June 2025).

18. Biller, B. M. K., Colao, A., De Martino, M. C., Isidori, A., et al. (2016). Complications of Cushing's syndrome: State of the art. https://core.ac.uk/download/54532161.pdf (accessed on 17th June 2025).

19. Bordoni, A., Dupont, D., Gille, D., Kachal, H., et al. (2015). Understanding the gastrointestinal tract of the elderly to develop dietary solutions that prevent malnutrition. https://core.ac.uk/download/286575279.pdf (accessed on 17th June 2025).

20. Bover, J., Carrero, J. J., Molina, P., Ureña Torres, P., Chauveau, P., & Mazzaferro, S. (2017). Vitamin D, a modulator of musculoskeletal health in chronic kidney disease. https://core.ac.uk/download/153367338.pdf (accessed on 17th June 2025).

21. Brandi, M. L., Cianferotti, L., & Marini, F. (2016). Epigenetic mechanisms in bone biology and osteoporosis: Can they drive therapeutic choices? https://core.ac.uk/download/301570886.pdf (accessed on 17th June 2025).

22. Broniec, G., Czapiewska, R., Dziewulska, A., Kiełt, P., et al. (2024). The significance of vitamin D in dentistry – Review. https://core.ac.uk/download/620863904.pdf (accessed on 17th June 2025).

23. Buckton, C., & Combet, E. (2014). Micronutrient deficiencies, vitamin pills and nutritional supplements. https://core.ac.uk/download/42357992.pdf (accessed on 17th June 2025).

24. Burton, L. A., & Sumukadas, D. (2010). Optimal management of sarcopenia. https://core.ac.uk/download/20453974.pdf (accessed on 17th June 2025).

25. Caffarelli, C., Cavati, G., Gennari, L., Gonnelli, S., et al. (2023). Dietary vitamin D intake in Italian subjects: Validation of a frequency food questionnaire (FFQ). https://core.ac.uk/download/643630089.pdf (accessed on 17th June 2025).

26. Cao, B., Hou, R., Jian, J., Mi, X., et al. (2014). Effects of antipsychotics on bone mineral density and prolactin levels in patients with schizophrenia: A 12-month prospective study. [No URL provided]

27. Chandna, P., Kochar, P. K. T., M. B., Siddesh, M. U., et al. (2016). Radiographic imaging of metabolic

bone disorders and their relative management. https://core.ac.uk/download/543134786.pdf (accessed on 17th June 2025).

28. Wu, Y., Chen, K., & Terkeltaub, R. (2016). Systematic review and quality analysis of emerging diagnostic measures for calcium pyrophosphate crystal deposition disease. *RMD open*, *2*(2), e000339. https://doi.org/10.1136/rmdopen-2016-000339(accessed on 17th June 2025).
29. Chodkowski, J. (2024). The impact of nutritional supplementation in selected chronic medical conditions: A review. https://core.ac.uk/download/636385561.pdf (accessed on 17th June 2025).
30. Cialfi, S., Ficociello, G., Talora, C., Uccelletti, D., et al. (2018). Yeast-based screen to identify natural compounds with a potential therapeutic effect in Hailey-Hailey disease. https://core.ac.uk/download/159268892.pdf (accessed on 17th June 2025).
31. Climstein, M., Hing, W., Pope, R., Simas, V., et al. (2017). Effects of water-based exercise on bone health of middle-aged and older adults: A systematic review and meta-analysis. https://core.ac.uk/download/196605036.pdf (accessed on 17th June 2025).
32. Coppo, R., Dal Canton, A., De Silvestri, A., Esposito, C., et al. (2014). Management of mineral metabolism in hemodialysis patients: Discrepancy between interventions and perceived causes of failure. https://core.ac.uk/download/226564108.pdf (accessed on 17th June 2025).
33. Covic, A., Mazzaferro, S., Muci, M. L., Pasquali, M., et al. (2017). Positioning novel biologicals in CKD-mineral and bone disorders. https://core.ac.uk/download/98344336.pdf (accessed on 17th June 2025).
34. D'Angelo, A., Cremasco, D., Del Prete, D., Tosetto, E., Anglani, F., Bonfante, L., Bertizzolo, L. M., et al. (2015). Nephrolithiasis, kidney failure and bone disorders in Dent disease patients with and without CLCN5 mutations. https://core.ac.uk/download/53528992.pdf (accessed on 17th June 2025).
35. Dalmaceno, C., & Moreira Neto, S. (2020). Vitamin D can influence the dental implants? https://core.ac.uk/download/337380136.pdf (accessed on 17th June 2025).
36. Davis, S. R., Gompel, A., Lumsden, M. A., Pinkerton, J. V., et al. (2017). Managing menopausal symptoms and associated clinical issues in breast cancer survivors. https://core.ac.uk/download/96884955.pdf (accessed on 17th June 2025).
37. De Vilder, E., & Vanakker, O. (2015). From variome to phenome: Pathogenesis, diagnosis and management of ectopic mineralization disorders. https://core.ac.uk/download/55848035.pdf (accessed on 17th June 2025).
38. Diamond, T. H., Eisman, J. A., Mason, R. S., Nowson, C., et al. (2004). Vitamin D in Australia: Issues and recommendations. http://hdl.handle.net/10536/DRO/DU:30002479 (accessed on 17th June 2025).
39. Fantauzzi, C. B., Iacobini, C., Menini, S., Pugliese, G., et al. (2017). Role of galectin-3 in bone cell differentiation, bone pathophysiology and vascular osteogenesis. https://core.ac.uk/download/141696866.pdf (accessed on 17th June 2025).
40. Furukawa, S., Leonard, J. I., & Vannordstrand, P. C. (2025). Systems identification and application systems development for monitoring the physiological and health status of crewmen in space. https://core.ac.uk/download/pdf/42869637.pdf (accessed on 17th June 2025).
41. He, H. F., Hu, Q. H., Li, Y. W., Lin, Y., et al. (2020). Efficacy of ultrasound-guided radiofrequency

ablation of parathyroid hyperplasia: Single session vs. two-session for effect on hypocalcemia. https://core.ac.uk/download/322850169.pdf (accessed on 17th June 2025).

42. Martín-Tereso, J., & Verstegen, M. W. (2011). A novel model to explain dietary factors affecting hypocalcaemia in dairy cattle. *Nutrition research reviews*, *24*(2), 228–243. https://doi.org/10.1017/S0954422411000126(accessed on 17th June 2025).

43. Meheust, A., McCartney, A. L., Neyrinck, A. M., Balsari, B., Ben, A., Stahl, B., Watzl, B., et al. (2010). Prebiotic effects: Metabolic and health benefits. https://core.ac.uk/download/9368.pdf (accessed on 17th June 2025).

44. Rowe, J., Stone, L. R., & Teeter, R. (2025). Digest of Russian space life sciences, issue 33. https://core.ac.uk/download/pdf/42807398.pdf (accessed on 17th June 2025).

45. Wang, B., & Yang, Y. (2018). PTH1R-CaSR cross talk: New treatment options for breast cancer osteolytic bone metastases. https://core.ac.uk/download/213444641.pdf (accessed on 17th June 2025).

JUVENILE IDIOPATHIC ARTHRITIS (JIA)

11

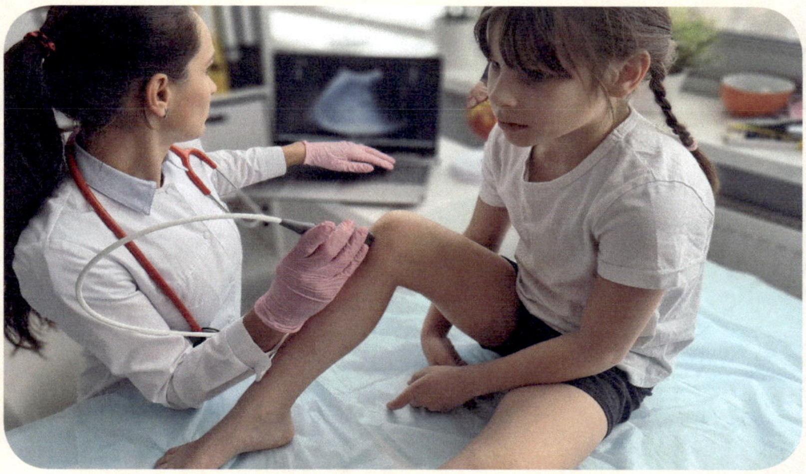

LEARNING OBJECTIVES

After studying this chapter, you will be able to:

1. Identify causes and risk factors
2. Explain symptoms and diagnosis
3. Focus on treatment options
4. Discuss living with juvenile idiopathic arthritis

Introduction

It is imperative to grasp juvenile idiopathic arthritis (JIA) due to its profound impacts on the kids and their families, both medical and psychosocial. JIA is characterized by joint inflammation, and that can lead to serious disability if left unaddressed. It is not merely a physical health issue; it has emotional implications as well, and most of the time it leads to anxiety and depression among child patients. There is some evidence for the potential role of a genetic factor, with susceptibility to JIA described in relation to specific variants, in particular in relation to the interleukin (IL)-10 cytokine family (Bryant et al., 2012). Because arthritis is such a prevalent long-term condition that affects millions, there is a requirement to understand the chronic pain and severe disability involved, as uncovered through Arthritis Australia's research into the lived experiences of the affected (Bates et al., 2014). Through exploration of these components, the intricacy of JIA and its expansive implications become clear (Figure 11.1).

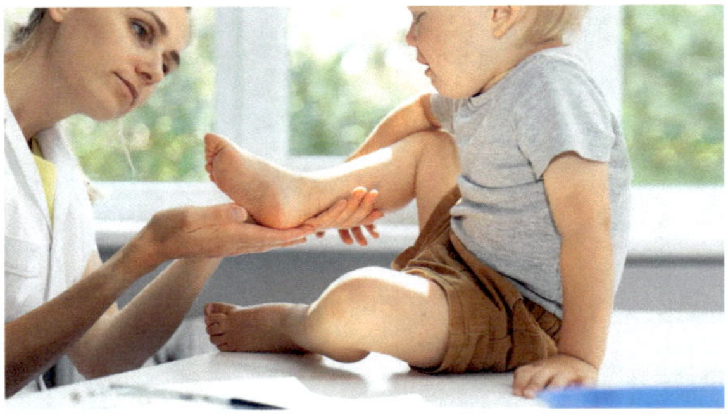

Figure 11.1. Juvenile Idiopathic Arthritis (JIA).

Source: https://images.everydayhealth.com/images/arthritis/juvenile-idiopathic-arthritis-jia-myths-and-facts-1440x810.jpg?sfvrsn=e1fce231_5.

11.1. Causes and Risk Factors

Learning Outcome

1. Understand genetic predisposition
2. Explain environmental triggers
3. Focus on immune system dysfunction
4. Discuss the role of infections
5. Explain the family history of autoimmune diseases
6. Know gender differences in incidence
7. Identify socioeconomic factors
8. Discuss ethnic variations in prevalence

Etiology and risk factors for JIA need to be identified for successful treatment and management. While the specific etiology is not known, several etiologic factors have been identified. Genetic causes play a major role; children with a family history of autoimmune diseases have a higher probability of developing JIA. Environmental triggers, such as viral infection and exposure to certain toxins, also induce or exacerbate inflammatory reactions in genetically susceptible subjects. Second, the interaction between environmental and immune dysregulation leads to defective immune response, further increasing the risk. Most importantly, the latest studies indicate the necessity for noncorticosteroid immunomodulatory drugs in the therapy of immune dysregulation disorders, with support from the changing insight into the complexities of JIA and potential therapies (Dick et al., 2018; Accorinti et al., 2018).

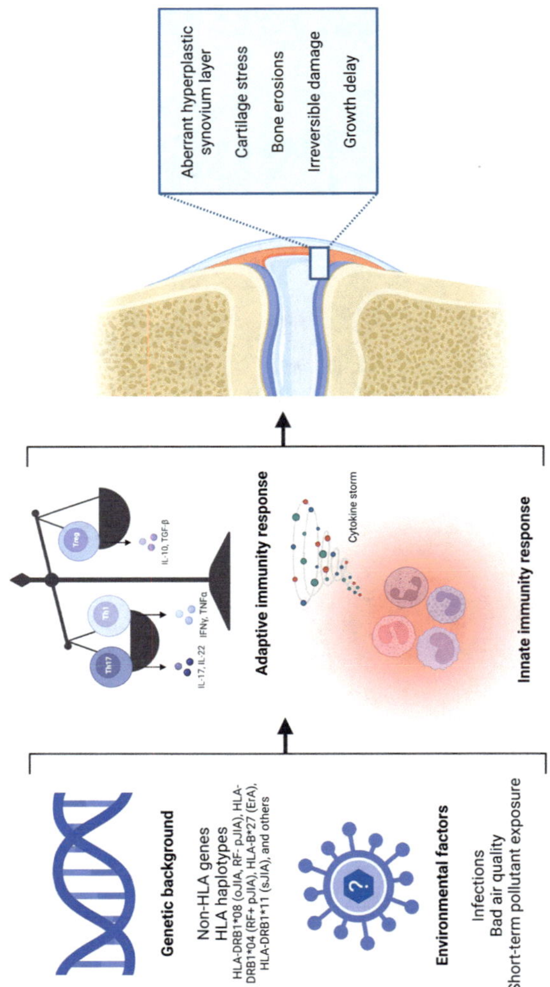

Figure 11.2. Genetic predispositions play a significant role; children with a family history of autoimmune diseases exhibit a higher likelihood of developing JIA.

Source: https://pub.mdpi-res.com/ijms/ijms-24-01846/article_deploy/html/images/ijms-24-01846-g001.png?1676006758.

Ultimately, the recognition of these risk factors may lead to early diagnosis and personalized therapeutic interventions (Figure 11.2).

11.1.1. Genetic Predisposition

An investigation into genetic predisposition reveals deep complexities in JIA development, a multifactorial disease with environmental and genetic causes. Genome-wide association studies have, in recent years, identified loci for autoimmune diseases, observing overlap between diseases, including JIA and rheumatoid arthritis. This is the understanding that patients with a documented family history of autoimmune conditions may be at a higher risk of developing JIA due to genetic predisposition and lack of pathogenic mechanisms (Richard-Miceli & Criswell, 2012). Furthermore, the implication of innate immune mechanisms, like the activation of macrophages and the engagement of cytokines like interferon gamma (IFN-γ), underscores the intricate interaction between genetic susceptibility and immune dysregulation in JIA pathogenesis (Bracaglia et al., 2018). These findings underscore the importance of continued research into genetic etiologies, which could lead to the opportunity for targeted diagnostic and therapeutic approaches based on the genetic profile of affected subjects.

11.1.2. Environmental Triggers

The role of environmental factors in the onset and evolution of JIA has been at the forefront of medical focus, particularly in light of its multifactorial etiology with involvement from genetics and the immune system. Research emphasizes that environmental influences, such as early exposure to antibiotics, can be likely to induce the development of JIA in genetically predisposed children. A systematic review found a dose-response relationship between antibiotic use and risk for JIA, which indicates that repeated purchases of antibiotics, particularly lincosamides and cephalosporins, are associated with a higher risk for this chronic disease (Niestradt et al.). Additionally, the overall conclusions of this study indicate the necessity for medical professionals to observe children exposed to antibiotics closely, as early interventions can prevent potential complications of JIA. Most importantly, it is important to recognize these environmental triggers given that JIA is a broad spectrum of diagnoses, hence requiring thorough investigations in this regard (Blanco et al., 2023).

11.1.3. Immune System Dysfunction

Dysregulation of the immune system is the key characteristic of JIA, which means an inappropriate immune response against the body's own joint structures. Immune system malfunction is reflected in chronic inflammation, pain, and potential long-term damage to joints. Macrohage activation syndrome (MAS), a severe JIA complication, is one illustration of the adverse effects of immune dysregulation. It is distinguished by an out-of-proportion inflammatory response leading to hypercytokinemia, predominantly with raised levels of IFN-γ, which is also highly incriminated in macophages found in affected organs (Bracaglia et al., 2018). MAS can present with intimidating features, such as prolonged fever, hepatosplenomegaly, and cytopenias, aggravating the clinical picture of JIA (Ramanan et al., 2016). The challenge is in distinguishing MAS from other conditions like systemic sepsis, and the necessity of making the early diagnosis with proper therapeutic strategies for improved prognosis in the patient. Management of these immune system abnormalities is crucial in handling the long-term effects of JIA in the children involved (Figure 11.3).

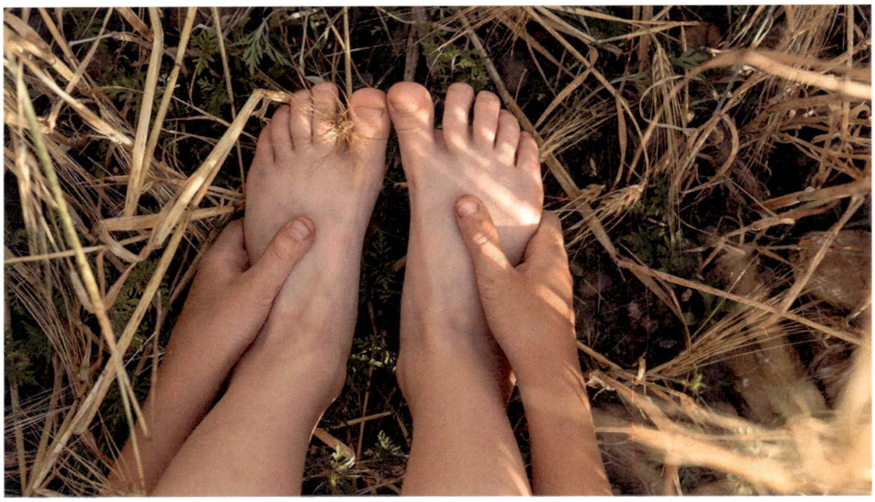

Figure 11.3. Immune system dysfunction is a central aspect of Juvenile Idiopathic Arthritis (JIA), characterized by an inappropriate immune response that targets the body's own joint tissues.

Source: https://post.healthline.com/wp-content/uploads/2022/12/child-holding-feet-1296-728-header.jpg.

11.1.4. Role of Infections

Pathogens have also been implicated as potential precipitants of the onset and triggering of JIA, highlighting the complex relationship between infection and immune dysregulation in JIA. Accumulating evidence suggests the role of specific pathogens in inflammatory mechanisms, which may render susceptible subjects at risk for subsequent autoimmune reactions. For instance, the activation of immune pathways during infections would result in the generation of autoantibodies, causing joint inflammation and destruction. Further, vitamins, being immune-modulating agents, plays a crucial role in children's immune responses. Evidence indicates that a significant proportion of pediatric patients with rheumatic disorders like JIA are susceptible to deficiency in vitamins, and thus the nutrient could potentially have relevance for both susceptibility to infection and disease activity (Burnham et al., 2011). It is important to comprehend such correlations when developing comprehensive management plans that address both prevention of infection as well as immune status in patients with JIA (Dick et al., 2018).

11.1.5. Family History of Autoimmune Diseases

The significance of family history of autoimmune disease as a determining factor in the etiology of JIA becomes evident. Etiologically, genetic predisposition has been identified by research as a primary causative factor in autoimmune diseases, thus suggesting that children who have a family history of such ailments are at a higher risk of developing JIA. Family presence of autoimmune diseases may lead to a shared immunological environment favoring increased inflammatory response, indicating a common immune dysregulation observed in patients with JIA. For instance, systemic JIA is accompanied by inflammatory processes like MAS, further complicating patient care (Didona et al., 2015). In addition, allergic conditions associated with chronic uveitis in JIA patients reflect the complexity of these conditions and also make a case for observation in children with a family history of autoimmune diseases (Bauer-Mehren et al., 2013) (Figure 11.4).

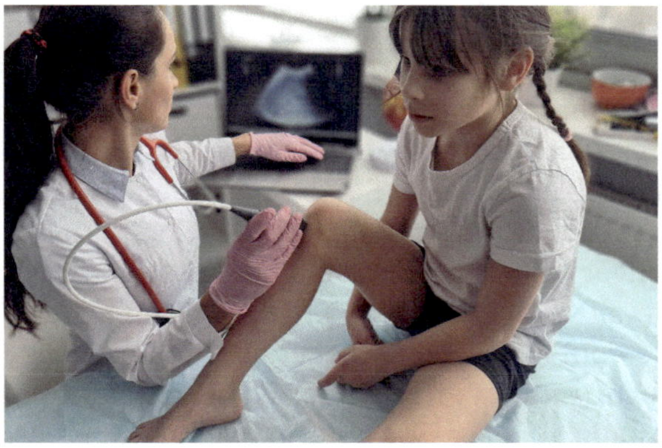

Figure 11.4. The significance of a family history of autoimmune diseases emerges as a critical factor in understanding the etiology of Juvenile Idiopathic Arthritis (JIA).

Source: https://images.ctfassets.net/yixw23k2v6vo/5gjoXXizTSSoikPuPrCtj3/81e4775b888d38424f9525264eef8338/girl-receives-knee-ultrasound-GettyImages-1456114101-3000x2000.jpg.

11.1.6. Gender Differences in Incidence

The prevalence of JIA has considerable gender variation, usually consistent with overall autoimmune disease trends. There is evidence to suggest that females are much more likely to develop JIA than males, and the disparity may be due to hormonal as well as genetic influences. Prevalence rates, for instance, indicate that autoimmune responses are more vigorous in females, possibly due to differences in immune system function. These inconsistencies not only influence the medical approaches used in treatment but also shape the psychosocial processes in JIA families. According to studies that analyze the lives of JIA families, healthy fathers and siblings of JIA children generally must manage complex emotional realities based on these gender differences. For example, fathers report inadequacy and social constraint, identifying the particular difficulty of having a daughter with a chronic illness, again reaffirming the need for tailored support networks in healthcare environments (Madill et al., 2007, 2008).

11.1.7. Socioeconomic Factors

Understanding the socioeconomic determinants that influence JIA is central to developing interventions and treatments that are effective. Studies have shown that children living in poor neighborhoods and non-White ethnic groups have a higher prevalence of complicating factors, as has been demonstrated through a cohort study where 28% and 31% of the participants were shown to comprise these groups.

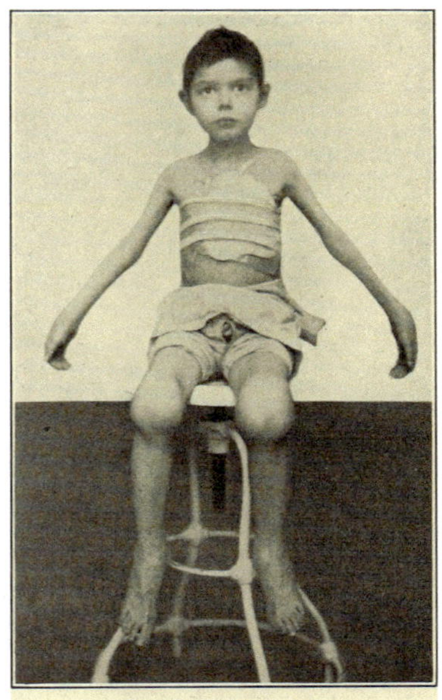

Figure 11.5. Understanding the socioeconomic factors influencing juvenile idiopathic arthritis (JIA) is crucial for developing effective treatment and intervention strategies.

Source: https://upload.wikimedia.org/wikipedia/commons/b/bd/Diseases_of_children_%281916%29_%2814579765477%29.jpg.

In addition, variation in insurance coverage has a significant impact on disease management; publicly insured children have more severe presentations, for instance, greater active joint counts and higher risk of polyarticular arthritis (Dallas et al., 2023). As much as there is an acute need for timely therapy upgrading, children with mixed sources of insurance demonstrate variation in access to care that may compromise outcomes. Addressing these socioeconomic disparities is key to facilitating equal access to healthcare and providing extensive healthcare to all JIA children (Figure 11.5).

11.1.8. Ethnic Variations in Prevalence

Ethnic variations in the incidence of JIA have important implications both in terms of diagnosis and treatment outcomes. Research has indicated that certain ethnic groups have increased rates of JIA, and that children who are non-White are overrepresented. An instance is where 31% of the cohort were children of diverse ethnic origins being diagnosed with non-infectious uveitis, an illness that is often associated with JIA. All these disparities may be attributed to a combination of genetic, environmental, and socio-economic health determinants causing health disparities. Further, awareness about such ethnic disparities is necessary in the delivery of optimal care strategies and access for all individuals equally. Interestingly, as in the context of AOSD discussion, individualized treatments have been reported to be significantly beneficial but can be heterogeneous in different populations (Baggio et al., 2018). It is crucial to address these differences, including in enhancing outcomes for all the involved children, irrespective of their ethnicity.

Test Your Knowledge

1. What infections have been associated as possible triggers of JIA?
2. What age group is most commonly affected by JIA?

11.2. Symptoms and Diagnosis

Learning Outcome

1. Identify common symptoms of JIA
2. Explain the types of JIA and their specific symptoms
3. Learn diagnostic criteria for JIA
4. Focus on the role of physical examinations
5. Know the importance of medical history
6. Discuss laboratory tests and imaging studies
7. Focus on differential diagnosis considerations
8. Identify challenges in diagnosing JIA
9. Know the early signs to watch for

Symptoms of JIA may be highly diverse among patients, making diagnosis even more challenging. Persistent pain, swelling, and stiffness of the joints, especially in the morning or following rest, are common presentations. Systemic manifestations like fever, rash, and lethargy can also occur as the disease progresses and can mimic other diseases, thereby creating diagnostic difficulty. Moreover, it has been observed that children with JIA are at risk of chronic uveitis, an acute complication that, if undiagnosed until late, causes loss of vision (Bauer-Mehren et al., 2013). It is worthwhile for a complete understanding of clinical associations, e.g., the possible association with allergy conditions, for proper risk stratification and management (Bauer-Mehren et al., 2013). Proper diagnosis generally requires a multidisciplinary approach through clinical assessment, laboratory tests, and radiologic studies to enable timely therapy and optimal results in the involved children.

11.2.1. Common Symptoms of Juvenile Idiopathic Arthritis

JIA is defined by a large number of symptoms that significantly impact the quality of life of said children. Although common grievances are joint pain, swelling, and stiffness, such symptoms are most evident in the morning or following rest. They can cause decreased mobility and impaired activities of daily living, highlighting the conditions disability affects as described in the latest research on the prevalence of arthritis (Bates et al., 2014) and its consequences of disability. Systemic findings , such as fever, rash, and fatigue, can occur with JIA, especially in systemic disease. With the growing integration of musculoskeletal ultrasound (MSUS) imaging into clinical practice, it enhances our ability to assess joint inflammation and damage and is a major contribution towards offering useful information for effective treatment planning (IAGNOCCO et al., 2016). Familiarity with these signs matters for early detection and appropriate management and improvement of children's experience of living with JIA (Figure 11.6).

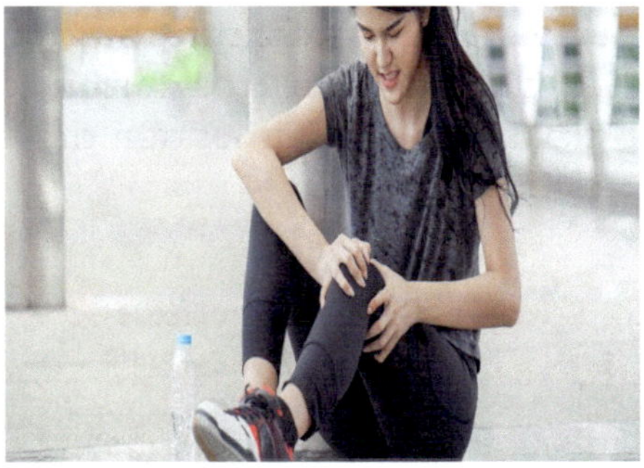

Figure 11.6. Commonly reported symptoms include persistent joint pain, swelling, and stiffness, particularly notable in the morning or after periods of inactivity.

Source: https://www.hopkinsmedicine.org/-/media/images/health/1_-conditions/arthritis/juvenile-rheumatoid-arthritis-hero.jpg?h=500&iar=0&mh=500&mw=1300&w=1125&hash=2C9A27E8DE038B6444C385DD96D9CC99.

11.2.2. Types of Juvenile Idiopathic Arthritis and their Specific Symptoms

JIA is characterized by numerous various subtypes, each with its own symptoms determining the course of the disease and the quality of life in children suffering from it. Oligoarticular JIA is one of the principal types and can typically involve four or fewer joints, being often characterized by chronic swelling of joints, typically the ankles and knees, and also causing eye inflammation , such as uveitis. Conversely, polyarticular JIA involves five or more joints and may manifest with systemic symptoms of fever and fatigue, resulting in a more variable outcome of the disease. Systemic JIA, being the most severe but rarest, involves systemic inflammation along with rash and fever as well as symptoms of arthritis (Bates et al., 2014). Furthermore, temporomandibular joint (TMJ) involvement has the potential to create orofacial pain and dysfunction with accompanying deformation over time, as longitudinal research has demonstrated (Collin et al., 2023). Identification of these diversified signs enables the formulation of specific treatment modalities for the unique presentations of JIA.

11.2.3. Diagnostic Criteria for Juvenile Idiopathic Arthritis

It is significant to learn the diagnostic criteria for JIA to have proper treatment protocols and improved patient outcomes. The classification of JIA relies heavily on a proper evaluation that distinguishes it from other rheumatic diseases; thus, it is crucial to have a proper diagnosis. Recent studies indicate that adults with a history of JIA may fulfill diagnostic criteria for certain adult rheumatic illnesses and thus must be regularly examined and reassigned from pediatric to adult status (Dzhus et al., 2017).

Moreover, even though standardized clinical examinations for the assessment of joint damage, such as temporomandibular joint disorders in JIA, exist, the validity of such criteria is doubtful, and more studies are needed (Berntson et al., 2019). Lastly, the establishment of strict diagnostic criteria is necessary to manage the late effects of JIA and develop personalized treatment plans based on evolving patient needs (Figure 11.7).

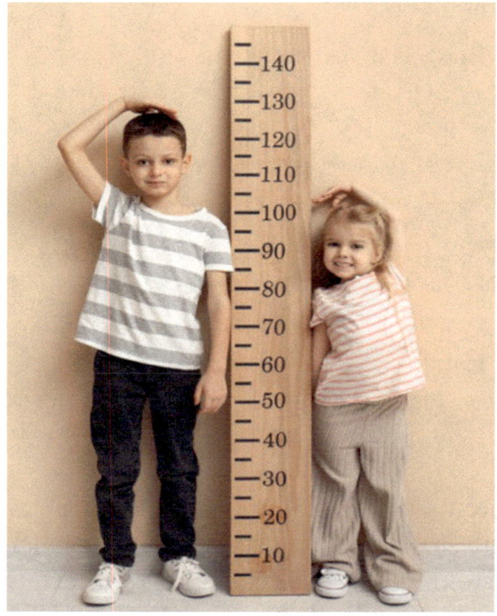

Figure 11.7. The classification of JIA relies heavily on a comprehensive assessment which distinguishes it from other rheumatic diseases, highlighting the importance of accurate diagnostic methods.

Source: https://www.emjreviews.com/wp-content/uploads/2025/03/AdobeStock_727563182.jpeg.

11.2.4. Role of Physical Examinations

Physical examination is an integral component of the diagnosis and management of JIA and is a fundamental starting point in defining and monitoring the disease course. Through complete clinical examination, the clinician is able to assess the function of joints, range of motion, and determine any complication associated with them, such as temporomandibular joint (TMJ) involvement, which is characterized by observation of a high prevalence of TMJ deformities in children with JIA (Collin et al., 2023). Also, while traditional clinical exams remain the foundation, imaging technology, particularly MSUS, has proven capable of supplementing physical examination findings and moving toward a more advanced method of evaluating joint inflammation and injury (Demirkaya et al., 2011). With the use of comprehensive physical examinations and new imaging modalities, health professionals can develop a broad plan for JIA diagnosis and treatment and ultimately achieve improved outcomes and quality of life for patients.

11.2.5. Importance of Medical History

The contribution of medical history to JIA cannot be overstated as it is a basic building block to effective diagnosis and treatment planning. A detailed medical history enables physicians to assess disease course, identify family patterns, and uncover comorbidities that may affect management. As an example, the development of a detailed history of joint symptoms and functional impairment can guide clinicians to tailor interventions, like multidisciplinary care plans highlighted in more recent research on children with JIA (Bernatsky et al., 2014). Additionally, institutionalization of national registries, like that focusing on idiopathic inflammatory myopathies, highlights the need to assemble systematic data to enrich studies and clinical care (Bohan et al., 2011). Thus, an extensive medical history gives clinicians the information they need to create individualized plans of treatment, which finally result in improved patient outcomes in this complex condition (Figure 11.8).

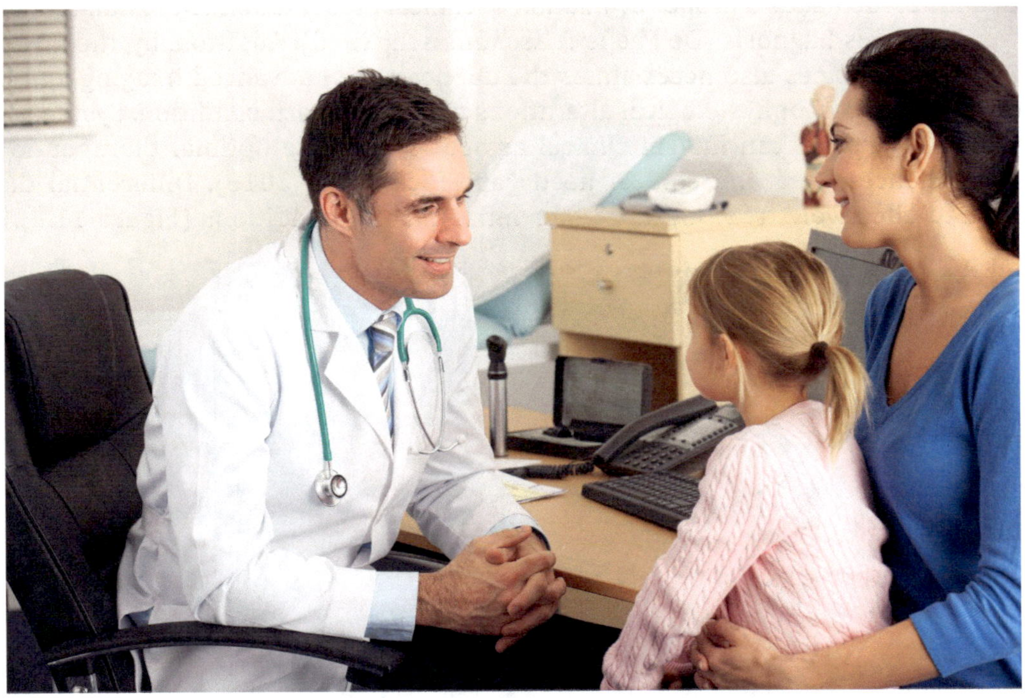

Figure 11.8. The importance of medical history in the context of Juvenile Idiopathic Arthritis (JIA) cannot be overstated, as it serves as a foundational element for effective diagnosis and treatment planning.

Source: https://juvenilearthritisnews.com/wp-content/uploads/2018/09/shutterstock_98521124-760x475@2x.jpg.

11.2.6. Laboratory Tests and Imaging Studies

In the diagnosis and management of JIA, laboratory tests and imaging studies play focal roles in determining disease activity and joint impairment. Panoramic radiography (PAN) and cone-beam computed tomography (CBCT) imaging techniques play pivotal roles in determining TMJ morphology, particularly with regard to the fact that TMJ deformity is common among patients with JIA and is correlated with functional disability, as documented in longitudinal studies (Collin et al., 2023). Laboratory tests, such as immunological biomarker analysis, are also relevant; however, findings affirm that even though certain proteins are identified in saliva, they do not vary significantly between JIA patients and healthy individuals, signifying minimal application for the aim of disease tracking (Collin et al., 2023). As the heterogeneity of JIA becomes clearer, enhanced diagnostic and imaging techniques will be crucial for efficient treatment of the disease, and continued research and development will be crucial in this area.

11.2.7. Differential Diagnosis Considerations

In differentially planning diagnosis in JIA, one should distinguish it from other inflammatory conditions that may lead to a similar presentation in children. Dermatomyositis and other idiopathic inflammatory myopathies (IIM) may have similar presentations, including arthralgia and weakness of the muscle, and it may therefore be difficult to diagnose. The heterogeneity of IIM, with well-defined pathological entities, demands a proper evaluation of clinical presentation and inflammation markers in an effort to avoid misdiagnosis (De Paepe & Zschüntzsch, 2015). Additionally, the involvement of cytokines in the pathologies also necessitates the application of advanced imaging and laboratory examination to define pathophysiological alterations unique for each condition. Systematic reviews and the opinion of experts can inform clinical advice to offer the optimal therapeutic practices, bridging the evidence-based and clinical need gap (Dick et al., 2018). Differential diagnosis is therefore vital to effectively treat JIA and other inflammatory conditions (Figure 11.9).

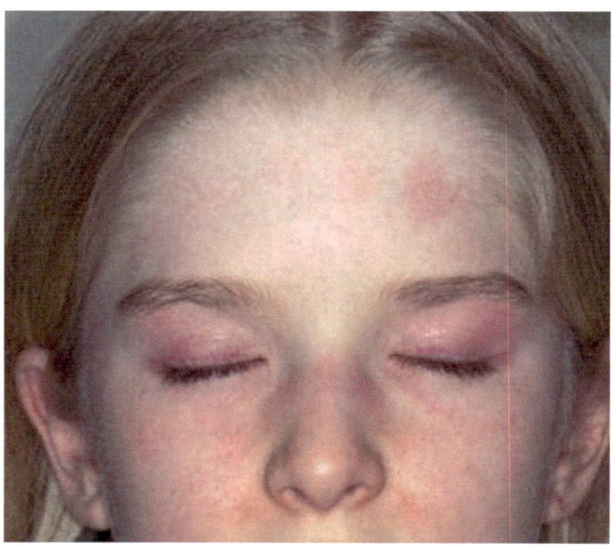

Figure 11.9. Juvenile dermatomyositis.

Source: https://img.medscapestatic.com/pi/meds/ckb/68/34668tn.jpg.

11.2.8. Challenges in Diagnosing Juvenile Idiopathic Arthritis

Diagnosis of JIA is fraught with many challenges that can delay and hinder effective treatment for the affected children. To begin with, the heterogeneous character of JIA makes it difficult to identify affected patients, as the manifestations may differ markedly between different patients and overlap with other childhood conditions. Besides, the majority of the healthcare professionals report an alarming uncertainty in the diagnosis and management of rheumatic disorders among children, with 77.9% reporting feelings of inadequacy in terms of their treatment expertise despite past experience (Cassidy et al., 2018). This feeling is aggravated by the absence of adequate training under undergraduate and postgraduate courses, leading to an inadequate pediatric rheumatology foundation (Cassidy et al., 2018). Additionally, diagnostic criteria have become complicated, whereby clinicians need to assess the latest guidelines, an effort that is overwhelming to those less familiar with the intricacies of the field. Finally, addressing such knowledge and confidence gaps is important to enhance diagnostic accuracy and patient outcomes in JIA.

11.2.9. Early Signs to Watch For

Early recognition of the early signs of JIA is critical in order to intervene early and control the condition. Parents and caregivers should look out for the following signs: chronic pain, swelling, and stiffness of the joint, particularly in the morning or after rest. Other indicators are range of motion limitation, tiredness, and fever and rash, which can be accompanied by joint symptoms. Early detection can determine long-term prognosis, with prompt treatment having the potential to prevent irreversible joint damage. Special attention should also be given to recognizing complications in areas , such as the temporomandibular joint (TMJ), as exemplified in the diagnostic criteria provided in the extended taxonomy for temporomandibular disorders, where injury is discovered during clinical evaluation that remains poorly supported (Berntson et al., 2019). Further, advanced care practices, including multidisciplinary assessments, can mitigate foot impairments that are experienced in JIA through early symptom identification for optimal treatment regimens (Brandon et al., 2013) (Figure 11.10).

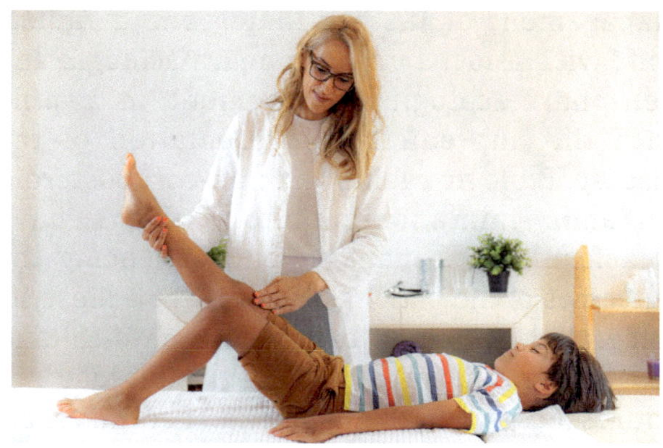

Figure 11.10. Early detection can significantly affect long-term outcomes, as timely treatment may prevent irreversible joint damage.

Source: https://www.wesleybaker.com/wp-content/uploads/2023/07/Understanding-Juvenile-Idiopathic-Arthritis-1024x683.jpg

Test Your Knowledge

1. What is the significance of morning stiffness in children with JIA?
2. Which laboratory tests are useful in diagnosing JIA?

11.3. Treatment Options

Learning Outcome

1. Understand the overview of treatment goals
2. Explain nonsteroidal anti-inflammatory drugs (NSAIDs)
3. Discuss disease-modifying antirheumatic drugs (DMARDs)
4. Focus on biologic therapies
5. Describe corticosteroids
6. Focus on physical therapy and rehabilitation
7. Explain the role of nutrition and lifestyle changes
8. Learn pain management strategies
9. Know the importance of multidisciplinary care

Management of JIA has undergone a radical shift with a focus on both pharmacologic and non-pharmacologic management in coping with the unpredictable presentation of the disease. Biologic agents and non-corticosteroid systemic immunomodulatory drugs have transformed the management, enhancing the outcomes of the patient as well as their lifestyle. Integrated models of care where physical and psychological expressions of the disease are addressed are now the trend. For instance, current research highlights the importance of specialist programmes, such as certain podiatric care, decreasing significantly foot-related impairments among JIA patients, as supported by the Juvenile Arthritis Disability Index (Manca et al., 2009). Additionally, best-practice agreement among experts emphasizes the importance of systematic evaluation and individually based treatment plans highly responsive to the distinctive needs of young patients in addressing issues of efficacy and safety (Dick et al., 2018). Such comprehensive treatment frameworks reflect the ongoing improvement in effectively managing JIA(Figure 11.11).

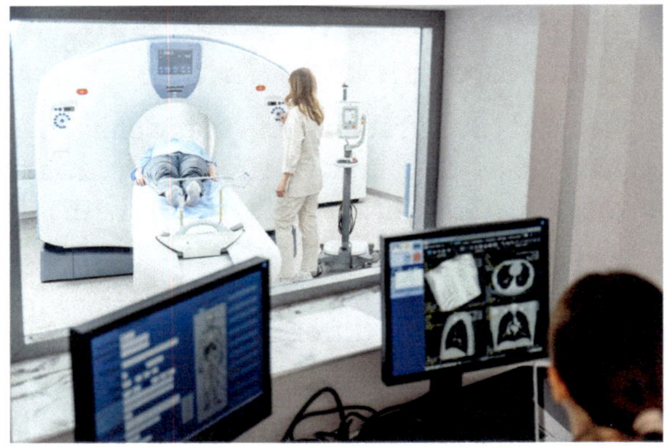

Figure 11.11. Biologic agents, along with non-corticosteroid systemic immunomodulatory therapies, have transformed the therapeutic landscape, enhancing patient outcomes and quality of life.

Source: https://www.britishjournalofnursing.com/media/csfbbb33/cancer-patient-undergoing-treatment-adada.jpeg.

11.3.1. Overview of Treatment Goals

An effective treatment regimen for JIA must pursue several interrelated goals directed towards improving the quality of life of such children. The primary one is to attain and maintain minimal disease activity or remission, thereby alleviating pain and preventing joint damage. This involves the use of both pharmacologic and non-pharmacologic treatment modalities tailored to the individual child's needs. Aside from that, preservation of physical function and normal growth and development are part and parcel of management because JIA can significantly impair general well-being as well as daily activities. Progress in imaging technology in the recent past has enabled monitoring of disease activity and treatment response, allowing for a better and more accurate management strategy (Avenarius et al., 2018). Besides, the knowledge about the disabling nature of arthritis, as revealed by recent studies, can inform health policies and improve the support services needed for full care (Bates et al., 2014). Last but not least, these goals seek to empower children and their families with an even-handed approach to the management of JIA.

11.3.2. Nonsteroidal Anti-inflammatory Drugs (NSAIDs)

NSAIDs are pivotal in the management of JIA in an effort to minimize pain and inflammation. They are both nonselective NSAIDs and COX-2 selective inhibitors that are employed to treat the symptomatic manifestation of JIA, which has the potential to have a devastating negative impact on a child's quality of life. Interestingly, while traditional nonselective NSAIDs , such as naproxen and meloxicam are favored, safety and efficacy of more recent ones , such as celecoxib have been in the limelight. A registry study demonstrated that the safety profile of celecoxib and the nonselective NSAIDs is the same with the same adverse effects in both groups (Beth S Gottlieb et al., 2014). However, it should be mentioned that while NSAIDs work effectively in symptom control, they may also be implicated in side effects, particularly cardiovascular events, and hence monitoring in children is worth it (Hilário et al., 2006; Altepeter et al., 2025). Thus, clinical use of NSAIDs in JIA must balance therapeutic benefit against potential risks (Figure 11.12).

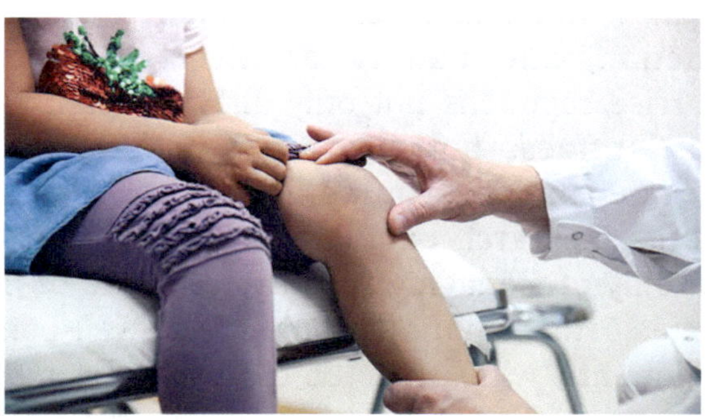

Figure 11.12. In the management of Juvenile Idiopathic Arthritis (JIA), Nonsteroidal Anti-Inflammatory Drugs (NSAIDs) play a pivotal role in alleviating pain and inflammation.

Source: https://images.everydayhealth.com/images/arthritis/rheumatoid-arthritis/stills-disease-juvenile-ra-jia-whats-the-difference-722x406.jpg?sfvrsn=87a73cdf_5.

11.3.3. Disease-modifying Antirheumatic Drugs (DMARDs)

Disease-modifying antirheumatic drugs (DMARDs) are important in the management of JIA, as DMARDs have the potential to significantly improve clinical outcomes compared to traditional treatments, such as non-steroidal anti-inflammatory drugs. Based on a systematic review, DMARDs like methotrexate have greater efficacy at alleviating JIA symptoms and improving the quality of life in children with JIA (Coeytaux et al., 2012). Clinically, the adoption of biological DMARDs (bDMARDs) has been impressive, with evidence showing most transitioning JIA patients being treated with these new therapies. Surprisingly, results show that 86% of patients were on DMARDs at transition to adult care, noting the continuation and success of treatments (Kosola et al., 2018). Despite concerns over adverse events, overall evidence contributes to an existing body of literature confirming safety and efficacy of DMARDs in treating JIA.

11.3.4. Biologic Therapies

With the development of biologic therapies, the treatment of JIA has evolved into a highly targeted approach with significant advantages for patients. Some examples are tumor necrosis factor (TNF) blockers and interleukin antagonists, which work by modulating specific mechanisms of the immune system to reduce inflammation and alleviate joint damage. Clinical trials demonstrated the efficacy of biologics to enhance the quality of life of children with JIA, particularly those who were partially responsive or inadequate responders to usual therapies, such as disease-modifying antirheumatic drugs (DMARDs). An outcome-directed evidence-based guideline has been created establishing the optimization of use of these agents in clinical practice, such as when to initiate therapy and assessing for safety and efficacy (Dick et al., 2018). Furthermore, the integration of these new treatments is an indicator of higher consensus among experts that enhances cooperative management practices aimed at patient care and system safety (Accorinti et al., 2018). This advancement underscores the importance of continued development and research in pediatric rheumatology (Figure 11.13).

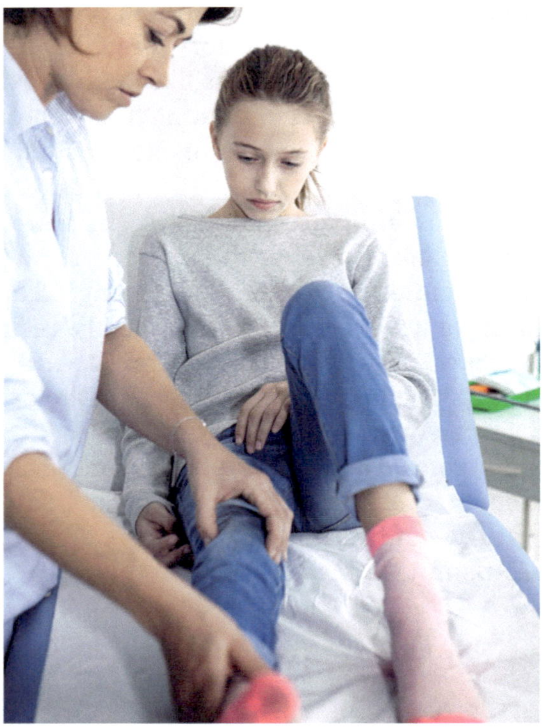

Figure 11.13. The advent of biologic therapies has revolutionized the treatment landscape for Juvenile Idiopathic Arthritis (JIA), offering targeted interventions that significantly improve patient outcomes.

Source: https://prdmspst.blob.core.windows.net/images/diseases/juvenile-idiopathic-arthritis-e2996c56-0c6c-49c5-9e53-9fa30145a46b-thumbnail.jpg.

11.3.5. Corticosteroids

Corticosteroids play a critical role in the management of JIA due to their anti-inflammatory and immunosuppressive properties, which have the ability to improve symptoms and hold long-term damage to joints. In first-line therapy, corticosteroids can potentially achieve rapid control of inflammation in cases of severe disease presentation. However, prolonged use of these drugs has implications for side effect induction, including growth retardation and osteoporosis, particularly with regards to children. Consensus recommendations today say that while corticosteroids remain cornerstones in the treatment of inflammatory disorders, there is growing awareness about the advisability of shifting to non-corticosteroid immunomodulatory medication to limit the risk of such side effects (Dick et al., 2018). In addition, a number of studies highlight that while corticosteroids in high doses are beneficial in the short term, a careful assessment of response to treatment is essential to maximize therapy in JIA to ensure individualized management techniques are employed (Alves et al., 2016).

11.3.6. Physical Therapy and Rehabilitation

The role of physical therapy and rehabilitation cannot be overemphasized in the management of JIA, with its aims being to enhance mobility, function, and quality of life. Customized exercise regimens not only alleviate pain and joint stiffness but also assist in developing an independent attitude among the affected youths. Research emphasizes the importance not only of managing the physical signs of JIA, but also the emotional and social well-being of patients, which may be quite compromised as a consequence of the disease (Ziff et al., 2016). Treatment may involve strength training, flexibility work, and water therapy that have been shown to be beneficial in symptom management and functional outcomes. In addition, physical therapy may play a crucial role in educating patients and their families on self-management habits, thereby ensuring long-term adherence to therapy (Boneparth et al., 2019). Integrative care is fundamental in reversing the disabling effect of JIA and enhancing the quality of life of individuals with this chronic disease (Figure 11.14).

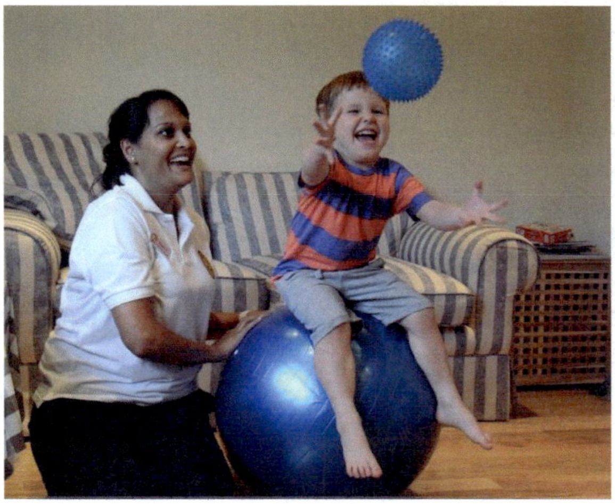

Figure 11.14. The role of physical therapy and rehabilitation is paramount in the management of Juvenile Idiopathic Arthritis (JIA), aiming to enhance mobility, function, and overall quality of life.

Source: https://www.central-health.com/wp-content/uploads/juvenile-idiopathic-arthritis.jpg.

11.3.7. Role of Nutrition and Lifestyle Changes

The interaction among nutrition, lifestyle change, and JIA is a subject of increased interest in pediatrics. Emerging evidence indicates that food choice can have a significant impact not only on the management of symptoms but also on the quality of life for these children. For instance, supplementation with omega-3 fatty acids has also been observed to be effective in reducing inflammatory responses, leading to improved joint health and functional activity in JIA patients (Bailey et al., 2023). Moreover, lifestyle modification , such as physical exercise, can also support overall health and keep the body weight healthy, particularly because of the observed growth issues in JIA children. However, existing literature indicates a need for high-quality studies to unravel the intricate association between diet and health outcomes in this population (Adamiak et al., 2017). It would seem that an integrative strategy combining both nutritional and lifestyle interventions is needed to optimize care in JIA patients.

11.3.8. Pain Management Strategies

Optimal pain management practice for JIA is essential to enhance the quality of life of the children and their families. This is normally applied through a multidisciplinary approach that can include drug and non-drug therapy, as tailored to the child's specific needs. Pharmacologically, non-steroidal anti-inflammatory drugs (NSAIDs) are prescribed most; however, parents have expressed a strong preference for interventions that maximize functional improvements and reduce pain intensity, as uncovered in studies of parents' preference for foot care in JIA (Bernatsky et al., 2014). Additionally, resilience-based interventions can play an important role in managing chronic pain. By highlighting the resilience and coping capacity of children and their families, health practitioners can foster more adaptive coping with the pain experience and thus optimize treatment outcomes. Addressing these multidimensional aspects of pain management is essential to building resilience and supporting overall well-being in children with JIA (Caes et al., 2017) (Figure 11.15).

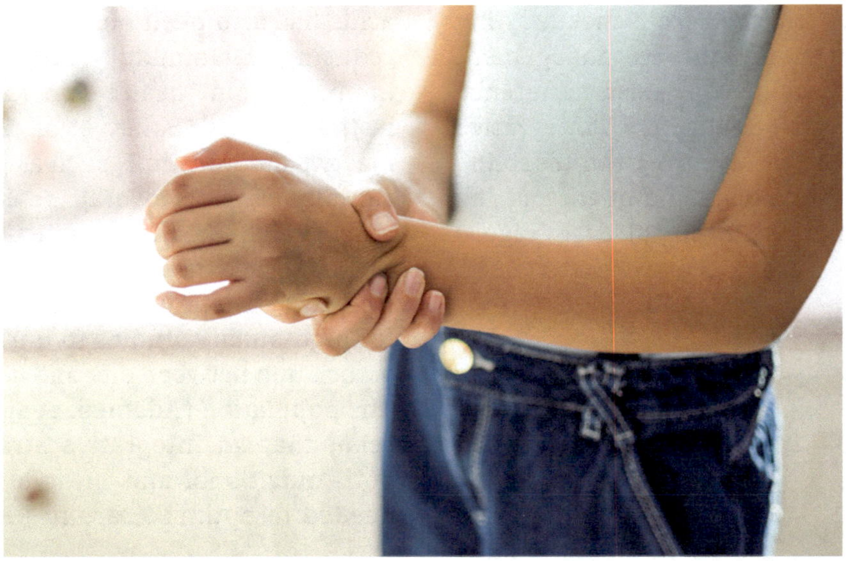

Figure 11.15. Effective pain management strategies for Juvenile Idiopathic Arthritis (JIA) are essential in enhancing the quality of life for affected children and their families.

Source: https://my.clevelandclinic.org/-/scassets/images/org/care-pages/pediatric/juvenile-idiopathic-arthritis-feature.jpg.

11.3.9. Importance of Multidisciplinary Care

The multidisciplinary approach to the treatment of JIA cannot be overemphasized, as it entails the integration of various forms of therapy in an attempt to optimize patient outcomes. A holistic treatment allows medical specialists, including rheumatologists, physical therapists, and podiatrists, to cater to the multi-faceted nature of the condition, particularly the often overlooked foot and ankle conditions associated with JIA. Evidence highlights that parents place more urgency on enhancing health outcomes like pain reduction and mobility, as opposed to logistical issues, indicating the need for advanced multidisciplinary foot care services (Bernatsky et al., 2014). Also, emerging research is such that combined care programs indeed play a significant role in clinical outcomes, significantly improving patients quality of life (Manca et al., 2009). Thus, adopting an inter-disciplinary methodology optimizes treatment efficacy while guaranteeing that healthcare delivery is also consistent with the aspirations and requirements of JIA-affected families, complementing the appeal for systemic change in pediatric rheumatology.

Test Your Knowledge

1. What are biologic therapies, and when are they used in JIA?
2. How is corticosteroid therapy used in JIA management?

11.4. Living with JIA

Learning Outcome

1. Understand psychological impact on children and families
2. Learn coping strategies for patients
3. Focus on support systems and resources
4. Provide educational accommodations for affected children
5. Discuss social implications and peer relationships
6. Explain transitioning to adult care
7. Know long-term health considerations
8. Identify advocacy and awareness efforts
9. Explain personal stories and testimonials

Living with JIA involves significant challenges beyond the physical symptoms that affect both the patient and his/her family life. Involvement of parents is significant as they feel the complexity of preferences for care, particularly foot care, which is a necessary part of a child's quality of life. There is evidence that parents place greater importance on quality-of-life benefits in the form of reduced pain and increased mobility, and not everyday issues like waiting times or affordability (Bernatsky et al., 2014). Additionally, prevalent consequences of arthritis highlight the need for support interventions and services that address the everyday living concerns of the affected families (Bates et al., 2014). This whole care emphasis stresses that symptom management is not sufficient unless effective; rather, it is essential to establish an environment in which children with JIA are able to do their best physically and emotionally and receive complete support, individually tailored to address their specific needs.

11.4.1. Psychological Impact on Children and Families

The psychosocial impact of JIA on families and children is considerable, impacting individual emotional well-being as well as family dynamics. The children with JIA experience isolation and unease because their condition could render them different from others, thus their family experiencing peculiarity in comparison to other families, as postulated by research exploring sibling perceptions. Siblings with good health can carry the emotional burdens, being insufficiently told and having to forego peer time in order to comply with their ill siblings' requirements, hence complicating social lives and relationships (Madill et al., 2007). Additionally, the doubled stress of a chronic condition can put pressure on parent relationships and increase family tensions, and this calls for increased support systems. When families navigate all these challenges, understanding the disability effects of arthritis becomes essential in order to inform the development of effective coping interventions and support (Bates et al., 2014) (Figure 11.16).

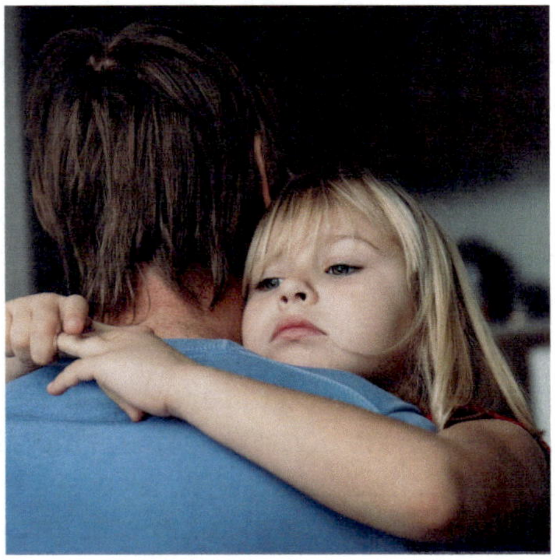

Figure 11.16. Children diagnosed with JIA often experience feelings of isolation and anxiety, as their condition may set them apart from peers, leading to a perception of their family as different from others

Source: https://images.ctfassets.net/yixw23k2v6vo/4HrCKZmtkaJHRHJQmpkDg5/cd9dff69ae66bf4c02d4e0380281f683/large-1-GettyImages-1135476957.jpg.

11.4.2. Coping Strategies for Patients

Lived experience with JIA necessitates the development of effective coping strategies in order to battle its physical and psychosocial challenges. Adolescents with JIA often encounter significant obstacles, including joint pain, decreased mobility, and emotional distress, that can undermine their functioning ability in daily life and in developing a social identity as an adolescent. However, research indicates that the majority of adolescents demonstrate excellent resilience by continuously working to take back control of their lives. They explain embracing behaviors like physical adaptation, open dialogue with physicians, and the formation of support networks to develop normalcy in their lives (Antonovsky et al., 2014). Further, as a reaction to the double burdens of physical ailments and emotional wellness, these adolescents utilize mechanisms that enhance acceptance and self-enhancement, thus enhancing the overall quality of their lives (Bruns et al., 2010). Such coping mechanisms are therefore essential in allowing patients to manage the demands of JIA living successfully.

11.4.3. Support Systems and Resources

Effective management of JIA relies significantly on robust support structures and systems. Identification of the diverse needs of individuals and families affected by JIA is essential, as the systems can become capable of providing emotional as well as practical support. For instance, peer support groups can establish feelings of belongingness and empathy among children with JIA so that they can learn from one another as well as exchange coping strategies. Also, occupational therapy, pain management clinics, and physiotherapy professional services are most critical in the facilitation of daily living and quality of life for such children. Based on studies by Arthritis Australia, awareness of the chronic disability impact of arthritis can contribute to better service delivery under such schemes as the National Disability Insurance Scheme, thereby assisting the patients and their families (Bates et al., 2014). Further, evidence-based approaches to aggregating clinical information can enable personalized interventions in JIA such that patients receive holistic care (Anjum et al., 2007) (Figure 11.17).

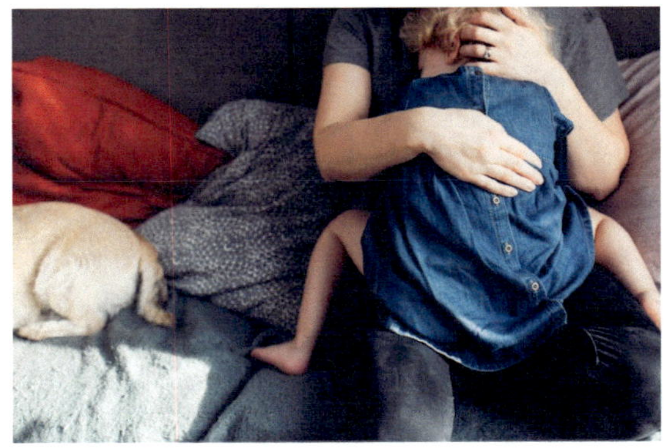

Figure 11.17. Effective management of Juvenile Idiopathic Arthritis (JIA) hinges significantly on robust support systems and resources.

Source: https://www.helpguide.org/wp-content/uploads/2023/02/Separation-Anxiety.jpeg.

11.4.4. Educational Accommodations for Affected Children

To kids with JIA, educational accommodations are central to their school success and well-being. These adaptations are needed to help relieve the physical and psychosocial burdens defined by adolescents living with JIA and typically have trouble finding balance between the desire for normalcy and the disease itself (Antonovsky et al., 2014). Supports could include flexible school attendance arrangements, the offering of additional test-taking time, and use of assistive technology, all intended to level the playing field created by chronic pain and mobility restrictions. As has been found in a study ordered by Arthritis Australia, understanding the children's specific needs is central to planning effective support services (Bates et al., 2014). By creating thoughtful educational adjustments, we not only adjust their learning process but also develop resilience, and therefore, affected children are able to excel in academics as well as manage their chronic diseases.

11.4.5. Social Implications and Peer Relationships

The social effects of JIA go far beyond the physical pain and impairment experienced by those affected children, with profound effects on their peer relationships and overall social integration. Healthy siblings in JIA-diagnosed families feel that their family life is not the same as that of others, leading them to withdraw and miss the experiences of everyday childhood life, such as spending good time with friends or engaging in group activities (Madill et al., 2007). This disruption has the potential to heighten the ambivalence of sibling relationships and can invoke complex emotional responses, particularly at the formative developmental years of late childhood and early adolescence. Moreover, evidence indicates greater recognition of JIAs contribution to disability is central in improving support services for affected families (Bates et al., 2014). Through the encouragement of a better understanding of such social problems, medical professionals and facilities can encourage all family members to make more intelligent emotional adaptations, eventually enhancing the quality of social interactions and peer relations (Figure 11.18).

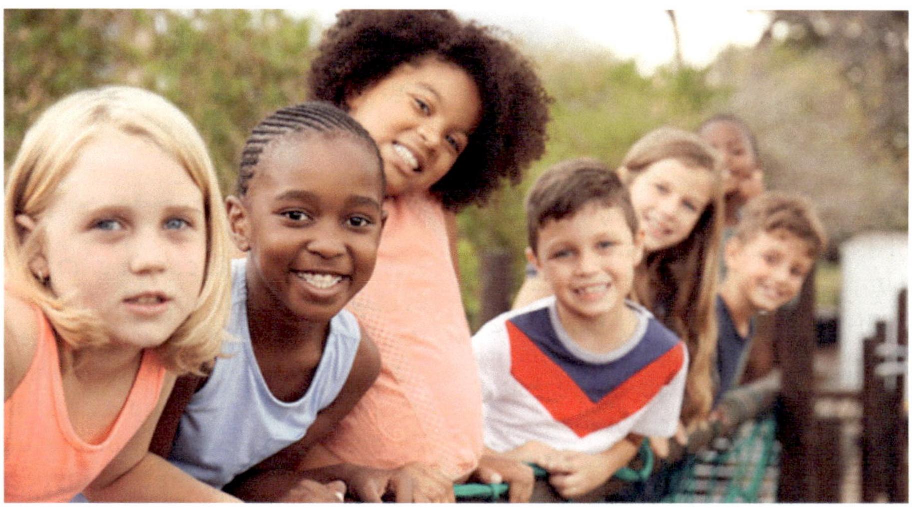

Figure 11.18. Healthy siblings in families with a JIA diagnosis often perceive their familial dynamic as distinct from peers, leading to feelings of isolation and a forfeit of typical childhood experiences, such as spending quality time with friends or engaging in shared activities.

Source: https://www.arthritis.org/getmedia/c8114b12-95c4-4d5c-adc6-5315ea813ddf/Diseases_Juvenile-Arthritis.jpg?width=600&height=325&ext=.jpg.

11.4.6. Transitioning to Adult Care

The process of transition between pediatric to adult care for JIA patients is met with huge challenges that have the potential to transform long-term health outcomes. Transitional care that is coordinated to enable adolescents is done through personalized education on physical activity and pain control, which is imperative at this developmental stage. EULAR guidelines emphasize the critical role of shared decision-making and patient engagement in their care in achieving readiness for this transfer, with the importance of proper patient education (Angevare et al., 2024). Furthermore, research reveals that an incredible 52% of patients fail transfers, many of which are due to reasons related to the clinic , such as an active joint count during transfer (Knauth et al., 2010). This points to the ultimate need to work toward addressing both disease care and psychosocial requirements in a bid to improve follow-up care compliance, wishing for improved health outcomes as these patients transition into young adulthood.

11.4.7. Long-term Health Considerations

Long-term care and medical needs for patients with JIA extend beyond short-term treatment regimens and symptoms, and a more integrated model of long-term care and management is required. Long-term, chronic inflammation of JIA can result in joint damage and functional impairment and in some cases affect mobility and quality of life as the young patient moves into adult life. Further, there are possible complications , such as serious eye disorders, for example, uveitis, which can happen, hence emphasizing the necessity of multidisciplinary intervention by ophthalmology and rheumatology professionals (Dick et al., 2018). An existing exploratory randomized controlled trial indicated the importance of a multidisciplinary foot-care program in treating specific complications , such as foot impairments, although outcomes indicated no statistically significant variations in outcomes from standard treatment (Brandon et al., 2013). Therefore, having effective long-term care practices that include regular monitoring, prompt referrals to numerous healthcare providers, and patient education is necessary to improve health status and minimize the residual effect of JIA (Figure 11.19).

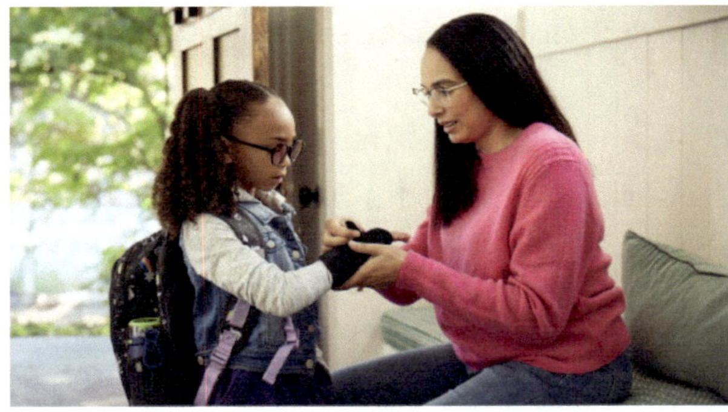

Figure 11.19. Chronic inflammation associated with JIA can lead to joint damage and functional impairments, which may affect mobility and overall quality of life as patients transition into adulthood.

Source: https://www.arthritis.org/getmedia/9ab73017-355d-4498-9478-07c3c36c5cd8/V1_JAAM_Thumbnail_600x325.jpg?width=600&height=326&ext=.jpg.

11.4.8. Advocacy and Awareness Efforts

Advocacy and education efforts play a vital role in improving the lives of individuals afflicted with JIA. The advocacy efforts are needed to inform medical practitioners, educators, and the general public about the complexities of this disease. By creating awareness of the daily challenges faced by young patients, advocacy groups can influence policy changes and campaign for the delivery of affordable healthcare services. For instance, research highlights the importance of identifying the effect of disability from arthritis, like in the efforts of Arthritis Australia focusing on maximizing support services among individuals with such conditions (Bates et al., 2014). Moreover, collective advocacy strategies, like the logic analysis model that is used in children's rehabilitation with pain, improve awareness and involvement among stakeholders like clinicians and families. Such interventions can eventually lead to evidence-based interventions that address the unique needs of persons living with JIA (Camden et al., 2020).

11.4.9. Personal Stories and Testimonials

Personal testimony and accounts are significant in understanding the lived experiences of children affected by JIA, the struggles and the triumphs that the children and their families go through.

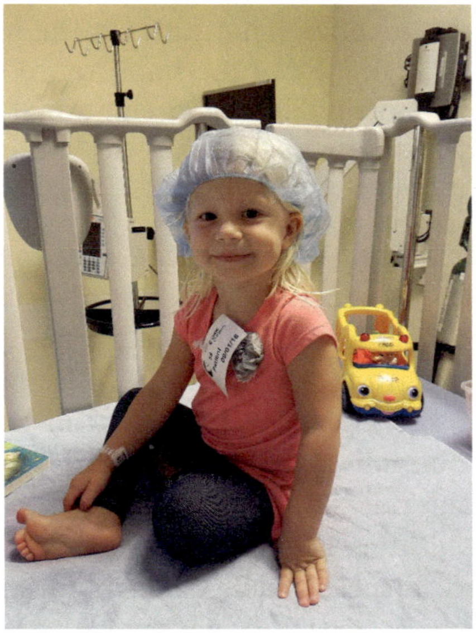

Figure 11.20. Personal stories and testimonials play a crucial role in understanding the lived experiences of those affected by Juvenile Idiopathic Arthritis (JIA), shedding light on the challenges and triumphs faced by children and their families.

Source: https://health.choc.org/wp-content/uploads/2019/07/mac-at-choc-e1562714941319.jpg.

Such accounts are likely to communicate the physical and emotional burden of the disease, painting the complexities of living with ongoing pain and mobility issues. As individuals and families prepare through treatment options, including emerging trends , such as hydrotherapy, patients' experiences can identify perceived benefits and limitations of such therapies for informing others to make informed choices in regard to care (Smith et al., 2018). Furthermore, experiences of adolescents using health monitoring technologies to track their symptoms can reveal empowerment and guardedness regarding self-tracking habits (Curtis et al., 2023). Ultimately, these individual experiences provide valuable insights into the patient journey together with advocating for more compassionate treatment and care for healthcare systems (Figure 11.20).

Test Your Knowledge

1. What physical activities are safe and beneficial for children with JIA?
2. How can schools and teachers accommodate children with JIA?

Summary

The impact of Juvenile Idiopathic Arthritis (JIA) extends beyond the individual diagnosed, affecting the entire family dynamic and necessitating a holistic approach to treatment and caregiving. Parents of children with JIA experience multifaceted challenges, including emotional strain and financial burdens, which significantly disrupt family life and relationships (Migowa et al., 2025). Acknowledging these difficulties is crucial for healthcare professionals, who must be attuned to the psychosocial needs of families navigating this chronic illness. Furthermore, recent findings suggest that combination therapies may lead to more significant clinical improvements in patients with JIA compared to monotherapy options, highlighting the importance of tailored interventions (Allaart et al., 2017). Therefore, addressing both medical and emotional aspects of care can enhance the overall quality of life for affected families, paving the way for improved management strategies and support systems crucial in the journey of living with JIA.

The complexity of JIA is underscored by its multifaceted impact on patients lives, especially concerning musculoskeletal health. A common yet often overlooked manifestation is foot and ankle problems, which significantly affect mobility and quality of life. Current interventions, though promising, rely on small, non-randomized studies that may not adequately represent the broader adult population with JIA, leaving a gap in robust clinical guidelines (Manca et al., 2009). Additionally, the lived experiences of individuals with arthritis highlight the condition as a leading cause of disability and chronic pain, raising questions about the effectiveness of existing support services (Bates et al., 2014). Integrating comprehensive care approaches, including innovative foot care programs, could enhance disease management and improve overall patient outcomes, emphasizing the need for holistic treatment strategies tailored to the unique challenges faced by young patients with JIA.

KEY TERMS FROM THIS CHAPTER

Adolescence	Adolescents
Biologic therapies	Chronic illness
Chronic inflammation	Corticosteroids
Diagnosis	Diagnostic criteria
Disability	Effective management
Genetic predisposition	Genetic susceptibility
Hypercytokinemia	Immune-modulating agents
Immune response	Interleukin
Juvenile Idiopathic Arthritis (JIA)	Macophages
Macrohage activation syndrome (MAS)	Macrophages

Critical Thinking Questions

1. **What is the most common type of Juvenile Idiopathic Arthritis (JIA)?**
   a. Systemic onset JIA
   b. Oligoarticular JIA
   c. Polyarticular RF-positive JIA
   d. Enthesitis-related arthritis
2. **Which of the following is a characteristic feature of systemic-onset JIA?**
   a. Morning stiffness only
   b. Daily (quotidian) fever spikes
   c. Rheumatoid factor positivity
   d. Uveitis
3. **Which autoantibody is most commonly positive in oligoarticular JIA?**
   a. Anti-dsDNA
   b. Anti-CCP
   c. ANA (antinuclear antibody)
   d. RF (rheumatoid factor)
4. **What is the primary treatment for mild oligoarticular JIA?**
   a. Methotrexate
   b. Biologics
   c. NSAIDs
   d. Steroids only
5. **Enthesitis-related arthritis (ERA) is most commonly associated with which HLA type?**
   a. HLA-DR4
   b. HLA-B27
   c. HLA-A1
   d. HLA-DQ2

Answers to Critical Thinking Questions

1. (b) 2. (b) 3. (c) 4. (c) 5. (b)

Short Answer Questions

1. What are the suspected causes of Juvenile Idiopathic Arthritis?
2. How does the immune system contribute to the development of JIA?
3. What are the common signs and symptoms of JIA?
4. How does JIA differ from adult rheumatoid arthritis?
5. What is the role of NSAIDs in managing JIA?
6. When are disease-modifying anti-rheumatic drugs (DMARDs) like methotrexate indicated?
7. How can JIA affect a child's growth and development?
8. What challenges do children with JIA face at school?

References

1. Accorinti, M., Acharya, N., Adan, A., Agrawal, R., et al. (2018). Guidance on noncorticosteroid systemic immunomodulatory therapy in noninfectious uveitis: Fundamentals of care for uveitis (FOCUS) initiative. https://core.ac.uk/download/156963570.pdf (accessed on 17th June 2025).

2. Dick, A. D., Rosenbaum, J. T., Al-Dhibi, H. A., Belfort, R., Jr, Brézin, A. P., Chee, S. P., Davis, J. L., Ramanan, A. V., Sonoda, K. H., Carreño, E., Nascimento, H., Salah, S., Salek, S., Siak, J., Steeples, L., & Fundamentals of Care for Uveitis International Consensus Group (2018). Guidance on Noncorticosteroid Systemic Immunomodulatory Therapy in Noninfectious Uveitis: Fundamentals Of Care for UveitiS (FOCUS) Initiative. *Ophthalmology*, *125*(5), 757–773. https://doi.org/10.1016/j.ophtha.2017.11.017(accessed on 17th June 2025).

3. Adamiak, A., Brooks, J., Andemariam, B., Douds, A., Annunziato, R., et al. (2017). UK guideline on transition of adolescent and young persons with chronic digestive diseases from pediatric to adult care. https://core.ac.uk/download/78863579.pdf (accessed on 17th June 2025).

4. Aji, N., Alshareefy, Y., et al. (2024). Advancements and progress in juvenile idiopathic arthritis: A review of pathophysiology and treatment. https://core.ac.uk/download/603360608.pdf (accessed on 17th June 2025).

5. Allaart, C. F., Bekkering, W. P., van den Berg, J. M., Brederije, M., et al. (2017). A comparison of three treatment strategies in recent onset non-systemic juvenile idiopathic arthritis: Initial 3-months results of the BeSt for Kids-study. https://core.ac.uk/download/154414697.pdf (accessed on 17th June 2025).

6. Alves, S. C., Fasano, S., & Isenberg, D. A. (2016). Current pharmacological treatment of idiopathic inflammatory myopathies. https://core.ac.uk/download/79552795.pdf (accessed on 17th June 2025).

7. Angevare, S., Anton, J., Ariza-Vega, P., Bini, M., et al. (2024). EULAR points to consider for patient education in physical activity and self-management of pain during transitional care. https://core.ac.uk/download/639218468.pdf (accessed on 17th June 2025).

8. Anjum, A., Bloodsworth, P., Branson, A., Hauer, T., et al. (2007). The requirements for ontologies in medical data integration: A case study. http://arxiv.org/abs/0707.0763 (accessed on 17th June 2025).

9. Antonovsky, A., Aujoulat, I., Barlow, J. H., Beresford, M., Casier, A., Christian, L., et al. (2014). Journeys of adjustment: The experiences of adolescents living with juvenile idiopathic arthritis. https://core.ac.uk/download/161123137.pdf (accessed on 17th June 2025).

10. Avenarius, D., de Horatio, L., Tanturri, L., Doria, A. S., Hemke, R., et al. (2018). Imaging in juvenile idiopathic arthritis–International initiatives and ongoing work. https://core.ac.uk/download/154910335.pdf (accessed on 17th June 2025).

11. Baggio, C., Bindoli, S., Galozzi, P., Oliviero, F., et al. (2018). Development and role in therapy of canakinumab in adult-onset Still's disease. https://core.ac.uk/download/168405209.pdf (accessed on 17th June 2025).

12. Bailey, K., Barker, K. L., Coe, S., Dawes, H., et al. (2023). An investigation into the relationship between nutritional status, dietary intake, symptoms and health-related quality of life in

children and young people with juvenile idiopathic arthritis: A systematic review and meta-analysis. https://core.ac.uk/download/587834701.pdf (accessed on 17th June 2025).

13. Balevic, S. J., Clark, S. J., Freed, G. L., Mater, M., et al. (2018). Prescribing for children with rheumatic disease: Perceived treatment approaches between pediatric and adult rheumatologists. http://deepblue.lib.umich.edu/bitstream/2027.42/141687/2/acr23273_am.pdf (accessed on 17th June 2025).

14. Bauer-Mehren, A., Cole, T. S., Frankovich, J., Iyer, A., et al. (2013). Profiling risk factors for chronic uveitis in juvenile idiopathic arthritis: A new model for EHR-based research. https://core.ac.uk/download/323067192.pdf (accessed on 17th June 2025).

15. Bernatsky, A., Gafni, A., Tong, A., Barron, A. C., Williams, A. E., Cahill, A. M., Arthritis and Musculoskeletal Alliance (ARMA), et al. (2014). An exploration of parents' preferences for foot care in juvenile idiopathic arthritis: A possible role for the discrete choice experiment. https://core.ac.uk/download/9376072.pdf (accessed on 17th June 2025).

16. Berntson, L., Billiau, A. D., Cedströmer, A. L., Dworkin, S. F., Helkimo, M., Küseler, A., Pedersen, T. K., et al. (2019). Temporomandibular joint damage in juvenile idiopathic arthritis: Diagnostic validity of diagnostic criteria for temporomandibular disorders. https://core.ac.uk/download/pdf/201590336.pdf (accessed on 17th June 2025).

17. Bohan, B., Brown, D., Chinoy, H., Christen-Zaech, S., Pilkington, C. A., et al. (2011). A national registry for juvenile dermatomyositis and other pediatric idiopathic inflammatory myopathies: 10 years' experience; the Juvenile Dermatomyositis National (UK and Ireland) Cohort Biomarker Study and Repository for Idiopathic Inflammatory Myopathies. https://core.ac.uk/download/10413.pdf (accessed on 17th June 2025).

18. Boneparth, A. D., CARRA Registry Investigators, Connelly, M., Schikler, K. N., et al. (2019). Demographic, clinical, and treatment characteristics of the juvenile primary fibromyalgia syndrome cohort enrolled in the Childhood Arthritis and Rheumatology Research Alliance Legacy Registry. https://core.ac.uk/download/323073272.pdf (accessed on 17th June 2025).

19. Bracaglia, C., Caiello, I., Chatel, L., De Min, M., et al. (2018). Neutralization of IFN-γ reverts clinical and laboratory features in a mouse model of macrophage activation syndrome. https://core.ac.uk/download/127587867.pdf (accessed on 17th June 2025).

20. Brandon, M., Friel, L., Gardner-Medwin, J., Hendry, G., et al. (2013). The effectiveness of a multidisciplinary foot care program for children and adolescents with juvenile idiopathic arthritis: An exploratory trial. https://core.ac.uk/download/293876502.pdf (accessed on 17th June 2025).

21. Bruns, A., Skarin, A., Hassett, A. L., Amine, B., Duarte-Salazar, C., Petersen, C., Gerhardt, C. A., et al. (2010). Burden of childhood-onset arthritis. https://core.ac.uk/download/pdf/8437352.pdf (accessed on 17th June 2025).

22. Bryant, A., BSPAR study group, Childhood Arthritis Prospective Study (CAPS), Childhood Arthritis Response to Medication Study (CHARMS), et al. (2012). Association of the IL-10 gene family locus on chromosome 1 with juvenile idiopathic arthritis (JIA). https://core.ac.uk/download/9652896.pdf (accessed on 17th June 2025).

23. Burnham, J. M., & von Scheven, E. (2011). Vitamin D supplementation in the pediatric rheumatology clinic. https://core.ac.uk/download/323072035.pdf (accessed on 17th June 2025).

24. Caes, L., Hynes, L., McGuire, B., Saetes, S., et al. (2017). Family resilience and adaptive coping in children with juvenile idiopathic arthritis: Protocol for a systematic review. https://core.ac.uk/download/132200315.pdf (accessed on 17th June 2025).

25. Camden, C., & Hurtubise, K. (2020). Using collaborative logic analysis evaluation to test the program theory of an intensive interdisciplinary pain treatment for youth with pain-related disability. https://core.ac.uk/download/362637045.pdf (accessed on 17th June 2025).

26. Cassidy, S., Coda, A., Grech, D., Hawke, F., et al. (2018). Confidence amongst multidisciplinary professionals in managing pediatric rheumatic disease in Australia. https://core.ac.uk/download/293884661.pdf (accessed on 17th June 2025).

27. Coeytaux, R. R., Kemper, A. R., Sanders, G. D., Van Mater, H., et al. (2012). Systematic review of disease-modifying antirheumatic drugs for juvenile idiopathic arthritis. https://core.ac.uk/download/pdf/8719762.pdf (accessed on 17th June 2025).

28. Collin, M. (2023). Orofacial aspects of juvenile idiopathic arthritis in children. https://core.ac.uk/download/570950848.pdf (accessed on 17th June 2025).

29. Richard-Miceli, C., & Criswell, L. A. (2012). Emerging patterns of genetic overlap across autoimmune disorders. Genome medicine, 4(1), 6. https://doi.org/10.1186/gm305(accessed on 17th June 2025).

30. Curtis, A., & Freeman, J. (2023). Putting the self in self-tracking: The value of a co-designed 'how might you' self-tracking guide for teenagers. https://core.ac.uk/download/603242378.pdf (accessed on 17th June 2025).

31. Dallas, J., Eckert, M., Huie, L., Roberts, H., et al. (2023). Insurance status and tumor necrosis factor inhibitor initiation among children with juvenile idiopathic arthritis in the CARRA Registry. https://core.ac.uk/download/614875704.pdf (accessed on 17th June 2025).

32. De Paepe, B., & Zschüntzsch, J. (2015). Scanning for Therapeutic Targets within the Cytokine Network of Idiopathic Inflammatory Myopathies. International Journal of Molecular Sciences, 16(8), 18683–18713. https://doi.org/10.3390/ijms160818683(accessed on 17th June 2025).

33. Demirkaya, E., Tok, F., & Özçakar, L. (2011). Musculoskeletal ultrasound in pediatric rheumatology. https://core.ac.uk/download/pdf/8622355.pdf (accessed on 17th June 2025).

34. Didona, D., Feola, A., Granata, G., Granata, F., et al. (2015). Macrophage activation syndrome as the onset of systemic lupus erythematosus: A case report and a review of the literature. https://core.ac.uk/download/153366215.pdf (accessed on 17th June 2025).

35. Dzhus, M. (2017). Juvenile idiopathic arthritis in adults: Long-term observation of Ukrainian patients. https://core.ac.uk/download/489786072.pdf (accessed on 17th June 2025).

36. Gottlieb, B. S., Lovell, D. J., Goldsmith, D. P., Giannini, E. H., Chalom, E. C., Brunner, H. I., Young, J. P., et al. (2014). Safety of celecoxib and nonselective nonsteroidal anti-inflammatory drugs in juvenile idiopathic arthritis: Results of the phase 4 registry. https://core.ac.uk/download/pdf/81275462.pdf (accessed on 17th June 2025).

37. Hilário, M. O. E., Len, C. A., & Terreri, M. T. R. A. (2006). Nonsteroidal anti-inflammatory drugs: Cyclooxygenase 2 inhibitors. https://core.ac.uk/download/37706683.pdf (accessed on 17th June 2025).

38. Iagnocco, A., & Naredo, E. (2016). One year in review: Ultrasound in arthritis. https://core.ac.uk/download/74318648.pdf (accessed on 17th June 2025).

39. Knauth, A., Ravelli, A., Duffy, C. M., Hazel, E., Reid, G. J., Stinson, J., Packham, J. C., et al. (2010). High rates of unsuccessful transfer to adult care among young adults with juvenile idiopathic arthritis. https://core.ac.uk/download/pdf/8377122.pdf (accessed on 17th June 2025).

40. Kosola, S., Luosujarvi, R., & Relas, H. (2018). Outcome of transition phase patients with juvenile idiopathic arthritis. https://core.ac.uk/download/287759991.pdf (accessed on 17th June 2025).

41. Madill, A., Baker, S., Banister, P., Barlow, J. H., Baumann, S. L., Britton, C., et al. (2008). Concealed concern: Fathers' experience of having a child with juvenile idiopathic arthritis. https://core.ac.uk/download/59279.pdf (accessed on 17th June 2025).

42. Madill, A., Banister, P., Bluebond-Langner, M., Britton, C., Charmaz, K., Dunn, J., Glaser, B. G., et al. (2007). Amplified ambivalence: Having a sibling with juvenile idiopathic arthritis. https://core.ac.uk/download/51906.pdf (accessed on 17th June 2025).

43. Manca, A., Mavidrou, A., Premkumar, A., Karmazyn, B., Wallace, C. A., Sherry, D. D., Turner, D. E., et al. (2009). Protocol for the Foot in Juvenile Idiopathic Arthritis trial (FiJIA): A randomized controlled trial of an integrated foot care programmed for foot problems in JIA. https://core.ac.uk/download/1396388.pdf (accessed on 17th June 2025).

44. Meira Blanco, G. C. (2023). The molecular basis of juvenile idiopathic arthritis and its correlation with other immune mediated diseases: A systematic review. https://core.ac.uk/download/590213891.pdf (accessed on 17th June 2025).

45. Migowa, A., Riang'a, R., Silim, H., Wamithi, M., et al. (2025). Experiences among parents caring for children with juvenile idiopathic arthritis at a tertiary referral hospital in Kenya. https://core.ac.uk/download/650947396.pdf (accessed on 17th June 2025).

46. Niestradt, H. (2025). Newly diagnosed juvenile idiopathic arthritis and childhood antibiotic use. https://core.ac.uk/download/pdf/86427517.pdf (accessed on 17th June 2025).

47. Ramanan, A. V., Sen, E. S., & Steward, C. G. (2016). Diagnosing hemophagocytic syndrome. https://core.ac.uk/download/83929215.pdf (accessed on 17th June 2025).

48. Bates, S. et al (2014). Arthritis and disability. https://core.ac.uk/download/pdf/30673486.pdf (accessed on 17th June 2025).

49. Smith, P. J. (2018). Evidence based hydrotherapy: A community of practice approach. https://core.ac.uk/download/334958611.pdf (accessed on 17th June 2025).

50. Ziff, M. (2016). Assessing quality of life needs in individuals with juvenile idiopathic arthritis and the potential role of occupational therapy. https://core.ac.uk/download/268401106.pdf (accessed on 17th June 2025).

THERAPEUTICS IN RHEUMATOLOGY

12

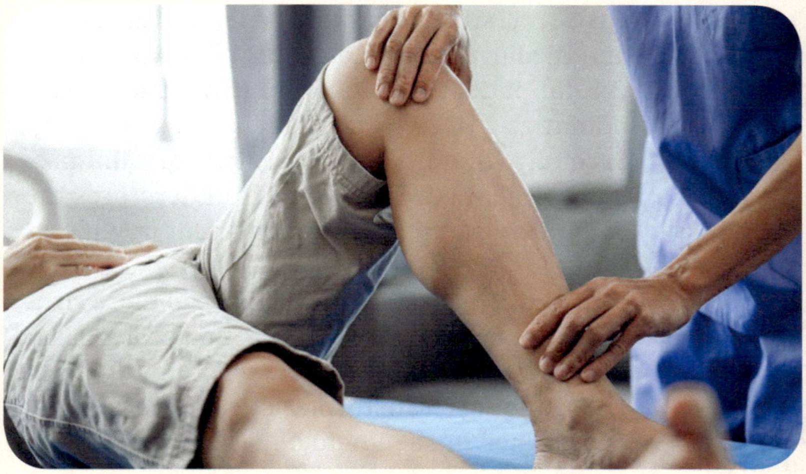

LEARNING OBJECTIVES

After studying this chapter, you will be able to:

1. Understand pharmacological treatments
2. Discuss non-pharmacological interventions
3. Focus on advances in research and technology
4. Identify challenges and barriers in rheumatologic care

Introduction

Rheumatology, an important medical specialty, is concerned with the diagnosis and treatment of various musculoskeletal and autoimmune disorders, among the most pertinent of which is psoriatic arthritis (PsA). The chronic inflammatory condition not only generates pain and joint destruction but can also generate significant disability, significantly affecting the lives of those affected. The emergence of tumor necrosis factor inhibitors (TNFi) has revolutionized treatment, with considerable clinical benefit for the majority of patients (Kraft et al., 2017). However, there remains a substantial resistant patient subgroup, demanding persistent research and exploration of alternative treatment modalities. Recent literature attests to the improved survival on drugs and efficacy of some anti-TNF drugs, i.e., adalimumab compared to others , such as etanercept and infliximab (Berardesca et al., 2018). As rheumatology progresses, awareness of such nuances is paramount in optimizing patient care and outcomes.

12.1. Pharmacological Treatments

Learning Outcome

1. Explain nonsteroidal anti-inflammatory drugs (NSAIDs)
2. Discuss disease-modifying antirheumatic drugs (DMARDs)
3. Focus on biologic response modifiers
4. Define corticosteroids
5. Focus on analgesics and pain management
6. Understand targeted synthetic DMARDs
7. Know combination therapy approaches
8. Discuss side effects and risks of pharmacological treatments

The pharmacological landscape of rheumatology has radically altered, and more so for autoimmune diseases , such as psoriatic arthritis (PsA) and systemic lupus erythematosus (SLE). TNFi have revolutionized the treatment pathway of PsA, with remarkable clinical efficacy and ability to inhibit radiographic progression, thus treating disability associated with severe disease. While TNFi have introduced better outcomes for the majority of patients, a great proportion is refractory or demonstrates diminishing gains with time, prefiguring the enduring need for new treatments (Kraft et al., 2017). In more recent developments, small molecule mimics of natural immunomodulators, such as ES-62 from parasitic worms, have proved to be protective against lupus nephritis through the inhibition of inflammatory processes and cytokines like IL-6. This research uncovers the potential for new classes of drugs that can treat the unmet needs of SLE patients, in which existing treatments do not do so satisfactorily (Harnett et al., 2015).

12.1.1. Nonsteroidal Anti-Inflammatory Drugs (NSAIDs)

In rheumatology, the Nonsteroidal Anti-Inflammatory Drugs (NSAIDs) are classed as cornerstone drugs due to their efficacy in managing signs and symptoms associated with inflammatory diseases , such as osteoarthritis (OA). NSAIDs work by blocking cyclooxygenase enzymes and, therefore, reducing the production of prostaglandins, which contribute to pain and inflammation. Though widely used—65% of U.S. OA patients receive NSAIDs—their side effects are of significant concern, particularly with chronic treatment. Some of these comprise gastrointestinal distress, renal disturbances, and cardiovascular incidents, all of which need careful patient monitoring and warning about potential side effects (Conway et al., 2021). Secondly, the ethical imperative to minimize pain without maximizing risks underscores the complexities of pain management regimens. Innovative approaches, such as fixed-dose combination analgesics, can mitigate these risks while enhancing the efficacy of analgesics (Laar et al., 2012). These considerations highlight the ongoing transformation of therapeutic approaches in rheumatology (Figure 12.1).

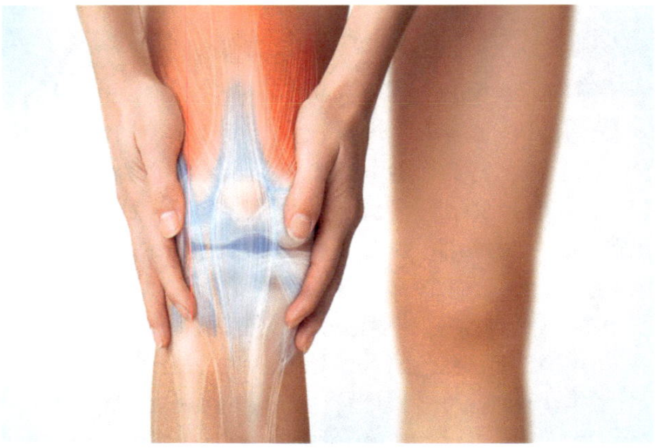

Figure 12.1. Nonsteroidal Anti-Inflammatory Drugs (NSAIDs) stand out as cornerstone treatments due to their efficacy in managing symptoms associated with inflammatory conditions , such as osteoarthritis (OA).

Source: https://creakyjoints.org/wp-content/uploads/2021/03/0221_nsaids-for-osteoarthritis-1024x683.jpg.

12.1.2. Disease-Modifying Antirheumatic Drugs (DMARDs)

In rheumatology, Disease-Modifying Antirheumatic Drugs (DMARDs) are responsible for managing chronic illness , such as rheumatoid arthritis (RA). They act directly on the disease process, with the aim of not only ameliorating symptoms but inducing remission and inhibiting long-term damage to joints. Current data emphasize the importance of initial treatment with DMARDs, particularly in subjects with high disease activity and with high titers of autoantibodies, as the optimal results are obtained from early treatment initiation (Aletaha et al., 2016). Among the different treatment plans that are available, the co-administration of conventional DMARDs and biologics , such as methotrexate and infliximab has been found to be superior to others in reducing functional impairment as well as radiographic disease progression among early RA patients (Pan et al., 2007). Hence, the strategic use of DMARDs is an important factor in redefining treatment strategies and improving prognostics for patients afflicted with rheumatic diseases.

12.1.3. Biologic Response Modifiers

Biologic response modifiers represent a significant shift in the rheumatology treatment paradigm, namely in diseases , such as rheumatoid arthritis (RA). These medications, acting on specific aspects of the immune system, have transformed treatment paradigms by offering more targeted interventions. Although traditional disease-modifying antirheumatic drugs do not block key inflammation pathways directly, biologics can do so and, by doing so, delay joint damage and improve patient outcomes. The use of these modifiers has brought about a paradigm shift in treatment, that of a treatment-to-target strategy aimed at treating strict remission or low disease activity. This is particularly relevant considering early treatment is directly linked with long-term prognosis, as noted by the need for new therapies to address the unmet needs of treatment-resistant patients (Aletaha et al., 2016). As continued research yields increased genetic and pathophysiologic insights, the future promise for biologics to offer additional improvement in therapeutic efficacy is an intriguing frontier in rheumatology (McInnes & Schett, 2017) (Figure 12.2).

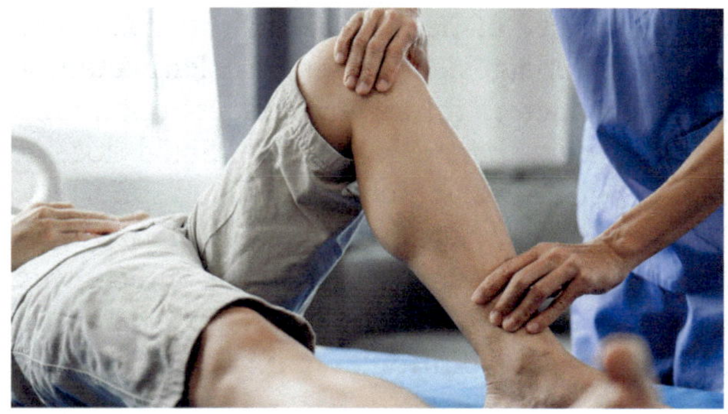

Figure 12.2. Biologic response modifiers represent a significant advancement in the treatment landscape of rheumatology.

Source: https://wakeresearch.com/wp-content/uploads/Orthopedics-1.jpg.

12.1.4. Corticosteroids

Corticosteroids occupy a central role in the therapeutic picture of rheumatology primarily due to their very potent anti-inflammatory and immunosuppressive properties. Corticosteroids are particularly valuable in managing inflammatory diseases, such as rheumatoid arthritis, systemic lupus erythematosus, and other autoimmune disorders. Their rapid onset renders corticosteroids very valuable in the context of an acute flare, bringing quick relief from the symptoms. Besides, novel corticosteroid formulations, for example, FX006, with extended-release properties maintain analgesic activity over prolonged durations, hence enhancing patient compliance and quality of life (Abhishek et al., 2018). However, the use of corticosteroids is not harmless as it carries potential side effects in the form of osteoporosis, hypertension, and diabetes, which need to be managed with correct handling techniques to prevent such complications. The challenge of balancing safety and effectiveness underscores the importance of individualized treatment regimens in rheumatology, where corticosteroids remain an anchor therapeutic modality with the caveat of being treated to their multi-dimensional side effect profiles (Abdallah et al., 2017).

12.1.5. Analgesics and Pain Management

In rheumatology, effective pain management is highly important in improving the quality of life of patients, particularly those afflicted with chronic illnesses like rheumatoid arthritis (RA). The heterogeneity of pain is because it has a complex pathophysiology, hence making the selection of proper analgesics challenging. Paracetamol and NSAIDs are employed commonly but turn into causative factors for adverse effects upon long-term use, deteriorating the condition of the patient unknowingly (Laar et al., 2012). Fixed-dose combination analgesics find newer evidence favoring their application, which can deliver synergistic effects while bringing down toxicity by low dose. Such methods are especially relevant as RA patients require individualized therapies that address both long-term management needs and chronic pain (Dinda et al., 2015). Therefore, an ever-evolving model of therapy involving low-dose combination therapies alongside intermittent therapy with NSAIDs may revolutionize pain relief outcomes in rheumatologic care (Figure 12.3).

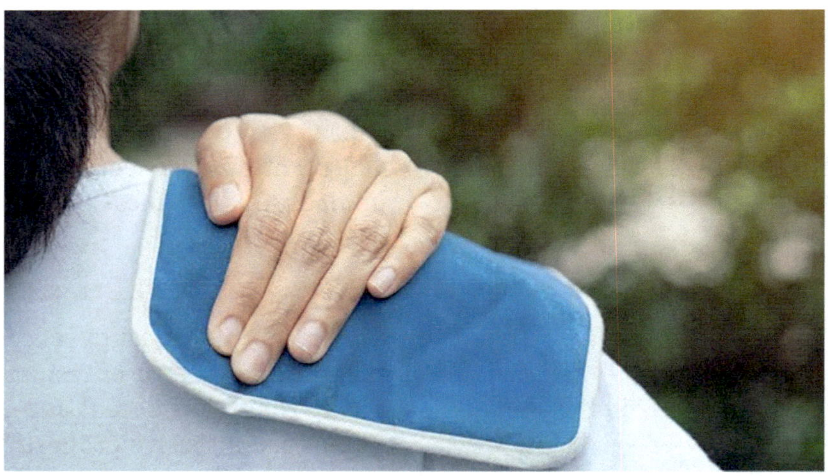

Figure 12.3. Effective pain management is essential for improving patients quality of life, particularly for those grappling with chronic conditions like rheumatoid arthritis (RA).

Source: https://images.everydayhealth.com/images/arthritis/rheumatoid-arthritis/rheumatoid-arthritis-pain-management-alt-722x406.jpg?sfvrsn=294d2c19_3.

12.1.6. Targeted Synthetic DMARDs

Over the past years, targeted synthetic disease-modifying antirheumatic drugs (DMARDs) have been exceedingly crucial elements in the treatment regimen of rheumatology, particularly for rheumatoid arthritis (RA). Targeted synthetic DMARDs are different from the traditional DMARDs in that they directly act on specific pathways accountable for the inflammatory process, offering a more specific therapeutic mechanism. Research has shown that these drugs, including Janus kinase inhibitors, significantly enhance disease management, especially in patients who respond poorly to conventional therapies (Aletaha et al., 2016). However, there are still challenges, especially among the elderly, who are likely to have non-uniform efficacy and retention. Registry analysis found that among RA patients >65 years, the primary cause of drug discontinuation was loss of efficacy, emphasizing the necessity of treatment with certain therapies according to both age and past treatment history (Atzeni et al., 2024). Therefore, ongoing research and development are necessary to optimize the use of targeted synthetic DMARDs across different groups of patients.

12.1.7. Combination Therapy Approaches

In rheumatology, combination treatment approaches are increasingly being perceived to provide greater treatment efficacy than that of monotherapy. These treatments address multiple mechanisms in the pathogenesis of autoimmune diseases, such as rheumatoid arthritis and gout, in order to improve outcomes in patients. One example is where the application of traditional disease-modifying antirheumatic drugs is combined with newer biological agents to attain significant reduction of disease activity alongside slowing down its progression (Aletaha et al., 2016). Furthermore, the establishment of new drugs, like leisured for gout, illustrates the evolving landscape of combination therapies that acknowledge the pharmacodynamic details of uric acid regulation without aggravating side effects (Girardet et al., 2016). This comprehensive strategy not only promotes a more complete control of the symptoms but also tries to achieve stringent remission or low disease activity, ultimately enhancing the quality of life of patients with chronic rheumatologic diseases. With further advances in research, the refinement of these strategies remains essential for filling up unmet therapeutic gaps (Figure 12.4).

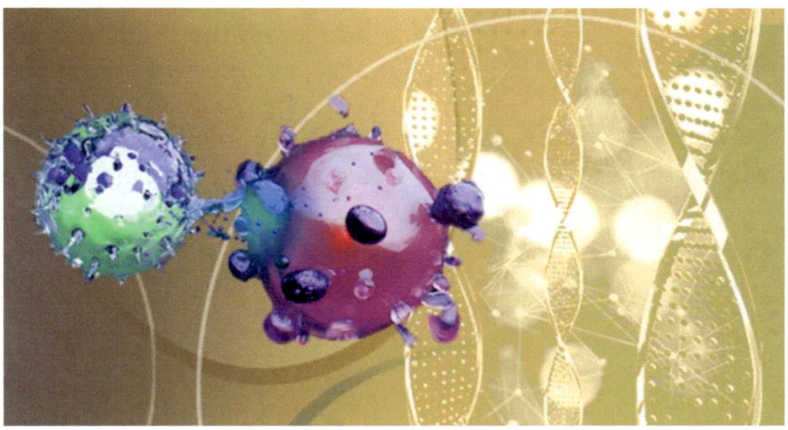

Figure 12.4. In the realm of rheumatology, combination therapy approaches are increasingly recognized for their potential to enhance treatment efficacy beyond that of monotherapy.

Source: https://opalbiopharma.com/wp-content/uploads/2024/11/Rituximabs_B-Cell_Depletion-jpg.webp.

12.1.8. Side Effects and Risks of Pharmacological Treatments

Pharmacological treatment in rheumatology, as crucial as it is for managing ailments like rheumatoid arthritis, exposes patients to significant risks and side effects that need to be carefully monitored.

Medications , such as nonsteroidal anti-inflammatory drugs (NSAIDs) and acetaminophen, which are used extensively to manage pain, have side effects, especially when administered in the long term or in excessive amounts, that can be poorly explained to patients (Laar et al., 2012). Additionally, the therapeutic profile of rheumatoid arthritis includes powerful drugs like methotrexate and biologics that, although effective, have serious complications. As scientists explore preventive treatments for at-risk individuals, including those with first signs of systemic autoimmunity, they must contend with balancing therapeutic benefits against side effects (Falahee et al., 2019). This highlights the importance of patient education and implementing a do ask, do tell policy that allows for free discussion of medication management to optimize safety and efficacy in rheumatological treatment.

Test Your Knowledge

1. What are the common side effects of long-term corticosteroid use in rheumatologic patients?
2. When should methotrexate therapy be discontinued in a patient planning pregnancy?

12.2. Non-Pharmacological Interventions

Learning Outcome

1. Understand physical therapy and rehabilitation
2. Discuss occupational therapy
3. Focus on dietary modifications and nutrition
4. Explain exercise and lifestyle changes
5. Learn complementary and alternative medicine
6. Focus on patient education and self-management
7. Understand psychological support and counseling
8. Know role of support groups
9. Discuss integrative approaches in rheumatology

Non-pharmacological treatments have gained popularity in the management of rheumatological conditions, as a substitute to conventional pharmacotherapy and to supplement the conventional method of disease management. Exercise therapy, manual therapy, and patient education are some of the interventions that are useful in pain relief and physical functioning improvement with no adverse effects unlike medication. It has been established through studies that exercise therapy and manual therapy are very effective in increasing pain levels and range of motion in patients with conditions like hip osteoarthritis, even despite the controversy in combined therapies (Bueno-Gracia et al., 2019). Furthermore, new trial designs , such as the REMAP-ILD platform could accelerate the evaluation of such interventions across different groups and conditions, a growing recognition of their application in holistic patient treatment (Kawano-Dourado et al., 2024). As rheumatology continues to evolve, the inclusion of non-pharmacological strategies can enhance improved outcomes and overall treatment regimen for patients.

12.2.1. Physical Therapy and Rehabilitation

Optimal physical therapy and rehabilitation are key aspects of rheumatologic management, particularly in optimizing patient outcomes and overall quality of life. Interventions are particularly critical for patients with osteoarthritis and JIA, where highly structured exercise protocols have been demonstrated to significantly minimize pain and maximize functional ability. For example, exercise modalities , such as strengthening and aerobic training have been found greater efficacy than no exercise in reducing pain and improving function in patients with knee osteoarthritis, as indicated by the cumulative evidence to support exercise intervention (Dziedzic et al., 2013). Additionally, in JIA, customized rehabilitation measures are essential to resist the multifaceted features of the disease, such as chronic inflammation and joint damage (Aji et al., 2024). Thus, the integration of targeted physical therapy not only facilitates physical healing but also assists in mental and emotional status of patients with chronic rheumatologic disorders (Figure 12.5).

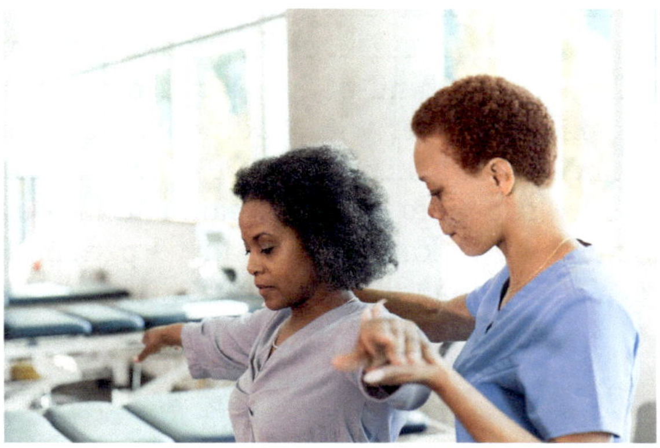

Figure 12.5. Effective physical therapy and rehabilitation play a pivotal role in the management of rheumatologic conditions, particularly in enhancing patient outcomes and improving quality of life.

Source: https://images.ctfassets.net/yixw23k2v6vo/2xY5FF15wkC80ceuoLKdFh/146b6deff500bf95dd416c19a3cfe04d/GettyImages-1366650744-3000x2000.jpg.

12.2.2. Occupational Therapy

Occupational therapy plays a critical role in the management of rheumatologic disorders with the goal of enhancing patients' functional daily activities and quality of life. With the application of specially tailored interventions, occupational therapists assist patients in learning to apply adaptive strategies and utilize assistive devices, both of which are crucial to overcome limitations based on joint stiffness and pain. Moreover, treatment that emphasizes skill development and environmental adaptation enables patients to regain independence in executing primary daily functions. The growing recognition of occupational therapy in multidisciplinary treatment protocols is a testament to the movement toward holistic patient care for rheumatology as evidence indicates that treatment can be more than just pharmacologic approaches. Today's evidence favors the effectiveness of occupational therapy for improving functional performance and activity engagement in patients, augmenting the entire goal of rheumatologic therapy. These integrative strategies emphasize the need for a comprehensive care model that is most responsive to the complex needs of individuals with chronic rheumatic diseases (Kinney, 2007; Gleasner, 2019).

12.2.3. Dietary Modifications and Nutrition

Dietary modification has emerged as central aspects of managing rheumatological diseases, particularly in the case of gout and rheumatoid arthritis (RA). Emerging data suggest that certain dietary habits play a significant role in determining the prognosis of the disease and inflammatory reactions. For instance, consumption of tart cherry juice has been linked to lowered serum urate and decreased inflammation, potentially lowering the frequency of gout attacks, as demonstrated in a recent trial employing a 12-month randomized controlled trial (Barker et al., 2020). In addition, excessive salt intake has previously been reported to exacerbate both hypertension and RA disease activity, as indicated by the positive correlation between urinary sodium-to-potassium ratio and the 28-Joint RA Disease Activity Score (Fujita et al., 2021). The evidence pointed towards the integration of dietary treatments into treatment regimens since it shows the possibility of nutrition being an effective adjunct to typical pharmacologic treatments in rheumatology (Figure 12.6).

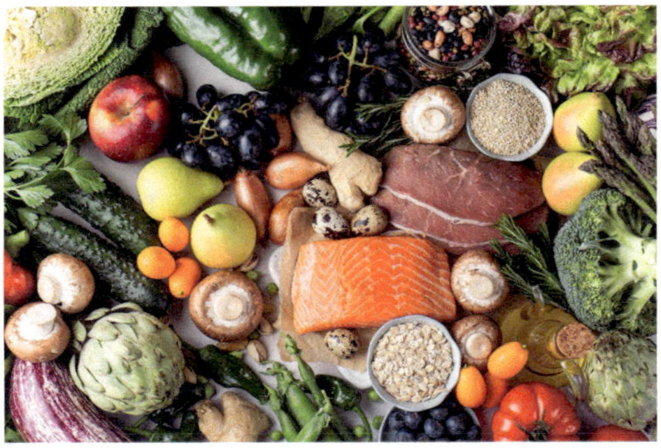

Figure 12.6. Dietary modifications have emerged as critical components in the management of rheumatological conditions, particularly concerning gout and rheumatoid arthritis (RA).

Source: https://www.rheumatologyadvisor.com/wp-content/uploads/sites/18/2023/11/Mediterranean.Diet_G_1390699821-1.jpg.

12.2.4. Exercise and Lifestyle Changes

The incorporation of exercise and lifestyle changes into the management of rheumatological conditions may have a significant influence on patient outcomes. Research indicates that structured exercise programs have been shown to alleviate pain and improve functioning among patients with osteoarthritis, providing evidence for their use in therapeutic measures through primary care settings (Gensichen et al., 2005). In addition, nonpharmacological methods that address lifestyle modifications, such as dietary changes and smoking cessation, have been shown to influence disease activity in conditions like psoriatic arthritis. This review also captures the encouraging evidence regarding physical exercise on both progression of disease and mental well-being, showing the value of integrative lifestyle interventions (Amarnani et al., 2023). With the advancement of rheumatologic care, emphasis on integrated methods encompassing exercise and lifestyle change will be crucial in maximizing quality of life in the patient and minimizing reliance on pharmacologic interventions. Promotion of such changes forms a significant therapeutic strategy in rheumatology.

12.2.5. Complementary and Alternative Medicine

In the recent years, integrating Complementary and Alternative Medicine (CAM) in the treatment of rheumatological diseases has gained significant attention. CAM entails a number of practices like acupuncture, herbal medicine, and mind-body practices that can be applied together with traditional medicinal treatments. For instance, the use of acupuncture has been shown to decrease pain and improve functionality in knee osteoarthritis patients, a prevalent rheumatological disease.

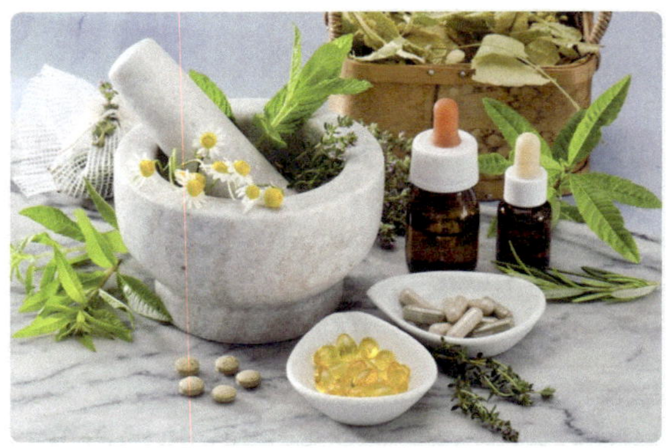

Figure 12.7. The integration of Complementary and Alternative Medicine (CAM) in the management of rheumatological conditions has gained significant attention.

Source: https://www.news-medical.net/image-handler/picture/2021/1/shutterstock_139839763.jpg.

One clinical trial that utilized a multimodal treatment package that combined exercise therapy, acupuncture, and functional electrical stimulation reported significant decrease in pain severity and better daily functioning in a patient with chronic knee osteoarthritis (Ansari et al., 2019). This indicates the potential for the efficacy of CAM modalities in treating symptoms when conventional treatments fail. As technology continues to develop, the inclusion of CAM in rheumatological practice may provide a patient with a more complete means of treating their disease (FitzGerald et al., 2013) (Figure 12.7).

12.2.6. Patient Education and Self-Management

An integral part of effective drugs in rheumatology is giving premium to patient education and self-management, which help individuals become participants in their health. Educating patients regarding their diseases—rheumatoid arthritis and osteoarthritis—helps healthcare professionals achieve high compliance with therapy and self-care regimens. For instance, intensive patient education is able to significantly improve outcomes for rheumatoid arthritis, which is likely to need early diagnosis and intervention in an effort to minimize cartilage and bone damage (Aletaha et al., 2016). Finally, an application of interventions like Arthritis Self-Management Programs (ASMPs) illustrates the benefit of formal education in a primary care environment, with improvements in quality of life and pain control (Gensichen et al., 2005). In general, creating a culture of educated self-management has the potential to allow patients to better manage the intricacies of their illness, resulting in improved health and less disease-induced disability.

12.2.7. Psychological Support and Counseling

Psychological support and counseling are an integral part of rheumatology treatment, particularly for patients suffering from chronic diseases, such as rheumatoid arthritis (RA). Uncertainty about disease progression and chronic pain are likely to affect a patient's mental well-being as well as the quality of life. Effective counseling empowers patients to enhance the knowledge and understanding of patients regarding treatment, which is multifaceted and complex. As evidence shows, educated patients are more likely to comply with treatment programs and healthy choices, where psychological support becomes absolutely essential to the situation (Al-Eidan et al., 2009). Additionally, as new medical methods evolve to involve preventive intervention among high-risk populations, counseling plays a vital role in fulfilling patient concerns and expectations regarding potential interventions. Patient understanding is central to successful treatment utilization and has the potential to increase the therapeutic relationship between providers and patients (Falahee et al., 2019) (Figure 12.8).

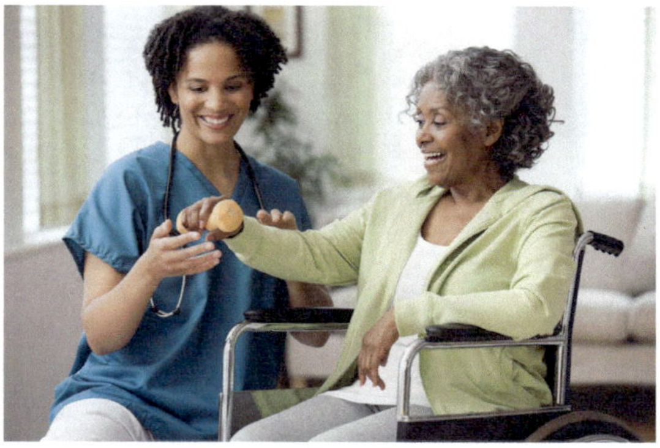

Figure 12.8. The provision of psychological support and counseling is an essential component of therapeutics in rheumatology, particularly for patients navigating chronic conditions , such as rheumatoid arthritis (RA).

Source: https://www.health.com/thmb/IExfyr2k6iq3z79mx1k8mV7zvBo=/1500x0/filters:no_upscale():max_bytes(150000):strip_icc()/rheumatoid-arthritis-treatment-GettyImages-93909438-71943186d8844b63aed80a21ddd48edc.jpg.

12.2.8. Role of Support Groups

Support groups play an important role in the general care of patients with rheumatological diseases, although they offer emotional relief as well as a feeling of belonging among individuals who share similar misfortune. Support groups enable patients to compare their experiences, coping strategies, and reaction to treatment, which can lead to better psychological status and therapeutic compliance. The psychosocial support gleaned from such interactions has a tendency to build resilience, reducing the feelings of isolation that are apt to accompany chronic illness like rheumatoid arthritis. There is evidence that disease beliefs and health status can be significantly influenced by support networks, and these can have an influence on inflammatory biomarkers and overall disease activity, as with studies examining miR-155 and its relationship to disease status in patients with rheumatoid arthritis (Elmesmari et al., 2016). Besides, understanding of immune pathways and therapeutic benefits can be optimized with shared knowledge in such forums, enhancing the therapeutic journey of the patient (McInnes & Schett, 2017).

12.2.9. Integrative Approaches in Rheumatology

Combination of different therapeutic strategies in rheumatology is becoming more a question of survival to achieve better patient outcomes. One prominent approach is the finding of new pharmacogenomic methods that possess the capability of identifying optimal and safe treatment by illuminating complex interactions between drugs, genes, and diseases.

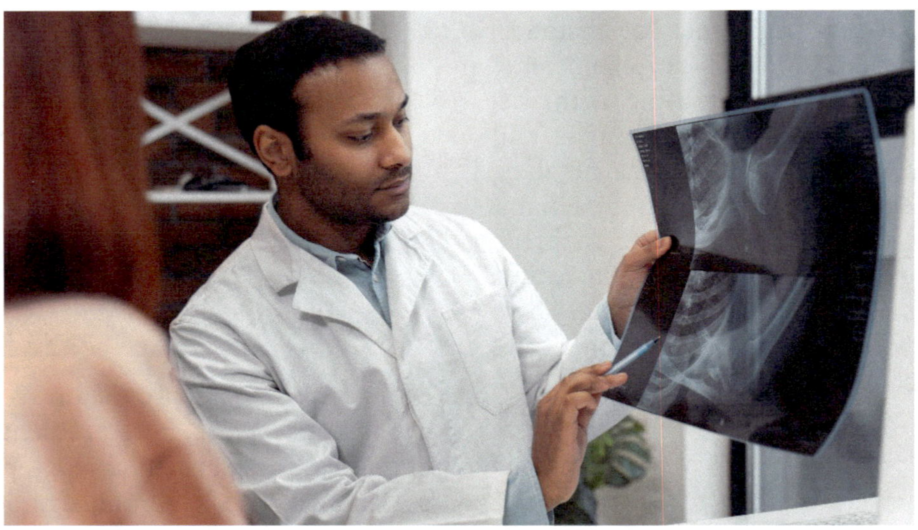

Figure 12.9. The integration of diverse therapeutic strategies in rheumatology is becoming increasingly vital for enhancing patient outcomes.

Source: https://tatamd.com/wp-content/uploads/2024/10/image-min-scaled.jpg.

Emphasized is that rheumatoid arthritis treatments are typically lacking in leading to remission without cytotoxicity, so innovative solutions become imperative (Bjourson et al., 2023). In addition, translational research can play an important role in bridging laboratory discoveries and clinic applications so that biomedical progress can be translated to therapeutic use more effectively (Boenink et al., 2015). Its integrative role not only aims to improve symptom management and quality of life for patients but to overcome the constraints of conventional treatments, paving the way for more personalized treatment regimens in rheumatology. Finally, this multidimensional approach creates a comprehensive understanding of disease management, which could revolutionize treatment practice in the field (Figure 12.9).

Test Your Knowledge

1. Describe the importance of patient education in managing rheumatoid arthritis.
2. What dietary modifications are recommended for patients with gout?

12.3. Advances in Research and Technology

Learning Outcome

1. Focus on genetic research in rheumatology
2. Understand biomarkers for disease monitoring
3. Know advances in imaging techniques
4. Focus on telemedicine in rheumatology
5. Explain artificial intelligence and machine learning
6. Discuss clinical trials and their importance
7. Describe personalized medicine approaches
8. Know innovations in drug development
9. Understand future research directions

There has been tremendous growth in research and technology over the past couple of decades that has significantly transformed rheumatology therapeutics, particularly disease management of juvenile idiopathic arthritis (JIA). Sophisticated research methods, including genome-wide studies and in vivo animal model usage, have been extremely useful in explaining JIAs multi-factorial etiology and hence directing more effective treatment strategies with an eye to preventing long-term joint damage (Aji et al., 2024). Besides, digital tool integration has changed the management of data in healthcare institutions to assist in mitigating data overload and personnel shortages. The application of frameworks like the balanced scorecard (BSC) allows healthcare organizations to quantify the impact of new technologies in a systematic way while ensuring constant improvement in patient care and facility efficiency (Grek et al., 2023). These advancements reflect a paradigm change in rheumatology that not only promotes short-term therapeutic efficacy but also long-term management paradigms that focus on patient outcomes (Bagnall et al., 2013).

12.3.1. Genetic Research in Rheumatology

The research of genetic research in rheumatology remains at the cornerstone of the creation of treatment modalities in diseases , such as rheumatoid arthritis (RA). By studying the complex interaction between genetic susceptibility, environment, and immune mechanisms, investigators aim to discover the precise mechanisms in RA that will enable individualized treatment. Genetic studies have determined numerous susceptibility loci of RA and propose that the genetic profile of the individual can be predicted or understood to formulate more effective therapy with fewer side effects. Furthermore, advancements in models of animals have given valuable information about RA pathophysiology, thereby enriching strategies of drug development. As emphasized in recent publications, integration of data obtained from animal models and human research is significant in constructing an integrated knowledge base for RAs etiology, thereby leading to improved clinical results as well as new therapeutic approaches (Talele et al., 2024; Apparailly et al., 2011). This model of genetic studies not only contributes to the improvement of patient care but also provides an avenue for developments in preventive treatments (Figure 12.10).

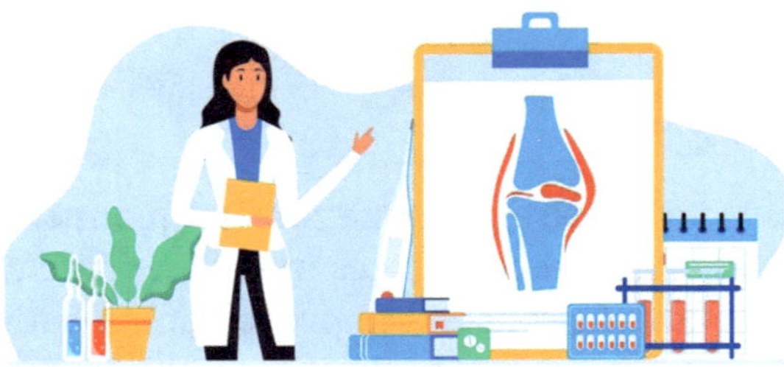

Figure 12.10. The exploration of genetic research in rheumatology is pivotal in advancing therapeutic strategies for conditions , such as rheumatoid arthritis (RA).

Source: https://www.news-medical.net/image-handler/picture/2021/5/shutterstock_1748836958-1.jpg.

12.3.2. Biomarkers for Disease Monitoring

The identification and validation of biomarkers for rheumatology monitoring of disease activity is of crucial significance towards the promotion of therapy methods. Biomarkers offer a way to understand the pathophysiology of the disease as well as to stratify patients by disease activity, prognosis, and response to treatment. For instance, studies have identified significant differences in miR-155 expression levels among RA patients, indicating that it can be used as a disease activity biomarker. Specifically, higher levels of miR-155 correlate with disease activity scores and consistently elevated levels in synovial fluid reveal that it plays a role within inflammatory processes (Elmesmari et al., 2016). Furthermore, understanding the manner in which miR-155 controls chemokine expression and receptor expression reveals its function in driving inflammatory cell recruitment within the synovium, thereby posing as a potential target for intervention (FitzGerald et al., 2013). Accordingly, the present studies on such biomarkers are essential to improving disease control in rheumatology.

12.3.3. Advances in Imaging Techniques

The new imaging technologies developed over the last few years have revolutionized the diagnostic and therapeutic landscape in rheumatology, particularly in diseases , such as rheumatoid arthritis (Cook et al., 2016). Accurate imaging techniques, e.g., magnetic resonance imaging (MRI) and ultrasound, allow for the early detection of joint inflammation and damage, a crucial point as early intervention can be a brake on long-term disability. Such techniques enable monitoring of disease activity and therapeutic response, guiding clinicians regarding the efficacy of therapy protocols. Visualization of structural changes in real-time, as described in studies, enables practitioners to adopt a treat-to-target approach, adjusting therapy in response to each patient's condition (Aletaha et al., 2016).

With the hope of improved outcomes with personalized medicine, the integration of advanced imaging modalities into routine clinical practice remains vital. Consequently, continued research to develop these imaging technologies will play a key role in resolving the unmet challenges of rheumatoid arthritis management (Figure 12.11).

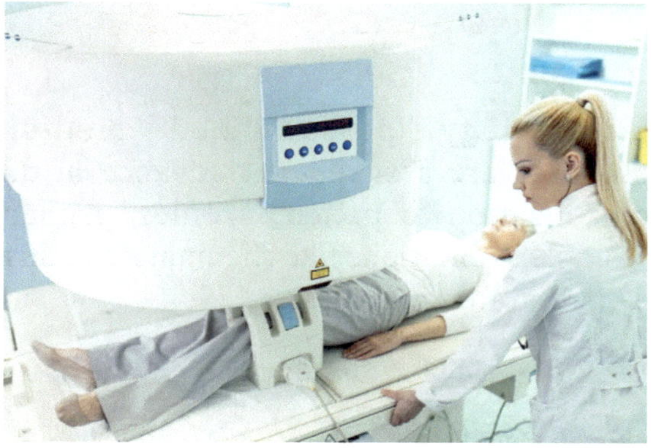

Figure 12.11. Precision imaging modalities, including magnetic resonance imaging (MRI) and ultrasound, allow for the early detection of joint inflammation and damage, which is crucial given that timely intervention can prevent long-term disability.

Source: https://doctorsclinicdubai.ae/wp-content/uploads/2024/11/Knee-MRI.webp.

12.3.4. Telemedicine in Rheumatology

The incorporation of telemedicine in rheumatology practice has changed the lives of patients, particularly in the context of recent global crises. Telemedicine, by facilitating remote consultation, has relieved the pressure on health systems while maintaining continuity of care in patients with rheumatic disease. The COVID-19 pandemic had an accelerated demand for telehealth, and this was seen as an immediate adoption among healthcare providers, as witnessed across various medical specialties. As highlighted, the majority of patients were content with telehealth care and stressed its use for follow-up visits and slight health conditions (Chandak et al., 2023). Telemedicine can also be an affordable method for clinical training and supervision, which would be of significant value in low-and-middle-income countries where healthcare facilities are limited (Khoza-Shangase et al., 2021). Thus, the integration of telemedicine into rheumatological practice not only enhances accessibility along with efficiency but also represents a critical component of current therapeutic practices in the field.

12.3.5. Artificial Intelligence and Machine Learning

The integration of Artificial Intelligence (AI) and Machine Learning (ML) into rheumatology is a game-changing process towards the enhancement of therapeutic strategies for patients with systemic autoimmune rheumatic diseases (SARDs). With the application of these technologies, clinicians can analyze large data sets, offering insights into disease patterns and possible patient outcomes at a level of precision never before seen. As noted, machine learning and AI is an untapped area...to infer patterns between patient information (Ventura et al., 2022).

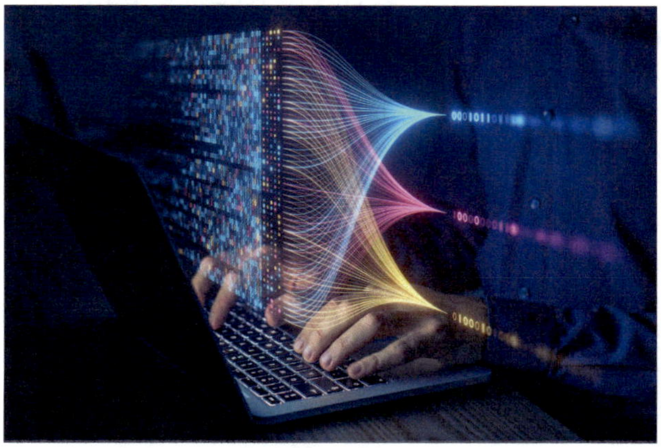

Figure 12.12. The integration of Artificial Intelligence (AI) and Machine Learning (ML) into rheumatology represents a transformative approach to enhancing therapeutic strategies for patients with systemic autoimmune rheumatic diseases (SARDs).

Source: https://media.licdn.com/dms/image/v2/D5612AQFovPb5M9mWEg/article-cover_image-shrink_720_1280/article-cover_image-shrink_720_1280/0/1701182676279?e=2147483647&v=beta&t=QyrqSSG-SBMJnfnesdUHCJRaOXX6yRpHNusy1vKFsoE.

This predictive role has the potential to revolutionally bridge the seronegative gap, allowing for more precise classifications and diagnoses in patients, hence maximizing clinical management and personalized treatment protocols. Moreover, the application of technology , such as the balanced scorecard (BSC) in e-health settings promotes effective translation of AI/ML technologies into practice, which ultimately enhances the quality of care, productivity of operations, and patient empowerment. The ongoing evolution of these technologies will necessarily shape the future of therapeutics in rheumatology (Grek et al., 2023) (Figure 12.12).

12.3.6. Clinical Trials and Their Importance

Clinical trials are crucial to treatment strategy development and validation in rheumatology, offering a scientific mechanism for the evaluation of new therapies' effectiveness and safety. Clinical trials provide researchers with the ability to quantify outcomes , such as symptom improvement, function, and quality of life for patients with chronic inflammatory conditions , such as psoriatic arthritis and rheumatoid arthritis. For instance, new evidence has demonstrated the groundbreaking impact of TNFi in the management of psoriatic arthritis, with significantly enhanced clinical effectiveness and radiographic progression (Kraft et al., 2017). Conversely, a significant part of such trials is the fulfillment of the unmet needs of failed patients of current treatments, as underpinned by evidence for an ongoing need for new pharmacotherapeutic drugs (Aletaha et al., 2016). Clinical trials are thus a key impetus for the rheumatology domain, informing clinical practice ultimately leading to enhanced patient outcomes.

12.3.7. Personalized Medicine Approaches

Rheumatology personalized medicine approaches are a significant advance in drug personalization to patient profiles, primarily for complex conditions like rheumatoid arthritis (RA) and systemic sclerosis (SSc).

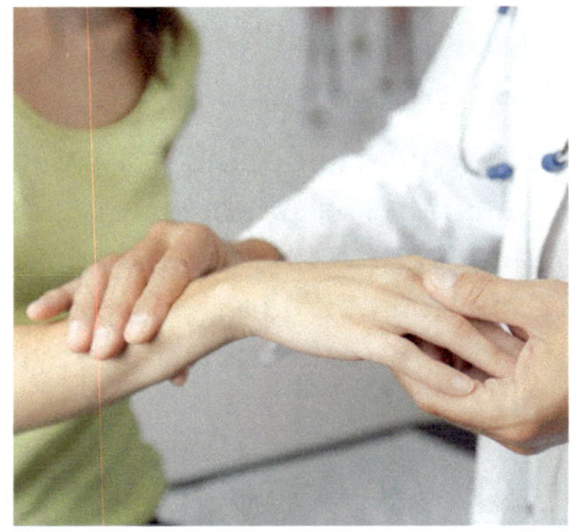

Figure 12.13. Personalized medicine approaches in rheumatology represent a significant advancement in tailoring treatments to individual patient profiles, particularly in complex diseases like rheumatoid arthritis (RA) and systemic sclerosis (SSc).

Source: https://www.attodiagnostics.com/assets/dynamic/practitioners/ra-autoimmune/pgx/hero.webp.

By fusing genetic, environmental, and clinical data, such approaches attempt to optimize the therapeutic strategy, allowing physicians to make informed decisions on the basis of individualized biomarkers and disease characteristics. For instance, current treatments in RA target early diagnosis and the administration of disease-modifying antirheumatic drugs in patients with high disease activity and autoantibodies with the goal of achieving a state of strict remission or low disease activity (Aletaha et al., 2016). Similarly, advances in understanding of SSc pathogenesis of GI involvement underscore the need for individualized therapies, since the manifestations can be highly diverse between patients, and recent studies point toward new therapeutic targets based on autoimmune mechanisms (Abraham et al., 2017). This individualized therapy trend not only optimizes treatment effectiveness but also overall patient outcome in rheumatology (Figure 12.13).

12.3.8. Innovations in Drug Development

Innovations in drug development are particularly significant in the field of rheumatology, where treatments often need to address multicategory and heterogonous patient responses. The greatest impact may have been the integration of personalized medicine, which adjusts treatments based on genetic and phenotypic factors that affect drug efficacy and safety. This approach not just enhances clinical advantages for patients but also poses regulatory and reimbursement challenges that must be met to advance clinical uptake. Further, the focus of translational research is essential in bridging the divide between laboratory results and clinical use with the ultimate objective of guaranteeing that scientific investigation properly translates into patient treatment. Nevertheless, there remains the necessity to critically examine the different perceptions of this translational gap, as highlighted in current literature, in a bid to reap the complete advantage of the progress made in the therapeutics of rheumatology science (Boenink et al., 2015; Sáinz de la Fuente et al., 2013).

12.3.9. Future Research Directions

With advancing rheumatology, studies in the future must focus more on identifying new targets of therapy, which will help address the complexities of autoimmune conditions. For instance, gastrointestinal involvement in SSc remains an ongoing challenge, with available treatments symptomatic as the underlying pathogenesis is not entirely understood (Abraham et al., 2017). Research into the pathogenic function of anti-muscarinic receptor autoantibodies may create new potential for targeted therapies, where the treatments are feasible. Similarly, psoriatic arthritis (PsA) indicates the need for new approaches beyond TNFi, particularly in those with suboptimal responses (Kraft et al., 2017). By placing focus on the pharmacokinetics of such therapies and the determinants of immunogenicity that govern their efficacy, scientists can set the stage for solutions in personalized medicine. Eventually, there will be a need for a multidisciplinary approach to optimize treatment strategies and improve outcomes for patients in rheumatology (Figure 12.14).

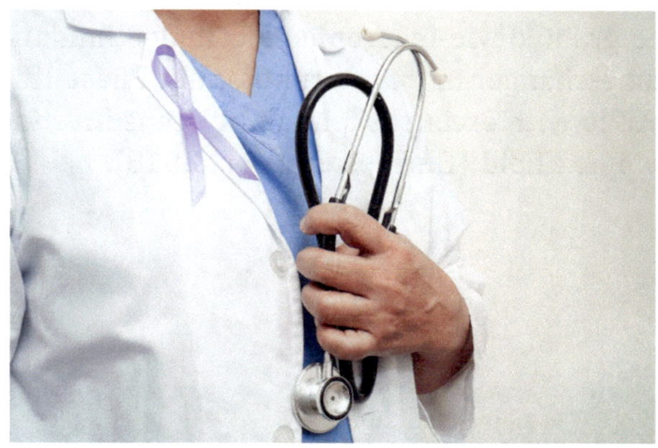

Figure 12.14. As the field of rheumatology continues to evolve, future research directions must emphasize the exploration of novel therapeutic targets that address the complexities of autoimmune diseases.

Source: https://bmidoctors.com/wp-content/uploads/2024/03/semaglutide-and-lupus-1-scaled.jpg.

Test Your Knowledge

1. How can wearable technology aid in disease monitoring in rheumatology?
2. What is the role of AI in early diagnosis and treatment planning for rheumatic diseases?

Summary

The therapeutics within the domain of rheumatology is constantly in flux, with constant learning of the underlying genetic and environmental determinants of autoimmune illnesses. Through recent research, as particularly emphasized, such advances as synovial tissue analysis have helped chart the unique characteristics of RA and PsA and thus guide more specific therapy. The identification of some genes, such as those mentioned in research studies on rat models, points out the heterogeneity and complexity of these conditions, which implies potential means to develop new therapies (Norin, 2017). Moreover, the results derived from enhanced biomarker studies and drug mechanisms point toward more directed therapeutic approaches in rheumatological disease management and improved patient outcomes (Codullo et al., 2011). This constant effort holds an enormous promise for rheumatology in the future, emphasizing the need for ongoing research in this crucial field.

The history of rheumatology therapeutics, and more so in the case of rheumatoid arthritis (RA) treatment, is marked by a firm emphasis on early diagnosis and precise application of treatment strategies. Proper management should be undertaken based on solid comprehension of the disease features, including increased disease activity as well as autoantibody presence, which are robust predictive risk factors for poor outcomes (Aletaha et al., 2016). The concomitant use of both traditional and biological disease-modifying antirheumatic drugs in a treatment-to-target approach has proven effective, allowing for maximum therapeutic success with improvement in patient outcomes. In recent times, mavrilimumab, a human monoclonal antibody directed against the granulocyte-macrophage colony-stimulating factor receptor alpha has emerged as a potential game-changer in long-term therapy. Phase IIb results demonstrate its sustained efficacy and safety profile with excellent tolerability, thus meeting the sustained need for efficacious treatment in this complex field (Burmester et al., 2018).

KEY TERMS FROM THIS CHAPTER

- Analgesic activity
- Balanced scorecard (BSC)
- Corticosteroids
- Dietary modification
- Gastrointestinal distress
- Machine Learning (ML)
- Molecule mimics
- Musculoskeletal
- Occupational therapists
- Optimal physical therapy
- Artificial Intelligence (AI)
- Complex pathophysiology
- Corticosteroids occupy
- Effective pain management
- Heterogeneity
- Medical specialty
- Monotherapy
- Natural immunomodulators
- Occupational therapy
- Pharmacological landscape

Critical Thinking Questions

1. **What is the mechanism of action of methotrexate in rheumatologic diseases?**
    a. TNF-alpha inhibition
    b. Inhibition of folate metabolism
    c. COX-2 inhibition
    d. IL-6 receptor blockade
2. **Which of the following is a TNF-alpha inhibitor?**
    a. Tocilizumab
    b. Rituximab
    c. Etanercept
    d. Abatacept
3. **Which disease-modifying anti-rheumatic drug (DMARD) is contraindicated in pregnancy?**
    a. Sulfasalazine
    b. Methotrexate
    c. Hydroxychloroquine
    d. Azathioprine
4. **Which of the following biologics targets the IL-6 receptor?**
    a. Tocilizumab
    b. Infliximab
    c. Anakinra
    d. Abatacept
5. **What is a common side effect of long-term corticosteroid therapy in rheumatic diseases?**
    a. Hypotension
    b. Hypoglycemia
    c. Osteoporosis
    d. Hyperkalemia

Answers to Critical Thinking Questions

1. (b) 2. (c) 3. (b) 4. (a) 5. (c)

Short Answer Questions

1. What is the difference between conventional DMARDs and biologic DMARDs?
2. What role does physical therapy play in managing chronic arthritis?
3. How can occupational therapy improve the quality of life for patients with rheumatic diseases?
4. What is the role of precision medicine in treating autoimmune rheumatic diseases?
5. How have biologics transformed the prognosis of rheumatoid arthritis?
6. What are the common barriers to early diagnosis of rheumatic diseases?
7. How does health inequity impact access to rheumatologic treatment?

References

1. Abdallah, K., Anderson, J., Andrews, S., Arrindell, J., et al. (2017). Managing toxicities associated with immune checkpoint inhibitors: Consensus recommendations from the Society for Immunotherapy of Cancer (SITC) Toxicity Management Working Group. https://core.ac.uk/download/155271511.pdf (accessed on 17th June 2025).
2. Abhishek, A., Altman, R., Bannuru, R., Bodick, N., Bodick, N., Da Costa, B., Dworkin, R., et al. (2018). Brief report: A phase IIb trial of a novel extended-release microsphere formulation of triamcinolone acetonide for intraarticular injection in knee osteoarthritis.
3. Abraham, D., Assandri, R., Assassi, S., Auluck, A., Bacher, P., Baron, M., Baron, M., et al. (2017). Review article: Pathogenesis and clinical manifestations of gastrointestinal involvement in systemic sclerosis. https://core.ac.uk/download/83049880.pdf (accessed on 17th June 2025).
4. Burmester, G. R., McInnes, I. B., Kremer, J. M., Miranda, P., Vencovský, J., Godwood, A., Albulescu, M., Michaels, M. A., Guo, X., Close, D., & Weinblatt, M. (2018). Mavrilimumab, a Fully Human Granulocyte-Macrophage Colony-Stimulating Factor Receptor α Monoclonal Antibody: Long-Term Safety and Efficacy in Patients With Rheumatoid Arthritis. *Arthritis & rheumatology (Hoboken, N.J.)*, *70*(5), 679–689. https://doi.org/10.1002/art.40420 (accessed on 17th June 2025).
5. Aji, N., Aji, N., Alshareefy, Y., Alshareefy, Y., et al. (2024). Advancements and progress in juvenile idiopathic arthritis: A review of pathophysiology and treatment. https://core.ac.uk/download/603360608.pdf (accessed on 17th June 2025).
6. Akpabio, A., Akpabio, A., Alpízar-Rodríguez, D., Berenbaum, F., Bhana, S., et al. (2021). Early experience of COVID-19 vaccination in adults with systemic rheumatic diseases: Results from the COVID-19 Global Rheumatology Alliance Vaccine Survey. https://core.ac.uk/download/492739380.pdf (accessed on 17th June 2025).
7. Al-Eidan, R., Al-Rashed, M., Al-Saffar, N., Angunawela, I., Anonymous, A., Arthur, H., Arthur, H., et al. (2009). Written information about individual medicines for consumers.
8. Aletaha, D., McInnes, I. B., & Smolen, J. S. (2016). Rheumatoid arthritis. https://core.ac.uk/download/77600864.pdf (accessed on 17th June 2025).
9. Allanore, Y., Bae, S., Bodukam, V., Clements, P. J., et al. (2017). Twenty-two points to consider for clinical trials in systemic sclerosis, based on EULAR standards. https://core.ac.uk/download/85210767.pdf (accessed on 17th June 2025).
10. Altepeter, T., Bray, K., Cheifetz, A. S., Chevalier, A., et al. (2025). Therapeutic drug monitoring of biologics: Current practice, challenges and opportunities–a workshop report. https://core.ac.uk/download/653314005.docx (accessed on 17th June 2025).
11. Amarnani, R., Bundy, C., Coates, L. C., Hailey, H., et al. (2023). Lifestyle modifications and nonpharmacologic interventions to improve outcomes in psoriatic arthritis: A systematic review. https://core.ac.uk/download/578153337.pdf (accessed on 17th June 2025).
12. Ansari, N. N., Hakakzadeh, A., Honarpishe, R., Ingle, G., et al. (2019). Multimodal impact of acupuncture, exercise therapy, and concurrent functional electrical stimulation on osteoarthritis of the knee: A case report. https://core.ac.uk/download/196345207.pdf (accessed on 17th June 2025).

13. Apparailly, F., Baumans, V., Desaintes, C., Di Santo, J. P., et al. (2011). Animal models for arthritis: Innovative tools for prevention and treatment. https://core.ac.uk/download/11279774.pdf (accessed on 17th June 2025).

14. Atzeni, F., Bazzani, C., Bugatti, S., Caporali, R., Cauli, A., Congia, M., Conti, F., et al. (2024). Retention rate of biologic and targeted synthetic anti-rheumatic drugs in elderly rheumatoid arthritis patients: Data from GISEA registry. https://core.ac.uk/download/614166083.pdf (accessed on 17th June 2025).

15. Bagnall, A., Day, R., & Kime, N. H. (2013). Systematic review of transition models for young people with long-term conditions: A report for NHS Diabetes. https://core.ac.uk/download/29018738.pdf (accessed on 17th June 2025).

16. Barker, M. E., Lamb, K. L., Lynn, A., Russell, J., et al. (2020). Effect of tart cherry juice on risk of gout attacks: Protocol for a randomized controlled trial. https://core.ac.uk/download/288393997.pdf (accessed on 17th June 2025).

17. Berardesca, E., Bernardini, N., Bianchi, L., Chimenti, S., et al. (2018). Use of biological drugs in patients with psoriasis and psoriatic arthritis in Italy: Results from the PSONG survey. https://core.ac.uk/download/154948747.pdf (accessed on 17th June 2025).

18. Bjourson, A. J., Gibson, D., McDonald, S., Rajan, R., et al. (2023). An AI approach to identifying novel therapeutics for rheumatoid arthritis. https://core.ac.uk/download/595736027.pdf (accessed on 17th June 2025).

19. Boenink, M., & Laan, A. L. van der. (2015). Beyond bench and bedside: Disentangling the concept of translational research. https://core.ac.uk/download/pdf/11486878.pdf (accessed on 17th June 2025).

20. Bueno-Gracia, E., Ceballos-Laita, L., Estébanez-de-Miguel, E., Fortún-Agúd, S., et al. (2019). Effects of non-pharmacological conservative treatment on pain, range of motion and physical function in patients with mild to moderate hip osteoarthritis: A systematic review. https://core.ac.uk/download/290001381.pdf (accessed on 17th June 2025).

21. Chandak, A., Holkar, M., Moghe, A., Washikar, P., et al. (2023). Use of telehealth during COVID-19 pandemic in India: Literature review. https://core.ac.uk/download/618286341.pdf (accessed on 17th June 2025).

22. Codullo, V., & McInnes, I. B. (2011). Synovial tissue response to treatment in psoriatic arthritis. https://core.ac.uk/download/pdf/8673459.pdf (accessed on 17th June 2025).

23. College of Health Professions. (2022). *College of Health Professions Research Newsletter: 2021–2022 Academic Year*. https://core.ac.uk/download/542932277.pdf (accessed on 17th June 2025).

24. Contreras, J. (2019). Utilization of mind-body practices for adults with fibromyalgia: 2017 National Health Interview Survey. https://core.ac.uk/download/231832574.pdf (accessed on 17th June 2025).

25. Conway, G. E., & Heffernan, S. M. (2021). Nutraceutical alternatives to pharmaceutical analgesics in osteoarthritis. https://core.ac.uk/download/392256349.pdf (accessed on 17th June 2025).

26. Cook, M. J., Diffin, J., Lunt, M., MacGregor, A. J., et al. (2016). Predictors and outcomes of sustained, intermittent or never achieving remission in patients with recent onset

inflammatory polyarthritis: Results from the Norfolk Arthritis Register. https://core.ac.uk/download/41994651.pdf (accessed on 17th June 2025).

27. Copley-Merriman, C., Costello, J., Khan, S., Krumbach, A., Reddy, P., Tanjinatus, O., Wells, A. F., et al. (2025). Health disparities in rheumatology in the United States. https://core.ac.uk/download/648103776.pdf (accessed on 17th June 2025).

28. DeHoratius, R. J., Ellis, L. A., Kafka, S., Kubacki, T., et al. (2019). Comparative analysis of US real-world dosing patterns and direct infusion-related costs for matched cohorts of rheumatoid arthritis patients treated with infliximab or intravenous golimumab. https://core.ac.uk/download/213445696.pdf (accessed on 17th June 2025).

29. Dinda, A., Julià, A., Livingston, A., Whittaker, A. L., Pulichino, A. M., Bolon, B., Gaskill, B. N., et al. (2015). Applying refinement to the use of mice and rats in rheumatoid arthritis research. https://core.ac.uk/download/42363811.pdf (accessed on 17th June 2025).

30. Du Pan, S. M., Finckh, A., & Gabay, C. (2007). A systematic review of infliximab in the treatment of early rheumatoid arthritis. https://core.ac.uk/download/pdf/8049451.pdf (accessed on 17th June 2025).

31. Dziedzic, K. S., Foster, N. E., Healey, E. L., Jordan, K. P., et al. (2013). Exercise for lower limb osteoarthritis: Systematic review incorporating trial sequential analysis and network meta-analysis. https://core.ac.uk/download/17030881.pdf (accessed on 17th June 2025).

32. Elmesmari, A., Fraser, A. R., Gilchrist, D., Kurowska-Stolarska, M., et al. (2016). MicroRNA-155 regulates monocyte chemokine and chemokine receptor expression in rheumatoid arthritis. https://core.ac.uk/download/42370682.pdf (accessed on 17th June 2025).

33. Escolar, M. L., Giugliani, R., & Zwaigenbaum, L. (2020). Development of a clinical algorithm for the early diagnosis of mucopolysaccharidosis III. https://core.ac.uk/download/348666604.pdf (accessed on 17th June 2025).

34. Faarvang, K. L., & da Silva, J. A. (2009). Competencies in rheumatology: a European framework. *Best practice & research. Clinical rheumatology, 23*(2), 145–160. https://doi.org/10.1016/j.berh.2008.12.001 (accessed on 17th June 2025).

35. Falahee, M., Finckh, A., Harrison, M., Raza, K., et al. (2019). Preferences of patients and at-risk individuals for preventive approaches to rheumatoid arthritis. https://core.ac.uk/download/pdf/196351786.pdf (accessed on 17th June 2025).

36. FitzGerald, O. R., Stephen, S., Opeyemi, S., Staunton, C., et al. (2013). Biomarkers of inflammatory arthritis and proteomics. https://core.ac.uk/download/288637789.pdf (accessed on 17th June 2025).

37. Fujita, Y., Hashimoto, M., Ikeda, K., Inagaki, K., et al. (2021). Urinary sodium-to-potassium ratio associates with hypertension and current disease activity in patients with rheumatoid arthritis: A cross-sectional study. https://core.ac.uk/download/541150528.pdf (accessed on 17th June 2025).

38. Gensichen, J., Joos, S., Körner, T., Muth, C., et al. (2005). Rationale, design and conduct of a comprehensive evaluation of a primary care-based intervention to improve the quality of life of osteoarthritis patients. *The PraxArt-Project: A Cluster Randomized Controlled Trial [ISRCTN87252339]; Study Protocol.* https://core.ac.uk/download/14504006.pdf (accessed on 17th June 2025).

39. Girardet, J. L., Hagerty, D. T., Hyndman, D., Iverson, C., et al. (2016). Lesinurad, a novel, oral compound for gout, acts to decrease serum uric acid through inhibition of urate transporters in the kidney. https://core.ac.uk/download/323066765.pdf (accessed on 17th June 2025).
40. Gleasner, R. M. (2019). Print journal analysis and journal removal projects. https://core.ac.uk/download/275886037.pdf (accessed on 17th June 2025).
41. Grek, V., & Hügle, T. (2023). Digital transformation of an academic hospital department: A case study on strategic planning using the balanced scorecard. https://core.ac.uk/download/592040502.pdf (accessed on 17th June 2025).
42. Harnett, M. M., Harnett, W., Pineda, M. A., Rodgers, D. T., et al. (2015). Drug-like analogues of the parasitic worm-derived immunomodulator ES-62 are therapeutic in the MRL/Lpr model of systemic lupus erythematosus. https://core.ac.uk/download/42361789.pdf (accessed on 17th June 2025).
43. Hider, S., Mallen, C., & Roddy, E. (2015). Mapping patients' experiences from initial symptoms to gout diagnosis: A qualitative exploration. https://core.ac.uk/download/599351412.pdf (accessed on 17th June 2025).
44. Irure Ventura, J., & López Hoyos, M. (2022). The past, present, and future in antinuclear antibodies (ANA). https://core.ac.uk/download/571642230.pdf (accessed on 17th June 2025).
45. Kawano-Dourado, L., Kulkarni, T., Richards, D., Ryerson, C. J., et al. (2024). Time to speed up scientific deliveries in fibrotic interstitial lung disease: Innovative clinical trial design to improve patient care. https://core.ac.uk/download/603241315.pdf (accessed on 17th June 2025).
46. Khoza-Shangase, K., Moroe, N., & Neille, J. (2021). Speech-language pathology and audiology in South Africa: Clinical training and service in the era of COVID-19. https://core.ac.uk/download/478006083.pdf (accessed on 17th June 2025).
47. Kinney, A. L. (2007). National scientific facilities and their science impact on non-biomedical research. http://arxiv.org/abs/0705.1797 (accessed on 17th June 2025).
48. Kraft, W. K., Mantravadi, S., & Ogdie, A. (2017). Tumor necrosis factor inhibitors in psoriatic arthritis. https://core.ac.uk/download/83049994.pdf (accessed on 17th June 2025).
49. Laar, M. van de, Langford, R., Mellinghoff, H. U., Merchante, M., et al. (2012). Tramadol/paracetamol fixed-dose combination in the treatment of moderate to severe pain. https://core.ac.uk/download/pdf/11486756.pdf (accessed on 17th June 2025).
50. McInnes, I. B., & Schett, G. (2017). Pathogenetic insights from the treatment of rheumatoid arthritis. *Lancet (London, England)*, *389*(10086), 2328–2337. https://doi.org/10.1016/S0140-6736(17)31472-1(accessed on 17th June 2025).
51. McInnes, I. B., Porter, D., & Siebert, S. (2017). Editorial: Choosing new targets for rheumatoid arthritis therapeutics: Too interesting to fail? https://core.ac.uk/download/80697149.pdf (accessed on 17th June 2025).
52. Nash, D. B. (2006). Annual report, 2005–2006. https://core.ac.uk/download/46965002.pdf (accessed on 17th June 2025).
53. Norin, U. (2017). Identification of genetic variants and their implications in autoimmunity. https://core.ac.uk/download/80515181.pdf (accessed on 17th June 2025).

54. Reynolds L A, Tansey E M. (eds), Clinical pharmacology in the UK, c. 1950–2000: influences and institutions, Wellcome Witnesses to Twentieth Century Medicine, vol. 33, London, Wellcome Trust Centre for the History of Medicine at UCL, 2008, pp. xxiv, 139 (paperback 978-085484-117-2).(accessed on 17th June 2025).

55. Sáinz de la Fuente, G. (2013). Personalized medicine, unmet need or business strategy? https://miami.uni-muenster.de/Record/aada0249-63a8-451c-acb3-8f2d63cdfead (accessed on 17th June 2025).

56. Shoji, A., Wells, A. F., Sarawate, C. A., Sarawate, C. A., Helmick, C. G., Lavernia, C. J., Krishnan, E., et al. (2012). Can racial disparities in optimal gout treatment be reduced? Evidence from a randomized trial. https://core.ac.uk/download/pdf/8718087.pdf (accessed on 17th June 2025).

57. Talele, C., Gohil, D., Kumari, M., Shah, N., & Sadhu, P. (2024). Comprehensive review of rheumatoid arthritis: Insights, challenges, and prospects. https://core.ac.uk/download/603897628.pdf (accessed on 17th June 2025).

INDEX

A

Abnormal immune 177, 178
Abnormalities 34, 36, 39
Acute myocardial infarction (AMI) 13
Adolescence 303
Adolescents 302, 303, 305, 308, 309
Aetiopathogenesis 69
Alleviate joint damage 297
American College of Rheumatology/European League Against Rheumatism (ACR/EULAR) 9
Amplifies autoimmune responses 147
Analgesic activity 315
Analgesic properties 236
Anatomical predisposition 204
Anifrolumab 35, 47
Ankylosing spondylitis 64, 65, 70, 71, 72, 75, 76, 80, 81, 82, 83, 84
Ankylosing spondylitis (AS) 60, 61
Anterior cruciate ligament (ACL) 227
Antibodies 31, 39, 42, 52, 53
Antibody-associated vasculitis (AAV) 183
Anti-inflammatory drugs 62, 75
Antineutrophil Cytoplasmic Antibodies (ANCA) 174
Antioxidants 239
Antirheumatic drugs 62, 75
Anti-topoisomerase 120, 121
Anxiety 285, 301
Apoptosis 268
Arthritis 1, 2, 3, 4, 5, 6, 7, 8, 9, 10, 11, 12, 13, 14, 15, 16, 17, 18, 19, 20, 21, 23, 24, 25, 26, 27, 285, 286, 287, 289, 290, 291, 292, 296, 297, 299, 301, 307, 308, 309, 310, 311, 27, 28
Arthropathies 14
Artificial Intelligence (AI) 325
Audiovestibular manifestations 118
Autoantibodies 30, 51, 52, 92, 93, 104, 108, 288
Autoantibody 86, 93, 109, 144, 153, 156, 157
Autoantibody production 86
Autoimmune diseases 2, 3, 5, 24, 30, 32, 34, 36, 40, 44, 55, 85, 87, 88, 91, 93, 94, 101, 102, 105, 286, 287, 288, 289, 112
Autoimmune dysfunction syndrome 97
Autoimmune illness 29, 35
Autoimmune reactions 288
Autoimmunity 30, 31, 33, 35, 53, 54, 116

B

Balanced scorecard (BSC) 323, 326
Behavior change 237, 246, 250
Biochemical processes 199
Biologic drugs 59
Biologic therapies 296, 297, 298, 300
Biologic treatments 14
Blockade therapy 59, 80
Body mass index (BMI) 226
Bone calcium 258

Bone destruction 71, 80
Bone health 256, 257, 258, 265, 266, 267, 268, 270, 277, 279
Bone marker (BM) 211
Bone matrix 258, 266
Bone metabolism 255, 256, 257, 258, 259, 260, 261, 262, 263, 264, 265, 266, 267, 268, 269, 270, 273, 274, 276, 279
Bone mineral density (BMD) 269
Bone tissue 258

C

Calcium balance 260
Calcium homeostasis 255, 256, 257, 258, 259, 260, 272, 280
Calcium metabolism disorders 260, 262
Calcium pyrophosphate crystal deposition disease (CPPD) 263
Calcium pyrophosphate dihydrate (CPPD) 199, 201, 205, 206, 207, 208, 216, 221
Calcium reabsorption 259
Calcium uptake mechanisms 256
Cardiovascular 13
Cardiovascular side effects 236
Cause disease flares 31
Cellular senescence 114, 115, 119, 139
Cerebral perfusion 34, 38
chemokines 147, 148, 149, 151, 152, 167
Chondrocytes 230, 253
Chronic arthropathies 207
Chronic autoimmune disease 2
Chronic autoimmune disorder 1
Chronic disease 227, 233, 248
Chronic illness 289, 306
Chronic inflammation 287, 304
Chronic kidney disease (CKD) 261, 262, 272, 279
Chronic musculoskeletal pain 228, 252
Chronic pain 1, 16, 17, 18, 225, 231, 235, 242, 243, 247
Clinical presentation 141, 142, 144, 146, 153, 164
Clinicopathological 142
Cognitive behavioral therapy 100
Community involvement 245
Complementary and Alternative Medicine (CAM) 320
Complex interplay 1, 4
complexity 142, 143, 144, 158
Complexity 3, 16, 226, 227, 235, 239, 246
Complex pathophysiology 316
Computed tomography (CT) 155
Cone-beam computed tomography (CBCT) 294
Connective tissue growth factor (CTGF) 117
Constant inflammation 1
Conventional crystal analysis (CCA) 263
Corticosteroids 158, 159, 298, 314, 315, 316
Corticosteroids occupy 315
Cosmetic complaints 119
Cryoglobulinaemia 181, 182, 183, 187, 190
Cryoglobulinemia 173
Crystal deposition 199, 201, 204, 205, 206, 207, 208, 210, 211, 221, 222
Crystal formation 201
Crystalline 206, 215
Crystalline deposits 10
Crystallization 204
Crystals 199, 200, 201, 202, 203, 205, 206, 207, 208, 209, 211, 212, 214, 215, 216, 218, 220, 221
Cycloplegic agents 67
Cyclosporine A (CsA) 97
Cytokines 59, 64, 66, 115, 132, 287, 294
Cytopenias 287

D

Decision aids (DAs) 244
Degenerative joint disease 226
Demographic aspects 2
Dent disease (DD) 267
Dermatomyositis 141, 142, 143, 144, 145, 146, 147, 148, 149, 150, 151, 160, 161, 162, 164, 165, 166, 167, 168, 169
Diagnosis 1, 7, 8, 9, 10, 11, 13, 19, 21, 25, 291, 294, 295
Diagnosis of Sjögren's syndrome 93
Diagnostic 9, 256, 260, 261, 262, 263, 266, 268, 269, 272, 274, 283
Diagnostic approach 141
Diagnostic assurance 10

Diagnostic criteria 261, 263, 291, 292, 295, 309
Diagnostic innovation 71
Diagnostic process 199
Diagnostic tools 72
Diclofenac demonstrating 13
Diclofenac sodium 232, 234
Dietary 257, 259, 262, 263, 265, 267, 269, 270, 283
Dietary cation–anion difference (DCAD) 257
Dietary modification 319
Diffuse inflammation 29
Disability 1, 4, 6, 12, 16, 18, 19, 20, 21, 22, 26, 225, 228, 231, 232, 235, 238, 244, 248, 285, 291, 294, 301, 302, 303, 310, 311, 252, 28
Disease 2, 3, 4, 5, 6, 7, 8, 9, 10, 11, 12, 13, 14, 15, 16, 17, 18, 19, 20, 21, 22, 23, 83, 25, 26, 62, 63, 64, 65, 66, 67, 68, 69, 71, 72, 73, 74, 75, 76, 77, 78, 79, 80, 82, 83, , 255, 256, 257, 260, 261, 262, 263, 264, 266, 267, 268, 272, 274, 275, 279, 280, 27, 282, 283
Disease Activity 14
Disease management 237, 290, 306
Disease-modifying antirheumatic drugs (DMARDs) 4, 12, 13, 14, 20, 96
Disease-modifying osteoarthritis drugs (DMOADs) 240
Disease progression 175, 179, 186
Distal muscle involvement 146
Dryness 87, 89, 90, 91, 92, 95, 96, 98, 100, 103, 104
Dual-energy computed tomography (DECT) 211
Dysfunction 286, 288, 292
Dysmotility 114, 118, 119, 120, 133
Dysphagia 157
Dysregulation 31, 33, 86, 87, 88, 102

E

Echocardiography 124, 126, 137
Ectopic mineralization 262, 267, 268
Effective interventions 144
Effective management 8, 261, 270, 275, 302
Effective pain management 316
Efficient management 72
Elastography 141, 155, 170
Electromyography (EMG) 145, 153
Electronic health records (EHRs) 8
Emotional distress 1
Endothelial dysfunction 177, 180
Endothelial progenitor cells (EPCs) 180
Enteropathic arthritis 60, 62
Enthesitis 60, 65, 70, 81
Environmental stimuli 3, 31
Eosinophilic granulomatosis 173, 175, 176, 182, 186, 187, 188, 191, 192, 194, 195
eosinophilic granulomatosis with polyangiitis (EGPA) 173, 175, 176, 187, 188, 192
Epigenetic action 265
Epithelial cells 256
Erectile dysfunction (ED) 122
Erythematosus 30, 31, 33, 34, 35, 37, 38, 39, 41, 43, 46, 48, 49, 50, 51, 53, 54, 55, 56, 88, 56, 57, 110, 111, 57
Estrogen 32
Ethnic variations 290
Etiologic rationale 96
Etiology 2, 3, 5
Extra-articular symptoms 59, 63
Extracellular matrix proteins 117
Extra-musculoskeletal 59

F

Fibrillation potentials 145
Fibroproliferative vasculopathy 114, 115
Fibrosis 113, 114, 115, 117, 118, 120, 121, 125, 126, 128, 132, 133, 134, 135, 138, 139
Fibrotic behavior 115

G

Gastrointestinal distress 314
Gastro-intestinal manifestations 120
Gastrointestinal manifestations 116
Gender variation 228, 289
Genetic causes 286
Genetic dispositions 31
Genetic etiologies 287
Genetic influences 289
Genetic loci 31
Genetic predisposition 2, 3, 286, 287, 288
Genetic susceptibility 2, 3, 4, 5, 227, 287

Gland pleomorphic adenoma 100, 110
Glandular dysfunction 86, 87, 94, 108
Glandular tissue 86
Gla-rich protein (GRP) 260, 282
Global collaboration 141
Glomerulonephritis 173, 181, 182, 183, 190, 195
Grasp inflammatory mechanisms 179
Guarantee active management 100
Gut microbiota 255, 259, 260, 279

H

Hand osteoarthritis 226, 235, 250, 251
hazardous 174
Health issue 1
Health-related quality 241, 243
Henoch-Schönlein purpura (HSP) 186
Hepatosplenomegaly 287
Heterogeneity 144, 146, 148, 161, 162, 316, 328
Heterogeneous series 60
High-resolution computed tomography (HRCT) 125, 127
Histopathological data 184
Holistic management 98
Holistic treatment 119
Holistic treatment strategies 306
Hormonal changes 226
Hormonal regulation 257
Hormones 3, 4
Human exocrine glands 87
Human immune responses 35
Human leukocyte antigen (HLA) 116
Hyperactivation 30
Hypercalcemia 255, 258, 259, 272, 273, 274, 275, 277, 280, 281, 282, 283
Hypercytokinemia 287
Hyperuricemia 200, 201, 202, 203, 204, 205, 210, 211, 213, 215, 218
Hypocalcemia 255, 256, 257, 259, 270, 272, 273, 274, 275, 277, 282
Hypophosphatemic rickets 266

I

Idiopathic inflammatory myopathies (IIM) 294
Immune cells 30, 33
Immune dysfunction 114
Immune dysregulation 286, 287, 288
Immune mechanisms 287
Immune-mediated disease 32
Immune-modulating agents 288
Immune response 286, 287, 288
Immune system 29, 30, 31, 52, 53, 61, 64, 65, 286, 287, 289, 297, 307
Immune system dysfunction 30, 31
Immune tolerance 29, 33
Immunological 2, 22
Immunologic components 30
Immunomodulatory 14, 264
Immunomodulatory agents 97
Immunomodulatory therapy 89
Immunosuppressants 158, 159, 162
Immunosuppressive therapy 144, 163, 172, 182, 191
Inadequacy 289, 295
Inclusion body myositis (IBM) 143
Infections 174, 178, 185, 186, 187
Inflammation 86, 87, 89, 90, 92, 96, 97, 101, 102, 105, 106
Inflammation symptoms 13
Inflammatory 2, 3, 5, 8, 11, 12, 13, 14, 15, 20, 23, 24, 25, 26, 27, 28
Inflammatory back pain (IBP) 63, 71
Inflammatory bowel diseases (IBD) 62
Inflammatory cell 148, 149
Inflammatory diseases 68, 79, 82
Inflammatory mechanisms 288
Inflammatory pathways 65
Influence 4, 6, 8, 9, 11, 19, 20, 21
Initial risk assessment 68
Insufficient calcium intake 261
Interferon gamma 287
Interleukin 285, 297
Interprofessional education (IPE) 98
Interstitial lung disease (ILD) 100, 143
Intervention 2, 5, 6, 7, 8, 9, 10, 11, 20, 21
Intravenous (IV) 14

J

Joint inflammation 285, 288, 291, 293
Joint trauma 2
Juvenile Arthritis Disability Index 296
Juvenile idiopathic arthritis (JIA) 285, 289, 309
Juvenile Idiopathic Arthritis (JIA) 285, 286, 288, 289, 293, 297, 298, 299, 300, 302, 305, 306, 307
Juvenile Spondyloarthritis (JSpA) 63

K

Keratoconjunctivitis 91, 102
Kidney damage 204

L

Labor force participation 243
Lengthy progression 144
Leukocytoclastic vasculitis 181
Levamisole-contaminated cocaine 171, 181, 192
Lifestyle modification 265
Local inflammation 8
Lymphocytic infiltrate 91
Lymphocytic infiltration 86, 87, 89

M

Machine Learning (ML) 325
Macophages 287
Macrohage activation syndrome (MAS) 287
Macrophages 287
Magnetic resonance imaging (MRI) 71, 72
Magnetic Resonance Imaging (MRI) 10
Major histocompatibility complex (MHC) 147
Mechanism 225, 252
Medical professionals 287, 303
Medical specialty 313
Mental health 228, 242, 247, 252
Meta-analyses 176
Metabolic bone disorder 261
Metabolic imbalance 30
Metabolic markers 260
Metabolic reprogramming 30
Microbial alterations 3
Microbial well-being 15
Microbiota 2, 3, 5, 8, 20, 27, 259
Microvascular changes 124, 125
Mineral dysregulation 262
Misdiagnosis 176, 185, 186
Molecular mechanisms 114, 117
Molecule mimics 314
Monosodium urate crystals 200, 201, 203, 205, 206, 208, 210
Monosodium urate (MSU) 200, 201
Monotherapy 317
Morbidity 113, 114, 115, 120, 121
Morphogenetic proteins 84,
Movement variability 227
Multidisciplinary assessments 295
Multi-factorial autoimmune 100
Multifactorial pathology 231
Multisystemic 117
Muscle 294
Muscle damage 141, 142, 145, 149, 155
Muscle fibers 142, 145, 148, 150, 151
Muscle inflammation 141, 142, 148, 151, 152, 153, 156, 160, 167
Muscle pathology 141, 148, 170
Muscular dystrophy 149, 150, 167
Musculoskeletal 313
Musculoskeletal complaints 9, 11
Musculoskeletal ultrasound 210, 223
Musculoskeletal ultrasound (MSUS) 291
Mutation-positive patients 262
Myofibroblast activation 114, 132
Myofibroblast function 114
Myofibroblasts 117
Myopathic 156, 157
Myopathies 141, 142, 143, 144, 145, 146, 147, 148, 149, 150, 151, 152, 153, 154, 155, 156, 157, 158, 159, 160, 161, 162, 163, 164, 165, 166, 167, 168, 169, 170
Myositis 141, 142, 143, 144, 145, 146, 147, 152, 153, 160, 164, 165, 166, 168, 169

N

Nailfold video capillaroscopy (NVC) 124
Natural bone mass 261
Natural immunomodulators 314
Necrotizing autoimmune myopathy (NAM) 144

Neurological 7
Neuropsychiatric symptoms 34
Nonconclusive evidence 150
Noncorticosteroid 286, 308
Nonhormonal medications 264
Nonpharmacological therapies 236
Non-steroidal anti-inflammatory drugs (NSAIDs) 210, 299
Nonsteroidal Anti-Inflammatory Drugs (NSAIDs) 314
Nuclear factor of activated T-cells (NFAT) 145, 148, 150, 151
Numerous diseases 262
Numerous physiological functions 259
Nutrient 288
Nutrient absorption 259, 265, 267
Nutrient-dense foods 98
Nutrition 258, 259, 270, 282
Nutritional therapy 8
Nutritionists 16

O

Obesity 2, 226, 227, 230, 238, 239, 241, 247, 249, 251
Obesity treatment 227
Observation 227
Occupational therapists 319
Occupational therapy 318, 319, 329
Ophthalmology 304
Optimal pain management 299
Optimal physical therapy 318
ositron emission tomography with computed tomography (PET/CT) 177
Osteoarthritis 7, 10, 23
Osteoarthritis (OA) 225, 227, 230, 231, 232, 233, 235, 236, 237, 238, 239, 243, 244, 245, 246
Osteoporosis 255, 256, 257, 258, 260, 261, 262, 263, 264, 265, 269, 270, 271, 275, 276, 280, 283
Otorhinolaryngologic 182
Otorhinolaryngologists 185

P

Panoramic radiography (PAN) 294
Parathyroid hormone 255, 259, 275, 280
Parathyroid hormone (PTH) 255, 275, 280
Particular therapy 176
Pathogen-associated molecules 33
Pathogenesis 3, 5, 9, 26, 27, 29, 31, 32, 33, 35, 45, 51, 57
Pathogenesis of Systemic Lupus Erythematosus 31, 32
Pathogens 288
Pathophysiological 86, 92
Pathophysiological alterations 294
Pathophysiologic mechanisms 60
Pathophysiology 3, 11, 29, 30, 32, 35, 113, 114, 115, 118, 119, 134, 171, 174, 175, 177, 179, 181, 190, 199, 200, 201, 205, 208, 211, 261, 262, 265
Patient education 304, 308
Patient journey 305
Patient management 13, 20, 93, 94, 104, 110
Periodontal disease 92, 104, 112
Peripheral arthritis 60, 70
Perivascular adipose tissue (PVAT) 180
Personal responsibilities 18
Pharmacological approach 98
Pharmacological landscape 314
Pharmacological treatment 317
Pharmacologic therapy 236
Phenotype 31, 231, 232
Phenotypes 147, 152, 159
Phosphatase 260, 266, 274
Physical adaptation 302
Physical disabilities 16
Physical pain 303
Physical therapy 75, 76, 78, 235, 236, 245
Physiological alterations 4
Pilocarpine 96, 97
Platelet-derived growth factor (PDGF) 117
Polyangiitis 173, 174, 175, 176, 177, 178, 182, 183, 184, 185, 186, 187, 188, 190, 191, 192, 193, 194, 195, 196
Polyarteritis nodosa 173, 193
Polymeric symptoms 98
Polymorphic amino acid 116
Polymorphisms 65, 66, 69, 82

Polymyositis 141, 142, 143, 144, 146, 148, 149, 151, 160, 161, 162, 165, 167, 168
Polymyositis (PM) 142, 143
Posterior reversible encephalopathy syndrome (PRES) 182, 187, 188
Post-traumatic osteoarthritis 225, 253
Potential 285, 286, 287, 288, 292, 295, 297, 303, 311
Potential enhancement 9
Pregnancy 91, 101, 110
primary Sjogren's Syndrome (pSS) 92
Probability 260
Prognostic algorithm 147
Proinflammatory cytokine 200
Proinflammatory cytokines 3
Pseudogout 199, 200, 201, 202, 203, 205, 206, 207, 208, 209, 210, 211, 212, 214, 215, 216, 217, 218, 219, 220, 221, 222, 223
Psoriatic arthritis 60, 66, 69, 70, 72, 82, 83
Psoriatic arthritis (PsA) 61
Psychological 1, 15, 17, 18, 20
Psychological effect 242
Psychosis 7
Psychosocial 285, 289, 301, 302, 304, 306
Public health 227
Pyrophosphate 199, 201, 202, 205, 206, 207, 208, 209, 211, 212, 214, 215, 216, 217, 218, 221, 222, 223

Q

quantitative magnetic resonance imaging (qMRI) 233

R

Radiographic changes 71
Radiographic disease 315
Radiographs 7, 73
Reactive oxidizing species (ROS) 115
Rehabilitation 236, 251
Renal manifestation 33
Retrospective analysis 142
Rheumatic diseases 60, 61, 67, 82
Rheumatic disorders 288, 295
Rheumatic illnesses 59
Rheumatic inflammatory disorders 71
Rheumatoid Arthritis (RA) 1, 2
Rheumatological cells 202
Rheumatology 63, 71, 72
Rheumatology professionals 304
Rigidity 232, 258
Rituximab 159, 168

S

Saliva production 92, 96, 97
Satellite cell activation 151
Scleroderma 113, 114, 115, 116, 117, 118, 119, 120, 121, 122, 123, 124, 125, 126, 127, 128, 129, 130, 131, 132, 133, 134, 135, 137, 138, 139, 140
Scleroderma fibrosis 115
Shared decision-making (SDM) 244
Single nucleotide polymorphisms (SNPs) 116
Skeletal health 258, 259, 264
Sleep disorders 1, 27
Social impact 242
Social isolation 1
Socioeconomic barriers 6
Socioeconomic disparities 290
Socio-economic health 290
Socioeconomic status 6
Soft tissue biomineralization 267
Spare respiratory capacity 30
Specific etiology 286
Specific therapeutic mechanism 316
Spondyloarthritides 59, 60, 61, 62, 63, 64, 65, 66, 67, 68, 69, 70, 71, 72, 73, 74, 75, 76, 77, 78, 79, 80, 81, 82, 84
Spondyloarthritis 60, 61, 62, 63, 64, 66, 67, 70, 71, 72, 73, 74, 78, 81
Spondyloarthritis International Society 60, 63, 72
Stem cell transplantation 113
Subsequent inflammation 202
Symptomatology 4, 118
Symptom management 95, 298, 301
Symptomology 93
Symptoms 291
Syndrome 85, 86, 87, 88, 89, 91, 92, 93, 94, 95, 96,

97, 98, 99, 100, 101, 103, 104, 105, 107, 110
Systemic acidosis 257
Systemic immunomodulatory drugs 296
Systemic lupus erythematosus 314, 315, 333
Systemic lupus erythematosus (SLE) 30, 33, 34, 314
Systemic Lupus Erythematosus (SLE) 29, 31, 32, 33, 36, 38, 40, 41, 42, 43, 44, 46, 47, 50

T

Temporomandibular disorders 295, 309
Temporomandibular joint (TMJ) 292, 295
Therapeutic difficulties 63
Therapeutic interventions 114, 121, 125, 287
Therapeutic options 96
Therapeutic rationale 117
Therapy 10, 11, 12, 13, 14, 15, 18, 20, 25, 28
Toll-like receptors (TLRs) 33
Tophaceous formation 204
Total joint replacements (TJRs) 226
Total knee arthroplasty (TKA) 236
T regulatory lymphocytes (Tregs) 29, 33
Triggering cutaneous 31
Tumor necrosis factor-alpha (TNFα) 59
Tumor necrosis factor inhibitors (TNFi) 13, 313
Tumor necrosis factor (TNF) 60, 297

U

Undifferentiated Spondyloarthritis (uSpA) 62, 63
Uric acid 200, 201, 202, 203, 210, 211, 212, 213, 214, 217, 218, 221

V

Vascular alterations 114, 116
Vascular injury 260
Vasculitic syndromes 183
Vasculitides 171, 172, 173, 174, 175, 176, 177, 178, 179, 180, 181, 182, 183, 184, 185, 186, 187, 188, 189, 190, 191, 192, 193, 194
Vasculitis development 179
Vasculopathy 115, 118
Ventricular function 124, 137
Vessel vasculitides 172, 173, 191, 192, 193
Vitamin D deficiency 264
Vulnerable 228

W

Worldwide public health 225

X

Xerostomia 91, 92, 96, 97, 98, 103, 104